Ancient and Traditional Foods, Plants, Herbs and Spices used in Cancer

The use of different foods, herbs and spices to treat or prevent disease has been recorded for thousands of years. Egyptian papyrus, hieroglyphics and ancient texts from the Middle East have described the cultivation and preparations of herbs and botanicals to "cure the sick." There are even older records from China and India. Some ancient scripts describe the use of medicinal plants which have never been seen within European cultures. Indeed, all ancient civilizations have pictorial records of different foods, herbs and spices being used for medical purposes. However, there are fundamental questions pertaining to the scientific evidence for the use of these agents or their extracts in modern medicine.

There have been considerable advances in scientific techniques over the last few decades. These have been used to examine the composition and applications of traditional cures. Modern science has also seen the investigation of herbs, spices and botanicals beyond their traditional usage. For example, plants which have been used for "digestion" or "medical ills" since time immemorial are now being investigated for anticancer properties or their toxicity, using high throughput screening. Techniques also include molecular biology, cellular biochemistry, physiology, endocrinology and even medical imaging. However, much of the material relating to the scientific basis or applications of traditional foods, herbs, spices and botanicals is scattered among various sources. The widespread applicability of foods or botanicals is rarely described and cautionary notes on toxicity are often ignored. These questions are explored in *Ancient and Traditional Foods, Plants, Herbs and Spices used in Cancer.*

Ancient and Traditional Foods, Plants, Herbs and Spices in Human Health

Series Editors:

Vinood B. Patel *University of Westminster, London*
Victor R. Preedy *King's College, London*
Rajkumar Rajendram *King Abdulaziz Medical City, Riyadh*

Each volume in the series provides an evidenced-based ethos describing the usage and applications of traditional foods and botanicals in human health. The content provides a platform upon which other scientific studies can be based. These may include the extraction or synthesis of active agents, *in vitro* studies, pre-clinical investigations in animals, and clinical trials.

The key benefits of each volume:

- Chapters provide a historical background on the usage of food and plant-based therapics.
- Chapters are based on the results of studies using scientific techniques and methods.
- Presents wide references to other foods, herbs, and botanicals reported to have curative properties.
- Chapters are self-contained, focused toward specific conditions.

Ancient and Traditional Foods, Plants, Herbs and Spices used in Cardiovascular Health and Disease
Edited by Rajkumar Rajendram, Victor R. Preedy, and Vinood B. Patel

Ancient and Traditional Foods, Plants, Herbs and Spices used in Diabetes
Edited by Rajkumar Rajendram, Victor R. Preedy, and Vinood B. Patel

Ancient and Traditional Foods, Plants, Herbs and Spices used in the Middle East
Edited by Rajkumar Rajendram, Victor R. Preedy, and Vinood B. Patel

Ancient and Traditional Foods, Plants, Herbs and Spices used in Cancer
Edited by Rajkumar Rajendram, Victor R. Preedy, and Vinood B. Patel

For more information about this series, please visit www.routledge.com/Ancient-and-Traditional-Foods-Plants-Herbs-and-Spices-in-Human-Health/book-series/ATFHSH

Ancient and Traditional Foods, Plants, Herbs and Spices used in Cancer

Edited by
Rajkumar Rajendram, Victor R. Preedy,
and Vinood B. Patel

CRC Press
Taylor & Francis Group
Boca Raton London New York

CRC Press is an imprint of the
Taylor & Francis Group, an **informa** business

First edition published 2024
by CRC Press
6000 Broken Sound Parkway NW, Suite 300, Boca Raton, FL 33487–2742

and by CRC Press
4 Park Square, Milton Park, Abingdon, Oxon, OX14 4RN

CRC Press is an imprint of Taylor & Francis Group, LLC

Library of Congress Cataloging-in-Publication Data
Names: Patel, Vinood B., editor. | Preedy, Victor R., editor. | Rajendram, Rajkumar, editor.
Title: Ancient and traditional foods, plants, herbs and spices used in cancer / edited by Vinood B. Patel, Victor R.
    Preedy, and Rajkumar Rajendram.
Description: First edition. | Boca Raton : CRC Press, 2023. | Includes bibliographical references. |
    Summary: "This book provides an evidenced-based approach in describing usage and applications
    of traditional foods and botanicals in prevention and treatment of cancer. Coverage includes the Mediterranean
    diet, traditionally prepared meat, Thai traditional herbs, diet-derived phytochemicals, traditional Chinese
    medicine, antioxidants in various plants including bergamot, blueberry ash, European mistletoe, fenugreek, flax
    seed, garlic, ginger, ginseng, grape skins, juniper, maidenhair tree, red belt conk, reishi, searocket, spreading
    sneezeweed, torch aloe, and turkey tail fungus. The chapters also provide a platform upon which other scientific
    studies can be based. These may include the extraction or synthesis of active agents, in vitro studies, pre-clinical
    investigations in animals and robust clinical trials"—Provided by publisher.
Identifiers: LCCN 2022061001 (print) | LCCN 2022061002 (ebook) | ISBN 9781032192536 (hardback) |
    ISBN 9781032200842 (paperback) | ISBN 9781003260028 (ebook)
Subjects: LCSH: Cancer—Diet therapy. | Cancer—Alternative treatment. | Cancer—Prevention.
Classification: LCC RC271.D52 A53 2023 (print) | LCC RC271.D52 (ebook) |
    DDC 616.99/40654—dc23/eng/20230414
LC record available at https://lccn.loc.gov/2022061001
LC ebook record available at https://lccn.loc.gov/2022061002

ISBN: 978-1-032-19253-6 (hbk)
ISBN: 978-1-032-20084-2 (pbk)
ISBN: 978-1-003-26002-8 (ebk)

DOI: 10.1201/9781003260028

Typeset in Times LT Std
by Apex CoVantage, LLC

Contents

SECTION I Overviews and Dietary Components

SECTION II Specific Agents, Items and Extracts

SECTION III Resources

Preface

The use of different foods, herbs and spices to treat or prevent disease has been recorded for thousands of years. Egyptian papyrus, hieroglyphics and ancient texts from the Middle East have described the cultivation and preparations of herbs and botanicals to "cure the sick". There are even older records from China and India. Aztec scripts describe the use of medicinal plants which have never been seen within European cultures. Indeed all ancient civilisations have pictorial records of different foods, herbs and spices being used for medical purposes. However, there are fundamental questions pertaining to the scientific evidence for the use of these agents in modern medicine.

There have been considerable advances in scientific techniques over the last few decades. These have been used to examine the composition and applications of traditional cures. Modern science has also seen the investigation of herbs, spices and botanicals beyond their traditional usage. For example, plants which have been used for "digestion" or "medical ills" since time immemorial are now being investigated for anti-cancer properties using high throughput screening. Techniques also include molecular biology, cellular biochemistry, physiology, endocrinology and even medical imaging. However, much of the material relating to the scientific basis or applications of traditional foods, herbs, spices and botanicals is scattered among various sources. The widespread applicability of foods or botanicals are rarely described and cautionary notes on toxicity are often ignored. This is addressed in *Ancient and Traditional Foods, Plants, Herbs and Spices used in Cancer*.

More scientifically vigorous trials are needed to ascertain the reported properties of many of these foods or plant based components or extracts. However, it is important to point out that the usage of any component or regimen requires scientifically vigorous trials and investigations. Treatments and pathways seen in modelling systems or *in vitro* need to be verified *in vivo*. Adverse effects also need to be investigated. The gold standard is randomised controlled trials and with due consideration of toxic and adverse effects; these chapters provide a framework only.

Each book has 3 sections

1. Overviews and diets
2. Specific agents, items and extracts
3. Resources

Each Chapter has a section on

Background
Other Foods, Herbs, and Spices And Botanicals Used in Cancer
Toxicity and Cautionary Notes
Summary Points

The section **Background** provides information on the earliest recorded use of the food or item in different text, when it was first mentioned and used for medical conditions. Cultural and traditional usage is also mentioned here. **Other Foods, Herbs, Spices And Botanicals used in cancer** is particularly important as it highlights the idea that there are other items that have been reported to be curative. **Toxicity and Cautionary Notes** provides information on adverse effects that may arise. **Summary Points** encapsulate the entire chapter in brief sets of simple sentences.

Ancient and Traditional Foods, Plants, Herbs and Spices Used in Cancer provides an evidenced based ethos in describing the usage and applications of traditional foods and botanicals. The chapters also provide a platform upon which other scientific studies can be based. These may include the extraction or synthesis of active agents, *in vitro* studies, pre-clinical investigations in animals and robust clinical trials.

Ancient and Traditional Foods, Plants, Herbs and Spices Used in Cancer is designed for research and teaching purposes. It is suitable for oncologists, cancer specialists, physicians, health scientists, healthcare workers, pharmacologists and research scientists. The audience also includes federal and state program directors. It is valuable as a personal reference book and also for academic libraries that cover the domains of health and medical sciences. Contributions are from leading national and international experts including those from world renowned institutions. It is suitable for undergraduates, postgraduates, lecturers and academic professors.

The Editors
Rajkumar Rajendram
Victor R Preedy
Vinood B Patel

Acknowledgements

We wish to acknowledge the professionalism and dedication of Tom Connelly who helped us throughout the preparation and production of this book.

We are also very grateful to Randy Brehm for her guidance and support, from when the ideas for this book were first raised to completion of the project.

The Editors

Editors

Dr. Rajkumar Rajendram, AKC, BSc (Hons), MBBS (Dist), MRCP (UK), FRCA, EDIC, FFICM, is a clinician scientist with a focus on internal medicine, anesthesia, intensive care and peri-operative medicine. Dr Rajendram's interest in traditional medicines began at medical school when he attended the Society of Apothecaries' history of medicine course. He subsequently graduated with distinctions from Guy's, King's and St. Thomas Medical School, King's College London in 2001. As an undergraduate he was awarded several prizes, merits and distinctions in pre-clinical and clinical subjects. Dr. Rajendram completed his specialist training in acute and general medicine in Oxford in 2010 and then practiced as a Consultant in Acute General Medicine at the John Radcliffe Hospital, Oxford. Dr. Rajendram also trained in anesthesia and intensive care in London and was awarded fellowships of the Royal College of Anaesthetists (FRCA) and the Faculty of Intensive Care Medicine (FFICM) in 2009 and 2013 respectively. He then moved to the Royal Free London Hospitals as a Consultant in Intensive Care, Anesthesia and Peri-operative Medicine. He has been a fellow of the Royal College of Physicians of Edinburgh (FRCP Edin) and the Royal College of Physicians of London (FRCP Lond) since 2017 and 2019 respectively. He is currently a Consultant in Internal Medicine at King Abdulaziz Medical City, National Guard Health Affairs, Riyadh, Saudi Arabia. Dr. Rajendram recognizes that integration of traditional medicines into modern paradigms for healthcare can significantly benefit patients. As a clinician scientist he has therefore devoted significant time and effort to nutritional science research and education. He is an affiliated member of the Nutritional Sciences Research Division of King's College London and has published more than 300 textbook chapters, review articles, peer-reviewed papers and abstracts.

Victor R. Preedy, BSc, PhD, DSc, FRSB, FRSPH, FRCPath, FRSC, is a staff member of the Faculty of Life Sciences and Medicine within King's College London. Professor Preedy is also a member of the Department of Nutrition and Dietetics (teaching), Director of the Genomics Centre of King's College London and Professor of Clinical Biochemistry (Hon) at King's College Hospital. Professor Preedy graduated in 1974 with an Honours Degree in Biology and Physiology with Pharmacology. He gained his University of London PhD in 1981. In 1992, he received his Membership of the Royal College of Pathologists and in 1993 he gained his second doctorate (DSc), for his outstanding contribution to protein metabolism in health and disease. Professor Preedy was elected as a Fellow to the Institute of Biology in 1995 and to the Royal College of Pathologists in 2000. Since then he has been elected as a Fellow to the Royal Society for the Promotion of Health (2004) and The Royal Institute of Public Health (2004). In 2009, Professor Preedy became a Fellow of the Royal Society for Public Health and in 2012 a Fellow of the Royal Society of Chemistry. Professor Preedy has carried out research when attached to Imperial College London, The School of Pharmacy (now part of University College London) and the MRC Centre at Northwick Park Hospital. He has collaborated with research groups in Finland, Japan, Australia, USA and Germany. Professor Preedy is a leading expert on the science of health and has a long-standing interest in dietary and plant-based components. He has lectured nationally and internationally. To his credit, Professor Preedy has published more than 700 articles, which include peer-reviewed manuscripts based on original research, abstracts and symposium presentations, reviews and numerous books and volumes.

Vinood B. Patel, BSc, PhD, FRSC, is currently Reader in Clinical Biochemistry at the University of Westminster and honorary fellow at King's College London. He presently directs studies on metabolic pathways involved in liver disease, particularly related to mitochondrial energy regulation and cell death. Research is being undertaken to study the role of nutrients, antioxidants, phytochemicals, iron, alcohol and fatty acids in the pathophysiology of liver disease. Other areas of interest are identifying new biomarkers that can be used for the diagnosis and prognosis of liver disease and understanding mitochondrial oxidative stress in Alzheimer's disease and gastrointestinal dysfunction in autism. Dr. Patel graduated from the University of Portsmouth with a degree in Pharmacology and completed his PhD in protein metabolism from King's College London in 1997. His postdoctoral work was carried out at Wake Forest University Baptist Medical School studying structural-functional alterations to mitochondrial ribosomes, where he developed novel techniques to characterize their biophysical properties. Dr. Patel is a nationally and internationally recognized researcher and has several edited biomedical books related to the use or investigation of active agents or components. These books include *The Handbook of Nutrition, Diet, and Epigenetics; Branched Chain Amino Acids in Clinical Nutrition; Cancer: Oxidative Stress and Dietary Antioxidants; Diet Quality: An Evidence-Based Approach; Toxicology: Oxidative Stress and Dietary Antioxidants;* and *Molecular Nutrition: Vitamins.* In 2014 Dr. Patel was elected as a Fellow to The Royal Society of Chemistry.

Contributors

Tayyiba Afzal
Department of Botany
PMAS Arid Agriculture University
Rawalpindi, Pakistan

Zainab Alsharea
Department of Clinical Pharmacy and
    Therapeutics
Applied Science Private University
Jordan

Abhay Aradhya
School of Osteopathic Medicine and Graduate
    School of Biomedical Sciences
Rowan University
Stratford, New Jersey, USA

Fereshteh Asgharzadeh
Department of Physiology Faculty of Medicine
Mashhad University of Medical Sciences
Mashhad, Iran

Gholamreza Askari
Food Security Research Center and
    Department of Community Nutrition School
    of Nutrition and Food Sciences
Isfahan University of Medical Sciences
Isfahan, Iran

Seyed Abdulmajid Ayatollahi
Phytochemistry Research Center
Shahid Beheshti University of Medical
    Sciences
Tehran, Iran

Mohammad Bagherniya
Food Security Research Center and
    Department of Community Nutrition School
    of Nutrition and Food Sciences
Isfahan University of Medical Sciences
Isfahan, Iran

Muna Barakat
Department of Clinical Pharmacy and
    Therapeutics
Applied Science Private University
Jordan

Sayan Basu
School of Osteopathic Medicine and
    Graduate School of Biomedical
    Sciences
Rowan University
Stratford, New Jersey, USA

Yamin Bibi
Department of Botany
PMAS Arid Agriculture University
Rawalpindi, Pakistan

Eamonn J. Brace
School of Osteopathic Medicine and Graduate
    School of Biomedical Sciences
Rowan University
Stratford, New Jersey, USA

Matthew James Cheesman
School of Pharmacy and Medical Sciences
Griffith University
Australia

Ian Edwin Cock
School of Environment and Science
Griffith University
Australia

Nathupakorn Dechsupa
Department of Radiologic Technology
Faculty of Associated Medical
    Sciences
Chiang Mai University
Thailand

Neziha Yagmur Diker
Department of Pharmaceutical Botany
Faculty of Pharmacy
Hacettepe University
Turkey

Zeynep Dogan
Department of Pharmacognosy
Faculty of Pharmacy
Hacettepe University
Turkey

Joseph J. Drabick
Department of Medicine Division of Hematology
    and Oncology
Penn State Cancer Institute
Pennsylvania State University College of Medicine
Hershey, Pennsylvania, USA

Thomas Efferth
Department of Pharmaceutical Biology
Institute of Pharmacy and Biochemistry
University of Johannes Gutenberg
Germany

Khaoula El Kinany
Department of Epidemiology and Public Health
Faculty of Medicine and Pharmacy of Fez
Sidi Mohamed Ben Abdellah University
Morocco

Soukaina El Kinany
Faculty of Sciences and Techniques
Moulay Ismail University
Errachidia, Morocco

Yujiang Fang
Department of Immunology and Microbiology
Des Moines University
Des Moines, Iowa, USA

Somayyeh Ghareghomi
Department of Biochemistry
Institute of Biochemistry and Biophysics (IBB)
University of Tehran
Tehran, Iran

Salar Hafez Ghoran
Phytochemistry Research Center
Shahid Beheshti University of Medical
    Sciences
Tehran, Iran

Michal Goga
Department of Botany
Institute of Biology and Ecology
Faculty of Natural Science
University of Pavol Jozef Šafárik
Slovakia

Gary S. Goldberg
School of Osteopathic Medicine and Graduate
    School of Biomedical Sciences
Rowan University
Stratford, New Jersey, USA

Amanda Greenspan
School of Osteopathic Medicine and Graduate
    School of Biomedical Sciences
Rowan University
Stratford, New Jersey, USA

Daniel Gyamfi
The Doctors Laboratory Ltd
United Kingdom

Shatha Khaled Haif
Department of Pharmacy
Princess Sarvath Community College
Amman, Jordan

Kelly L. Hamilton
School of Osteopathic Medicine and Graduate
    School of Biomedical Sciences
Rowan University
Stratford, New Jersey, USA

Eliza Hasen
Department of Clinical Pharmacy and
    Therapeutics
Applied Science Private University
Jordan

Mohamed-Elamir F. Hegazy
Department of Chemistry of
    Medicinal Plants
National Research Centre
Egypt

Tyler J. Hellmig
School of Osteopathic Medicine and Graduate
    School of Biomedical Sciences
Rowan University
Stratford, New Jersey, USA

Ali Hosseini
Department of Pharmacognosy
School of Pharmacy
Shiraz University of Medical Sciences
Shiraz, Iran

Katarzyna Jachimowska
School of Osteopathic Medicine
    and Graduate School of
    Biomedical Sciences
Rowan University
Stratford, New Jersey, USA

Cheng Jiang
Department of Pharmacology
Pennsylvania State University College of Medicine
Hershey, Pennsylvania, USA

Monika Joshi
Department of Medicine Division of Hematology
    and Oncology
Penn State Cancer Institute
Pennsylvania State University College of
    Medicine
Hershey, Pennsylvania, USA

Jiraporn Kantapan
Department of Radiologic Technology
Faculty of Associated Medical Sciences
Chiang Mai University
Thailand

Nattiya Kapol
Department of Health
Consumer Protection and Pharmacy
    Administration
Faculty of Pharmacy
Silpakorn University
Thailand

Martin Kello
Department of Pharmacology
Faculty of Medicine
University of Pavol Jozef Šafárik
Slovakia

Prashant Kesharwani
Department of Pharmaceutics
School of Pharmaceutical Education and
    Research
Jamia Hamdard, India

Vahap Murat Kutluay
Department of Pharmacognosy
Faculty of Pharmacy
Hacettepe University
Turkey

Clara Bik-San Lau
Institute of Chinese Medicine and State
    Key Laboratory of Research on Bioactivities
    and Clinical Applications of Medicinal
    Plants
Chinese University of Hong Kong
Shatin, New Territories, Hong Kong

Christopher Laugier
School of Osteopathic Medicine and Graduate
    School of Biomedical Sciences
Rowan University
Stratford, New Jersey, USA

Hae-Jeung Lee
Department of Food and Nutrition
College of Bionanotechnology
Gachon University
Republic of Korea

Hayden Young Lee
Department of Immunology and Microbiology
Des Moines University
Des Moines, Iowa, USA

Vuanghao Lim
Advanced Medical and Dental Institute
Universiti Sains Malaysia
Penang, Malaysia

Junxuan Lü
Department of Pharmacology
Pennsylvania State University College of
    Medicine
Hershey, Pennsylvania, USA

Asma Ismail Mahmod
Department of Clinical Pharmacy and
    Therapeutics
Applied Science Private University
Jordan

Maryam Moradi Binabaj
Cellular and Molecular Research Center
Sabzevar University of Medical Sciences
Sabzevar, Iran

Heba K. Nabih
Department of Medical Biochemistry
National Research Centre
Egypt

Preecha Nootim
Department of Thai Traditional and Alternative
    Medicine
Ministry of Public Health
Thailand

Saumil Parikh
School of Osteopathic Medicine and Graduate
    School of Biomedical Sciences
Rowan University
Stratford, New Jersey, USA

Seon-Joo Park
Department of Food and Nutrition
College of Bionanotechnology
Gachon University
Republic of Korea

Vinood B. Patel
School of Life Sciences
University of Westminster
United Kingdom

Victor R. Preedy
School of Life Course and Population Sciences
Faculty of Life Science and Medicine
King's College London
United Kingdom

Arcadius Puwein
Department of Biotechnology
Assam Don Bosco University
India

Rajkumar Rajendram
College of Medicine
King Saud bin Abdulaziz University for
    Health Sciences
Riyadh, Saudi Arabia

Amirhossein Sahebkar
Applied Biomedical Research Center
Biotechnology Research Center
Pharmaceutical Technology Institute
Department of Biotechnology School of
    Pharmacy
Mashhad University of Medical Sciences
Mashhad, Iran

Nozlena Abdul Samad
Advanced Medical and Dental Institute
Universiti Sains Malaysia
Penang, Malaysia

Iclal Saracoglu
Department of Pharmacognosy
Faculty of Pharmacy
Hacettepe University
Turkey

Farnaz Shahdadian
Department of Clinical Nutrition
School of Nutrition and Food Science
Food Security Research Center
Isfahan University of Medical Sciences
Isfahan, Iran

Anshul Sharma
Department of Food and Nutrition
College of Bionanotechnology
Gachon University
Republic of Korea

Yongquan Shen
School of Osteopathic Medicine and Graduate
    School of Biomedical Sciences
Rowan University
Stratford, New Jersey, USA

Fatemeh Taktaz
Department of Biology
Faculty of Sciences
University of Hakim Sabzevari
Sabzevar, Iran

Wamidh H. Talib
Department of Clinical Pharmacy and
    Therapeutics
Applied Science Private University
Jordan

Trien Trey Tang
Department of Microbiology and Immunology
Des Moines University
Des Moines, Iowa, USA

Shiny C. Thomas
Department of Biotechnology
Assam Don Bosco University
India

Teodora Todorova
Institute of Biodiversity and Ecosystem Research
Bulgarian Academy of Sciences
Sofia, Bulgaria

Xiaoxuan (Farrah) Wu
School of Osteopathic Medicine and Graduate
    School of Biomedical Sciences
Rowan University
Stratford, New Jersey, USA

Yoke Keong Yong
Department of Human Anatomy
Faculty of Medicine and Health Sciences
Universiti Putra Malaysia
Selangor, Malaysia

Grace Gar-Lee Yue
Institute of Chinese Medicine and State Key
    Laboratory of Research on Bioactivities and
    Clinical Applications of Medicinal Plants
Chinese University of Hong Kong
Shatin, New Territories, Hong Kong

Kulsoom Zahara
Department of Botany
PMAS Arid Agriculture University
Rawalpindi, Pakistan

Btissame Zarrouq
Department of Epidemiology and Public Health
Faculty of Medicine and Pharmacy of Fez
Sidi Mohamed Ben Abdellah University
Morocco

Section I

Overviews and Dietary Components

1 Ginsenosides and Hepatic Cancer
A Review of Preclinical and Clinical Studies

Anshul Sharma, Seon-Joo Park and Hae-Jeung Lee

ABBREVIATIONS

AFP	alpha fetoprotein
Akt	protein kinase B
ALT	alanine transaminase
AP-1	activator protein-1
ARHGAP9	rho GTPase activating protein 9
AST	aspartate aminotransferase
Atg7	autophagy related 7
Bax	Bcl-2 associated X apoptosis regulator
Bcl-2	B-cell lymphoma-2
Bclaf1	Bcl-2 associated transcription factor 1
CA4P	combretastatin A4 phosphate
CCl_4	carbon tetrachloride
CD	cluster of differentiation
Cdc25A	cell division cycle 25 A
CDK2	cyclin-dependent kinases 2
CRISPR	clustered regularly interspaced short palindromic repeats
CTX	cyclophosphamide
DEN	dimethylnitrosamine
DNMT	DNA methyltransferase
EGF	epidermal growth factor
EGFR	EGF receptor
ERK	extracellular signal–regulated kinase
ERS	endoplasmic reticulum stress
Fas	first apoptosis signal
FasL	Fas ligand
GRP78	glucose-regulated protein 78
GSK-3β	glycogen synthase kinase-3beta
HCC	hepatocellular carcinoma
HIF-1α	hypoxia-inducible factor-1alpha
HMGB1	high mobility group box 1
IC_{50}	half maximal inhibitory concentration
iCCA	intrahepatic cholangiocarcinoma
IFN-γ	interferon gamma
IL	interleukin
JNK	c-Jun N-terminal kinase

DOI: 10.1201/9781003260028-2

KRG	Korean red ginseng
LDH	lactate dehydrogenase
LPS	lipopolysaccharide
MAPK	mitogen-activated protein kinase
miR-21	microRNA-21
MMP	matrix metalloproteinase
mTOR	mammalian target of rapamycin
MyD88	myeloid differentiation primary response 88
NF-κB	nuclear factor kappa B subunit
NHE1	Na$^+$/H$^+$ exchanger 1
NOD	nonobese diabetic
PARP	poly adenosine diphosphate–ribose polymerase
PI3K	phosphoinositide 3-kinase
PPD	protopanaxadiol
PPT	protopanaxatriol
PTEN	phosphatase and tensin homolog
RCT	randomized controlled trial
ROS	reactive oxygen species
SCID	severe combined immunodeficiency
shRNA	short hairpin small interfering RNA
SIRT2	sirtuin 2
STAT3	signal transducer and activator of transcription 3
TACE	transcatheter arterial chemoembolization
TAE	transcatheter arterial embolization
TLR4	toll-like receptor 4
TNF-α	tumor necrosis factor alpha
VEGF	vascular endothelial growth factor

1.1 INTRODUCTION

Ginseng is a root that gets its name from the Chinese term *jen-shen*, which refers to its man-like shape. It has a long history and is currently one of the world's most extensively used medical herbs (Qi et al. 2011). Ginseng refers to herbal treatments made from the roots of various plants, primarily Asian, or Korean (*Panax ginseng* C. A. Meyer); American or North American ginseng (Xiyangshen, *P. quinquefolius* L.); Japanese ginseng (*P. japonicus* C. A. Meyer); and Vietnamese ginseng (*P. vietnamensis* Ha et Grushv.) (Ratan et al. 2021). Sanchi (Sanqi, Tienqi, or Tienchi) is a Chinese herbal medicine made from the roots of *P. notoginseng* (Burkill) F.H. Chen, also known as radix notoginseng (Yun 2001). The genus *Panax*, which was named after the Russian botanist Carl Anton Von Meyer, means "all-healing" in Greek (Waminal et al. 2012).

1.1.1 Botanical Description

Ginseng is a member of the Araliaceae plant family, and each species has its own unique physiological effects. Ginseng is farmed in a number of places, including South Korea, China, the United States, and Canada, and it requires specific climatic and soil conditions to thrive (Baeg and So 2013). Ginseng is a perennial herb that grows to be 60–80 cm tall. Its roots are fleshy, aromatic, bifurcated, and grayish white to amber-yellow in color, and 5–6 cm long. The surface of the root is wrinkled and divided, and it has a slight sweet flavor at first, followed by a bitter aftertaste. Ginseng has a simple, long, and deep red stalk, a pink blossom, and a red fruit that looks like a little berry. It has leaves that are compound, digitated, round, and thin. There are a total of five leaflets, with the three terminal leaflets being larger than the two lateral leaflets (Yun 2001). Many studies have been conducted to investigate the health benefits of the ginseng plant's fruits, flower buds, stems, leaves, seeds, and berries, as well as the root (Qi et al. 2011).

1.1.2 GINSENOSIDES

Ginseng contains an array of components including ginsenosides with many health-promoting effects (Chen et al. 2021). Ginsenosides are a form of triterpenoid saponin that is related to steroids. Over 200 saponins are found in ginseng plants (Ratan et al. 2021). They are connected to a sugar chain that can be separated into two classifications, oleanane and dammarane, depending on their structural differences (Ratan et al. 2021). Dammarane type ginsenosides are divided into PPD and PPT ginsenosides based on the position of the sugar moieties at carbon positions 3 and 6, respectively. PPD ginsenosides consist of Ra1, Rb1, Ra2, Rb2, Rg3, Rb3, Rd, Rc, and so on, whereas PPT ginsenosides include Rg1, Rh1, Rg2, Rf, Re, and so on. Additionally, 20 (S) and 20 (R) types have also been identified for PPD and PPT ginsenosides, because of the differences in the chiral carbon (C-20) substitution groups. Ginsenosides are annotated alphabetically using Rx and Fx, where R and F signify roots and leaves (folia) of the ginseng plant, respectively, and x (x = 0, a1, b1, c, d, etc.) denotes the order of the ginsenoside based on polarity in thin-layer chromatograms, beginning with the most hydrophilic (Wee et al. 2011; Kim et al. 2017).

1.2 BACKGROUND

Historically, the root of this herbal plant has been used for over 4000 years as a universal remedy and to promote long life (Attele et al. 1999). It has been used for millennia as a hemostatic herb (Yang et al. 2014) and is effective in treating cough, vomiting, and other symptoms. Ginseng is the most valuable medicinal herb in Korea, Japan, and China, and has long been employed as a tonic, curative, and anti-aging agent in traditional medicine (Park et al. 2012). In traditional Chinese beliefs (Leung and Wong 2013), ginseng is said to be an aphrodisiac and to improve sexual behavior. *Panax ginseng* is the most commonly used medication, accounting for 16.6% of the 3,944 remedies listed in the Korean Clinical Pharmacopoeia (Dongeuibogam), which was compiled in 1610 (Yun 2001). According to pre-modern herbal literature written during China's Ming dynasty, ginseng can cure anxiety, despair, and boost cognition (Ong et al. 2015). South Korea appears to have the biggest global proportion, accounting for over a third of all ginseng clinical studies (59), followed by the United States (38) and China (25) (Chen et al. 2021).

1.3 GINSENOSIDES AGAINST HEPATIC CANCER

According to the World Health Organization, over 1 million people will die from liver cancer by 2030 (Anstee et al. 2019). The majority of primary liver malignancies (85%) are hepatocellular carcinoma, with iCCA accounting for the remaining 15% (Yang et al. 2019). Globally, HCC is the sixth most frequent cancer and the fourth main cause of cancer deaths. Despite meticulous surveillance, most HCC patients are in late-stage disease, when curative treatments are rare (Yang et al. 2019). A major case-control study found that ginseng users had a lower risk of cancer than non-users for the duration of their use and lifetime consumption (Yun and Choi 1995).

1.3.1 PRECLINICAL STUDIES

The effects of several ginsenosides on hepatocellular carcinoma using *in vitro* and *in vivo* models are shown in Tables 1.1–1.5.

TABLE 1.1

Preclinical Studies on the Effects of Ginsenoside Rd on Liver Carcinoma

Cell/Animal Model	Type/Dose	Outcome	Reference
HepG2	Rd-0, 10, 50, 100, 200 µM, 24 or 48 hours	Dose- and time-dependent inhibition of the invasion and migration. Dose-dependent reduction of MMP-1, −2, and −7. ⊥ p-ERK, p-p38 MAPK, p-JNK, AP-1 activation	Yoon et al. 2012
HepG2	Rd-2, 10, 20 µM, CA4P-0.05, 0.2, 0.5 µM, 24 hours	CA4P + Rd ⊥ proliferation, ↑ apoptosis	Yang et al. 2021
BALB/c mice	CA4P-5 mg/kg, twice a week, Rd-20 mg/kg, every day	Body weight no change and reduced tumor volume. ⊥ proliferation, ↑ apoptosis, ↑ necrosis, ↓ p-PI3K, ↓ p-mTOR, ↓ p-Akt, ↓ HIF-1α protein	

Note: ⊥ = inhibited; ↑ = increased; ↓ = decrease.

1.3.1.1 Ginsenoside Rd

Ginsenoside Rd inhibited tumor invasion and metastasis in hepatic cancer cells (Yoon et al. 2012). A 48-hour exposure to 100 µM ginsenoside Rd decreased the number of migrating HepG2 cells. Also, Rd at 50 and 100 µM reduced HepG2 migration by 45% and 58%, respectively. These effects may result from the inhibition of MMP activation, induction of focal adhesion formation, and blocking of the MAPK signaling pathway by ginsenoside Rd (Yoon et al. 2012). These findings suggest that Rd may be a candidate therapeutic agent against malignant tumors, including liver cancer.

Recently, the combination of Rd and CA4P (a vascular disrupting agent) inhibited proliferation and activated apoptosis of HepG2 cells. This combination reduced tumor growth and the expression of HIF-1α *in vivo* through synergistic inhibition of the PI3K/Akt and the mTOR signaling pathways (Table 1.1) (Yang et al. 2021).

1.3.1.2 Ginsenoside Rg3

Ginsenoside Rg3 is trace constituent of ginseng that has anticancer activity against numerous cancers, including hepatic cancer. Rg3 consists of two stereo isomeric forms: 20(R)-ginsenoside Rg3 [20(R)-Rg3] and 20(S)-ginsenoside Rg3 [20(S)-Rg3] (Wu et al. 2014). In SMMC-7721 and HepG2 cells, Rg3 effectively inhibited HCC growth and increased apoptosis by activating the endogenous mitochondria-mediated caspase-dependent apoptosis pathway (Zhang et al. 2012). In another study, Rg3 treatment inhibited Hep1–6 and HepG2 cell growth by triggering apoptosis via caspase-dependent signaling. *In vivo*, Rg3 with CTX was more effective than CTX alone in reducing Hep1–6 tumor growth (Table 1.2) (Jiang et al. 2011).

TAE and TACE are reported to cause necrosis in hyper-vascular tumor tissue by restricting arterial supply to malignant tissues. However, hypoxia may also enhance the expression of angiogenic factors, including VEGF and insulin-like growth factor 2, thereby increasing the proliferation and metastasis of residual tumor cells, thus limiting the effectiveness of TAE or TACE (Strebel and Dufour 2008). Chemical-based anti-angiogenic factors offer new possibilities, but they have their own set of limitations. To combat angiogenesis, Zhou and colleagues used plant-based ginsenoside Rg3. A combination of Rg3 and TAE reduced metastasis and prolonged survival by lowering VEGF expression in HCC rat tumors (Zhou et al. 2014). A previous study on white rabbits described the efficacy of Rg3 injected into the hepatic artery combined with TAE as a therapeutic treatment for liver cancer. Rg3 combined with TAE enhanced tumor cell apoptosis and inhibited angiogenesis. This combination also demonstrated antitumor effects *in vitro* (Table 1.2) (Yu et al. 2013).

TABLE 1.2

Preclinical Studies on the Effects of Ginsenoside Rg3 on Liver Carcinoma

Cell/Animal Model	Type/Dose	Outcome	Reference
SMMC-7721, HepG2	Rg3–0, 25, 50, 75, 100 µg/mL, 24 hours, 48 hours	Significant time- and concentration-dependent inhibition of cell proliferation, ↑ apoptosis, ↑ caspase-3, ↑ Bax, ↓ Bcl-2	Zhang et al. 2012
Hep1–6, HepG2	Rg3–0, 50, 100, 200 µg/mL, 24 hours	↓ Proliferation in concentration- and time-dependent manner, ↓ mitochondrial membrane potential, ↑ Bax, ↓ Bcl-2	Jiang et al. 2011
C57BL/6 mice	Intra-tumor injection of Rg3 daily, 3.0 mg/kg, 10 days	Extended survival time, ⊥ tumor growth by >50%	
Buffalo rats	Rg3–1 mg/kg, 8 weeks	Rg3 + TAE reduced body weight, tumor diameter, and metastasis, ↓ microvessel density, ↓ VEGF overexpression, ↓ CD31	Zhou et al. 2014
HepG2	Rg3–25, 50, 75, 100 mg/L, for 12, 24, 36, 48 hours	⊥ Cell proliferation, ↓ VEGF expression	Yu et al. 2013
White male rabbits	Rg3–6.0 mg/kg, TAE or a mixture, 2 weeks	Reduced tumor volume with Rg3 and TAE. ↓ CD31, ↓ VEGF, ↑ caspase-3, ↑ Bax, ↓ Bcl-2	
Specific pathogen-free (SPF) KM mice	20(S)-Rg3 and 20(R)-Rg3 (3 mg/kg, BW) on day 2, once a day, 10 consecutive days	Significant inhibition of tumor growth, ↑ lymphocyte proliferation, ↑ IFN-γ, ↑ IL-2	Wu et al. 2014
HepG2	20(S)-Rg3 or 20(R): Rg3–0, 7.81, 15.63, 31.25, 62.5, 125, 250, 500 µg/mL, 48 hours	⊥ Proliferation, DNA methylation control = 3.56% ± 0.125%, R-type 3.36% ± 0.082%, S-type 2.66% ± 0.111%. ↑ DNMT1, ↓ DNMT3a, ↓ DNMT3b	Teng et al. 2017
HepG2, MHCC-97L	Rg3–1.2, 2.5, 5 µg/mL, 24 hours	Suppressed the migration and invasion of liver cancer cells by upregulating ARHGAP9 protein expression	Sun et al. 2019
BABL/c nude mice	Rg3–2.5, 5, 10 mg/kg/day, 21 days	Inhibited HepG2 and MHCC-97L tumor growth in mouse model	
HepG2, Huh7	Sorafenib-2.5, 5, 10, 15, 20 µM + Rg3–50, 100 µg/mL, 48 hours	Dose-dependent cytotoxicity in HepG2 and Huh7 cells, ↑ apoptosis, ↑ PTEN, ↑ Bax, ↑ cleaved-caspase-3, ↓ p-PDK, ↓ p-Akt	Lu et al. 2018
BALB/c nude mice	Sorafenib-30 mg/kg + Rg3–5 mg/kg once a day	Significant reduction in tumor volume and weight, ↑ PTEN, ↓ p-Akt	

(Continued)

TABLE 1.2
(Continued)

Cell/Animal Model	Type/Dose	Outcome	Reference
Bel-7402 and HCCLM3	Rg3–0, 10, 25, 50, 100 μM, 24 hours	↓ Cell viability, ↑ apoptosis from 2.9% to 16.22%, ↑ cleaved-caspase-3, ↑ cell cycle arrest at G1 phase, ↓ NHE1, ↓ EGF, ↓ EGFR, ↑ HIF-1α, ⊥ inhibited ERK1/2 activation	Li et al. 2018
BALB/c nude mice	Rg3–10 mg/kg BW IP once every 2 days, 3 weeks	Suppressed tumor growth, ↑ cleaved-caspase-3, ↓ NHE1, ↓ EGF, ↓ EGFR, ↑ HIF-1α, ↓ p-ERK1/2	
HepG2	0.25, 0.5, 1 mg/mL of UA+Rg3-LIP, 48 hours	↓ Cell proliferation, ↑ apoptosis, cell cycle arrest G0/G1 phase	Wang et al. 2021
Bel-7402, HCCLM3	Rg3–10, 20, 40, 80, 160, 240 μM, 48 hours	Dose-dependent cell proliferation inhibition, Bel-7402, $IC_{50} = 287.6$ μM, HCCLM3 $IC_{50} = 462.1$ μM, cell cycle arrest at G1 phase, ↓ CDK2, ↓ cyclin D1, ↓ SIRT2	Zheng et al. 2021

Note: ⊥ = inhibited; ↑ = increased; ↓ = decreased.

Another study evaluated the effects of Rg3 stereo forms on tumor growth and immunity using an H22-bearing mouse model. A significant inhibition of tumor growth (40.9% and 23.6%, respectively) was observed using 20 (R)-Rg3 and 20(S)-Rg3. Furthermore, cellular immunity improved significantly, although 20(R)-Rg3 was more effective compared with 20(S)-Rg3 (Wu et al. 2014). Likewise, Teng and coworkers determined the effects of Rg3 R and S types on human HCC, particularly on DNA methylation. The S type lowered cell growth and DNA methylation, and modified cytosine methylation in the promotor regions of Bcl-2, P53, and VEGF. Downregulated expression of DNA methyltransferases (3a/3b) was also observed. In contrast to the earlier study, the S type exhibited more profound inhibitory effects compared with the R type (Teng et al. 2017).

ARHGAP9 must be characterized to properly comprehend its role as a biomarker or therapeutic target at various stages of tumor growth and metastasis (Song et al. 2021). Rho GTPases can regulate cell proliferation, cell adhesion, and the actin cytoskeleton, all of which are important to tumor growth and metastasis (Vega and Ridley 2008). Sun and colleagues described the inhibitory effects of ginsenoside, Rg3, on cancer cells by upregulating ARHGAP9 protein expression. This resulted in considerable suppression of MHCC-97L and HepG2 invasion and migration *in vitro* and prevented the formation of HepG2 and MHCC-97L tumors *in vivo* (Sun et al. 2019).

Another study evaluated the synergistic effect of Rg3 and sorafenib against HCC. By regulating the PTEN/Akt signaling pathway, the combination of Rg3 and sorafenib markedly inhibited HCC cell proliferation and promoted apoptosis compared with sorafenib alone. This combination also reduced tumor volume *in vivo* (Lu et al. 2018).

NHE1 is a widely expressed, acid-extruding membrane transporter that is upregulated and associated with oncogenesis. It is also a candidate therapeutic target for HCC (Yang et al. 2011). The role of Rg3 as an antitumor agent was recently shown using *in vitro* and *in vivo* models of HCC by downregulating NHE1 expression. EGF can stimulate NHE1. Rg3 treatment inhibited tumor growth by lowering EGF, EGF receptor, HIF-1α, and phosphorylated ERK1/2 expression. These results suggest a multitargeting function of Rg3 against HCC (Li et al. 2018). Ursolic acid has been shown to suppress HepG2 proliferation (Yie et al. 2015) and enhance the apoptosis rate in HCC (Kim et al. 2019). In this line, a study demonstrated that the combined use of Rg3 and urosolic acid-loaded liposomes led to a decrease in cell viability, an increase in apoptosis, and a stop in the cell cycle at G0/G1 (Wang et al. 2021). Another study found that Rg3 slows down HCC growth by lowering levels of sirtuin 2 (Zheng et al. 2021).

1.3.1.3   Ginsenoside Rh1

Ginsenoside Rh1 is a single-sugar 20(S) type that exhibits antioxidant, immunomodulatory, anticancer, and estrogenic properties (Tam et al. 2018). Yoon and coworkers demonstrated that Rh1 inhibited HepG2 cell invasion and migration. Rh1 inhibited MMP-1 transcriptional activity, reduced expression and stability of the AP-1 dimer, c-Fos, c-Jun, and inhibited MAPK signaling pathways in HepG2 cells stimulated by phorbol myristate acetate (Yoon et al. 2012) (Table 1.3).

1.3.1.4   Ginsenoside Rh2

Ginsenoside Rh2 suppressed DNA synthesis in SK-Hep-1 cells by boosting p27kip1 (a versatile cyclin-dependent kinase inhibitor) expression and thereby downregulating cyclin E-dependent kinase activity, resulting in G1/S cell cycle arrest (Lee et al. 1996). Chen and coworkers studied

TABLE 1.3
Preclinical Studies on the Effects of Ginsenosides Rh1 and Rh2 on Liver Carcinoma

Cell/Animal Model	Type/Dose	Outcome	Reference
HepG2	Rh1–10, 50, 100, 200 µM, 24 hours	⊥ Invasion and migration, ↓ MMP-1 expression, ⊥ p-ERK1/2, p-p38 MAPK, and p-JNK1/2, ⊥ AP-1 activation	Yoon et al. 2012
SK-Hep-1	Rh2–0.25–100 µmol/L	⊥ G1/S, ↓ Cdc25A ↓ cyclin E, ↑ p27kip1, ⊥ DNA synthesis	Lee et al. 1996
Male Kun-Ming mice	Rh2, Rh2-O 10 mg/kg once daily, 15 days	No change in body weight, ⊥ tumor growth, ↑ apoptosis, ↓ Bcl-2, ↑ Bax, ↑ cleaved-caspase 9/3, ↑ IL-2, ↑ TNF-α, ↓ VEGF	Chen et al. 2017
HepG2	Rh2–10–160 µ/mol, 24, 48, 72 hours	⊥ Cell growth dose- and time-dependent, ⊥ AP-1 transcription factor, ⊥ MMP3 expression and protein inhibit migratory ability. Effective 80 µ/moL	Shi et al. 2014
HepG2, SMMC-7721	Rh2–5, 10, 20, 40, 100 µM, 48 hours	↓ Cell viability, ⊥ proliferation, ↓ EGFR levels, ↑ microRNA 491 level	Chen and Qiu 2015
Male NOD/SCID mice	Rh2–1 mg/kg BW, twice/week, 1 month	⊥ Tumor growth	
HepG2	Rh2–50, 100, 150, 200 µmol/L, 24, 48, 72 hours	⊥ of cell growth dose- and time-dependent, cell cycle arrest at Go/G1 phase, ↑ apoptosis, activated GSK-3β, ↓ cyclin D1, ↓ Bcl-2, ↓ MMP3, ↑ Bax	Shi et al. 2016

(Continued)

TABLE 1.3
(Continued)

Cell/Animal Model	Type/Dose	Outcome	Reference
BALB/c mice	Rh2–20 mg/kg, once a day, 20 days	Nucleus atypia, condensation of nuclei in tumor tissue. ↑ GSK-3β expression, ↓ cyclin D1, ↓ Bcl-2, ↓ MMP3,↑ Bax	
HepG2, Huh7	Rh2–0.01, 0.1, 1 mg/mL, 24 hours	Dose-dependent inhibition of cell growth, ↓ tumor sphere-like structure formation, ↓ β-catenin, ↑ Atg7, ↑ microtubule-associated protein 1A/1B-light chain 3 (LC3) II/I	Yang et al. 2016
Female NOD/SCID mice	Rh2–1mg/kg BW, twice/week, 4 weeks	⊥ tumor growth	

Note: ⊥ = inhibited; ↑ = increased; ↓ = decreased.

the antitumor and immunomodulatory effects of Rh2 and its octyl ester derivative (Rh2-O) using the H22-bearing mouse model. The tumor inhibitory rates of Rh2-O and Rh2 were 50.6% and 28.2%, respectively. Both activated caspases, which led to apoptosis, and changed cell immunity by boosting the production of IL-2 and TNF-α. Both Rh2-O and Rh2 caused a marked decrease in VEGF, although the ester derivative had a greater effect (Chen et al. 2017). Rh2 inhibited the capacity of HepG2 cells to migrate by engaging histone deacetylase, which inhibits AP-1 transcription factors (Shi et al. 2014). A recent study discovered that miR-491 inhibits HCC progression by suppressing the EGFR signaling pathway. Thus, treatment with Rh2 may raise the levels of miR-491 while also lowering the levels of EGFR (Chen and Qiu 2015) (Table 1.3).

In a study, ginsenoside Rh2 downregulates β-catenin by activating GSK-3 to reduce tumor weight *in vivo*. The IC_{50} values of Rh2 on HepG2 and HepG2-β-catenin cells treated *in vitro* for 48 and 72 hours were 100 and 58.12 μmol/l, and 129.2 and 83.33 μmol/l, respectively (Shi et al. 2016). Another intriguing study looked at the link between autophagy and β-catenin and found that Rh2 inhibited β-catenin, enhanced autophagy in HCC, and had antitumor properties. The authors also discovered that inhibiting autophagy with shRNA against Atg7 prevented Rh2-mediated β-catenin modification (Yang et al. 2016) (Table 1.3).

1.3.1.5 Ginsenoside R1

Saponin R1, also known as notoginsenoside R1, is a novel, active triterpene saponin molecule discovered from the roots of *Panax notoginseng* with antioxidative, anti-inflammatory, neuroprotective, pro-apoptotic, and antiproliferative activities (He et al. 2012).

HCC cell invasion and migration are increased by miR-21 overexpression, whereas miR-21 deficiency has antiproliferative and apoptotic effects (Najafi et al. 2015). Using miR-21 as a therapeutic target, Li et al. exhibited antihepatoma activity of saponin R1 via miR-21 downregulation (Li et al. 2020). In HCC cells, R1 treatment inhibited cell growth and invasion while promoting apoptosis. These effects were caused by downregulating miR-21, which inactivated the PI3K/Akt signaling pathway (Li et al. 2020) (Table 1.4).

TABLE 1.4

Preclinical Studies on the Effects of Ginsenosides R1 and Rk3 on Liver Carcinoma

Cell/Animal Model	Type/Dose	Outcomes	Reference
MHCC97H, HepG2, Huh7, BEL7402, PLC/PRF/5 (PLC), SMMC7721	Notoginsenoside-R1- 5, 10, 20, 40, 80, 160 μM, 48 hours miR-21 Transfection + 40 μM, 48 hours	⊥ Viability, ↑ apoptosis, ↑ caspase 3/7 activity, ↑ LDH release, ↓ miR-21 expression, ⊥ PI3K/Akt pathway activation	Li et al. 2020
Caco-2	Rk3–5, 10, 15, 20, 25, 30, 35, and 40 μM + 1 μg/mL LPS and 30 μM Rk3, 24 hours	↓ Dose-dependent cell viability. Restored TJ protein expression	Qu et al. 2021
DEN- and CCl$_4$-induced male C57BL/6J mice	L-Rk3 group (30 mg/kg, i.g.), and H-Rk3 group (60 mg/kg, i.g.), 22 weeks	↓ Tumor nodules in the liver, ↓ cyclin B1, ↓ ALT, ↓ AST, ↓ HMGB1, serum and liver AFP levels, ↓ TNF-α, ↓ NF-κB, ↓ MyD88, ↑ IL-10, ↑ Bax, ↓ Bcl-2, ↓ TLR4 protein expression	

Note: ⊥ = inhibited; ↑ = increased; ↓ = decreased.

1.3.1.6   Ginsenoside Rk3

Ginsenoside Rk3 is a rare but potent molecule produced from Rg1 that can be found in heat-treated ginseng at a lower molecular weight. Rk3 has a number of health benefits (Qu et al. 2021).

A study published recently looked at the effects of ginsenoside Rk3 on HCC growth, inflammation, and gut microbiota in the CCl$_4$- and DEN-induced spontaneous HCC mouse models. Ginsenoside Rk3 was discovered to reduce HCC development, liver damage, cirrhosis, fibrosis, and inflammation by targeting the TLR4 pathway through the gut-liver axis. Furthermore, ginsenoside Rk3 ameliorated intestinal flora dysbiosis, promoting beneficial microbiota and successfully preventing HCC recurrence. These data show that Rk3 may be an effective therapeutic and preventive agent for HCC (Qu et al. 2021) (Table 1.4).

1.3.1.7   Ginsenoside Compound K

Compound K (CK, also known as M1 or IH-901) is a novel, active metabolite generated by the glycosylation of ginsenosides Rb1, Rc, and Rb2 by human gut microbiota and reported to have various health-enhancing effects (Sharma and Lee 2020). An earlier study found that IH-901 induced apoptosis in HepG2 cells through a mitochondrial-mediated mechanism, which resulted in caspase-9 activation and concomitant activation of the mitochondrial apoptosis pathway. Caspase-8 was discovered to cleave BH3-interacting domain death agonist (Bid), causing it to move to the mitochondria and activate the mitochondrial pathway (Table 1.5) (Oh and Lee 2004).

IH-901 was tested against human SMCC7721 cells and shown to have growth inhibitory and apoptotic effects via a mitochondrial-mediated mechanism that resulted in caspase-9 and caspase-3 activation and mitochondrial cytochrome c release (Ming et al. 2007). Another study investigated CK's effects on HCC cells *in vitro* and *in vivo* (Ming et al. 2011). CK treatment significantly reduced adhesion, colony formation, and invasion *in vitro*. The growth of spontaneous HCC metastatic nodules was inhibited *in vivo* following the treatment of a mouse model with CK (Table 1.2). They also discovered that downregulating MMP2/9 and nuclear export of NF-κB p65 were associated with CK-induced metastatic suppression (Ming et al. 2011). Wang and colleagues found that CK inhibits the proliferation of HepG2 cells by down-regulating the NF-κB component p50 and selectively targeting annexin A2. Furthermore, cas-pase 9 and 3 expressions were increased. This study discovered for the first time that annexin A2 is a target for CK (Table 1.5) (Wang et al. 2019).

CK reduced the proliferation of highly metastatic MHCC97-H cells. Also, CK supplementation caused DNA damage and reduced the potential of the mitochondrial membrane. Overall, CK sup-presses cell growth and triggers apoptosis in HCC cells through Fas- and mitochondria-mediated caspase-dependent pathways (Table 1.5) (Zheng et al. 2014).

TABLE 1.5

Preclinical Studies on the Effects of Ginsenoside Compound K on Liver Carcinoma

Cell/Animal Model	Type/Dose	Outcomes	Reference
HepG2	IH-901–10, 20, 40, 60 μmol/L	↑ Antiproliferative effects, ↓PARP, ↑apoptosis, ↑ caspase-3, -8, -9, ↑ cytochrome c	Oh and Lee 2004
SMMC7721	IH-901–25, 50, 75, 100 μM, 12, 24, 48, 72 hours	⊥ Proliferation, dose- and time-dependent, ↑ cell cycle arrest at the G0-G1 phase. ↑ Bax, ↑ P53	Ming et al. 2007
MHCC97-H	CK-25, 50, and 75 μM	Significant ⊥ cell growth, ⊥ colony formation, ⊥ cell adhesion	Ming et al. 2011
BALB/c (nu/nu)	50 and 100 μg/mL	Significant ⊥ of cell growth and metastasis	
HepG2	CK (6 μM), etoposide (25 μg/mL) or Phorbol myristate acetate (PMA, 100 ng/mL)	Targeting annexin A2, ↓ NF-κB, ↑ caspase-9, ↑ caspase-3	Wang et al. 2019
MHCC97-H	CK-25, 50, 75, and 100 μM, 48 hours	Dose- and time-dependent reduction of HCC IC_{50} (48 hours) = 49.8 ± 2.5 μM. ↑ G0/G1 cell cycle arrest, ↑ Fas/FasL expression, ↑ cleaved-caspase-8, ↓ pro-caspase-9 and −3, ⊥ p-Akt, ↑ Bax/Bcl-2 ratio	Zheng et al. 2014
HepG2, SMMC-7721, Hep3B, Huh7	CK-20, 40, 60 μM, 48 hours	↑ ERS, ↓ p-STAT3, ↑ GRP78 IC_{50} of CK for HepG2, SMMC-7721, Hep3B, and Huh7 cells: 40.45, 48.36, 45.55, and 41.93 μM	Zhang et al. 2018
Bel-7404, Huh7	CK-20, 40, 60, 80 μM, 24, 48, and 72 hours	↓ Bclaf1, ↓ HIF-1α, ↓ HIF-1α-mediated glycolysis pathway, IC_{50} of CK in Bel-7404 cells: 24 hours – 63.78, 48 hours – 38.52, and 72 hours – 28.88 μM. In Huh7 cells: 24 hours – 64.00, 48 hours – 38.54, and 72 hours – 28.31 μM, respectively	Zhang et al. 2020
SD rats	CK (low-dose, 2.5 mg/kg; high-dose, 5 mg/kg)	⊥ Hepatocellular carcinoma	

Note: ⊥ = inhibited; ↑ = increased; ↓ = decreased.

In HepG2 and SMMC-7721 cells, CK treatment reduced STAT3's DNA-binding capacity. The application of CRISPR/Cas9 technology to suppress STAT3 aided in the promotion of CK-induced ERS and apoptosis. Overall, CK promoted ERS and apoptosis in human liver cancer cells through decreasing phosphorylated-STAT3 levels (Zhang et al. 2018).

Recent research has focused on the mechanism by which CK regulates HIF1α-mediated glycolysis *in vitro* and *in vivo* to limit the proliferation of human liver cancer cells. CK reduces the expression of Bcl-2-associated transcription factor 1 in hypoxic liver cancer cells by inhibiting HIF1α-mediated glycolysis and suppressing cell growth. CK blocked cell growth by arresting the cell cycle at the G0/G1 stage (Zhang et al. 2020) (Table 1.5).

1.3.2 CLINICAL STUDIES

Due to their low bioavailability, the application of ginsenosides has been constrained to cells and laboratory animals, and just a few human studies have been documented. Earlier research looked at the link between ginseng and cancer. In one epidemiological study (Yun et al. 2001), patients who consumed KRG had a lower risk of cancer than those who did not. Furthermore, individuals who consumed ginseng had a lower risk of developing liver cancer than those who did not. In a clinical study of 26 Egyptian HCC patients, the pharmacological potential of KRG extract was tested (Abdel-Wahhab et al. 2011). The liver function of these individuals was tested at 6 and 11 weeks after they received oral KRG supplementation. When compared to the control group, patients who received KRG had significantly lower serum ALT and AST levels. Additionally, after 6 weeks of KRG administration, an oral dose of the extract resulted in higher serum albumin levels. These data indicate that KRG may be effective in the treatment of HCC. Ginsenosides have been used as adjuvants for TACE treatment against HCC. A single-center, open-label, randomized, controlled trial involving 228 patients with advanced HCC showed that combining ginsenoside Rg3 capsules with TACE improved overall survival compared to TACE alone (Table 1.6) (Zhou et al. 2016).

Furthermore, in a recent study, two meta-analyses were undertaken to examine if combined TACE and ginsenosides therapy had a better effect on HCC, and subgroup analyses were performed to optimize the ginsenosides and TACE combination. Rg3 was shown to be the best choice for HCC treatment when combined with TACE (Zhu et al. 2021).

TABLE 1.6
Clinical Studies on the Effects of the Ginsenosides on Liver Carcinoma

Participants/ Country	Treatment	Ginsenosides	Outcomes	Reference
26 people with HCC/Egypt	KRG extract capsule (900 mg/d) 11 wk	Rg3, Rh2, Rh1, Rh4, Rs1, or Rs2, Rs3, Rs4, Rg5, Rg2, F4, notoginsenoside R4, IH-901	↑ α-fetoprotein	Abdel-Wahhab et al. 2011
228 patients with advanced HCC/China	Rg3 capsule + TACE or TACE alone	Rg3	Rg3 + TACE may prolong overall survival	Zhou et al. 2016
18 RCTs with 1308 HCC patients/China	Total ginsenoside, Rg3, Rh2 and CK + TACE	Rg3, Rh2, CK	Rg3 + TACE best combination	Zhu et al. 2021

Note: ↑ = increase.

1.4   OTHER KOREAN FOODS USED IN CANCER

Kimchi is a Korean fermented vegetable preparation that contains dietary fiber, quercetin, lactic acid bacteria, vitamin C, minerals, and capsaicin, among other things. In Korea, about 200 types of kimchi are prepared based on the raw components utilized, the processing methods employed, the geographical regions and the harvest seasons. The most essential ingredients in kimchi include garlic, ginger, with and without red pepper and salted fish, spring onion, radish, and *Baechu* cabbage. However, other vegetables are utilized depending on seasonal availability in different areas (Patra et al. 2016). Kimchi has many health-promoting benefits, including anticancer activity (Kim et al. 2015). Another fermented food is *doenjang* (soybean paste), which has been utilized as a flavor and protein source for generations. It has been demonstrated to have anticancer properties (Lim et al. 1999).

1.5   TOXICITY AND CAUTIONARY NOTES

Ginseng has been linked to mild toxicity in humans, with only a few reported side effects. A two-year human investigation found adverse effects linked to long-term ginseng intake at doses of up to 15 g per day. Fourteen individuals out of 133 had morning diarrhea, uneasiness, decreased appetite, skin eruption, sleeplessness, hypertension, edema, and depression, which is known as ginseng abuse syndrome (Siegel. 1979). Furthermore, research based on a review of the literature suggests that ginseng is rarely connected to major side effects similar to placebo or drug interactions (Coon and Ernst 2002; Shergis et al. 2013). However, further research is needed to assess high- and long-term doses as well as their relationship to adverse events or drug interactions.

1.6   SUMMARY POINTS

- Ginsenosides' anti–liver cancer activities are mostly mediated through cytotoxicity, antiproliferation, anti-invasion, and metastasis, inducing apoptosis, anti-angiogenesis, miRNA activity downregulation, and activation of tumor suppressor genes.
- Ginsenosides enhanced the efficiency of existing drugs such as sorafenib, cyclophosphamide (Rg3), and combretastatin A4 phosphate (Rd), showed synergetic effects on inhibiting proliferation, promoting apoptosis, and reducing tumor volume by modulation of signaling pathways.
- Ginsenoside Rk3 decreased HCC development, liver damage, cirrhosis, fibrosis, and inflammation by targeting the TLR4 pathway through the gut-liver axis and ameliorated intestinal flora dysbiosis.
- In people with advanced hepatocellular cancer, Rg3 eased symptoms of transcatheter arterial chemoembolization and helped them live longer.
- More human studies using ginsenosides with improved bioavailability, including large epidemiological investigations and well-designed clinical trials, are needed to show that ginsenosides have anti–hepatic cancer effects.

REFERENCES

Abdel-Wahhab, Mosaad A, Khaled Gamil, Ahmed A El-Kady, Aziza A El-Nekeety, and Khayria M Naguib. 2011. Therapeutic effects of Korean red ginseng extract in Egyptian patients with chronic liver diseases. Journal of Ginseng Research 35 (1):69–79.

Anstee, Quentin M, Helen L Reeves, Elena Kotsiliti, Olivier Govaere, and Mathias Heikenwalder. 2019. From NASH to HCC: Current concepts and future challenges. Nature Reviews Gastroenterology & Hepatology 16 (7):411–428.

Attele, Anoja S, Ji An Wu, and Chun-Su Yuan. 1999. Ginseng pharmacology: multiple constituents and multiple actions. Biochemical Pharmacology 58 (11):1685–1693.

Baeg, In-Ho, and Seung-Ho So. 2013. The world ginseng market and the ginseng (Korea). Journal of Ginseng Research 37 (1):1–7.

Chen, Fang, Yong Sun, Shi-Lian Zheng, Yan Qin, David Julian McClements, Jiang-Ning Hu, and Ze-Yuan Deng. 2017. Antitumor and immunomodulatory effects of ginsenoside Rh2 and its octyl ester derivative in H22 tumor-bearing mice. Journal of Functional Foods 32:382–390.

Chen, Weijie, Peifen Yao, Chi Teng Vong, Xiuzhu Li, Zhejie Chen, Jianbo Xiao, Shengpeng Wang, and Yitao Wang. 2021. Ginseng: A bibliometric analysis of 40-year journey of global clinical trials. Journal of Advanced Research 34:187–197.

Chen, Weiwen, and Yurong Qiu. 2015. Ginsenoside Rh2 targets EGFR by up-regulation of miR-491 to enhance anti-tumor activity in hepatitis B virus-related hepatocellular carcinoma. Cell Biochemistry and Biophysics 72 (2):325–331.

Coon, Joanna Thompson, and Edzard Ernst. 2002. *Panax ginseng*: A systematic review of adverse effects and drug interactions. Drug Safety 25 (5):323–344.

He, Nian-Wu, Yan Zhao, Ling Guo, Jun Shang, and Xing-Bin Yang. 2012. Antioxidant, antiproliferative, and pro-apoptotic activities of a saponin extract derived from the roots of *Panax notoginseng* (Burk.) FH Chen. Journal of Medicinal Food 15 (4):350–359.

Jiang, Jian-Wen, Xin-Mei Chen, Xin-Hua Chen, and Shu-Sen Zheng. 2011. Ginsenoside Rg3 inhibit hepatocellular carcinoma growth via intrinsic apoptotic pathway. World Journal of Gastroenterology: WJG 17 (31):3605–3613.

Kim, Bohkyung, Jia-Le Song, Jae-Hyun Ju, Soon-Ah Kang, and Kun-Young Park. 2015. Anticancer effects of kimchi fermented for different times and with added ingredients in human HT-29 colon cancer cells. Food Science and Biotechnology 24 (2):629–633.

Kim, Geon-Hee, Sang-Yeon Kan, Hyeji Kang, Sujin Lee, Hyun Myung Ko, Ji Hyung Kim, and Ji-Hong Lim. 2019. Ursolic acid suppresses cholesterol biosynthesis and exerts anti-cancer effects in hepatocellular carcinoma cells. International Journal of Molecular Sciences 20 (19):4767.

Kim, Ji Hye, Young-Su Yi, Mi-Yeon Kim, and Jae Youl Cho. 2017. Role of ginsenosides, the main active components of *Panax ginseng*, in inflammatory responses and diseases. Journal of Ginseng Research 41 (4):435–443.

Lee, Kwang Youl, Jeong Ae Park, Eunah Chung, You Hui Lee, Shin Kim II, and Seung Ki Lee. 1996. Ginsenoside-Rh2 blocks the cell cycle of SK-HEP-1 cells at the G1/S boundary by selectively inducing the protein expression of p27kip1. Cancer Letters 110 (1–2):193–200.

Leung, Kar Wah, and Alice ST Wong. 2013. Ginseng and male reproductive function. Spermatogenesis 3 (3):e26391.

Li, Xiao, Jiaywei Tsauo, Chong Geng, He Zhao, Xuelian Lei, and Xiao Li. 2018. Ginsenoside Rg3 decreases NHE1 expression via inhibiting EGF-EGFR-ERK1/2-HIF-1 α pathway in hepatocellular carcinoma: A novel antitumor mechanism. The American Journal of Chinese Medicine 46 (08):1915–1931.

Li, Yuan, Zhong Li, Yunhao Jia, Bo Ding, and Jinsong Yu. 2020. In vitro anti-hepatoma activities of notoginsenoside R1 through downregulation of tumor promoter miR-21. Digestive Diseases and Sciences 65 (5):1364–1375.

Lim, Sun Young, Kun Young Park, and Sook-Hee Rhee. 1999. Anticancer effect of doenjang in vitro sulforhodamine B (SRB) assay. Journal of the Korean Society of Food Science and Nutrition 28 (1):240–245.

Lu, Mingxia, Zhenghua Fei, and Ganlu Zhang. 2018. Synergistic anticancer activity of 20 (S)-Ginsenoside Rg3 and Sorafenib in hepatocellular carcinoma by modulating PTEN/Akt signaling pathway. Biomedicine & Pharmacotherapy 97:1282–1288.

Ming, Yan-lin, Gang Song, Liang-hua Chen, Zhi-zhong Zheng, Zhong-yan Chen, Gao-liang Ouyang, and Qing-xuan Tong. 2007. Anti-proliferation and apoptosis induced by a novel intestinal metabolite of ginseng saponin in human hepatocellular carcinoma cells. Cell Biology International 31 (10):1265–1273.

Ming, Yan-lin, Zhong-yan Chen, Liang-hua Chen, Dejian Lin, Qing-xuan Tong, Zhi-zhong Zheng, and Gang Song. 2011. Ginsenoside compound K attenuates metastatic growth of hepatocellular carcinoma, which is associated with the translocation of nuclear factor-κB p65 and reduction of matrix metalloproteinase-2/9. Planta Medica 77 (5):428–433.

Najafi, Z, M Sharifi, and G Javadi. 2015. Degradation of miR-21 induces apoptosis and inhibits cell proliferation in human hepatocellular carcinoma. Cancer Gene Therapy 22 (11):530–535.

Oh, Seon-Hee, and Byung-Hoon Lee. 2004. A ginseng saponin metabolite-induced apoptosis in HepG2 cells involves a mitochondria-mediated pathway and its downstream caspase-8 activation and Bid cleavage. Toxicology and Applied Pharmacology 194 (3):221–329.

Ong, Wei-Yi, Tahira Farooqui, Hwee-Ling Koh, Akhlaq A Farooqui, and Eng-Ang Ling. 2015. Protective effects of ginseng on neurological disorders. Frontiers in Aging Neuroscience 7:129.

Park, Ho Jae, Dong Hyun Kim, Se Jin Park, Jong Min Kim, and Jong Hoon Ryu. 2012. Ginseng in traditional herbal prescriptions. Journal of Ginseng Research 36 (3):225–241.

Patra, Jayanta Kumar, Gitishree Das, Spiros Paramithiotis, and Han-Seung Shin. 2016. Kimchi and other widely consumed traditional fermented foods of Korea: A review. Frontiers in Microbiology 7:1493.

Qi, Lian-Wen, Chong-Zhi Wang, and Chun-Su Yuan. 2011. Isolation and analysis of ginseng: Advances and challenges. Natural Product Reports 28 (3):467–495.

Qu, Linlin, Xiaoxuan Ma, and Daidi Fan. 2021. Ginsenoside Rk3 suppresses hepatocellular carcinoma development through targeting the gut-liver axis. Journal of Agricultural and Food Chemistry 69 (35):10121–10137.

Ratan, Zubair Ahmed, Mohammad Faisal Haidere, Yo Han Hong, Sang Hee Park, Jeong-Oog Lee, Jongsung Lee, and Jae Youl Cho. 2021. Pharmacological potential of ginseng and its major component ginsenosides. Journal of Ginseng Research 45 (2):199–210.

Sharma, Anshul, and Hae-Jeung Lee. 2020. Ginsenoside compound K: Insights into recent studies on pharmacokinetics and health-promoting activities. Biomolecules 10 (7):1028.

Shergis, Johannah L, Anthony L Zhang, Wenyu Zhou, and Charlie C Xue. 2013. *Panax ginseng* in randomised controlled trials: A systematic review. Phytotherapy Research 27 (7):949–965.

Shi, Qingqiang, Jing Li, Ziqiang Feng, Lvcui Zhao, Lian Luo, Zhimei You, Danyang Li, Jing Xia, Guowei Zuo, and Dilong Chen. 2014. Effect of ginsenoside Rh2 on the migratory ability of HepG2 liver carcinoma cells: Recruiting histone deacetylase and inhibiting activator protein 1 transcription factors. Molecular Medicine Reports 10 (4):1779–1785.

Shi, Qingqiang, Xueping Shi, Gei Zuo, Wei Xiong, Haixing Li, Pei Guo, Fen Wang, Yi Chen, Jing Li, and Di-Long Chen. 2016. Anticancer effect of 20 (S)-ginsenoside Rh2 on HepG2 liver carcinoma cells: Activating GSK-3β and degrading β-catenin. Oncology Reports 36 (4):2059–2070.

Siegel, Ronald K. 1979. Ginseng abuse syndrome: problems with the panacea. Jama 241 (15):1614–1615.

Song, Wenping, Jinhua Chen, Shuolei Li, Ding Li, Yongna Zhang, Hanqiong Zhou, Weijiang Yu, Baoxia He, Wenzhou Zhang, and Liang Li. 2021. Rho GTPase activating protein 9 (ARHGAP9) in human cancers. Recent Patents on Anti-cancer Drug Discovery 17(1):55–65.

Strebel, Bruno M, and Jean-François Dufour. 2008. Combined approach to hepatocellular carcinoma: a new treatment concept for nonresectable disease. Expert Review of Anticancer Therapy 8 (11):1743–1749.

Sun, Meng-Yao, Ya-Nan Song, Miao Zhang, Chun-Yan Zhang, Li-Jun Zhang, and Hong Zhang. 2019. Ginsenoside Rg3 inhibits the migration and invasion of liver cancer cells by increasing the protein expression of ARHGAP9. Oncology Letters 17 (1):965–973.

Tam, Dao Ngoc Hien, Duy Hieu Truong, Thi Thanh Hoa Nguyen, Le Nhat Quynh, Linh Tran, Hong Duong Nguyen, Bahaa eldin Shamandy, Thi Minh Huong Le, Dang Khoa Tran, Dina Sayed, Van Vinh Vu, Shusaku Mizukami, Kenji Hirayama, Nguyen Tien Huy 2018. Ginsenoside Rh1: A systematic review of its pharmacological properties. Planta Medica 84 (03):139–152.

Teng, Siying, Yi Wang, Pingya Li, Jinhua Liu, Anhui Wei, Haotian Wang, Xiangkun Meng, Di Pan, and Xinmin Zhang. 2017. Effects of R type and S type ginsenoside Rg3 on DNA methylation in human hepatocarcinoma cells. Molecular Medicine Reports 15 (4):2029–2038.

Vega, Francisco M, and Anne J Ridley. 2008. Rho GTPases in cancer cell biology. FEBS Letters 582 (14):2093–2101.

Waminal, Nomar Espinosa, Hye Mi Park, Kwang Bok Ryu, Joo Hyung Kim, Tae-Jin Yang, and Hyun Hee Kim. 2012. Karyotype analysis of *Panax ginseng* C.A. Meyer, 1843 (*Araliaceae*) based on rDNA loci and DAPI band distribution. Comparative Cytogenetics 6 (4):425–441.

Wang, Bin, Qiaoqiao Xu, Chenjian Zhou, and Yu Lin. 2021. Liposomes co-loaded with ursolic acid and ginsenoside Rg3 in the treatment of hepatocellular carcinoma. Acta Biochimica Polonica 68 (4):711–715.

Wang, Yu-Shi, Hongyan Zhu, He Li, Yang Li, Bing Zhao, and Ying-Hua Jin. 2019. Ginsenoside compound K inhibits nuclear factor-kappa B by targeting Annexin A2. Journal of Ginseng Research 43 (3):452–459.

Wee, Jae Joon, Kyeong Mee Park, and An-Sik Chung. 2011. Biological activities of ginseng and its application to human health. In: Herbal Medicine: Biomolecular and Clinical Aspects, ed. Iris F. F. Benzie and Sissi Wachtel-Galor, 2nd edition. Boca Raton (FL): CRC Press/Taylor & Francis.

Wu, Rihui, Qin Ru, Lin Chen, Baomiao Ma, and Chaoying Li. 2014. Stereospecificity of Ginsenoside Rg3 in the promotion of cellular immunity in hepatoma H22-bearing mice. Journal of Food Science 79 (7):H1430–H1435.

Yang, Ju Dong, Pierre Hainaut, Gregory J Gores, Amina Amadou, Amelie Plymoth, and Lewis R Roberts. 2019. A global view of hepatocellular carcinoma: Trends, risk, prevention and management. Nature Reviews Gastroenterology & Hepatology 16 (10):589–604.

Yang, Xiaochen, Xingjiang Xiong, Heran Wang, and Jie Wang. 2014. Protective effects of panax notoginseng saponins on cardiovascular diseases: A comprehensive overview of experimental studies. Evidence-Based Complementary and Alternative Medicine 2014: 204840.

Yang, Xinxiu, Meng Gao, Mengqi Miao, Cuihua Jiang, Dongjian Zhang, Zhiqi Yin, Yicheng Ni, Jing Chen, and Jian Zhang. 2021. Combining combretastatin A4 phosphate with ginsenoside Rd synergistically inhibited hepatocellular carcinoma by reducing HIF-1α via PI3K/AKT/mTOR signalling pathway. Journal of Pharmacy and Pharmacology 73 (2):263–271.

Yang, Xuekang, Desheng Wang, Wei Dong, Zhenshun Song, and Kefeng Dou. 2011. Expression and modulation of Na+/H+ exchanger 1 gene in hepatocellular carcinoma: A potential therapeutic target. Journal of Gastroenterology and Hepatology 26 (2):364–370.

Yang, Zhiqing, Tingting Zhao, Hongli Liu, and Leida Zhang. 2016. Ginsenoside Rh2 inhibits hepatocellular carcinoma through β-catenin and autophagy. Scientific Reports 6 (1):19383.

Yie, Yinyi, Shunyu Zhao, Qin Tang, Fang Zheng, Jingjing Wu, LiJuan Yang, ShiGuan Deng, and Swei Sunny Hann. 2015. Ursolic acid inhibited growth of hepatocellular carcinoma HepG2 cells through AMPKα-mediated reduction of DNA methyltransferase 1. Molecular and Cellular Biochemistry 402 (1):63–74.

Yoon, Ji-Hae, Yeo-Jin Choi, Seon-Woo Cha, and Seong-Gene Lee. 2012. Anti-metastatic effects of ginsenoside Rd via inactivation of MAPK signaling and induction of focal adhesion formation. Phytomedicine 19 (3–4):284–292.

Yu, Yang, Chunle Zhang, Lingjun Liu, and Xiao Li. 2013. Hepatic arterial administration of ginsenoside Rg3 and transcatheter arterial embolization for the treatment of VX2 liver carcinomas. Experimental and Therapeutic Medicine 5 (3):761–766.

Yun, Taik Koo. 2001. Brief introduction of Panax ginseng CA Meyer. Journal of Korean Medical Science 16 (Suppl):S3–S5.

Yun, Taik-Koo, and Soo-Yong Choi. 1995. Preventive effect of ginseng intake against various human cancers: a case-control study on 1987 pairs. Cancer Epidemiology and Prevention Biomarkers 4 (4):401–408.

Yun, Taik Koo, Soo Yong Choi, and Hyo Yung Yun. 2001. Epidemiological study on cancer prevention by ginseng: are all kinds of cancers preventable by ginseng? Journal of Korean Medical Science 16 (Suppl):S19–S27.

Zhang, Chunle, Lingjun Liu, Yang Yu, Bin Chen, Chengwei Tang, and Xiao Li. 2012. Antitumor effects of ginsenoside Rg3 on human hepatocellular carcinoma cells. Molecular Medicine Reports 5 (5):1295–1298.

Zhang, Silin, Meilan Zhang, Jiaxin Chen, Jiaqi Zhao, Jielin Su, and Xuewu Zhang. 2020. Ginsenoside compound K regulates HIF-1α-mediated glycolysis through Bclaf1 to inhibit the proliferation of human liver cancer cells. Frontiers in Pharmacology 11: 583334.

Zhang, Xuan, Silin Zhang, Qitong Sun, Wenjun Jiao, Yan Yan, and Xuewu Zhang. 2018. Compound K induces endoplasmic reticulum stress and apoptosis in human liver cancer cells by regulating STAT3. Molecules 23 (6):1482.

Zheng, Qiyu, Zhidong Qiu, Zhiyuan Sun, Lingling Cao, Fuqiang Li, Da Liu, and Donglu Wu. 2021. In vitro validation of network pharmacology predictions: Ginsenoside Rg3 inhibits hepatocellular carcinoma cell proliferation via SIRT2. Natural Product Communications 16 (4):1934578X211004826.

Zheng, Zhi-Zhong, Yan-Lin Ming, Liang-Hua Chen, Guo-Hua Zheng, Shao-Song Liu, and Qing-Xi Chen. 2014. Compound K-induced apoptosis of human hepatocellular carcinoma MHCC97-H cells in vitro. Oncology Reports 32 (1):325–331.

Zhou, Bo, Jianhua Wang, and Zhiping Yan. 2014. Ginsenoside Rg3 attenuates hepatoma VEGF overexpression after hepatic artery embolization in an orthotopic transplantation hepatocellular carcinoma rat model. OncoTargets and Therapy 7:1945–1954.

Zhou, Bo, Zhiping Yan, Rong Liu, Peng Shi, Sheng Qian, Xudong Qu, Liang Zhu, Wei Zhang, and Jianhua Wang. 2016. Prospective study of transcatheter arterial chemoembolization (TACE) with ginsenoside Rg3 versus TACE alone for the treatment of patients with advanced hepatocellular carcinoma. Radiology 280 (2):630–639.

Zhu, He, Si-Yu Wang, Jin-Hao Zhu, Hui Liu, Ming Kong, Qian Mao, Wei Zhang, and Song-Lin Li. 2021. Efficacy and safety of transcatheter arterial chemoembolization combined with ginsenosides in hepatocellular carcinoma treatment. Phytomedicine 91:153700.

2 Patients with Cancer and Use of Thai Traditional Herb

Nattiya Kapol and Preecha Nootim

ABBREVIATIONS

CBD	cannabidiol
CI	confidence interval
CYP	cytochrome
CYP2C9	cytochrome P450 family 2 subfamily C member 9
CYP3A4	cytochrome P450 family 3 subfamily A member 4
THC	tetrahydrocannabinol

2.1 INTRODUCTION

Cancer is a major health problem worldwide and is the leading cause of death in Thailand. According to the World Health Organization, there were approximately 187,677 new cases of cancer in 2020, which is equivalent to 161.7 people per 100,000 diagnosed, and approximately 99.8 people per 100,000 died in Thailand in 2020 (World Cancer Research Fund International 2022). Despite the constant development in new cancer treatments such as chemotherapy, radiotherapy, and target therapy, some cancers are not curable. Difficulties in cancer treatment can be caused by drug resistance (Król et al. 2010), cancer metastasis, lack of effective biomarkers, and other factors (Chakraborty and Rahman 2012). These situations influence some patients and caregivers to seek alternative treatment. Herbs are the most commonly used alternative treatment for patients with cancer, particularly in Thailand. Patients with cancer use herbs for self-medication and as prescribed by Thai traditional medicine practitioners. Herbs as treatments for cancer have long been documented in Thai traditional textbooks. Knowledge of some herbs is also disseminated from senior to junior Thai traditional medicine practitioners. However, owing to the lack of scientific evidence on the effectiveness and safety of herbs, Thai traditional medicine practitioners are hesitant to use them on patients (Nootim et al. 2020). Currently, clinical research on herbs has received support from the government, and the number of studies is increasing. However, some research was not published or published in domestic journals. Therefore, this chapter reviews the knowledge and findings of studies on Thai traditional herbs used in patients with cancer.

2.2 BACKGROUND

Cancer has long been mentioned in Thai culture. According to Thai traditional theory, cancer is caused by an imbalance of four elements in the human body, which include earth, water, wind and fire, and three elements of the universe, namely *vata* (wind), *pitta* (bile) and *kapha* (phlegm) (Endo and Nakamura 1995; Lumlerdkij et al. 2018). If one or two elements are not balanced, benign neoplasms develop; if all elements are not balanced, malignant tumors develop. The basic

DOI: 10.1201/9781003260028-3

principle of cancer treatment is to either increase or decrease the imbalanced elements. Cancer treatment in Thai traditional theory focuses on holistic therapy including physical care, mental care, food, and herbs. In addition to the patients' physical health, their mental and social health should be also attended.

According to the Thai traditional theory, there are four concepts of herbal uses for cancer treatment including *ru, lom, ruksa,* and *bumrung*. First, *ru* refers to the draining or reducing of waste in the body. Wastes can be urine, excretions, sweat, or undigested food (Lumlerdkij et al. 2018). Second, *lom* means preventing disease from spreading to other organs. Third, *ruksa* means treatment. Finally, *bumrung* indicates boosting human immunity. Herbs are used in each concept according to their taste. The specifics of each concept and the recommended herbs are shown in Table 2.1. Thai traditional textbooks classify herbs based on their taste. Bitter and sour herbs help drain or reduce waste and toxic substances in the human body. Bland herbs help drain urine. Hot and spicy herbs support blood circulation and reduce flatulence or other complications of diseases. Cool, aromatic herbs nourish the heart. Herbs that are drunk are used as antidotes and to fight cancer. Healthcare providers must be familiar with herbal

TABLE 2.1
Thai Traditional Concepts and Herbs Used in Cancer Treatment

Concept	Taste	Herbs	Indication
Ru refers to draining or reducing waste in human body. This concept aims to clean and refresh the human body in order to prevent waste from interfering with the next treatment step.	Bitter	• *Azadirachta indica* • *Solanum torvum* • *Phyllanthus niruri* L. • Benja Amarit formulation	Drain waste and toxic substances in human body
	Sour	• Limeade (*Citrus aurantifolia* (Christm.) Swingle) • Triphala formulation	
	Bland	• *Orthosiphon aristatus* (Blume) Miq. • *Pluchea indica* (L.) Less • *Cymbopogon citratus* • *Thunbergia laurifolia*	Increase the amount of urine
Lom refers to disease control in order to prevent disease spread to other organs. This concept is to treat disease-related side effects before moving on to other treatments.	Hot and spicy	• Ginger (*Zingiber officinale*) • Cinnamon (*Cinnamomum* spp.) • *Ocimum sanctum*	Improve circulation, regulate digestion, relieve intestinal gas
Ruksa refers to treatment based on symptoms and causes.	Drunken	• *Smilax cerbularia* subsp. *Corbularia* • *Smilax glabra* • *Rhinacanthus nasutus* Kurz (root) • *Stemona collinsae* Craib. (root)	Use as antidote, fight cancer
Bumrung is used when symptoms have improved. This concept aims to alleviate unpleasant symptoms, boost immunity, improve appetite, and rejuvenate.	Cool aroma	• Lotus pollen (*Nelumbo nucifera* Gaertn.) • Ya-hom-thep-pa-jit formulation • *Anethum graveolens* L. • *Cuminum cyminum* L. • *Nigella sativa* L. • *Lepidium sativum* L.	Nourish the heart

Source: Department of Thai Traditional and Alternative Medicine (2018).

flavors to treat patients with cancer effectively (Department of Thai Traditional and Alternative Medicine 2018).

2.3 HERBAL MEDICINES IN PATIENTS WITH CANCER

Herbal medicines are commonly used by patients with cancer worldwide. A recent systematic review and meta-analysis (Asiimwe et al. 2021) included studies from 44 countries and presented that the pool prevalence of herbal medicine use in patients with cancer was 22% (95% confidence interval [CI], 18%–25%). The largest pooled prevalence was found in Palestine (69%, 95% CI 59%–77%), followed by China (58%, 95% CI 45%–71%), and it was 12% in Thailand (95% CI 0%–38%). In Thailand, patients with early-stage cancer are treated using Western medicine. Patients usually seek alternative medicines when they are in stages III and IV (Nootim et al. 2020). Similarly, the guidelines for Thai traditional medicine use in patients with cancer recommend herbal use as a supplement for patients with end-stage cancer (Department of Thai Traditional and Alternative Medicine 2018). However, some of these patients reject Western medicines and use herbal medicines alone for treatment (Teerachaisakul et al. 2020). Patients with cancer use herbal medicines to treat disease, relieve cancer-related symptoms, and treat the side effects of anticancer drugs, radiotherapy, or chemotherapy (Nootim et al. 2020; Puataweepong et al. 2012). Moreover, herbs are used in the treatment of cancer to enhance overall well-being and slow cancer progression (Kanimozhi et al. 2021).

The Ministry of Public Health of Thailand encourages and supports the use of herbal medicines for Thai people. They announced the National List of Herbal Medicine 2021 (Ministry of Public Health 2021a), which included 94 herbal medicines. Some items are used for the treatment of cancer and side effects of cancer treatment. Other herbs that can be used for cancer treatment have been included in Thai traditional textbooks as single herbs and herbal formulations. However, the cancer treatment concept of the Thai traditional theory is to balance several elements in the human body. As a result, herbal medicines for cancer therapy are usually in the form of formularies because they contain many herbs that can aid in elemental balancing or synergy of the plants (Itharat 2010).

Herbs for cancer treatment in the National List of Herbal Medicine and Thai traditional textbooks can be identified into two groups. These are herbs that treat disease and herbs that treat cancer-related symptoms. Examples of formularies for cancer treatment are presented in Table 2.2. These formularies are composed of several herbs and some are indicated for specific cancer (Department of Thai Traditional and Alternative Medicine 2018).

TABLE 2.2
Herbal Formulations for Cancer Treatment and Their Components

Herbal Formulation	Component
Benja Amarit	– *Wrightia arborea* 10 g
	– *Cyperus rotundus* 60 g
	Each of the following components weighs 15 g.
	– *Zingiber ligulatum* Roxb.
	– *Piper nigrum* L.
	– *Piper retrofractum* Vahl
	– *Dischidia major*
	– *Gymnopetalum integrifolim* Kurz.
	– *Plumbago indica*

(Continued)

TABLE 2.2
(Continued)

Herbal Formulation	Component
	– *Tribulus terrestris*
	– *Cinnamomum bejolghota*
	– *Cinnamomum porrectum* Kosterm
	Each of the following components weighs 22.50 g.
	– *Piper sarmentosum* Roxb.
	– *Piper interruptum* Opiz
	Each of the following components weighs 7.5 g.
	– *Aegle marmelos*
	– *Siphonodon celastrineus*
	– *Ligusticum chuanxiong*
	– *Iris germanica*
	– *Atractylodes lancea*
	– *Angelica sinensis* (Oliv.) Diels
	– *Artemisia annua*
	– *Anethum graveolens* L.
	– *Cuminum cyminum* L.
	– *Foeniculum vulgare* Miller subsp. var. vulgare
	– *Nigella sativa* L.
	– *Lepidium sativum* L.
	– *Terminalia bellirica* (Gaertn.) Roxb.
	– *Terminalia chebula* Retz.
	– *Terminalia arjuna* Wight and Arn.
	– *Rhinacanthus nasutus* Kurz
	– Potassium nitrate
	– Alum
	– *Coriandrum sativum*
	– *Kaempferia galanga* L.
	– Borax
Yodya Mareng	– *Acanthus ebracteatus* Vahl
	– *Cordia globifera* W.W. Sm.
	– *Dioscorea membranacea* Pierre ex Prain & Burkill
	– *Eupatorium capillifolium* (Lam.) Small ex Porter & Britton
	– *Hydnophytum formicarum* Jack
	– *Levisticum officinale* W.D.J. Koch
	– *Orthosiphon aristatus* (Blume) Mig.
	– *Polyalthia cerasoides* (Roxb.)
	– *Rhinacanthus nasutus* (L.) Kurz
	– *Salacia chinensis* L.
	– *Smilax corbularia* Kunth
Samhannachan	– *Betula alnoides* Buch. Ham.
	– *Ficus foveolata* Wall
	– *Ochna integerrima* (Lour.) Merr.
	– *Coptosapelta flavescens* Korth.
	– *Litsea cubeba* (Lour.) Pers.
	– *Suregada multiflorum* (A. Juss) Baill.
	– *Caesalpinia sappan* L.
	– *Andrographis paniculata* (Burm.f.) Wall. ex Nees
	– *Coscinium fenestratum* (Goetgh.) Colebr
	– *Bauhinia strychnifolia* Craib

Source: Department of Thai Traditional and Alternative Medicine (2018).

2.4 HERBAL FORMULATION FOR CANCER TREATMENT

Benja Amarit ("ben-ja-aum-ma-rit"), a traditional Thai medicine formulation, has been practically used in combination with the standard treatment for patients with liver cancer in Thai traditional hospitals. The components and preparation of Benja Amarit were traditionally documented in a few Thai traditional textbooks with the same core components. In a Thai traditional textbook, three herbs including pepper, ginger, and long pepper were added to Benja Amarit to balance the vata (wind) element. The components of Benja Amarit are shown in Figure 2.1. Benja Amarit formulation has a

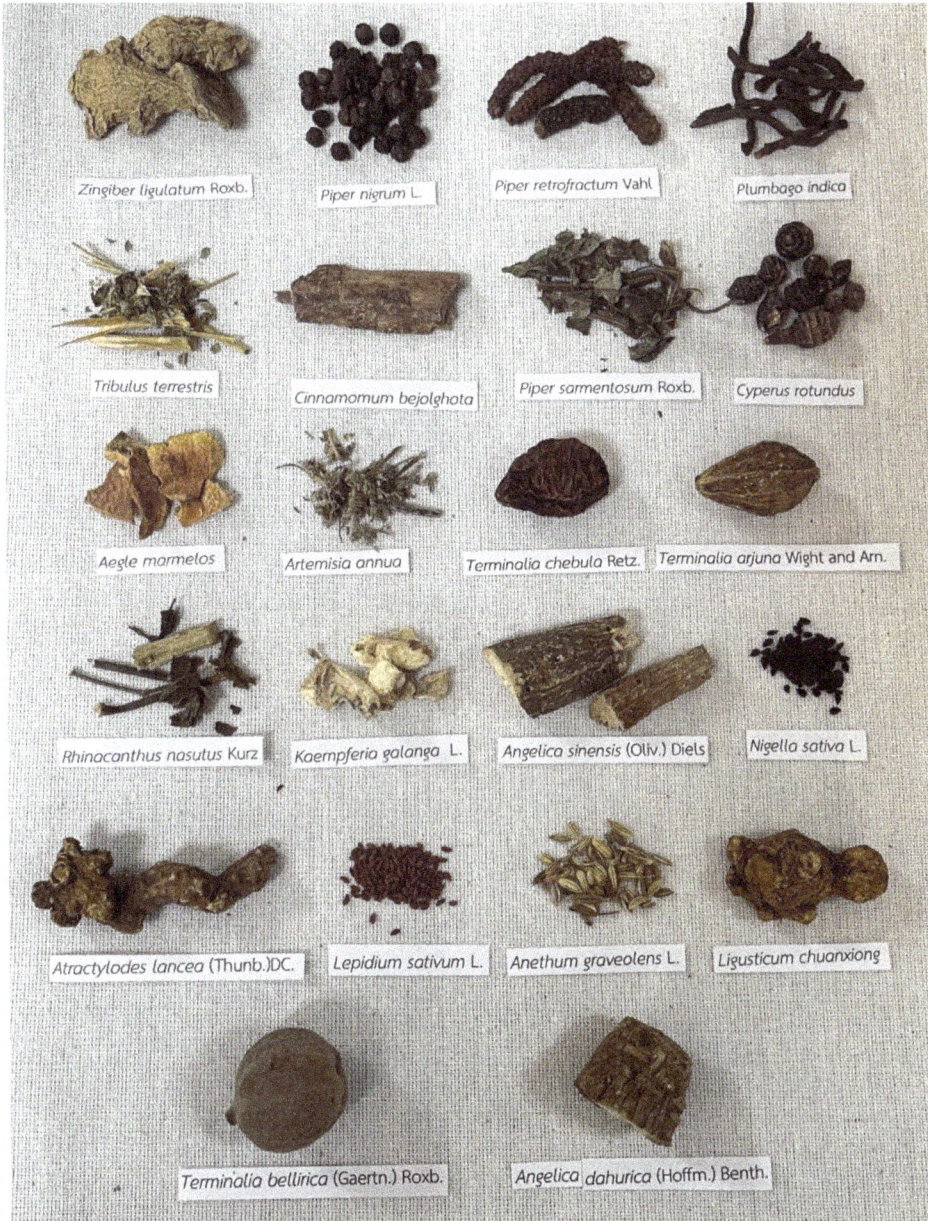

FIGURE 2.1 Components of Benja Amarit formulation.

potent laxative effect. The goal of this formulation is to remove waste from the liver in patients with liver cancer (Termsiririrkkul 2014). All components are ground into powder for this formulation. Patients with cancer can mix this powder with lemon juice, bergamot juice, or honey and take it two times a day before meals (Department of Thai Traditional and Alternative Medicine 2018).

Yodya Mareng ("yod-ya-ma-reng") is a traditional formulation prescribed to patients with liver cancer at the Khampramong Temple, Sakon Nakhon, Thailand (Poonthananiwatkul et al. 2015). The formulation includes 11 herbs and is made as a decoction in liquid form. Additionally, a freeze-dried extract capsule of the decoction is available for patients with cancer who have restrictions on liquid intake. This formulation has not been studied in a randomized controlled trial. It is only used by patients with cancer at the Khampramong Temple, which provides many herbal medicines to patients. Therefore, the effects of a single herb or formulation cannot be evaluated. In an observational survey conducted on day 4 of admission and at the end of the admission, cancer-related symptoms decreased. The incidence of the 13 most common symptoms, such as pain, dyspepsia, abdominal pain and fatigue, was significantly reduced.

Samhannachan ("sa-mhan-na-chan") (Thongdeeying et al. 2017) is one of the drug formulations given to treat patients with cancer at Khampramong Temple, Sakon Nakhon, Thailand. Samhannachan is used adjunctly with Yodya Mareng. Its formulation is composed of 10 herbs (Figure 2.2).

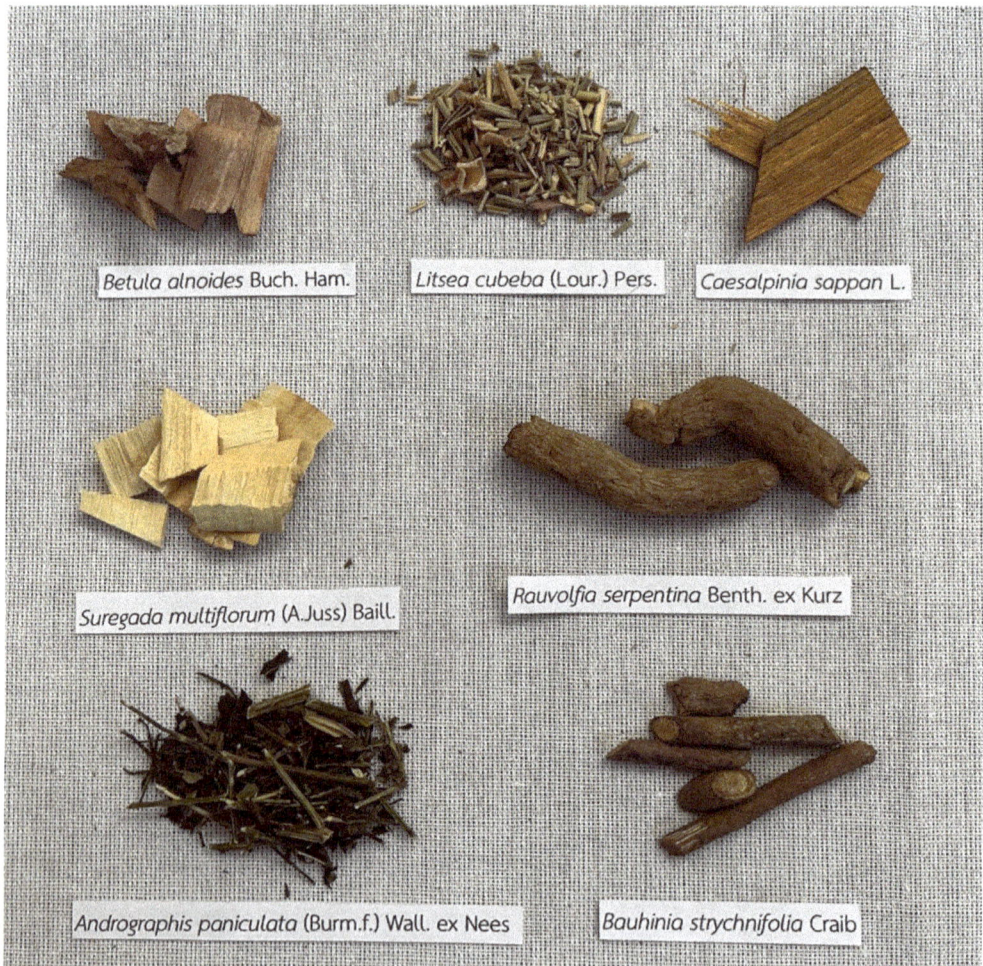

FIGURE 2.2 Components of Samhannachan formulation.

All ingredients are boiled to create a liquid decoction that can be consumed before meals. The goal of this formulation is to reduce body inflammation. This formulation has not been analyzed in a clinical study. Only one *in vivo* study in Thailand (Thongdeeying et al. 2017) investigated the cytotoxic activity of Samhanachan extracts and its ingredients. The results revealed that the ethanolic and water extracts of Samhanachan had low potent activity against lung cancer cells. However, the extract of *Coscinium fenestratum* had high potent activity against lung cancer cells. This finding proposed that *C. fenestratum* is the active plant ingredient for this formulation.

2.5 HERBAL FORMULATION FOR CANCER-RELATED SYMPTOM RELIEF

Herbal formulations are also used for the treatment of cancer-related symptoms. Most of them help relieve any symptoms, such as fever, thirst, and indigestion. Some formulations are shown in Table 2.3.

TABLE 2.3

Herbal Formulations for Cancer-Related Symptom Relief and Their Components

Herbal Formulation	Component	Indication
Chantaleela	Each of the following components weighs 12 g. – *Angelica dahurica* Benth. – *Atractylodes lancea* (Thunb.) DC. – *Artemisia annua* L.	Fever, seasonal fever
	– *Gymnopetalum cochichinense* (Lour.) Kurz – *Santalum album* L. – *Pterocarpus santalinus* L.f. – *Tinospora crispa* (L.) Miers ex Hook.f.&Thoms. – *Eurycoma longifolia* Jack Mix with 3 g Camphor (*Dryobalanops aromatica* Gaertn.)	
Keawhom	Each of the following components weighs 5 g. – *Pogostemon cablin* (Blanco) Benth. – *Limnophila rugosa* (Roth) Merr. – *Cordyline fruticosa* (L.) A. Chev – *Eupatorium fortunei* Turcz. – *Vetiveria zizanioides* (L.) Nash – *Kaempferia galanga* L. – *Dracaena loureiroi* Gagnep. – *Tarenna hoaensis* Pit. – *Angiopteris evecta* (G. Forst.) Hoffm. – *Ludisia discolor* (Ker Gawl.) A. Rich. – *Tacca chantrieri* André – *Sophora exigua* Craib – *Cyathea podophylla* (Hook.) Copel. – *Mimusops elengi* L. – *Mammea siamensis* T. Anderson – *Mesua ferrea* L. – *Nelumbo nucifera* Gaertn. – *Rauvolfia serpentina* Benth. ex Kurz	Fever, thirst, aphthous ulcer

(Continued)

TABLE 2.3
(Continued)

Herbal Formulation	Component	Indication
Thadbanjob	– *Neopicrorhiza scrophulariiflora* (Pennell) D.Y. Hong 8 g	Antiflatulence, indigestion
	– *Terminalia chebula* Retz. 16 g	
	Each of the following components weighs 4 g.	
	– *Zingiber ligulatum* Roxb.	
	– *Atractylodes lancea* (Thunb.) DC.	
	– *Terminalia chebula* Retz. var chebula	
	– *Angelica sinensis* (Oliv.) Diels	
	– *Angelica dahurica* Benth.	
	– *Nigella sativa* L.	
	– *Cuminum cyminum* L.	
	– *Pimpinella anisum* L.	
	– *Trachyspermum ammi* (L.) Sprague	
	– *Lepidium sativum* L.	
	– *Myristica fragrans* Houtt.	
	– *Syzygium aromaticum* (L.) Merr. & L.M. Perry	
	– *Cinnamomum bejolghota* (Buch.-Ham.) Sweet	
	– *Amomum krervanh* Pierre ex Gagnep	
	– *Coriandrum sativum* L.	
	– *Piper retrofractum* Vahl	
	– *Pogostemon cablin* (Blanco) Benth.	
	– *Kaempferia galanga* L.	
	– *Cinnamomum camphora* (L.) J. Presl.	

Source: Department of Thai Traditional and Alternative Medicine (2018).

2.6   ANTIPYRETIC AND ANTIFEVER HERBAL MEDICINES

Chantaleela ("chan-ta-lee-la"), a formulation used in Thai traditional folk medicine for fever relief, is on Thailand's National List of Herbal Medicinal Products. The components of Chantaleela are shown in Figure 2.3. Powder and tablet preparations are available. In the case of fever, adults can take 1–2 g of the formulation dissolved in water every 3–4 hours (Department of Thai Traditional and Alternative Medicine 2018). Although Chantaleela has long been used in Thai traditional medicine, no randomized controlled trials have been conducted to investigate its effects on cancer. However, a clinical trial with 24 healthy volunteers investigated the effects of Chantaleela on platelet aggregation (Itthipanichpong et al. 2010). Participants received a 250 mg tablet of Chantaleela every 8 hours for a total of three doses. The results revealed that there was no change in platelet aggregation and no adverse events were found.

Keawhom ("keaw-hom") is a formulation used to treat exanthematous fevers such as chickenpox, measles and herpes zoster. It is composed of 18 Thai traditional plants (Sukkasem 2015). The formulation is a household Thai traditional remedy in powder form. Keawhom is used topically and orally to treat exanthematous fever. The powder should be dissolved in jasmine-scented water for oral administration. For topical use, the powder is dissolved in water used to wash rice and applied to the body to relieve fever (Department of Thai Traditional and Alternative

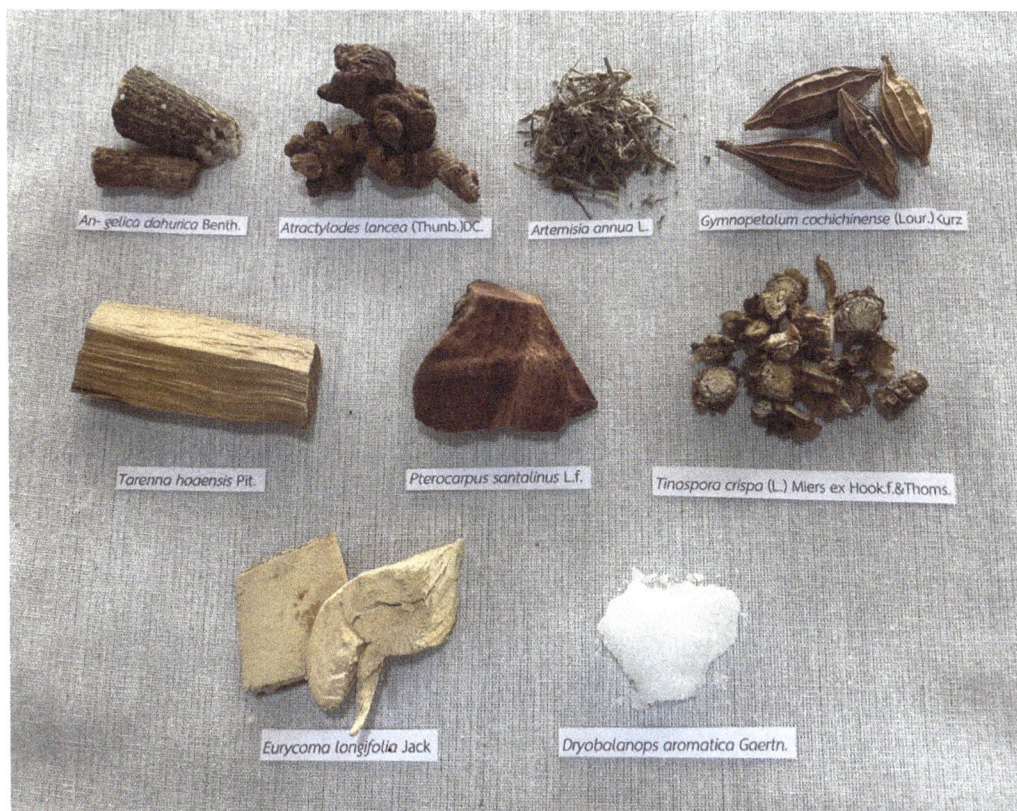

FIGURE 2.3 Components of Chantaleela formulation.

Medicine 2018). However, no clinical studies on the effects of Keawhom formulation have been conducted.

2.7 ANTIFLATULENCE AND DYSPEPSIA HERBAL MEDICINES

Thadbanjob ("thad-ban-job") is a Thai traditional medicine and has been recorded in Thai traditional textbooks for a long time. Currently, Thadbanjob is on Thailand's National List of Herbal Medicinal Products. It is available in powder and capsule forms as antiflatulent and indigestion treatment. In powder form, patients can dissolve 1 g of thadbanjob in an aqueous adjuvant and take it three times a day before meals or for flatulence (Department of Thai Traditional and Alternative Medicine 2018).

2.8 EVIDENCE-BASED HERBAL MEDICINES

Although herbal medicines have been widely used by patients with cancer in Thailand, clinical trials to support their efficacy and side effects are limited. The lack of scientific evidence supporting the efficacy of herbal medicines affects their acceptance by Western physicians. Therefore, the national policy in Thailand encourages researchers to conduct clinical studies of herbal medicines. However, many studies on the anticancer effect of single herbs and herbal formularies are still being conducted *in vitro* and *in vivo*.

Currently, the clinical studies related to the efficacy of herbal medicines in cancer treatment have been increasing. These studies include the use of herbal medicines in cancer treatment directly, relief of complications from cancer, or reduction of adverse events from cancer treatment. This review provides evidence-based information on the use of herbal medicines in Thai patients with cancer.

2.9   HERBAL MEDICINES FOR CANCER TREATMENT

There have been studies on cancer treatment using both single herbs and formulations.

Lingzhi mushroom (*Ganoderma lucidum*) is a food supplement marketed worldwide. Preclinical studies have indicated *G. lucidum* inhibited the growth of tumor cells through the immune system. A systematic review and meta-analysis showed that patients who received *G. lucidum* along with chemo/radiotherapy had improved immune function indicators and quality of life when compared with controls (Jin et al. 2016). Therefore, the anticancer effect and safety of lingzhi were investigated in a phase III clinical trial in Thailand. Thirty Thai patients with advanced liver cancer received either the water extract and spores of lingzhi or the placebo. Consequently, patients who received lingzhi had a median survival of 105.93 ± 6.2 days in comparison to 92.63 ± 9.3 days in the placebo group and no significant difference was found ($p = 0.065$). No serious adverse events were reported in this study (Leerapun et al. 2012).

Benja Amarit: The clinical evidence of Benja Amarit was initially determined in a prospective study that evaluated its safety and effectiveness. A total of 96 Thai patients with liver cancer received 300 mg Benja Amarit capsules twice a day, 1–4 capsules at a time for 6 months. The results showed that the quality of life scores of patients were increased after taking Benja Amarit formula continuously for 2 months ($p < 0.05$). Moreover, the survival rate during the 1-year follow-up was 27.08% and no serious adverse events were reported (Yossathera et al. 2017). With these findings, a clinical trial of Benja Amarit is ongoing to further determine the effects of this formulation. Moreover, an *in vivo* study demonstrated its anticancer activity against human hepatocellular carcinoma and colon cancer cells (Yapasert et al. 2020).

N040 is an herbal formula composed of nine herbs that have been proven to be effective in cancer cells *in vivo*. A clinical trial phase 1b trial was conducted to investigate its effects on advanced cervical cancer. Thirty-two patients received one capsule of N040 two times a day for 6 months. One capsule contained 267.50 mg of N040 extract. The findings revealed 1-year survival rate of 62.5%. Percent neutrophils, blood urea nitrogen, and alkaline phosphatase levels were increased in patients, but the levels were within the normal range. However, the quality of life was the same before and after N040 therapy (Teerachaisakul et al. 2018).

Benjakul is a formulation prescribed by folk healers to balance elements in patients with cancer. Benjakul is composed of five herbs, namely *Piper chaba* fruits, *Piper sarmentosum* root, *Piper rostratum* stem, *Plumbago indica* root and *Zingiber officinale* rhizome. The ethanolic extract of Benjakul formulation showed cytotoxic activity against three human cancer cell lines which were lung cancer, cervical cancer, and liver cancer cell lines (Ruangnoo et al. 2012). An experimental study (Chantor et al. 2017) evaluated its effectiveness and safety in patients with stage 4 non–small cell lung cancer. Only one patient volunteered and met the criteria for this study. The patient received two capsules of 100 mg Benjakul formulation three times a day for 6 months. However, the patient stopped taking this formulation at 5.9 months because the disease progressed. This study showed that the disease was stable at weeks 4–20 after taking Benjakul. The progression-free survival was 5.9 months, and the overall survival was 6.7 months. Sweating and feeling hot were reported as side effects of Benjakul. There was no toxicity on renal function, but liver function and lipid profile increased. Furthermore, the patient's quality of life improved from "good" to "very good" by week 8 and so on.

2.10   HERBAL MEDICINES FOR COMPLICATION TREATMENT

Ginger (*Zingiber officinale*) has been used as a spice in Thai foods and beverages. According to Thai traditional textbooks and the National List of Essential Medicine, ginger is also used to treat gastrointestinal disorders such as flatulence, nausea, and vomiting. Ginger contains various compounds. Its most bioactive compound is 6-gingerol, an anti-emetic agent (de Lima et al. 2018). A clinical randomized trial was conducted to determine the efficacy of 6-gingerol as an anti-emetic in patients with solid tumors receiving moderately to highly emetogenic chemotherapy. Thai patients were randomized to receive 6-gingerol 10 mg or placebo twice daily for 12 weeks. The emesis-free rate was significantly higher in the 6-gingerol group than in the placebo group ($p = 0.001$) (Konmun et al. 2017).

Patients with gastrointestinal and urinary tract cancer were given a ginger powder drink four times a day after chemotherapy to test the anti-emetic effect of ginger. A study reported that patients who received a ginger powder drink had a lower incidence of nausea and vomiting (Utane and Maneesorn 2019).

Moreover, a randomized controlled trial investigated the effects of ginger tea in patients with colon cancer who received FOLFOX4 (5-fluorouracil, leucovorin, and oxaliplatin) chemotherapy. These patients had decreased blood cell count. The experimental group received ginger tea 4 g/day and compared with the control group that received the placebo. As a result, the mean white blood cell count was significantly higher in the experimental group (7.97×10^3 cell/mm^3) than in the control group (7.25×10^3 cell/mm^3; $p = 0.031$) (Cheepcharoenrat et al. 2021).

Cannabis (*Cannabis sativa* L.) is legally regulated in Thailand for medical and research purposes since 2019. Previously, cannabis was categorized as a class 5 narcotic in Thailand. The Narcotic Act 2019 allows the medical use of cannabis for patients. The Ministry of Public Health published a list of medical cannabis indications with strong evidence. Chemotherapy-induced nausea and vomiting, as well as palliative care, are cancer-related indications. Furthermore, the Department of Thai Traditional and Alternative Medicine announced 16 cannabis-based formulations for patients suffering from pain, insomnia, flatulence, and other symptoms (Ministry of Public Health 2021b). Patients can obtain cannabis oil from a hospital-based medical cannabis clinic. After the legalization of cannabis, a cross-sectional study (Sukrueangkul et al. 2022) surveyed the attitudes toward the medical use of cannabis in 565 Thai patients with cancer. The results revealed that patients with a positive attitude have a higher demand for medical cannabis than other groups. After completing modern treatment, 45.3% of the patients with cancer decided to use cannabis.

Many studies have investigated the effectiveness and safety of cannabis for the treatment of cancer-related symptoms (Aviram et al. 2022; Johnson et al. 2010; Lynch et al. 2014). The current number of studies in Thailand is limited, but some studies have begun. The effects of cannabis sublingual oil were studied retrospectively using medical records of patients with end-stage cancer. In the clinic, patients received tetrahydrocannabinol (THC) 1.7% w/v cannabis sublingual oil 1–4 drops per day. In these patients with end-stage cancer, cannabis sublingual oil helped relieve pain, anorexia, insomnia, and anxiety significantly. The utility score of patients has increased after taking cannabis. Furthermore, the incidence of adverse events was 30.1% and most events were manageable (Kraikosol et al. 2021). Recently, the safety and efficacy of cannabis were examined in 14 patients with stage IV cancer (Thanasitthichai et al. 2020). The patients received cannabis extract (THC:CBD, 1:1) 1–4 mg/day sublingually for 3 months. All 12 patients with insomnia reported sleep improvement, and 50% of the patients with moderate to severe pain had improved pain scores.

Harag (in Thai), a five-root formulation, is made of the roots of *Harrisonia perforate* (Blanco) Merr., *Capparis micracantha* DC, *Clerodendrum indicum* (L.) Kuntze, *Ficus racemosa* L. and *Tiliacora triandra* (Colebr.) Diels. D. A quasi-experimental study examined the effects of Harag herbal poultice for pain relief in patients with end-stage liver cancer. The experimental group applied Harag herbal poultice in the painful area (abdominal pain) twice daily for 3 days, whereas the control group did not receive Harag herbal poultice. The results revealed that pain scores were lower in the experimental group than in the control group (Nootim et al. 2020).

2.11   HERBS REDUCE CHEMOTHERAPY-RELATED ORAL MUCOSITIS

Tiliacora (*Tiliacora triandra* (Colebr.) Diels) is a plant mostly found in northeast Thailand and Lao PDR. According to an *in vitro* study (Rattana et al. 2016), the main compound of *T. triandra* leaves is oxoanolobine and its extracts have activity against lung and oral cavity cancer cell lines. The effectiveness of Tiliacora extract was studied in humans. The effects of cold-pressed Tiliacora extract to reduce mucositis in patients with leukemia treated with chemotherapy were evaluated in a quasi-experimental research in Thailand. Patients with leukemia who received chemotherapy in the experimental group were encouraged to use cold-pressed Tiliacora extract for 14 days, whereas the control group was provided 0.9% normal saline. The results revealed that the pain score for mucositis in the intervention group was significantly lower than that of the control group from days 9 to 14 (Luanratanakorn et al. 2021).

Coconut oil is an edible oil derived from matured coconut kernels. Coconut oil has been shown to reduce the severity of oral mucositis induced by chemotherapy (Chadayan 2020; Kannan et al. 2021). In Thailand, a randomized controlled trial examined the effects of coconut oil on stomatitis in patients with cancer receiving chemotherapy. Fifty-five patients with colorectal cancer were included. The experimental group received the oral health self-care programme and a coconut oil gargle twice daily (morning and bedtime) for 7 days and compared with the control group without coconut oil gargle intervention. As a result, the stomatitis score was significantly improved in the experimental group (Suwanpiwat et al. 2017).

Gynura procumbens is a medicinal plant commonly found in Asia. *G. procumbens* has been studied *in vivo* and *in vitro* since 1995 and has been shown to have antitumor activity (Tan et al. 2016). A randomized crossover study was conducted to assess the effects of an oral self-care programme with *G. procumbens* in patients with cancer who received chemotherapy in Thailand. The experimental group started applying oral *G. procumbens* 24 hours after chemotherapy, whereas the control group received a placebo. The patients applied the gel until days 14–21 or until the absence of lesions in the oral cavity. Patients who received *G. procumbens* had significantly lower pain scores for oral mucositis and lower severity score than those who received the placebo gel (Chabuakam et al. 2014).

2.12   TOXICITY AND CAUTIONARY NOTES

Thai patients with cancer use herbs alone or in combination with anticancer drugs during cancer treatment. As a result, they are at risk of drug-herb interactions that may affect the effectiveness and safety of anticancer drugs. Thai herbal formularies contain various herbs, which may increase the possibility of drug-herb interactions. Patients with cancer may be unaware of the herbs used in the formulation. Patients who use herbal formulations in addition to anticancer drugs may experience side effects or therapeutic failure of anticancer drugs. Anticancer drugs from the Thailand National List of Essential Medicine and herbs from Thai Herbal Pharmacopoeia were reviewed to determine potential drug-herb interactions. A total of 565 potential drug-herb interactions were found, in which 90% involve cytochrome P450 (CYP) inhibition (Jiso et al. 2022).

The Benja Amarit formulation contains several herbs that inhibit CYP3A4, such as *Aegle marmelos, Angelica sinensis, Atractylodes lancea, Piper nigrum*, and so on. *P. nigrum* has been reported to be an CYP3A4 and CYP2C9 inhibitor. The use of *P. nigrum* with some anticancer drugs such as doxorubicin, paclitaxel, nilotinib will increase anticancer drug concentrations and cause more adverse events. Furthermore, when *P. nigrum* is combined with tamoxifen, ifosfamide, or cyclophosphamide, the active metabolites of anticancer drugs are reduced, leading to therapeutic failure (Jiso et al. 2022). Although some herbs can help patients with cancer, drug-herb interactions can be hazardous. Health professionals should educate patients with cancer about drug-herb interactions and regularly monitor the effects of drug treatment.

2.13 SUMMARY POINTS

- This chapter focuses on the use of herbal medicines among patients with cancer in Thailand.
- According to the Thai traditional theory, cancer is caused by an imbalance of elements in the human body.
- Based on Thai traditional theory, there are four concepts of herbal uses for cancer treatment, including *ru, lom, ruksa,* and *bumrung.*
- Herbal medicines for cancer treatment are usually in the form of formularies because they contain many herbs that aid in elemental balancing or the synergy of the plants.
- Herbs for cancer treatment were classified in Thai traditional textbooks into herbs that treat disease and herbs that treat cancer-related symptoms.
- In Thailand, Benja Amarit, Yodya Mareng, and Samhanachan are herbal formulations used for cancer treatment.
- Chantaleela, Keawhom, and Thadbanjob are herbal formulations for the treatment of cancer-related symptoms.
- Evidence-based herbal medicines are limited.
- Herbal medicines that have been investigated in clinical trials include lingzhi mushroom, Benja Amarit, N040, Benjakul, ginger, cannabis, Harag, Tiliacora, coconut oil, and *Gynura procumbens.*

REFERENCES

Asiimwe, J. B., P. B. Nagendrappa, E. C. Atukunda, M. M. Kamatenesi, G. Nambozi, C. U. Tolo, P. E. Ogwang, and A. M. Sarki. 2021. Prevalence of the use of herbal medicines among patients with cancer: A systematic review and meta-analysis. Evidence-Based Complementary and Alternative Medicine 2021:9963038. doi:10.1155/2021/9963038

Aviram, J., G. M. Lewitus, Y. Vysotski, M. A. Amna, S. Ouryvaev, S. Procaccia, I. Cohen, A. Leibovici, L. Akria, D. Goncharov, N. Mativ, A. Kauffman, A. Shai, G. Bar-Sela, and D. Meiri. 2022. The effectiveness and safety of medical cannabis for treating cancer related symptoms in oncology patients. Frontiers in Pain Research 3. doi:10.3389/fpain.2022.861037

Chabuakam, N., P. Kunsara, and P. Putwatana. 2014. The effects of an oral self-care program with Gynura Procumbens on chemotherapy related oral mucositis in patients with cancer. Nursing Journal of the Ministry of Public Health 25, no. 1 (January–April): 110–123.

Chadayan, C. 2020. Effectiveness of coconut oil pulling on oral mucositis among cancer patients in a selected hospital at Madurai. Indian Journal of Applied Research 10, no. 5 (May): 64–65.

Chakraborty, S., and T. Rahman. 2012. The difficulties in cancer treatment. Ecancermedicalscience 6: ed16–ed16. doi:10.3332/ecancer.2012.ed16

Chantor, P., H. Rattanabanjerdkul, and A. Itharat. 2017. Case studies of Benjakul recipes in treating stage 4 non–small cell lung cancer. Thammasat Medical Journal 17, no. 2 (April–June): 172–181.

Cheepcharoenrat, N., C. Thongborn, K. Komolmethchai, P. Vejkama, and P. Khanngein. 2021. Effects of ginger tea drinking to blood cell counts of FOLFOX4 chemotherapy patients in colon cancer. Journal of Health Science 30, no. 5 (September–October): 935–943.

de Lima, R. M. T., A. C. dos Reis, A. P. M. de Menezes, J. V. de Oliveira Santos, J. W. G. de Oliveira Filho, J. R. de Oliveira Ferreira, M. V. O. B. de Alencar, A. M. O. F. da Mata, I. N. Khan, A. Islam, S. J. Uddin, E. S. Ali, M. T. Islam, S. Tripathi, S. K. Mishra, M. S. Mubarak, and A. A. de Carvalho Melo-Cavalcante. 2018. Protective and therapeutic potential of ginger (*Zingiber officinale*) extract and [6]-gingerol in cancer: A comprehensive review. Phytotherapy Research 32, no. 10 (October): 1885–1907. doi:10.1002/ptr.6134

Department of Thai Traditional and Alternative Medicine. 2018. Handbook of integrated palliative care for end-stage patients. Bangkok: Best Step Advertising Co., Ltd.

Endo, J., and T. Nakamura. 1995. [Comparative studies of the tridosha theory in Ayurveda and the theory of the four deranged elements in Buddhist medicine]. Kagakushi Kenkyu 34, no. 193: 1–9.

Itharat, A. 2010. Research on Thai medicinal plants for cancer treatment. Journal of Basic and Applied Pharmacology 32, no. 1: 39.

Itthipanichpong, R., A. Lupreechaset, S. Chotewuttakorn, P. Akarasereenont, T. Onkoksoong, T. Palo, S. Kongpatanakul, S. Chatsiricharoenkul, P. Thitilertdecha, P. Punpeng, and T. Laohapand. 2010. Effect of Ayurved Siriraj herbal recipe Chantaleela on platelet aggregation. Journal of the Medical Association of Thailand 93, no. 1 (Janurary): 115–122.

Jin, X., J. R. Beguerie, D. M. Sze, and G. C. Chan. 2016. Ganoderma lucidum (Reishi mushroom) for cancer treatment. The Cochrane Database of Systematic Reviews 4, no. 4 (April): Cd007731. doi:10.1002/14651858. CD007731.pub3

Jiso, A., P. Khemawoot, P. Techapichetvanich, S. Soopairin, K. Phoemsap, P. Damrongsakul, S. Wongwiwatthananukit, and P. Vivithanaporn. 2022. Drug-herb interactions among Thai herbs and anti-cancer drugs: A scoping review. Pharmaceuticals 15, no. (2): 146. doi:10.3390/ph15020146

Johnson, J. R., M. Burnell-Nugent, D. Lossignol, E. D. Ganae-Motan, R. Potts, and M. T. Fallon. 2010. Multicenter, double-blind, randomized, placebo-controlled, parallel-group study of the efficacy, safety, and tolerability of THC:CBD extract and THC extract in patients with intractable cancer-related pain. Journal of Pain and Symptom Management 39, no. 2 (February): 167–179. doi:10.1016/j. jpainsymman.2009.06.008

Kanimozhi, T., K. Hindu, Y. Maheshvari, Y. Khushnidha, M. Kumaravel, K. Srinivas, M. Manickavasagam, and K. Mangathayaru. 2021. Herbal supplement usage among cancer patients: A questionnaire-based survey. Journal of Cancer Research and Therapeutics 17, no. 1: 136–141. doi:10.4103/jcrt. JCRT_612_18

Kannan, N., S. Asokan, K. R. Gopal, S. Poddar, and A. Bhaumik. 2021. Randomized controlled trial for comparative assessment of effect of artificial saliva versus virgin coconut oil on salivary proteolytic activity & radiation mucositis in patients undergoing radiotherapy for head and neck cancers. Malaysian Journal of Medicine and Health Sciences 17, no. supplement 4 (June): 52–56.

Konmun, J., K. Danwilai, N. Ngamphaiboon, B. Sripanidkulchai, A. Sookprasert, and S. Subongkot. 2017. A phase II randomized double-blind placebo-controlled study of 6-gingerol as an anti-emetic in solid tumor patients receiving moderately to highly emetogenic chemotherapy. Medical Oncology 34, no. 4: 69. doi:10.1007/s12032-017-0931-4

Kraikosol, W., A. Chaocharoen, P. Laemluang, N. Musigawong, and P. Kwankhao. 2021. Effects and safety of cannabis sublingual oil THC 1.7% w/v formula in patients with end stage cancers in medical cannabis clinic, Chao Phya Abhiabhubejhr Hospital. Journal of The Department of Medical services 46, no. 3 (July–September): 50–59.

Król, M., K. M. Pawłowski, K. Majchrzak, K. Szyszko, and T. Motyl. 2010. Why chemotherapy can fail? Polish Journal of Veterinary Sciences 13, no. 2: 399–406.

Leerapun, A., S. Thongsawat, T. Chitapanarax, P. Nitisuwanraksa, and R. Phuackchantuck. 2012. Phase III: Study of efficacy and safety of Ganoderma lucidum in patients with unresectable progressive liver cancer. Thailand: Department of Thai Traditional and Alternative Medicine, Ministry of Public Health.

Luanratanakorn, S., S. Kueareenuntawoot, and N. Sangsai. 2021. Effects of cold-pressed Tiliacora extract in reducing mucositis among leukemia patients treated with chemotherapy at Uttaradit Hospital. Health Science Clinical Research 36, no. 1 (January–June): 28–40.

Lumlerdkij, N., J. Tantiwongse, S. Booranasubkajorn, R. Boonrak, P. Akarasereenont, T. Laohapand, and M. Heinrich. 2018. Understanding cancer and its treatment in Thai traditional medicine: An ethnopharmacological-anthropological investigation. Journal of Ethnopharmacology 216: 259–273. 10.1016/j. jep.2018.01.029.

Lynch, M. E., P. Cesar-Rittenberg, and A. G. Hohmann. 2014. A double-blind, placebo-controlled, crossover pilot trial with extension using an oral mucosal cannabinoid extract for treatment of chemotherapy-induced neuropathic pain. Journal of Pain and Symptom Management 47, no. 1 (January): 166–173. doi:10.1016/j.jpainsymman.2013.02.018

Ministry of Public Health. 2021a. Announcement of national drug system development committee: National list of essential medicine in herbal medicine. Royal Thai Government Gazette.

Ministry of Public Health. 2021b. Medical cannabis. www.medcannabis.go.th/ (accessed May 18, 2022).

Nootim, P., N. Kapol, W. Bunchuailua, P. Poompruek, and P. Tungsukruthai. 2020. Current state of cancer patient care incorporating Thai traditional medicine in Thailand: A qualitative study. Journal of Integrative Medicine 18, no. 1 (January): 41–45. doi:10.1016/j.joim.2019.12.004

Nootim, P., A. Rachderm, and W. Raksaithong. 2020. Effectiveness of Harag herbal poultice for relieving abdominal pain as per Thai traditional medicine practice guidelines for end-stage liver cancer patients at the Thai traditional and integrated medicine hospital, Bangkok. Journal of Thai Traditional & Alternative Medicine 18, no. 1 (January–April): 5–18.

Poonthananiwatkul, B., R. H. M. Lim, R. L. Howard, P. Pibanpaknitee, and E. M. Williamson. 2015. Traditional medicine use by cancer patients in Thailand. Journal of Ethnopharmacology 168: 100–107. doi:10.1016/j.jep.2015.03.057

Puataweepong, P., N. Sutheechet, and P. Ratanamongkol. 2012. A survey of complementary and alternative medicine use in cancer patients treated with radiotherapy in Thailand. Evidence-Based Complementary and Alternative Medicine 2012: 670408. doi:10.1155/2012/670408

Rattana, S., B. Cushnie, L. Taepongsorat, and M. Phadungkit. 2016. Chemical constituents and in vitro anti-cancer activity of Tiliacora triandra leaves. Pharmacognosy Journal 8, no. 1 (January–February): 1–3. doi:10.5530/pj.2016.1.1

Ruangnoo, S., A. Itharat, I. Sakpakdeejaroen, R. Rattarom, P. Tappayutpijarn, and K. Kumarn. 2012. In vitro cytotoxic activity of Benjakul herbal preparation and its active compounds against human lung, cervical and liver cancer cells. Journal of the Medical Association of Thailand 95, no. 1 (January): S127–S134.

Sukkasem, K. 2015. Biological activities of Thai traditional remedy called Kheaw-Hom and its plant ingredients. M.S. thesis. Thammasat University, Thailand.

Sukrueangkul, A., S. Phimha, N. Panomai, W. Laohasiriwong, and C. Sakphisutthikul. 2022. Attitudes and beliefs of cancer patients demanding medical cannabis use in North Thailand. Asian Pacific Journal of Cancer Prevention 23, no. 4 (April): 1309–1314. doi:10.31557/apjcp.2022.23.4.1309

Suwanpiwat, A., W. Petpichetchian, and K. Maneewat. 2017. Effects of co-applying oral health self-care programme and coconut oil gargle on stomatitis in cancer patients treated with chemotherapy. Thai Journal of Nursing Council 32, no. 1 (January–March): 18–31.

Tan, H., K. Chan, P. Pusparajah, L. Lee, and B. Goh. 2016. Gynura procumbens: An overview of the biological activities. Frontiers in Pharmacology 7: 52. doi:10.3389/fphar.2016.00052

Teerachaisakul, M., T. Khuayjarernpanishk, W. Worakunphanich, K. Bancheun, A. Chaiyasat, and T. Kamoltham. 2018. Safety and preliminary efficacy of herbal formulary "N040" in advanced cervical cancer: A clinical trial phase 1b. Journal of Thai Traditional & Alternative Medicine 16, no. 3 (September–December): 380–389.

Teerachaisakul, M., T. Nakaphan, R. Klinhom, C. Silarangsri, K. Bancheun, T. Chamyenura, N. Rochanapraphun, and P. Stienrut. 2020. Herbal use and symptom experiences of cancer patients: A cross-sectional survey in cancer patients with MORSANG Herbal Medicine Formularies. Journal of Thai Traditional & Alternative Medicine 18, no. 1 (January–April): 19–30.

Termsiririrkkul, R. 2014. Benja Amarit . . . Drug formulation for liver cancer treatment? https://shorturl.asia/OmRb5. (accessed April 1, 2022).

Thanasitthichai, S., C. Simasatikul, A. Srisubat, W. Krongkaew, B. Kunin, R. Seedadard, L. Chuensanit, P. Sailamai, S. Naewvong, R. Buasom, J. Krairittichai, N. Suwanpidokkul, C. Bodhibukkana, P. Prayakprom, and V. Khaowroongrueng. 2020. Safety and efficacy evaluation of the 1st legalized pharmaceutical grade medical cannabis for palliative cancer in Thailand. Journal of the Department of Medical Services 45, no. 3 (July–September): 116–122.

Thongdeeying, P., J. Kitsiripipat, S. Ruangnoo, P. Pibanpaknitee, and A. Itharat. 2017. Cytotoxic activity of Samhannachan recipe and its ingredients against lung cancer cell. Thammasat Medical Journal 17, no. 4 (October–December): 565–573.

Utane, M., and J. Maneesorn. 2019. Effect of ginger powder drinking on nausea and vomiting in cancer patient's receiving chemotherapy in male surgical ward 2. Chiangrai Medical Journal 11, no. 2: 52–59.

World Cancer Research Fund International. 2022. Global cancer data by country. www.wcrf.org/cancer-trends/global-cancer-data-by-country/ (accessed June 8, 2022).

Yapasert, R., B. Sripanidkulchai, M. Teerachaisakul, K. Banchuen, and R. Banjerdpongchai. 2020. Anticancer effects of a traditional Thai herbal recipe Benja Amarit extracts against human hepatocellular carcinoma and colon cancer cell by targeting apoptosis pathways. Journal of Ethnopharmacology 254: 112732. doi:10.1016/j.jep.2020.112732

Yossathera, K., W. Worakunphanich, M. Teerachaisakul, and P. Stienrut. 2017. Traditional Thai medicine formula "Benja Amarit" in liver cancer patients: A safety and quality of life. Journal of Thai Traditional & Alternative Medicine 15, no. 3 (September–December): 301–311.

3 Association between Traditional Dairy Products and Cancer
A Literature Review

*Khaoula El Kinany, Soukaina El Kinany
and Btissame Zarrouq*

ABBREVIATIONS

BC	breast cancer
CLA	conjugated linoleic acid
CRC	colorectal cancer
CUP	Continuous Update Project
ER+	estrogen receptor positive
ER−	estrogen receptor negative
IGF1R	insulin-like growth factor 1 receptor
LAB	lactic acid bacteria
PR+	progesterone receptor positive
WCRF	World Cancer Research Fund
WHO	World Health Organization

3.1 INTRODUCTION

Cancer is a leading cause of death worldwide, accounting for nearly 19.3 million incident cases and 10 million deaths in 2020, or nearly one in six deaths (World Health Organization 2022; International Agency for Research on Cancer 2020). Breast, lung, and colorectal cancers were the most commonly diagnosed cancers worldwide, accounting for 11.7%, 11.4%, and 10% of all incident cases diagnosed in 2020, respectively (International Agency for Research on Cancer 2020). Lung cancer was the leading cause of cancer death (almost 1.8 million deaths [18%]), followed by colorectal (9.4%) and liver (8.3%) cancers (International Agency for Research on Cancer 2020).

Several studies have provided solid evidence that lifestyle factors including smoking, overweight, physical inactivity, and changing reproductive patterns associated with urbanization and economic development are likely to be determinants of cancer risk (Torre et al. 2015).

According to the World Cancer Research Fund (WCRF) Third Expert Report, the consumption of foods containing dietary fiber, carotenoids, dithiolthiones, isothiocyanates, flavonoids, and phenols protects against several types of cancer (World Cancer Research Fund and American Institute for Cancer Research 2018). As reported by the World Health Organization (WHO), 30%–50% of all cancer cases are preventable through major modifiable risk factors such as a healthy diet, being physically active, and maintaining a healthy weight (World Health Organization 2022).

DOI: 10.1201/9781003260028-4

Recently, several nutrigenetics studies have attempted to identify and characterize gene variants linked to different nutrient responses, as well as to link this variation to cancer risk (gene-diet interactions) (da Cruz et al. 2020; El Asri et al. 2020). The accumulation of genetic changes resulting from the interaction of genetic and environmental factors is thought to be a multi-step process in the molecular pathogenesis of cancer (Theodoratou et al. 2017).

The human microbiota is made up of 10–100 trillion symbiotic microbial cells harbored primarily bacteria in the gut (Turnbaugh et al. 2007). The gut microbiota is largely influenced by an individual's diet (Huybrechts et al. 2020). Commensal bacteria can invade the gut wall and surrounding tissue and cause inflammation when the gut microbiota balance is disrupted (Akbar et al. 2022). Hence, chronic inflammation has been shown to be a driver of tumor development (Huybrechts et al. 2020; Akbar et al. 2022).

Regarding dietary factors, milk and dairy products have a high nutritional value (especially lactose, calcium, protein, and vitamin D). Dairy products are an interesting source of other important minerals such as potassium, phosphorus, zinc, and iodine (Górska-Warsewicz et al. 2019). Also they play an essential role in human development and nutrition throughout life, especially during childhood (FAO 2013).

The effect of milk and dairy fat on human health is not entirely clear. Dairy products are components that could hypothetically increase or reduce the risk of cancer (World Cancer Research Fund and American Institute for Cancer Research 2018). Currently, controversy has arisen over the benefits versus harms of milk fat, including concerns about long-term effects (Górska-Warsewicz et al. 2019). According to the CUP (Continuous Update Project) expert panel, there is no significant relationship between total dairy consumption (milk, cheese, and yogurt) and an increased overall risk of cancer mortality (Farvid et al. 2017; Tong et al. 2017), although there is limited evidence regarding the consumption of dairy products and calcium-rich diets and increased risk of prostate cancer (World Cancer Research Fund and American Institute for Cancer Research 2018). On the other hand, in the same report, after summarizing the results of numerous studies, they concluded that there is strong evidence of a decreased risk of colorectal cancer (CRC) with the consumption of dairy products (total dairy products, milk, cheese and dietary calcium) (World Cancer Research Fund and American Institute for Cancer Research 2018).

The quality of milk, which is the original product of traditional dairy products, is supposed to be microbiologically controlled. However, spoilage microorganisms and foodborne pathogens can easily contaminate milk from a variety of sources, including animal feces, soil, air, feed, water, equipment, animal hides, and people (Owusu-Kwarteng et al. 2020). As a result, a variety of factors and their interactions influence the prevalence of pathogenic and spoilage microorganisms in milk and milk products including the health of the dairy herd, the cleanliness of the dairy farm environment, milking and pre-storage conditions, available storage facilities and technologies, farm management practices, geographic location, and season (Owusu-Kwarteng et al. 2020). Traditional dairy products are typically sold directly to consumers without any microbiological quality assurance. Pathogens can contaminate milk in a variety of ways, including roaming the land in search of pasture and water in small rural dairies where livestock are fed grass, crop residues, and cultivated fodder, and containers in which farmers store the milk (Owusu-Kwarteng et al. 2020).

We conducted a literature review to summarize the most recent epidemiological evidence on the link between traditional dairy products and cancer. Understanding how traditional dairy products consumption affects the occurrence of various cancers could lead to useful prevention strategies.

3.2 DEFINITION OF TRADITIONAL DAIRY PRODUCTS

Milk has been consumed by humans since the dawn of agriculture. There is a wide variety of traditional dairy products, which are distinguished by their names and manufacturing processes all over the world (Leksir et al. 2019). These products are also distinguished by their taste (Leksir et al. 2019).

The main traditional dairy products cited are as follows:

Lben is a traditional North African drink usually prepared from cow's milk, but other types of milk can be used, such as goat's milk, sheep's milk, camel's milk, or a mixture of two of these types (Tantaoui-Elaraki and El Marrakchi 1987). A mixture of two of these types of milk is fermented for 24–48 hours at about 18–24°C depending on the season (Tantaoui-Elaraki and El Marrakchi 1987). The curd after coagulation is stirred in a goat skin bag (*chekoua*), which is vigorously stirred back and forth (Tantaoui-Elaraki and El Marrakchi 1987).

Zebda beldi is raw butter, with a strong diacetyl flavor, separated from the lben after churning the spontaneously coagulated milk (Benkerroum 2013). Zebda beldi is a dairy product common to all North African countries (Benkerroum 2013).

Smen is obtained from salted raw butter (8%–10%) and matured in the dark under cool, anaerobic conditions (13–15°C) (Benkerroum 2013; Benkerroum and Tamime 2004).

Raib is spontaneously curdled raw milk. It is prepared from cow's milk, without draining and without churning (Hamama 1992).

Jben is prepared by placing the coagulated milk in a cloth at room temperature and draining the whey (Hamama 1992).

Arish or *Kariesh* is made from the remaining curd after removing the top layer of cream from the spontaneously coagulated milk (*raib*) in an earthenware pot (*matared*) (Benkerroum 2013).

Kefir is a fermented milk with a Caucasian and Tibetan origin that is made by incubating kefir grains with raw milk or water (Sharifi et al. 2017).

Klila is prepared by moderately heating the *lben* until it becomes curdled, then draining it in a muslin cloth (Leksir et al. 2019).

Labaneh is a fermented milk product prepared from yogurt that has been filtered through cloth bags to remove water and water-soluble compounds, primarily whey protein, resulting in a relatively thick consistency, while maintaining a distinctive sour taste (Atamian et al. 2014).

Zabadi is prepared from milk enriched with skim milk powder, dried whey, or soybean flour, heat-treated and inoculated with the yogurt starter culture, then stored at 30 to 35°C until coagulation occurs (4–24 hours) (el-Neshawy and el-Shafie 1988).

Rigouta is obtained from heated whey (80–90°C) in order to coagulate the proteins (albumins and globulins); the product is then drained into a straw basket, cloth, or plastic or metal container (Ghrairi et al. 2004).

Khoa is an Indian heat-dried dairy product, is the base for preparation of a variety of sweet meat products (Murtaza et al. 2017).

Chhana is a coagulated milk product obtained by direct acidification of hot milk, used for a variety of sweets (Murtaza et al. 2017).

Rasgulla is made from milk casein with an attractive white color, a spongy and porous structure, and a spherical shape (Sarkar, Salauddin, and Chakraborty 2021).

Sandesh is a traditional Indian dairy product that is used as a sweet dairy dessert and is made by acid and heated coagulation of milk (Murtaza et al. 2017).

Paneer is obtained by acid and heated coagulation of milk. It is a non-fermentative, non-rennet, non-melting, and unripened type of cheese (Khan and Pal 2011).

Dahi is made from pasteurized or boiled cow's milk by natural acidification or using lactic acid or bacterial cultures (Murtaza et al. 2017).

Shrikhand is a semi-soft, sweetish-sour whole milk product made from lactic fermented curd (Pal 2018).

3.3 ASSOCIATIONS BETWEEN TRADITIONAL DAIRY PRODUCTS AND CANCERS

3.3.1 BREAST CANCER

In order to provide more scientific preventive strategies for breast cancer (BC) dietary choices, there is now an urgent need for a detailed analysis of the available research data to provide reliable evidence of the association between consumption of traditional dairy products and BC risk.

A meta-analysis has provided evidence that consuming dairy products are inversely associated with the risk of developing BC (Zang et al. 2015). A Polish case-control study found that increasing total dairy consumption by one serving per week significantly reduced the risk of BC among premenopausal women (Wajszczyk et al. 2021). Cottage cheese consumption reduced BC risk by 20% in postmenopausal women, with an $OR_{trend} = 0.80$ for an increase of one serving per week (Wajszczyk et al. 2021). Similarly, a pooled analysis of 21 cohort studies found that ricotta (cottage cheese) intake was inversely associated with the risk of ER-negative BC (Wu et al. 2021).

The findings of a recent meta-analysis showed that total dairy products can lower the incidence rate of BC, particularly estrogen receptor-positive (ER+) and progesterone receptor-positive (PR+) BC, but this trend is not statistically significant (He et al. 2021). Fermented dairy products can lower the BC risk in postmenopausal women while having no effect on premenopausal women (He et al. 2021).

Several nutrients present in dairy products may be responsible for the observed association include calcium, vitamin D, conjugated linoleic acid (CLA), butyric acid, and vaccenic acid, as well as whey protein and the composition of microorganisms in fermented products (Wajszczyk et al. 2021). It has been shown that lactobacillus acidophilus, a lactic acid bacterium classified as a probiotic found in yogurt, can modulate immune responses against BC in mouse models (Bourrie, Willing, and Cotter 2016), and balance gut microbiota, thereby reducing the risk of cancer (Merenstein et al. 2010).

Little research has been published on the association between traditional dairy products and the occurrence of BC. Nonetheless, the relationship between dairy intake and the BC onset is largely inconsistent (Moorman and Terry 2004). Therefore, studies evaluating the association between intake of traditional dairy products and BC risk are needed.

3.3.2 LUNG CANCER

A meta-analysis of prospective cohort studies showed non-significant association between dairy products consumption and lung cancer risk (Yu et al. 2016). Yang et al. found that the dairy products intake (including all types: total dairy, milk, cheese, yogurt, and calcium) was not significantly associated with lung cancer risk (Yang et al. 2016).

Lung cancer is a complex and heterogeneous disease with diverse genetic origins (Gazdar and Zhou 2018). The mechanism of a possible relationship between dairy consumption and lung cancer risk is still unknown. Studies have suggested associations between lung cancer and insulin-like growth factor 1 receptor (IGF1R) (Nurwidya et al. 2016), and low vitamin D intake (Feng et al. 2017; Cheng et al. 2013), indicating that these factors may play a role in carcinogenesis.

3.3.3 COLORECTAL CANCER

The relationship between dairy products consumption and CRC risk was widely studied in the literature. A systematic review and meta-analysis of prospective studies concluded that there was no association between consumption of fermented milk and CRC risk (Ralston et al. 2014). Similarly,

TABLE 3.1

Association between Traditional Dairy Products and Breast Cancer Risk

Author/Country	Studied Population	Study Type	Dairy Products	OR/RR/HR[*]	95%CI[**]
Wajszczyk B et al./Poland (Wajszczyk et al. 2021)	1699 women	Case-control study	Cottage cheese (Spearman's *r*)	$OR_{trend} = 0.80$	($p < 0.001$)
			>1.5 to ≤2.5 portions/ week	$OR_{trend} = 0.57$	0.33–0.99
				$OR_{trend} = 0.48$	0.29–0.80
			>2.5 portions/week		
Wu Y et al./USA; Canada; Japan; Australia; Netherlands; Italy; Sweden (Wu et al. 2021)	1 million women who were followed for a maximum of 8–20 years	A pooled analysis of 21 cohort studies	Cottage/ricotta cheese ≥25 g/d (referent class <1 g/d)	$RR_{trend} = 0.85$	0.76–0.95
He et al./Sweden; USA; France; Finland; Netherlands; Korea; Norway; China; UK; Italy; Mexico; Brazil; Poland; Japan; Uruguay; India; Iran (He et al. 2021)	Whole population: 1,019,232 participants/ Fermented dairy products: 496,747 participants	Meta-analysis	Fermented dairy products in postmenopausal population	$HR = 0.96$	0.93–0.99

[*] OR/RR/HR: Odds ratio/relative risk/hazard ratio.
[**] CI: Confidence interval.

a meta-analysis study found that cottage cheese and fermented dairy products were not associated to CRC risk (D. Aune et al. 2012). On the other hand, the NutriNet-Santé prospective cohort study reported a significant association between cottage cheese consumption and an increased CRC risk (Deschasaux-Tanguy et al. 2022).

A Jordanian study found a significant positive association between CRC incidence and *labaneh* consumption, specifically the frequency of consumption of ≥5 servings of *labaneh* per week. However, lower consumption (<5 servings per week) of *labaneh* did not show a significant association with CRC (Tayyem et al. 2016). A Moroccan study including 225 CRC cases and 225 controls concluded that CRC cases consumed less traditional *jben* fresh cheese compared to controls (Imad et al. 2020). Of note, the consumption of traditional products was low in this study population

A large Moroccan case-control study suggested a protective effect of traditional Moroccan dairy products namely *lben* (OR= 0.77, 95% CI 0.67–0.88), *raib* (OR= 0.86, 95% CI 0.76–0.96) and *jben* (OR= 0.77, 95% CI 0.67–0.88) on CRC risk (El Kinany et al. 2020). Hence, consumption of total traditional dairy products was inversely related to CRC risk (OR = 0.84, 95% CI 0.77–0.95).

Traditional milk processing in developing countries, particularly Morocco, entails a variety of operations such as heat treatments, fermentation, and the use of antimicrobial additives to prevent overgrowth of surviving pathogens and to improve the milk safety. The dairy production are based on the fermentation with lactic acid bacteria (LAB) (Benkerroum 2013). Food allergies and inflammatory bowel disease have both been successfully treated with LAB (Zhong, Zhang, and Covasa 2014). LAB has also shown a variety of properties in the prevention of CRC by inhibiting the initiation or progression of the disease via multiple pathways (Zhong, Zhang, and Covasa 2014). LAB has the potential to boost immunity, improve gastrointestinal function, increase obesity resistance, and boost antioxidant capacity, as well as lower blood glucose intake and cholesterol concentration

(Nowak, Paliwoda, and Błasiak 2019; Mathur, Beresford, and Cotter 2020). According to recent studies, anticancer proprieties of LAB are due to the following active substances: extracellular polysaccharides (EPS) (Zhou et al. 2017), peptidoglycan (Fichera, Fichera, and Milone 2016), nucleic acid (Liu et al. 2021), bacteriocin (Norouzi et al. 2018), and S-layer protein (Zhang et al. 2020).

3.3.4 PROSTATE CANCER

Prostate cancer is the second most common cancer in men and the fourth most common cancer overall. There were more than 1.4 million new cases of prostate cancer in 2020 ('Prostate Cancer Statistics | World Cancer Research Fund International' 2022).

According to the 2020 WCRF report, dietary choices may play an important role in developing prostate cancer, especially a higher consumption of dairy products ('Prostate Cancer | What Causes Prostate Cancer?' 2022). In fact, vis-à-vis the lack of data concerning the association between traditional dairy products and front of prostate cancer, there is an abundance of epidemiologic and ecologic studies exploring the relation between this type of cancer and other dairy products. Hence, the finding that a high intake of dairy foods, milk, low-fat milk, cheese, and total, dietary, and dairy calcium was positively associated with total prostate cancer risk, and

TABLE 3.2

Association between Traditional Dairy Products and Colorectal Cancer Risk

Author/Country	Studied Population	Study Type	Dairy Products	OR/RR/HR*	95% CI**
Tayyem R et al./Jordan (Tayyem et al. 2016)	220 CRC cases/281 healthy controls	Case-control study	Cooked yogurt (*jammed*) ≥2 servings per week (referent class ≤1 serving per week)	$OR_{trend} = 0.54$	0.09–3.23
			Labaneh ≥1 serving per day (referent class ≤1 serving per week)	$OR_{trend} = 1.91$	1.03–3.52
Imad F et al./Morocco (Imad et al. 2020)	225 CRC cases/225 healthy controls	Case-control study	*Lben* 4–7 times per week (referent class never)	OR = 1.04	0.30–3.20
			Jben 4–7 times per week (referent class never)	OR = 0.60	0.10–2.60
El Kinany K et al./ Morocco (El Kinany et al. 2020)	1453 CRC cases/1453 healthy controls	Case-control study	*Lben* >23.3 mL/day (referent class ≤23.3 mL/day)	$OR_{trend} = 0.77$	0.67–0.88
			Raib >0.0 mL/day (referent class ≤0.0 mL/day)	$OR_{trend} = 0.86$	0.76–0.96
			Saykok >20.0 mL/day (referent class ≤20.0 mL/day)	$OR_{trend} = 0.89$	0.80–1.00
			Jben >0.0 mL/day (referent class ≤0.0 mL/day)	$OR_{trend} = 0.77$	0.67–0.88

* OR/RR/HR: Odds ratio/relative risk/hazard ratio.
** CI: Confidence interval.

increased prostate cancer mortality risk, was substantiated by many systematic reviews and meta-analyses published since 2004 (Qin et al. 2004; Gao, LaValley, and Tucker 2005; Qin et al. 2007; Dagfinn Aune et al. 2015; Lu et al. 2016). Experimental studies have been suggested that drinking milk may result in increase of estrone and progesterone levels in the blood, which might affect prostate cancer development (Maruyama, Oshima, and Ohyama 2010; Li et al. 2003). In addition, milk protein casein may stimulate the proliferation of prostate cancer cells (Park et al. 2014).

However, the evidence that a higher consumption of dairy products increases the risk of prostate cancer steel limited, since other meta-analysis of 45 observational studies showed no evidence of an association between dairy products, dietary calcium, and vitamin D use and an increased risk of prostate cancer (Huncharek, Muscat, and Kupelnick 2008). On the other hand, another meta-analysis established that high intake of whole milk revealed a significant inverse association with total prostate cancer risk (Dagfinn Aune et al. 2015).

In summary, the total evidence generated to date about the association between prostate cancer and dairy products is still not conclusive (López-Plaza et al. 2019), especially that only a small number of experimental studies have been conducted to explore this topic (Sargsyan and Dubasi 2021).

3.4 TOXICITY AND CAUTIONARY NOTES

Milk and milk products are important components of the diet of people in developing countries. The safety risks associated with the consumption of raw milk and dairy products vary widely between developed and developing countries. The microbial safety characteristics of traditional dairy products and fermented milk products can be influenced by several factors, including the health status of the dairy herd, the level of hygiene of the dairy farm environment, milking conditions and pre-storage, and available storage facilities and technologies. The consumption of unpasteurized raw milk and its products has been shown to pose a real threat to health due to possible contamination with human pathogens such as *Mycobacterium bovis, Coxiella burnetii, Escherichia coli, Bacillus cereus*, and *Listeria monocytogenes*, which are of particular food safety concern due to their ability to cause disease in humans through the production of various forms of enterotoxins and emetic toxins. To ensure consumer safety, various precautionary measures should be implemented during milk production, handling, and processing.

3.5 CONCLUSION

The association between traditional dairy consumption and cancer risk has been moderately explored in numerous reports and studies, but limitations may reduce the validity of previously published results. We need more high-quality prospective studies to fully confirm the relationships between traditional dairy consumption and cancer risk.

Up to now, there is currently not sufficient evidence to justify a reduction in daily dairy product consumption. That is why organizations like the World Cancer Research Fund/American Institute for Cancer Research have reported that there is not sufficient evidence to recommend reducing modern or traditional dairy consumption to reduce the risk of cancer ('Summary-of-Third-Expert-Report-2018.Pdf' 2022).

3.6 SUMMARY POINTS

- Dietary patterns are major components that could influence and contribute to risk for cancer.
- Traditional dairy products are rich in calcium, vitamin D, and probiotics.

- Traditional dairy products are beneficial and could prevent against colorectal cancer.
- People involved in the traditional dairy products manufacturing lack adequate knowledge of good hygiene practices.
- The impact of traditional dairy products on cancer risk should be investigated further in order to understand the mechanisms behind their actions.

REFERENCES

Akbar, Noor, Naveed Ahmed Khan, Jibran Sualeh Muhammad, and Ruqaiyyah Siddiqui. 2022. 'The Role of Gut Microbiome in Cancer Genesis and Cancer Prevention'. *Health Sciences Review* 2 (March): 100010. doi:10.1016/j.hsr.2021.100010

Atamian, Samson, Ammar Olabi, Omar Kebbe Baghdadi, and Imad Toufeili. 2014. 'The Characterization of the Physicochemical and Sensory Properties of Full-Fat, Reduced-Fat and Low-Fat Bovine, Caprine, and Ovine Greek Yogurt (Labneh)'. *Food Science & Nutrition* 2 (2): 164–173. doi:10.1002/fsn3.89

Aune, D., R. Lau, D. S. M. Chan, R. Vieira, D. C. Greenwood, E. Kampman, and T. Norat. 2012. 'Dairy Products and Colorectal Cancer Risk: A Systematic Review and Meta-Analysis of Cohort Studies'. *Annals of Oncology: Official Journal of the European Society for Medical Oncology* 23 (1): 37–45. doi:10.1093/annonc/mdr269

Aune, Dagfinn, Deborah A. Navarro Rosenblatt, Doris S. M. Chan, Ana Rita Vieira, Rui Vieira, Darren C. Greenwood, Lars J. Vatten, and Teresa Norat. 2015. 'Dairy Products, Calcium, and Prostate Cancer Risk: A Systematic Review and Meta-Analysis of Cohort Studies'. *The American Journal of Clinical Nutrition* 101 (1): 87–117. doi:10.3945/ajcn.113.067157

Benkerroum, Noreddine. 2013. 'Traditional Fermented Foods of North African Countries: Technology and Food Safety Challenges With Regard to Microbiological Risks'. *Comprehensive Reviews in Food Science and Food Safety* 12 (1): 54–89. doi:10.1111/j.1541-4337.2012.00215.x

Benkerroum, Noreddine, and A. Y Tamime. 2004. 'Technology Transfer of Some Moroccan Traditional Dairy Products (Lben, Jben and Smen) to Small Industrial Scale'. *Food Microbiology* 21 (4): 399–413. doi:10.1016/j.fm.2003.08.006

Bourrie, Benjamin C. T., Benjamin P. Willing, and Paul D. Cotter. 2016. 'The Microbiota and Health Promoting Characteristics of the Fermented Beverage Kefir'. *Frontiers in Microbiology* 7. www.frontiersin.org/article/10.3389/fmicb.2016.00647.

Cheng, Ting-Yuan David, Andrea Z. LaCroix, Shirley A. A. Beresford, Gary E. Goodman, Mark D. Thornquist, Yingye Zheng, Rowan T. Chlebowski, Gloria Y. F. Ho, and Marian L. Neuhouser. 2013. 'Vitamin D Intake and Lung Cancer Risk in the Women's Health Initiative'. *The American Journal of Clinical Nutrition* 98 (4): 1002–1011. doi:10.3945/ajcn.112.055905

da Cruz, Raquel Santana, Elaine Chen, Megan Smith, Jaedus Bates, and Sonia de Assis. 2020. 'Diet and Transgenerational Epigenetic Inheritance of Breast Cancer: The Role of the Paternal Germline'. *Frontiers in Nutrition* 7. www.frontiersin.org/article/10.3389/fnut.2020.00093.

Deschasaux-Tanguy, Mélanie, Laura Barrubés Piñol, Laury Sellem, Charlotte Debras, Bernard Srour, Eloi Chazelas, Gaëlle Wendeu-Foyet, et al. 2022. 'Dairy Product Consumption and Risk of Cancer: A Short Report from the NutriNet-Santé Prospective Cohort Study'. *International Journal of Cancer* n/a (n/a). doi:10.1002/ijc.33935

El Asri, Achraf, Btissame Zarrouq, Khaoula El Kinany, Laila Bouguenouch, Karim Ouldim, and Karima El Rhazi. 2020. 'Associations between Nutritional Factors and KRAS Mutations in Colorectal Cancer: A Systematic Review'. *BMC Cancer* 20 (1): 696. doi:10.1186/s12885-020-07189-2

El Kinany, Khaoula, Meimouna Mint Sidi Deoula, Zineb Hatime, Hanae Abir Boudouaya, Inge Huybrechts, Achraf El Asri, Abdelatif Benider, et al. 2020. 'Consumption of Modern and Traditional Moroccan Dairy Products and Colorectal Cancer Risk: A Large Case Control Study'. *European Journal of Nutrition* 59 (3): 953–963. doi:10.1007/s00394-019-01954-1

el-Neshawy, A. A., and N. M. el-Shafie. 1988. 'Quality of Zabadi Made from Cow's Milk Fortified with Whey and Soy Proteins'. *Die Nahrung* 32 (10): 939–943. doi:10.1002/food.19880321005

FAO. 2013. *Milk and Dairy Products in Human Nutrition*. Rome, Italy: FAO. www.fao.org/documents/card/fr/c/5067e4f2-53f8-5c9a-b709-c5db17d55c20/.

Farvid, Maryam S., Akbar F. Malekshah, Akram Pourshams, Hossein Poustchi, Sadaf G. Sepanlou, Maryam Sharafkhah, Masoud Khoshnia, et al. 2017. 'Dairy Food Intake and All-Cause, Cardiovascular Disease, and Cancer Mortality'. *American Journal of Epidemiology* 185 (8): 697–711. doi:10.1093/aje/kww139

Feng, Qianqian, Han Zhang, Zhengqin Dong, Yang Zhou, and Jingping Ma. 2017. 'Circulating 25-Hydroxyvitamin D and Lung Cancer Risk and Survival'. *Medicine* 96 (45): e8613. doi:10.1097/MD.0000000000008613

Fichera, Giuseppe A., Marco Fichera, and Giuseppe Milone. 2016. 'Antitumoral Activity of a Cytotoxic Peptide of *Lactobacillus casei* Peptidoglycan and Its Interaction with Mitochondrial-Bound Hexokinase'. *Anti-Cancer Drugs* 27 (7): 609–619. doi:10.1097/CAD.0000000000000367

Gao, Xiang, Michael P. LaValley, and Katherine L. Tucker. 2005. 'Prospective Studies of Dairy Product and Calcium Intakes and Prostate Cancer Risk: A Meta-Analysis'. *Journal of the National Cancer Institute* 97 (23): 1768–1777. doi:10.1093/jnci/dji402

Gazdar, Adi F., and Caicun Zhou. 2018. '4 – Lung Cancer in Never-Smokers: A Different Disease'. In *IASLC Thoracic Oncology (Second Edition)*, edited by Harvey I. Pass, David Ball, and Giorgio V. Scagliotti, 23–29.e3. Philadelphia: Elsevier. doi:10.1016/B978-0-323-52357-8.00004-4

Ghrairi, T., M. Manai, J. M. Berjeaud, and J. Frère. 2004. 'Antilisterial Activity of Lactic Acid Bacteria Isolated from Rigouta, a Traditional Tunisian Cheese'. *Journal of Applied Microbiology* 97 (3): 621–628. doi:10.1111/j.1365-2672.2004.02347.x

Górska-Warsewicz, Hanna, Krystyna Rejman, Wacław Laskowski, and Maksymilian Czeczotko. 2019. 'Milk and Dairy Products and Their Nutritional Contribution to the Average Polish Diet'. *Nutrients* 11 (8): 1771. doi:10.3390/nu11081771

Hamama, Abed. 1992. *Moroccan Traditional Fermented Dairy Products. Applications of Biotechnology to Fermented Foods: Report of an Ad Hoc Panel of the Board on Science and Technology for International Development.* US: National Academies Press. www.ncbi.nlm.nih.gov/books/NBK234690/.

He, Yujing, Qinghua Tao, Feifei Zhou, Yuexiu Si, Rongrong Fu, Binbin Xu, Jiaxuan Xu, Xiangyuan Li, and Bangsheng Chen. 2021. 'The Relationship between Dairy Products Intake and Breast Cancer Incidence: A Meta-Analysis of Observational Studies'. *BMC Cancer* 21 (1): 1109. doi:10.1186/s12885-021-08854-w

Huncharek, Michael, Joshua Muscat, and Bruce Kupelnick. 2008. 'Dairy Products, Dietary Calcium and Vitamin D Intake as Risk Factors for Prostate Cancer: A Meta-Analysis of 26,769 Cases from 45 Observational Studies'. *Nutrition and Cancer* 60 (4): 421–441. doi:10.1080/01635580801911779

Huybrechts, Inge, Semi Zouiouich, Astrid Loobuyck, Zeger Vandenbulcke, Emily Vogtmann, Silvia Pisanu, Isabel Iguacel, et al. 2020. 'The Human Microbiome in Relation to Cancer Risk: A Systematic Review of Epidemiologic Studies'. *Cancer Epidemiology, Biomarkers & Prevention* 29 (10): 1856–1868. doi:10.1158/1055-9965.EPI-20-0288

Imad, Fatima Ezzahra, Houda Drissi, Nezha Tawfiq, Karima Bendahhou, Abdellatif Benider, and Driss Radallah. 2020. 'Facteurs de Risque Alimentaires du Cancer Colorectal au Maroc: Étude Cas Témoin'. *The Pan African Medical Journal* 35 (February): 59. doi:10.11604/pamj.2020.35.59.18214

International Agency for Research on Cancer. 2020. 'All Cancers Source: Globocan 2020'. https://gco.iarc.fr/today/data/factsheets/cancers/39-All-cancers-fact-sheet.pdf.

Khan, Shahnawaz Umer, and Mohammad Ashraf Pal. 2011. 'Paneer Production: A Review'. *Journal of Food Science and Technology* 48 (6): 645–660. doi:10.1007/s13197-011-0247-x

Leksir, Choubaila, Sofiane Boudalia, Nizar Moujahed, and Mabrouk Chemmam. 2019. 'Traditional Dairy Products in Algeria: Case of Klila Cheese'. *Journal of Ethnic Foods* 6 (1): 7. doi:10.1186/s42779-019-0008-4

Li, Xiang-Ming, Davaasambuu Ganmaa, Li-Qiang Qin, Xiu-Fan Liu, and Akio Sato. 2003. '[The effects of estrogen-like products in milk on prostate and testes]'. *Zhonghua Nan Ke Xue = National Journal of Andrology* 9 (3): 186–190.

Liu, Chaoran, Jiaqi Zheng, Xuan Ou, and Yuzhu Han. 2021. 'Anti-Cancer Substances and Safety of Lactic Acid Bacteria in Clinical Treatment'. *Frontiers in Microbiology* 12 (October): 722052. doi:10.3389/fmicb.2021.722052

López-Plaza, Bricia, Laura M. Bermejo, Cristina Santurino, Iván Cavero-Redondo, Celia Álvarez-Bueno, and Carmen Gómez-Candela. 2019. 'Milk and Dairy Product Consumption and Prostate Cancer Risk and Mortality: An Overview of Systematic Reviews and Meta-Analyses'. *Advances in Nutrition (Bethesda, Md.)* 10 (suppl_2): S212–S223. doi:10.1093/advances/nmz014

Lu, Wei, Hanwen Chen, Yuequn Niu, Han Wu, Dajing Xia, and Yihua Wu. 2016. 'Dairy Products Intake and Cancer Mortality Risk: A Meta-Analysis of 11 Population-Based Cohort Studies'. *Nutrition Journal* 15 (1): 91. doi:10.1186/s12937-016-0210-9

Maruyama, Kazumi, Tomoe Oshima, and Kenji Ohyama. 2010. 'Exposure to Exogenous Estrogen through Intake of Commercial Milk Produced from Pregnant Cows'. *Pediatrics International: Official Journal of the Japan Pediatric Society* 52 (1): 33–38. doi:10.1111/j.1442-200X.2009.02890.x

Mathur, Harsh, Tom P. Beresford, and Paul D. Cotter. 2020. 'Health Benefits of Lactic Acid Bacteria (LAB) Fermentates'. *Nutrients* 12 (6): E1679. doi:10.3390/nu12061679

Merenstein, D. J., K. H. Smith, M. Scriven, R. F. Roberts, M. E. Sanders, and S. Petterson. 2010. 'The Study to Investigate the Potential Benefits of Probiotics in Yogurt, a Patient-Oriented, Double-Blind, Cluster-Randomised, Placebo-Controlled, Clinical Trial'. *European Journal of Clinical Nutrition* 64 (7): 685–691. doi:10.1038/ejcn.2010.30

Moorman, Patricia G., and Paul D. Terry. 2004. 'Consumption of Dairy Products and the Risk of Breast Cancer: A Review of the Literature'. *The American Journal of Clinical Nutrition* 80 (1): 5–14. doi:10.1093/ajcn/80.1.5

Murtaza, Mian Anjum, Ajit J. Pandya, George F. W. Haenlein, and M. Mohamed H. Khan. 2017. 'Traditional Indian Dairy Products'. In *Handbook of Milk of Non-Bovine Mammals*, 343–367. John Wiley & Sons, Ltd. https://doi.org/10.1002/9781119110316.ch4.3. https://onlinelibrary.wiley.com/doi/abs/10.1002/9781119110316.ch4.3

Norouzi, Zohreh, Ali Salimi, Raheleh Halabian, and Hossein Fahimi. 2018. 'Nisin, a Potent Bacteriocin and Anti-Bacterial Peptide, Attenuates Expression of Metastatic Genes in Colorectal Cancer Cell Lines'. *Microbial Pathogenesis* 123 (October): 183–189. doi:10.1016/j.micpath.2018.07.006

Nowak, Adriana, Anna Paliwoda, and Janusz Błasiak. 2019. 'Anti-Proliferative, Pro-Apoptotic and Anti-Oxidative Activity of Lactobacillus and Bifidobacterium Strains: A Review of Mechanisms and Therapeutic Perspectives'. *Critical Reviews in Food Science and Nutrition* 59 (21): 3456–3467. doi:10.1080/10408398.2018.1494539

Nurwidya, Fariz, Sita Andarini, Fumiyuki Takahashi, Elisna Syahruddin, and Kazuhisa Takahashi. 2016. 'Implications of Insulin-Like Growth Factor 1 Receptor Activation in Lung Cancer'. *The Malaysian Journal of Medical Sciences: MJMS* 23 (3): 9–21.

Owusu-Kwarteng, James, Fortune Akabanda, Dominic Agyei, and Lene Jespersen. 2020. 'Microbial Safety of Milk Production and Fermented Dairy Products in Africa'. *Microorganisms* 8 (5): 752. doi:10.3390/microorganisms8050752

Pal, Mahendra. 2018. 'Shrikhand: A Delicious Fermented Dairy Product of India'. *Beverage & Food World* 45 (7). https://www.researchgate.net/publication/327107250_Shrikhand_A_Delicious_Fermented_Dairy_Product_of_India.

Park, Sung-Woo, Joo-Young Kim, You-Sun Kim, Sang Jin Lee, Sang Don Lee, and Moon Kee Chung. 2014. 'A Milk Protein, Casein, as a Proliferation Promoting Factor in Prostate Cancer Cells'. *The World Journal of Men's Health* 32 (2): 76–82. doi:10.5534/wjmh.2014.32.2.76

'Prostate Cancer | What Causes Prostate Cancer?' 2022. *WCRF International*. Accessed April 29. www.wcrf.org/diet-activity-and-cancer/cancer-types/prostate-cancer/.

'Prostate Cancer Statistics | World Cancer Research Fund International'. 2022. *WCRF International*. Accessed April 29. www.wcrf.org/cancer-trends/prostate-cancer-statistics/.

Qin, Li-Qiang, Jia-Ying Xu, Pei-Yu Wang, Takashi Kaneko, Kazuhiko Hoshi, and Akio Sato. 2004. 'Milk Consumption Is a Risk Factor for Prostate Cancer: Meta-Analysis of Case-Control Studies'. *Nutrition and Cancer* 48 (1): 22–27. doi:10.1207/s15327914nc4801_4

Qin, Li-Qiang, Jia-Ying Xu, Pei-Yu Wang, Jian Tong, and Kazuhiko Hoshi. 2007. 'Milk Consumption Is a Risk Factor for Prostate Cancer in Western Countries: Evidence from Cohort Studies'. *Asia Pacific Journal of Clinical Nutrition* 16 (3): 467–476.

Ralston, Robin A., Helen Truby, Claire E. Palermo, and Karen Z. Walker. 2014. 'Colorectal Cancer and Nonfermented Milk, Solid Cheese, and Fermented Milk Consumption: A Systematic Review and Meta-Analysis of Prospective Studies'. *Critical Reviews in Food Science and Nutrition* 54 (9): 1167–1179. doi:10.1080/10408398.2011.629353

Sargsyan, Alex, and Hima Bindu Dubasi. 2021. 'Milk Consumption and Prostate Cancer: A Systematic Review'. *The World Journal of Men's Health* 39 (3): 419–428. doi:10.5534/wjmh.200051

Sarkar, Tanmay, Molla Salauddin, and Runu Chakraborty. 2021. 'Rasgulla–the Ethnic Indian Sweetmeat Delicacy and Its Evolutionary Journey through Contemporary Research'. *Journal of Ethnic Foods* 8 (1): 11. doi:10.1186/s42779-021-00091-7

Sharifi, Mohammadreza, Abbas Moridnia, Deniz Mortazavi, Mahsa Salehi, Marzieh Bagheri, and Abdolkarim Sheikhi. 2017. 'Kefir: A Powerful Probiotics with Anticancer Properties'. *Medical Oncology (Northwood, London, England)* 34 (11): 183. doi:10.1007/s12032-017-1044-9

'Summary-of-Third-Expert-Report-2018.Pdf'. 2022. Accessed April 29. www.wcrf.org/wp-content/uploads/2021/02/Summary-of-Third-Expert-Report-2018.pdf.

Tantaoui-Elaraki, A., and A. El Marrakchi. 1987. 'Study of Moroccan Dairy Products: Iben and Smen'. *MIRCEN Journal of Applied Microbiology and Biotechnology*. https://scholar.google.com/scholar_lookup?title=Study+of+Moroccan+dairy+products%3A+iben+and+smen&author=Tantaoui-Elaraki%2C+A.&publication_year=1987.

Tayyem, R. F., H. A. Bawadi, I. Shehadah, S. S. AbuMweis, L. M. Agraib, T. Al-Jaberi, M. Al-Nusairr, D. D. Heath, and K. E. Bani-Hani. 2016. 'Meats, Milk and Fat Consumption in Colorectal Cancer'. *Journal of Human Nutrition and Dietetics: The Official Journal of the British Dietetic Association* 29 (6): 746–756. doi:10.1111/jhn.12391

Theodoratou, Evropi, Maria Timofeeva, Xue Li, Xiangrui Meng, and John P. A. Ioannidis. 2017. 'Nature, Nurture, and Cancer Risks: Genetic and Nutritional Contributions to Cancer'. *Annual Review of Nutrition* 37 (August): 293–320. doi:10.1146/annurev-nutr-071715-051004

Tong, Xing, Guo-Chong Chen, Zheng Zhang, Yu-Lu Wei, Jia-Ying Xu, and Li-Qiang Qin. 2017. 'Cheese Consumption and Risk of All-Cause Mortality: A Meta-Analysis of Prospective Studies'. *Nutrients* 9 (1): 63. doi:10.3390/nu9010063

Torre, Lindsey A., Freddie Bray, Rebecca L. Siegel, Jacques Ferlay, Joannie Lortet-Tieulent, and Ahmedin Jemal. 2015. 'Global Cancer Statistics, 2012'. *CA: A Cancer Journal for Clinicians* 65 (2): 87–108. doi:10.3322/caac.21262

Turnbaugh, Peter J., Ruth E. Ley, Micah Hamady, Claire M. Fraser-Liggett, Rob Knight, and Jeffrey I. Gordon. 2007. 'The Human Microbiome Project'. *Nature* 449 (7164): 804–810. doi:10.1038/nature06244

Wajszczyk, Bożena, Jadwiga Charzewska, Dariusz Godlewski, Brunon Zemła, Elżbieta Nowakowska, Maciej Kozaczka, Małgorzata Chilimoniuk, and Dorothy R. Pathak. 2021. 'Consumption of Dairy Products and the Risk of Developing Breast Cancer in Polish Women'. *Nutrients* 13 (12): 4420. doi:10.3390/nu13124420

World Cancer Research Fund, and American Institute for Cancer Research. 2018. 'Diet, Nutrition, Physical Activity and Cancer: A Global Perspective Continuous Update Project Expert Report'. www.wcrf.org/wp-content/uploads/2021/02/Summary-of-Third-Expert-Report-2018.pdf.

World Health Organization. 2022. 'Cancer'. www.who.int/news-room/fact-sheets/detail/cancer, www.who.int/activities/improving-treatment-for-snakebite-patients.

Wu, You, Ruyi Huang, Molin Wang, Leslie Bernstein, Traci N. Bethea, Chu Chen, Yu Chen, et al. 2021. 'Dairy Foods, Calcium, and Risk of Breast Cancer Overall and for Subtypes Defined by Estrogen Receptor Status: A Pooled Analysis of 21 Cohort Studies'. *The American Journal of Clinical Nutrition* 114 (2): 450–461. doi:10.1093/ajcn/nqab097

Yang, Yang, Xu Wang, Qinghua Yao, Liqiang Qin, and Chao Xu. 2016. 'Dairy Product, Calcium Intake and Lung Cancer Risk: A Systematic Review with Meta-Analysis'. *Scientific Reports* 6 (February): 20624. doi:10.1038/srep20624

Yu, Yi, Hui Li, Kaiwu Xu, Xin Li, Chunlin Hu, Hongyan Wei, Xiaoyun Zeng, and Xiaoli Jing. 2016. 'Dairy Consumption and Lung Cancer Risk: A Meta-Analysis of Prospective Cohort Studies'. *OncoTargets and Therapy* 9. Dove Press: 111. doi:10.2147/OTT.S95714

Zang, Jiajie, Meihua Shen, Sufa Du, Tianwen Chen, and Shurong Zou. 2015. 'The Association between Dairy Intake and Breast Cancer in Western and Asian Populations: A Systematic Review and Meta-Analysis'. *Journal of Breast Cancer* 18 (4): 313–322. doi:10.4048/jbc.2015.18.4.313

Zhang, Tao, Daodong Pan, Yujie Yang, Xiaoxiao Jiang, Jiaxin Zhang, Xiaoqun Zeng, Zhen Wu, Yangying Sun, and Yuxing Guo. 2020. 'Effect of Lactobacillus Acidophilus CICC 6074 S-Layer Protein on Colon Cancer HT-29 Cell Proliferation and Apoptosis'. *Journal of Agricultural and Food Chemistry* 68 (9): 2639–2647. doi:10.1021/acs.jafc.9b06909

Zhong, Li, Xufei Zhang, and Mihai Covasa. 2014. 'Emerging Roles of Lactic Acid Bacteria in Protection against Colorectal Cancer'. *World Journal of Gastroenterology* 20 (24): 7878–7886. doi:10.3748/wjg. v20.i24.7878

Zhou, Xingtao, Tao Hong, Qiang Yu, Shaoping Nie, Deming Gong, Tao Xiong, and Mingyong Xie. 2017. 'Exopolysaccharides from *Lactobacillus plantarum* NCU116 Induce C-Jun Dependent Fas/Fasl-Mediated Apoptosis via TLR2 in Mouse Intestinal Epithelial Cancer Cells'. *Scientific Reports* 7 (1). Nature Publishing Group: 14247. doi:10.1038/s41598-017-14178-2

4 Traditional Chinese Medicine and Treatment Response in Cancer

Kulsoom Zahara, Yamin Bibi and Tayyiba Afzal

ABBREVIATIONS

CYP3A   cytochrome P450 isoforms
EGCG   epigallocatechin-3-gallate
FDA   US Food and Drug Administration
INBM   integrated network-based medicine
IU   international unit
PSA   prostate-specific antigen
SHH   sonic hedgehog homology
TCM   traditional Chinese medicine

4.1 BACKGROUND

Complementary and alternative medicines are widely used in combination with conventional anti-cancer practices in order to decrease side effects and improve their efficacy. However, many physicians of modern medicine criticize these practices (Wang 2003).

Cancer treatment with traditional Chinese medicine (TCM) has a long history. Discussions of cancer appeared in classical works, such as *The Yellow Emperor's Inner Canon* and *The Classic of Medical Problems*, more than 2000 years ago (Hua 2007). Concepts of diagnosis and treatment, such as strengthening body resistance and eliminating pathogens, treating both the manifestation and root cause, treating the same disease with different methods, and treating different diseases with the same methods, have been proven by clinical practice (Li 2006). These concepts have become characteristics and advantages of TCM for cancer prevention and treatment, as demonstrated by modern technology and methods. Heritage has laid the foundation for the innovation and development of cancer treatment with TCM, attracting more and more international attention and cooperation (McCulloch et al. 2006).

Cancer treatment with TCM remains the most ancient living tradition; the word "tumor" was discovered on 3500-year-old oracle bone inscriptions. The wholism of interconnection and mutual restraint inside the human body and the concept of treatment according to syndrome differentiation have been reflected in the cognition of cancer etiology and the principles of diagnosis and treatment with TCM (Gan et al. 2010).

The diagnosis and treatment of tumors was discussed in the literature of ancient Chinese medicine, where there is a wealth of content. Apart from descriptions of symptoms, prognosis, and differential diagnosis, we can also find summaries of cancer pathogenesis and treatment strategy, revealing that our ancestors recognized that cancer etiology involved exopathogens, environment, emotional maladjustment, and improper diet: "With discomfort, improper diet, cold temperature from time to time, pathogens prevail and accumulation has left" (*The Yellow Emperor's Inner Canon*, English translation). Chinese ancestors emphasized that cancer

DOI: 10.1201/9781003260028-5

stemmed from an endogenous cause – "The form of ulcer is sore, swollen, all because of the cumulative toxicity of five viscera and six bowels, not exclusively for RongWei congestion" (*The Central Treasury Canon*, English translation) – and that the tumor is a partial consequence of systemic disease. These theories represent the formulation of TCM treatment strategies for cancer: the combination of partial and systemic therapy, strengthening body resistance and eliminating pathogens, treatment of the body, and the regulation of emotion (Li et al. 2013). Treatment methods, such as strengthening body resistance, heat-clearing and detoxifying, activating blood and removing stasis, and softening and resolving hard masses, were also developed from these theories. *Indispensable Medical Reading* (Li 2006) first proposed cancer treatment by different stages: "In the early stage of the disease, the vital qi is strong, the evil qi is light and easily attacked; in the middle stage, the evil qi is deeper, the vital qi becomes weak and should be attacked or benefit; in the end, the evil qi is strong, the vital qi is weaker and should be well benefit."

Some ancient classical prescriptions and medicine are still in use today, such as Xiaojin dan, the Xihuang pill, the Dahuangzhechong pill, the Liushen pill, and Pianzaihuang. This chapter enlists the evidence of herbal medicine as adjuvants in conventional cancer therapies (Zhong et al. 2012).

4.2 PROSTATE CANCER

Prostate cancer is characterized by a very long dormant period and has very limited strategies for treatment if diagnosed at an advanced stage. That's why most patients look toward herbal medicines with the hope that they are viable option with very little side effects. This belief is strongly endorsed by various Asian societies; therefore it needs to be validated with a scientific approach. Recent studies have revealed that inflammation may have some vital role in the formation of prostate carcinoma. It is observed that vitamin supplements are widely used by patients diagnosed with prostate cancers. In smokers daily use of >100IU of vitamin E showed a 56% reduction in risk in prostate cancer relative to non-users (Mao et al. 2014).

4.2.1 Green Tea, Soy, and *Scutellaria baicalensis*

In a study conducted on polyphenolic compounds of green tea, soy, and *Scutellaria baicalensis* revealed that green tea (epigallocatechin-3-gallate (EGCG)) successfully inhibits metalloproteinase *in vitro* and arrest DU145 and LNCaP prostate cancer cells at their G0-G1 phase of the cell cycle, although this suppressive effect is achieved at very high concentration. In a similar study on patients with androgen-independent metastatic prostate carcinoma, when administered with green tea, one patient gained a >50% prostate-specific antigen (PSA) response that lasted for about a month. However, that patient also showed some toxicity effect during this study, including fatigue, nausea, and diarrhea. Another study on soy isoflavones observed that they successfully inhibited 5α-reductase activity (an enzyme that converts testosterone to androgen dihydrotestosterone) (Zhang and Xu 1998).

S. baicalensis is reported to have very high percentage of baicalin, which is reported to have an inhibitory effect on eicosanoid synthesis (a mediator of prostate tumor cell proliferation). It restricts the proliferation of androgen-independent PC-3 and DU145 prostate cancer cells. Baicalin is reported to drastically suppress prostate cancer at a clinically achievable concentration. In most studies, tomato products are being used as a source of lycopenes. It is observed that oxidative damage in prostate cancer patients was successfully recovered after dietary intervention. However, it is not clear yet whether this effect is caused by lycopenes or whether a more complex metabolite in food causes this effect (Zhou et al. 2005).

4.2.2 PC-SPES

From the mid-1990s an extract with the name PC-SPES has been sold as a dietary supplement for prostate health. This name is derived from PC ("prostate cancer") and *spes* ("hope"). This formulation contains a mixture of eight plants: *Glycyrrhiza uralensis, Ganoderma lucidum, Panax notoginseng, Scutellaria baicalensis, Serenoa repens, Rabdosia rubescens, Dendranthema morifolium*, and *Isatis indigotica*. These plants were selected on the basis of traditional Chinese medicine. The healing potential of PC-SPES appeared to be promising, but unfortunately, this formulation was withdrawn from the market due to contamination reported by the US Food and Drug Administration (FDA) (Xu et al. 2011).

4.3 LUNG CANCER

The lungs are one of the main sites for metastasis of tumors from other body tissues, and lung cancer is one of the most lethal cancers. Conventional chemotherapy has very little survival benefits as it cause severe toxicity of carcinogens (e.g., vinorelbine, paclitaxel, etoposide, and paclitaxel). A large number of medicinal plants have been used in various medicine systems to treat lung cancer, including *Draba nemorosa* (Brassicaceae), *Platycodon grandiflorum* (Campanulaceae), *Tussilago farfara* (Compositae), *Morus alba* (Moraceae), *Stemona japonica* (Stemonaceae), *Prunus armeniaca* (Rosaceae), and *Perilla frutescens* (Labiatae) (Liu et al. 1995).

It is observed that the percentage of patients that are using herbal formulations along with conventional methods is as high as 77%. These herbal formulations are utilized to mitigate the toxicity caused by conventional therapies and even used sometimes to increase their anticancer effect. Although, it is important to keep in mind that some complementary and alternative medicines may reduce the efficacy of conventional therapies or cause adverse effects (Piao et al. 1991).

4.3.1 Shenqi Fuzheng

Shenqi Fuzheng is an injection made from two important herbs from the Chinese system of medicine: *Radix astragali* (root) and *Radix codonopsis* (root). This formulation was approved by the State Food and Drug Administration of China in 1999 as an antitumor injection. Many trials approved the efficacy of this injection along with platinum-based chemotherapy for treating non–small cell lung cancer (NSCLC) (Tang et al. 1994).

4.3.2 Dixiong (地芎汤, a Chinese Herbal Decoction)

It is observed that administration of the Dixiong decoction reduces pneumonitis after radiation therapy. It diminishes lung injury and also improves quality of life for the patient (Sun et al. 2006).

4.3.3 Liangxue Jiedu Huoxue Decoction

This is a Chinese herbal formulation made from seven herbs: *Rhizoma chuanxiong, Fructus forsythiae*, peach seed, *Flos carthami, Radix astragali, Radix rehmanniae*, and *Cortex moutan*. Studies suggest that this formulation can reduce the occurrence of radiation pneumonitis (Lin and Zhang 2008).

4.3.4 Astragalus Polysaccharide (APS): *Astragalus propinquus*

When tested on patients with Non Small Cell Lung Cancer (NSCLC) and platinum-based chemotherapy, astragalus appears to be more effective than chemotherapy alone. Astragalus injection in combination with chemotherapy is appeared to have an inhibitory effect on tumors and also decreases the toxicity caused by chemotherapy in patients (Xu et al. 2014).

4.3.5   BZYQD

Bu-Zhong-Yi-Qi-Tang is a famous anticancer medicine that is derived from eight plants (Table 4.1). Studies suggested that combination therapy of BZYQD and cisplatin-based chemotherapy causes the initiation of apoptosis and autophagy. BZYQD is useful not only for the improvement of daily activity of chronic fatigue syndrome but also for the enhancement of antitumor effects of other drugs (Sun et al. 2005).

4.3.6   Huang-Lian-Jie-Du-Tang

Huang-Lian-Jie-Du-Tang is a famous Chinese formulation that is reported to cause apoptosis in Hepatocellular Carcinoma (HCC) cells (see Table 4.2). This arrests the cell cycle and stimulates a mitochondrion-mediated apoptosis by limiting the activity of NF-κB (Wang et al. 1999).

4.4   BREAST CANCER

Several *in vitro* studies have shown that vitamins and selenium have some anticancer activities. In a randomized study, 2972 patients with breast carcinoma were administered 200 mg of vitamin A (fenretinide) on a daily basis. After 97 months, a significant reduction was observed in premenopausal women. Another study conducted by Lesperance et al. (2002) also reported the fact that an uptake of vitamin E long term has some impact on breast cancer reduction (Chen and Zhang 2014).

TABLE 4.1
Plants Used in the Preparation of Bu-Zhong-Yi-Qi Decoction (BZYQD)

Pharmaceutical Name	Part Used	Amount (g)
Astragalus membranaceus (Fisch.) Bge. var. *mongholicus* (Bge.) Hsiao	Root	18
Glycyrrhiza uralensis Fisch.	Root and rhizome	9
Codonopsis pilosula (Fisch.) Nannf.	Root	6
Angelica sinensis (Oliv.) Diels	Root	3
Citrus reticulate Blanco	Pericarp	6
Cimicifuga heracleifolia Kom.	Rhizome	6
Bupleurum chinense DC.	Root	6
Atractylodes macrocephala Koidz.	Rhizome	9

TABLE 4.2
Huang-Lian-Jie-Du-Tang

Herb Component	Ratio
Coptis chinensis Franch.	1
Scutellaria baicalensis Georgi.	1
Phellodendron amurense Ruprecht	1
Gardenia jasminoides Ellis	1

4.4.1 PHYTOESTROGENS

Plants like soy, linseed, wheat, flaxseed, fruits, and vegetables are reported to have high percentages of lignans and isoflavones. Both lipophilic lignans and water-soluble isoflavones are classes of phytoestrogens. Phytoestrogens derived from soy are often recommended to women with breast cancer during tamoxifen therapy. Soy is reported to have a very high percentage of isoflavones, chiefly daidzein and genistein that are very much similar to 17β-estradiol and impose a weak estrogenic effect. However, we do not have any clear evidence to support the use of phytoestrogens for easing climacteric symptoms or in the treatment of breast cancer (Miu and Shen 2009).

4.4.2 TRADITIONAL CHINESE MEDICINE (TCM)

Various studies on traditional Chinese medicine have revealed a large array of anti–breast cancer agents. These agents were of six classes: artesunate, quinone, terpenoids, flavonoids and polyphenols, coumarins, and alkaloids. Compounds that fall in these categories has been used as dietary supplements for decades, although *in vivo* and clinical studies are still required to confirm their clinical applications (Lin and Fu 1998).

4.4.3 JIA-WEI-XIAO-YAO-SAN (JWXYS)

This is a herbal formulation of ten plants: Herba Menthae (Bo-He), Poriae Cocos (Fu-Ling), Radix Angelicae Sinensis (Dang-Gui), Radix Bupleuri (Chai-Hu), Fructus Gardeniae (Zhi-Zi), Rhizoma Atractylodis, Cortex Moutan Radicis, Radix Glycyrrhizae Uralensis, Rhizoma Zingiberis Recens, Radix Paeoniae Alba. This formulation is reported to treat climacteric syndrome, anxiety, insomnia, and dyspepsia (Me and Chen 2003).

4.5 PANCREATIC CANCER

Pancreatic cancer develops when uncontrolled cell growth begins in a part of the pancreas. Symptoms include jaundice and abdominal pain, but these might not appear until the later stages. There are two types of tumors that grow in the pancreas: exocrine and neuroendocrine. About 93% of all pancreatic tumors are exocrine tumors, and the most common kind of pancreatic cancer is called adenocarcinoma. Pancreatic adenocarcinoma is what people usually mean when they say they have pancreatic cancer. The most common type begins in the ducts of the pancreas and is called ductal adenocarcinoma (He 2009)

The rest of the pancreatic tumors are neuroendocrine tumors (NETs), also called pancreatic NETs (PNETs), an islet cell tumor or islet cell carcinoma. Some NETs produce excessive hormones. They are named based on the type of hormone the cell makes; for instance, insulinoma would be a tumor in a cell that makes insulin.

Cyclopamine is an alkaloids isolated from *Veratrum californicum*. It is reported to have inhibitory effect on SHH signaling (sonic hedgehog homology). This pathway plays a major role in cancer stem cell behavior. Cyclopamine successfully inhibits the SMO protein of the SHH pathway by direct binding with its 7-helix. The cyclopamine and SMO protein complex affect the binding of the 12-transmembrane receptor patched-1 (PTCH-1) and ultimately change its structure. It is also important to know that cyclopamine not only weakens the conversion of the bone marrow precursor cell into cancer cells but also inhibits tumor formation. After administration of cyclopamin in a patient, the cancer cell network becomes weaker and unstable due to angiopoietin-1 expression (factor under the regulation of SHH). This inhibitory effect of cyclopamine on cancer cells suggests that this medicinal plant should be explored further in future in order to obtain a more targeted anti-cancer drug (Luo et al. 2008).

4.5.1 Kanglaite (KLT): Coix Lacryma-Jobi

The injection of KLT is thought to be an alternative option for malignant cancer therapy. Studies confirmed that synergistic treatment of KLT injection and radio chemotherapy is appeared to be much more effective than radio chemotherapy alone. This combination therapy also improve patients' quality of life.

4.5.2 SPES and PC-SPES

SPES and PC-SPES are two important Chinese herbal formulations. Both of these drugs induce apoptosis in pancreatic cancer cells.

SPES is combination of 15 herbs: *Patrinia heterophylla, Cervus nippon, Rabdosia rubescens, Pyrola rotundifolia, Zanthoxylum nitidum, Panax ginseng, Stephania sinica, Ganoderma japonicum, Lycoris radiata, Stephania delavayi, Agrimonia pilosa, Glycyrrhiza glabra, Cistanche deserticola, Corydalis bulbosa*, and *Serenoa repens*.

PC-SPES is a powdered formulation of seven medicinal herbs: *Glycyrrhiza glabra, Dendranthema morifolium, Rabdosia rubescens, Isatis indigotica, Scutellaria baicalensis, Panax ginseng*, and *Ganoderma lucidum*.

4.5.3 Zyflamend

This is a combination of ten standardized concentrated herbal extracts (holy basil, barberry, huzhang, oregano, turmeric, ginger, baikal skullcap, rosemary, green tea and Chinese goldthread). This herbal formulation is reported to inhibit pancreatic cells by inhibiting NF-κB signaling pathways.

4.5.4 MK615

A Japanese medicinal formulation normally called UME is a concentrated extract of apricot that has been reported to have antipyretic agents. A study conducted by Hattori et al. indicates that it successfully restricts the propagation of human pancreatic cancer cells.

4.6 LIVER FIBROSIS AND CANCER

Liver fibrogenesis is a major ailment of the liver which arises due to stimulation of hepatic stellate cells (HSCs). This disease results in decreased degradation of extracellular materials. Unfortunately, the reported cases of hepatocellular carcinoma (HCC) are increasing day by day, and there is no clinically satisfactory therapy for it. In China, Japan, and other parts of Asia, herbal practices are being considered as possible solutions for liver fibrosis and HCC. In different studies, these medicinal herbs – Yi Guan Jian (YGJ), Inchin-ko-to (TJ-135), Fufang-Liu-Yue-Qing, Inchin-ko-to (TJ-135), and Danggui Buxue Tang (DBT) – were tested and the mechanism of action of their compounds (oxymatrine, curcumin and salvianolic acid B [SAB]) was explained.

In traditional Chinese medicine, a combination of ten herbs including membranaceus, *Spatholobus suberectus, Salvia miltiorrhiza* (sage), and Astragalus known as "king herb" were tested in different clinical studies for their antifibrotic action. When administered on 60 patients with hepatitis B, 22 patients showed a beneficial effect on their liver (Zuo 2007).

4.6.1 Yi Guan Jian (mYGJ)

Yi Guan Jian is commonly used formulation of traditional Chinese medicine and is mostly given to patients with fibrosis and cirrhosis. Its decoction is prepared by mixture of six herbs (see Table 4.3). Studies revealed that mYGJ enhances the bone marrow–derived mesenchymal stem cell differentiation into hepatocytes and biliary cells. It is suggested that Yi Guan Jian might have some effect

TABLE 4.3

Plants Used in the Preparation of Yi Guan Jian (mYGJ)

Glehnia littoralis F. Schmidt ex Miq.

Ophiopogon japonicus (Thunb.) Ker Gawl.

Angelica sinensis (Oliv.) Diels.

Rehmannia glutinosa (Gaertn.) Libosch. ex Fisch. & C. A. Mey.

Lycium barbarum L.

Melia toosendan Siebold & Zucc.

in stromal-cell derived factor-1 which ultimately enhanced differentiation of bone marrow–derived mesenchymal stem cells.

4.6.2 TJ-9

There is a herbal medicine called (kampo yaku) Sho saiko-to (TJ-9), a combination of seven herbs that is being used extensively to treat liver diseases. In a randomized study, a hepatitis B patient received a 7.5 g dose of aqueous TJ-9 extract along with conventional methods. When compared with control (patients without TJ-9 treatment), patients with TJ-9 administration show significantly low development of hepatocellular carcinoma (HCC). Unfortunately, this drug is contraindicated because some patients are reported to attain interstitial pneumonia after its administration. Therefore, a well-designed future trial is needed (He and Wang 1995).

4.7 COLORECTAL CANCER

Colorectal cancer, also known as bowel cancer, colon cancer, or rectal cancer, is any cancer that affects the colon and rectum. Colorectal cancer is the third most common cancer in the United States and the second cause of cancer-related deaths. Various herbal formulations are being used, including St. John's wort, echinacea, kava, and grape seed.

4.7.1 *Hypericum perforatum* (St. John's Wort)

It was observed that usage of St. John's wort by patients showed increased expression of CYP3A (cytochrome P450 isoforms). CYP3A ultimately results in effective metabolism of irinotecan (responsible for DNA damage when interacted with topoisomerase). Therefore, it could be used for treating metastatic carcinoma.

4.7.2 Fu-Pi-Yi-Wei Decoction

This decoction is reported to decrease the side effects of conventional therapy and, in some cases, it is reported to increase the effectiveness of chemotherapy. It also improves the immune system of patients (Table 4.4).

4.7.3 Fu-Zheng and Qu-Xie Capsules

Qu-Xie capsules and Fu-Zheng capsules, when tested on patients, appeared to have limiting effect on metastasis. Like other formulations, they also improve life quality of patients with stage 2 and 3 cancer after radical resection (Table 4.5).

TABLE 4.4
Plants Used in Preparation of Fu-Pi-Yi-Wei

Dendrobium (Shi-Hu)	*Poria cocos* (Fu-Ling)
Atractylodes lancea (Cang-Shu)	Amonnan compact = Soland.
Coix seed (Yi-Yi-Ren)	Ex Maton (Dou-Kou)
Pinellia ternata (Ban-Xia)	*Gynostemma pentaphyllum* (Jiao-Gu-Lan)
Dioscorea opposita numb. (Shan-Yao)	*Paeonia lactiflora* (Bai-Shao)
Agastache rugosa (Huo-Xiang)	

TABLE 4.5
Plants Used in the Preparation of Fu-Zheng and Qu-Xie Capsules

Fu-Zheng Capsule	**Qu-Xie Capsule**
Panax ginseng (Ren-Shen)	*Croton tiglium* L. (Ba-Dou)
Poria cocos (Fu-Ling)	*Evodia rutaecarpa* (Wu-Zhu-Yu)
Atractylodes macrocephala (Bai-Shu)	*Zingiber officinale* (Gan-Jiang)
Glycyrrhiza uralensis (Gan-Cao)	*Cinnamomum cassia* (Rou-Gui)
Myristica fragrans (Rou-Dou-Kou)	*Aconitum carmichaelii* Debx. (Chuan-Wu)
Citrus reticulata Blanco	*Pinellia ternata* (Ban-Xia)
Aucklandia lappa Decne. (Mu-Xiang)	*Citrus reticulata* Blanco (Chen-Pi)
Hordeum vulgare L. (Mai-Ya)	
Gallus gallus domesticus Brisson (Ji-Nei-Jin)	

4.7.4   PHY906

PHY906 is a Chinese herbal formula containing three herbs (*Paeonia lactiflora* Pall, *Scutellaria baicalensis* Georgi, and *Ziziphus jujuba* Mill). In Asia and especially in China, this herbal formulation is named Huang Qin Tang. Extensive research has shown that this formulation has a synergistic effect in radiotherapy and chemotherapy.

4.7.5   Pi-Shen

This formulation is a decoction made from three plants (*Astragalus membranaceus* [Huang-Qi], *Codonopsis pilosula*, and *Atractylodes macrocephala* Koidz. [Bai-Shu]). It is reported to reduce the toxicity of chemotherapy and radiotherapy.

4.8   FUTURE DIRECTIONS OF TRADITIONAL CHINESE MEDICINE IN CANCER PREVENTION AND TREATMENT

4.8.1   Basic Research

Through the interaction of seed and soil, we explore the mechanisms of TCM therapeutic methods, such as strengthening body resistance, heat clearing and detoxifying, activating blood, and removing stasis, which serve to expand the basis of scientific connotation and materials. Research on the mechanisms of TCM in fields of immune regulation, inflammatory microenvironment, and the biological behavior of cancer stem cells is predicted. The rapid development of genome sequencing technology, nanoscience, and information science will help us further explore the mechanism of TCM on multiple targets, balance adjustment, and palliative effects. For example, we apply high content analysis technology to screen anticancer TCM and find the basis of materials in more effective ways. The Cancer Genome Atlas will be used in research for the detection of a connection between TCM symptom patterns and genomes. It can also help identify multiple target effects caused by TCM intervention, in order to predict effects and guide a timely adjustment of treatment (Saif et al. 2014).

4.8.2 EFFICACY EVALUATION AND DRUG DEVELOPMENT OF TCM

According to the advantages and characteristics of TCM, new drug development will focus on improving quality of life and cancer-related symptoms. Based on general evaluation criteria and methods, patient outcomes will be incorporated into efficacy assessment, which is currently confined to a doctor's evaluation. It is necessary to develop new drugs for the prevention of tumor recurrence and metastasis after surgery, to relieve the adverse reactions caused by targeted therapy, and improve progression-free survival of advanced cancer patients during maintenance treatment.

The reevaluation of drugs once they have been released into the marketplace is very necessary in order to locate the population who can benefit from the treatment, improve combination regimens, and monitor short- and long-term efficacy and adverse reactions. According to new discoveries in clinical practice and basic research, we can continue research by expanding the indications of the marketed drug, as the same disease might be treated in different ways and different diseases might be treated in the same way.

In future, a new generation of medicine will be developed. Leung et al. proposed integrated network-based medicine (INBM), which considers the interactive nature of the human body and its environment. TCM offers us a blueprint for building a personalized approach to cancer.

4.8.3 EVIDENCE-BASED MEDICAL RESEARCH OF TCM IN ONCOLOGY

Clinical research methods, interventions, outcome measures, quality control, and other aspects in clinical study need to be improved in order to achieve high-level evidence. We also need to pay more attention to translational research, including the effect on the metabolism of active pharmaceutical ingredients and efficacy predictors. For example, a clinical trial designed with Bayesian or factorial analysis will include fewer patients, a reduced study period, reduced cost, will quickly filter the best treatment options, and detect the efficacy of individualized therapy in comprehensive treatment.

We look forward to further results of clinical studies of TCM in cancer prevention and rehabilitation. TCM has been proven to prevent tumor recurrence and metastasis in postoperative cancer patients, prolong disease-free progression for advanced cancer patients, delay resistance to targeted therapy, and promote physical and psychological rehabilitation of cancer patients.

As evidence is continually updated, experts will continue to discuss syndrome differentiation, differentiation methods, treatment principles, treatment options, recommended drugs, and recommended levels in order to reach consensus. TCM oncology guidelines corresponding to the National Comprehensive Cancer Network, the European Society for Medical Oncology, or other internationally recognized oncology clinical practice guidelines can be developed and published.

As modern medical concepts adjust from curing to preventing disease and improving the body, the advantages of TCM become more obvious than they have been in the past. Focusing on the characteristics and advantages of TCM in cancer treatment, we can make use of advanced methods

TABLE 4.6

Chinese Herbal Medicines and Their Effect on Cancer Metastasis

Suppressive Effects on Carcinogenesis and Cancer Metastasis	Herbal Medicine
Inhibits the androgen receptor (AR) signaling pathway	*Wedelia chinensis*
To reduce risk of breast cancer	Isoflavone
Inhibition of cancer cell growth	Alkaloids
Decreases serum testosterone concentrations ($p < 0.05$); decreases serum concentrations of prostate-specific antigen	PC-SPES
Antiproliferation	Flavonoids and polyphenols
Anticancer effect in lung cancer patients	*Platycodon grandiflorum*
MCF-7 cell apoptosis	Terpenoids
Impair the proliferation of androgen-independent PC-3 and DU145 prostate cancer cells in culture	Baicalein
Decrease the proliferation of human breast cancer cells from expressing a high ERα:ERβ ratio	Artemisunate
Preventive effect on liver fibrosis	Inchin-ko-to (TJ-135)
Suppressive effect on hepatic fibrogenesis and carcinogenesis	Curcumin
Reduces/limits the progression of hepatocellular carcinoma	Sho saiko-to (TJ-9)
Maintain homeostasis and prevent various metabolic disorders	Vitamins A-D and retinoid
Arrest LNCaP and DU145 prostate cancer cells at the G0-G1 phase of the cell cycle	Epigallocatechin-3-gallate (EGCG)
SMO antagonists; deregulation of sonic hedgehog homology (SHH)	GDC-0449, IPI-926, XL-139 and PF-04449913
Inhibit SHH signaling by directly binding to the 7-helix bundle of the SMO protein; arrest the growth of pancreatic tumors	Cyclopamine
200 mg/day significantly reduces the recurrence of local breast cancer in premenopausal women	Vitamin A (fenretinide)
Leads to malabsorption or maldigestion in cancer patients; balanced and healthy diet	Vitamin E

and technologies in various disciplines with international cooperation and communication in order to improve the development of clinical and basic research of TCM in oncology.

4.9   SUMMARY

- This chapter focuses on traditional Chinese medicine used in cancer treatment.
- Traditional Chinese medicine (TCM) has a long history. The earliest use of TCM dates back more than 2000 years.
- Cancer treatment with TCM remains the most ancient living tradition; the word "tumor" was discovered on 3500-year-old oracle bone inscriptions.
- Some ancient classical prescriptions and medicine are still in use today, such as Xiaojin dan, the Xihuang pill, the Dahuangzhechong pill, the Liushen pill, and Pianzaihuang.
- TCM has been proven to prevent tumor recurrence and metastasis in postoperative cancer patients, prolong disease-free progression for advanced cancer patients, delay resistance to targeted therapy, and promote physical and psychological rehabilitation of cancer patients.
- Focusing on the characteristics and advantages of TCM in cancer treatment, we can make use of advanced methods and technologies in various disciplines with international cooperation and communication in order to improve the development of clinical and basic research of TCM in oncology.

REFERENCES

Chen, Z. F., and Zhang, J. H. 2014. Meta research of TCM treatment for precancerous lesions of esophageal cancer. Traditi Chin Med Res. 12:20–21.

Gan, T., Wu, Z., Tian, L., and Wang Y. 2010. Chinese herbal medicines for induction of remission in advanced or late gastric cancer. Cochrane Database Syst Rev. (1):CD005096.

He, H. B., and Wang, F. 1995. The idea and method of treatment of Bile Reflex Gastritis with Zheng-dan decoction. Med Philos. 16:599–600. (In Chinese.)

He, Y. 2009. Objective to Tanreqing Injection for Sputum Retention after lung cancer operation. J Emerg Tradit Chin Med. 2:194. (In Chinese.)

Hua, T. 2007. People's Medical Publishing House, Beijing (Han Dynasty). The Central Treasury Canon.

Li, S. G., Chen, H. Y., and Ou-Yang, C. S. 2013. The efficacy of Chinese herbal medicine as an adjunctive therapy for advanced non–small cell lung cancer: A systematic review and meta-analysis. PLoS One. 8(2):e57604.

Li, Z. Z. 2006. *Indispensable Medical Reading*. People's Medical Publishing House, Beijing (Ming Dynasty).

Lin, H. S., and Zhang, Y. 2008. Evidence-based medical study of TCM on non small cell lung cancer. World Sci Technol. 10:121–125. (In Chinese.)

Lin, Y., and Fu, J. 1998. Effect of Fei'an decoction on the symptomatic relief in postoperative pulmonary carcinoma. J Guangzhou Univ Tradit Chin Med. 2:21–23.

Liu, J.X., Shi, Z. M., and Xu, Z. Y. 1995. Studies on late primary adenocarcinoma of lung treated by methods of nourishing yin to replenish fluid and warming Yang to benefit Qi. J Tradit Chin Med. 36:155–158.

Luo, X. B., Li, L., and Liu, N. M. 2008. Effect observation of TCM treatment for breast cancer patients after operation. J Emerg Tradit Chin Med. 17:770–771.

Mao, C. G., Tao, Z. Z., Wan, L. J., Han, J. B., Chen, Z., and Xiao, B. K. 2014. The efficacy of traditional Chinese medicine as an adjunctive therapy in nasopharyngeal carcinoma: A systematic review and meta-analysis. J BUON. 19:540–548.

McCulloch, M., See, C., and Shu, X. J. 2006. Astragalus-based Chinese herbs and platinum-based chemotherapy for advanced non–small-cell lung cancer: Meta-analysis of randomized trials. J Clin Oncol. 24:419–430.

Me, H., and Chen, Z.C. 2003. The effect of shenfu injection on human immune function at lung cancer patients. Guizhou Med J. 27:796.

Miu, C. R., and Shen, H. 2009. Meta-analysis of effectiveness of Chinese medicinal herbs in treating precancerous lesions of gastric cancer. J Liaoning Univ Tradit Chin Med. 11:35–37.

Piao, B. K., Tang, W. X., Zhang, Z. Q., Lin, H. S., Duan, F. W., and Yu, G. Q. 1991. The clinical observation of Feiliuping paste curing advanced lung cancer–and clinical analysis of 339 cases. J Tradit Chin Med. 4:21–23.

Saif, M. W., Li, J., and Lamb, L. 2014. First-in-human phase II trial of the botanical formulation PHY906 with capecitabine as second-line therapy in patients with advanced pancreatic cancer. Cancer Chemother Pharmacol. 73:373–380.

Sun, G. Z., Yu, G. Q., and Zhang, P. T. 2005. Clinical and mechanism research on Fu Zheng Pei Ben serial formulas' application on gastric cancer treatment. J Zhejiang Univ Tradit Chin Med. 33:695–700. (In Chinese.)

Sun, Y., Lin, H. S., and Zhu, Y.Z. 2006. A randomized, prospective, multi-centre clinical trial of NP regimen (vinorelbine + cisplatin) plus Gensing Rg3 in the treatment of advanced non–small cell lung cancer patients. Chin J Lung Cancer. 9:254–258.

Tang, W. X., Zhang, Z. Q., Lin, H. S., Hou, W., and Piao, B. K. 1994. The clinical observation of the TCM treatment of NSCLC. J Tradit Chin Med. 5: 283–285.

Wang, B. 2003. Ancient Books of TCM Publishing House, Beijing 2003(Tang Dynasty). The Yellow Emperor's Inner Canon.

Wang, W., Xu, L., and Shen, C. 1999. Effects of traditional Chinese medicine in treatment of breast cancer patients after mastectomy: A meta-analysis. Cell Biochem Biophys. doi:10.1007/s12013-014-0348-z

Xu, L., and Liu, J. X. 1997. Effect of yifei kangliu yin on lung cancer metastasis and immune function. Chin J Integr Med. 17:401–403. (In Chinese.)

Xu, W., Yang, G., and Xu, Y. 2014. The possibility of traditional Chinese medicine as maintenance therapy for advanced nonsmall cell lung cancer. Evid Based Complement Alternat Med. 2014:278917.

Xu, Z. Y., Jin, C.J., and Zhou, C. C. 2011. Treatment of advanced non–small-cell lung cancer with Chinese herbal medicine by stages combined with chemotherapy. J Cancer Res Clin Oncol. 137:1117–1122.

Zhang, D. Z., and Xu, J. D. 1998. Clinical and experimental researches on improving radiation sensibility for lung cancer patients. Chin J Surg Integr Tradit West Med. 4:71–75.

Zhong, L. L., Chen, H. Y., Cho, W. C., Meng, X. M., and Tong, Y. 2012. The efficacy of Chinese herbal medicine as an adjunctive therapy for colorectal cancer: A systematic review and meta-analysis. Complement Ther Med. 20:240–252.

Zhou, D. H., Lin, L. Z., and Zhou, Y. Q. 2005. Effect of Chinese herbal medicine in prolonging median survival time in patients with non–small-cell lung cancer. J Guangzhou Univ Tradit Chin Med. 7:255–258.

Zuo, M. H., Li, Q. W., and Sun, T. 2007. Malignancy intestinal obstruction cases of clinical observation by enema with Chinese medicine. China J Tradit Chin Med Pharm. 22:654–655. (In Chinese.)

5 Plant-Derived Natural Products and Cancer Hallmarks

Wamidh H. Talib, Muna Barakat, Shatha Khaled Haif,
Zainab Alsharea, Eliza Hasen and Asma Ismail Mahmod

5.1 INTRODUCTION

Cancer is a general concept that is used to verify a large group of associated diseases marked mainly by continuous uncontrolled growth of abnormal cells (Hassanpour and Dehghani 2017). It has been classified as one of the leading causes of death in the world. In 2020, the numbers of cancer incidence and mortality were about 19.3 million new cases and 10.0 million deaths (Sung et al. 2021). Interestingly, cancer hallmarks were recognized by Hanahan and Weinberg in 2011, they demonstrated the ten main alterations in cell physiology leading a healthy normal cell to convert into a neoplastic one (Hanahan and Weinberg 2011). Many phytochemicals have shown an impact on different stages of tumor genesis and interrupted the cycle of cancer progression (Orlikova and Diederich 2012; Talib et al. 2020). Hence, the anticancer activity of natural products is mediated by various mechanisms, including apoptosis induction, inhibition of signal transduction, angiogenesis, invasion, and metastasis (Efferth and Oesch 2021; Majolo et al. 2019). In this chapter, we have summarized ten natural products targeting multiple cancer hallmarks, demonstrating their mechanisms, formulation, and clinical studies.

5.2 HALLMARKS OF CANCER

5.2.1 GENOMIC INSTABILITY

Genomic instability is a feature of many cancer cells. Several pathways like telomerase damage, centrosome amplification, epigenetic alterations, and DNA damage can promote genomic instability (Ferguson et al. 2015). During the cell cycle of a normal cell, checkpoints maintain the integrity of the genome, and any dysfunction in their work may give the chance of aneuploidy nuclei to develop abnormal cells (Rusin, Zajkowicz, and Butkiewicz 2009; Talib 2018). The checkpoints are controlled by several oncogenes and tumor suppressor genes; however, cancer cells can alter these genes' functions to stimulate uncontrolled growth (Talib 2018).

5.2.2 SUSTAINED PROLIFERATIVE SIGNALING

The main characteristic of cancer cells is their ability to sustain chronic proliferation, and this can be achieved by deregulating the expression of growth-promoting signals (Hanahan and Weinberg 2011). The following signaling pathways are the essential targets to inhibit sustained proliferation in cancer; hypoxia-inducible factor-1 (HIF-1), NF-κBs, PI3K/AKT, insulin-like growth factor receptor (IGF-1R), cyclin-dependent kinase (CDK), and estrogen receptor signaling (Yaswen et al. 2015).

DOI: 10.1201/9781003260028-6

5.2.3 EVASION OF ANTIGROWTH SIGNALING

The evasion of antigrowth signals is another strategy adopted by cancer cells to keep proliferation. Blocking tumor suppressor genes that are controlling the antigrowth signals, as well as mutations in these genes, have been observed in cancer cells (Talib 2018). The most known mutated tumor suppressor gene is p53, followed by ataxia-telangiectasia mutated (ATM), cyclin-dependent kinase inhibitor 2A (CDKN2A), phosphatase and tensin homolog (PTEN), adenomatous polyposis coli (APC), breast cancer gene 1 & 2 (BRCA1 & BRCA2), retinoblastoma (RB), and Wilms tumor (WT1) (Yaswen et al. 2015).

5.2.4 RESISTANCE TO APOPTOSIS

Cancer cells stimulate the overexpression of anti-apoptotic proteins and suppress the normal programmed cell death (Hanahan and Weinberg 2011). They can limit or circumvent apoptosis via many pathways such as altering the function of TP53 tumor suppressor, upregulation of anti-apoptotic regulators (Bcl-2 and Bcl-xL), promoting survival signals (Igf1/2), decreasing the expression of proapoptotic factors (Bax, Bim, Puma), and suppressing the signals of the extrinsic ligand-induced death pathway (Hanahan and Weinberg 2011).

5.2.5 REPLICATIVE IMMORTALITY

One of the special characteristics of cancer cells is the limitless replicative potential. Telomerase is a specialized reverse transcriptase that extends the ends of shortening chromosomes in dividing cells (Bodnar et al. 1998; Talib 2018). Activation of this enzyme is the key to keeping continuous cell division in several types of cancer (Hanahan and Weinberg 2011). Interestingly, replicative immortality can be modulated by suppressing many targets including telomerase, mTOR, CDK4/6, CDK 1/2/5/9, Akt, and PI3K (Yaswen et al. 2015).

5.2.6 DYSREGULATED METABOLISM

Modifying energy metabolism has been proven to be a cancer-associated trait, which involves the activation of many oncogenes and mutated suppressor genes (Hanahan and Weinberg 2011). To increase glucose uptake and lactate production, different glycolytic enzymes are stimulated including hexokinase 2 (HK2), 6-phosphofructo-2-kinase/fructose-2,6-biphosphatase 3 (PFKFB3), and pyruvate kinase isoform M2 (PKM2) (Talib 2018). Besides, overexpression of other metabolic regulators such as hypoxia-inducible factor 1 (HIF-1) and MYC oncogene was observed in cancer cells (Bensinger and Christofk 2012; Dang et al. 2008).

5.2.7 TUMOR-PROMOTING INFLAMMATION

There is a particular association between chronic inflammation and cancer development (Chakraborty et al. 2020; Hou, Karin, and Sun 2021). Many factors play a crucial role in triggering cancer-related inflammation including cytokines (interleukins, TNF-α, TGF-β, and granulocyte macrophage colony stimulating factor), chemokines, and transcription factors (NF-κB, STAT3, HIF 1-α) (Chakraborty et al. 2020).

5.2.8 Angiogenesis

During malignancy, tumor cells start to trigger an "angiogenic switch," which involves the activation of angiogenic factors to mediate vascularization (Chakraborty, Njah, and Hong 2020). The formation of new blood vessels provides the dividing cancer cells with oxygen and nutrients, which are essential to sustain cell proliferation (Chakraborty, Njah, and Hong 2020). Many transmembrane proteins and pathways regulate the angiogenesis process, including vascular endothelial growth factor (VEGF), VEGF receptor 2 (VEGFR2), Tie-angiopoietin pathways, platelet-derived growth factor (PDGF), epidermal growth factor (EGF), and hepatocyte growth factor (HGF) (Bergers and Benjamin 2003; Chakraborty, Njah, and Hong 2020).

5.2.9 Tissue Invasion and Metastasis

Cancer metastasis is a multi-step process that begins with local invasion of cancer cells into the surrounding tissues, followed by intravasation into the nearby vessels, extravasation to distant places and organs, and in the last step adaptation to a new microenvironment and starting a micro-metastasis that will progress into a secondary tumor (Hanahan and Weinberg 2011). Tumor cell metastasis is initiated by the disruption of cell-cell adhesion which is composed of tight junctions, adherens junctions, gap junctions, desmosomes, and hemidesmosomes (Martin et al. 2013).

5.2.10 Immune Evasion

Cancer cells use different strategies to evade immune surveillance including modifying immune checkpoint pathways, recruiting immunosuppressive cells (e.g., regulatory T cells and myeloid-derived suppressor cells), and impairing components of the immune system (e.g. suppress infiltrating CTLs and NK cells by overexpression of TGF-β or other immunosuppressive factors) (Hanahan and Weinberg 2011). Figure 5.1 summarizes the main cancer hallmarks.

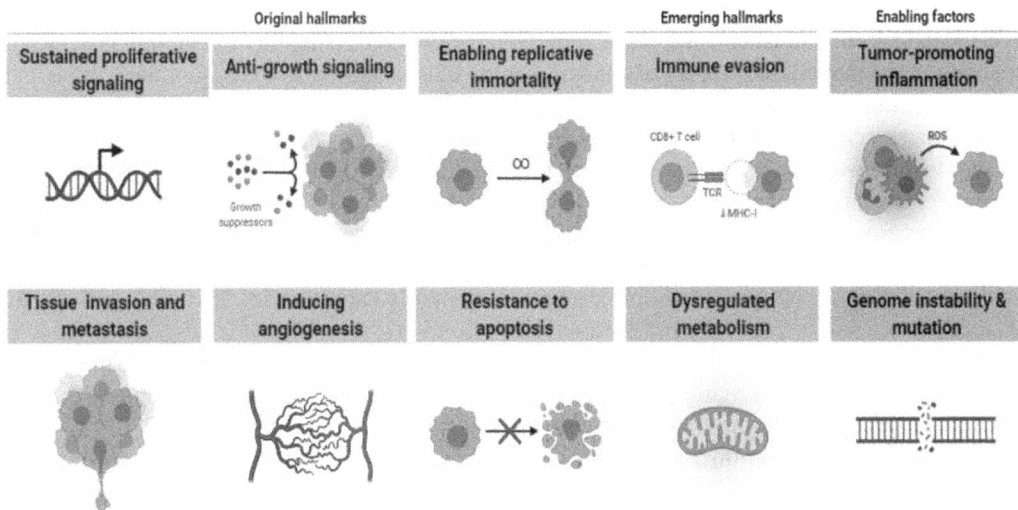

FIGURE 5.1 Cancer hallmarks.

5.3 NATURAL PRODUCTS TARGETING MULTIPLE CANCER HALLMARKS

5.3.1 CURCUMIN

Curcumin is also called diferuloylmethane (1,7-bis(4-hydroxy-3-methoxyphenyl)-1,6-heptadiene-3,5-dione), which is the key natural biphenolic active compound of turmeric and derived from the rhizome of perennial *Curcuma longa* and other *Curcuma* species (PubChem 2021). Turmeric (containing curcumin) has been highlighted as one of the important natural products in the scientific, medical, and culinary fields. Medically, it has been used as traditional therapy for many diseases for thousands of years in Asian countries due to many properties, including anti-inflammatory, antioxidant, antidiabetic, antimicrobial (i.e., bacterial, fungal, protozoal, and viral), antifibrotic, immunomodulatory, and anticarcinogenic. These activities mainly result from the ability of polyphenols to target various signaling tracks in the cells to exert therapeutic effects. Accordingly, turmeric shows a significant potential in the management of inflammatory illnesses, degenerative eye conditions, metabolic syndrome, and cancer.

In the context of cancer, curcumin is considered one of the candidates for cancer treatment with and without drug combinations (Giordano and Tommonaro 2019) as curcumin targets genetic transcription, growth, inflammatory cytokines, apoptosis, protein kinases, and survival/proliferative proteins (Giordano and Tommonaro 2019). It has been reported that curcumin is capable of inhibiting a number of cell cycle proteins, such as cyclins (e.g., cyclin D1, cyclin D3) and cyclin-dependent kinase 2, which contribute directly to tumor development (Sa and Das 2008). It also inhibits the cell cycle by inducing suppressor angiogenesis by affecting many factors such as MMP-2, MMP-9, and VEGF (Wang and Chen 2019). Different transcription pathways are inhibited by curcumin, especially NF-κB, catenin, pk65, Notch-1, and mTOR, which lead to tumor suppression and apoptosis induction. As well, its anti-apoptotic effect was reported via modulation of anti-apoptotic protein Bcl-2 and proapoptotic protein (Bax) expression with alleviation of oxidative stress. Studies revealed the ability of curcumin to induce epigenetic alternation through the inhibition of DNA methyltransferases, regulation of histone acetyltransferases and deacetylases, modulation of microRNAs (miRNA), and interaction with many other transcription factors, activation of tumor suppression gene: p53 and PTEN (Wang et al. 2021).

Nowadays, the clinical potential of curcumin is becoming well-known mainly due to its antioxidant and anti-inflammatory properties. However, the poor bioavailability of curcumin is considered one of the major issues for its administration; this also contributes to its poor absorption and facilitated elimination (including metabolism). Accordingly, targeting bioavailability improvement is one of the essential steps in the curcumin formulation. For instance, it was reported that the concomitant administration of piperine (a key element in black pepper) with curcumin blocks the curcumin metabolism, enhancing the extent of absorption and bioavailability (to reach 2000%). Several delivery systems have been designed to enhance curcumin efficacy and bioavailability, including micelles, liposomes, phospholipid complexes, microemulsions, nano-emulsions, emulsions, solid lipid nanoparticles, nanostructured lipid carriers, biopolymer nanoparticles, and microgels (Stohs et al. 2020).

The advantages of curcumin use have been recognized globally. Different dosage forms of curcumin are available in the market, including tablets, capsules, chewable (e.g., gummies), liquids, powders, strips, ointments, beverages, and cosmetics (Gupta, Patchva, and Aggarwal 2013). In 2018, the US Food and Drug Administration (FDA) had approved the safety and tolerability profile of the curcumin for clinical use even at doses 4000 and 8000 mg/day, up to 12,000 mg/day of 95% concentration of three different curcuminoids (FDA 2018). Therefore, curcumin is considered a promising natural product in the clinical field in multiple domains, and the evidence behind its benefits is still growing and enriching the scientific database.

5.3.2 GENISTEIN

Genistein is a soy-derived isoflavone [5,7-dihydroxy-3-(4-hydroxyphenyl) chromen-4-one or 7-hydroxyisoflavone]. Because of the structural and functional reassembly to estradiol, genistein is also classified as a phytoestrogen. It was isolated in 1899 from dyer's broom, *Genista tinctorial* (Fabaceae), and is used abundantly in the Asian countries, especially Japan and China (average consumption 25–50 mg/day). In addition, legumes (*Lupinus*, commonly known as lupins) are considered an important source of genistein and have valuable health benefits similar to soybeans.

Literature has reported several biological activities of genistein, including anthelmintic, antioxidant, anti-inflammatory, and anticancer activity. Notably, genistein confers a preventive and potential therapeutic effect for cancer due to its antioxidant, anti-inflammatory, anti-angiogenic, proapoptotic, and antiproliferative activities (Tuli et al. 2019). The main anticancer activity of genistein involves induction of apoptosis by enhancing caspase-9 and/or caspase-3, inhibiting the NF-κB pathway, modulating the levels of Bax/Bcl-2 and p38 MAPK signaling pathway, inducing induction of ER stress with upregulation of the expression of glucose-regulated protein 78 (GRP78) and CCAAT/enhancer-binding protein homologous, and protein activating of the apoptotic protease activator factor 1 from the mitochondria. The anti-inflammatory effect of genistein is mainly related to the reduction in the expression of cytokines interleukin-1 beta (IL-1β), IL-6, and IL-8 from tumor necrosis factor alpha (TNF-α) released by cells. Moreover, genistein has the ability to inhibit the cell cycle at different phases depending on the type of tumor and mechanism of action. Mostly, genistein's arrest activity is mediated by mRNA and TERT (Tuli et al. 2019). While the antiproliferative effect is mediated by complex cellular activities including inhibition of mTOR, p70S6K1, 4E-BP1, NF-κB, Bcl-2, DNA methylation, crosstalk between ERα and IGF-IR pathway, topoisomerase II, MMP-2, VEGF, HDAC4/5/7, DVL, survivin, phospho MEK. On the other hand, it induces many other processes involving p-ERK, pCREB, BDNF, Bax, ERα expression, TAM-dependent anti-estrogen therapeutic sensitivity, p53, and DKK1. The inhibition of MMP-2 and "DMBA-induced metastatic transition" is potentiating the antimetastatic activity of genistein (Tuli et al. 2019).

Notwithstanding the bioactivity of genistein, it has poor bioavailability and aqueous solubility, which is considered one of the major limitations of its application. One of the proposed methods to solve this issue is methylation of the free hydroxymethyl group of genistein, which promotes its metabolic stability and membrane penetration ability. Besides, studies showed that the treatment of soybeans with fermentation could enhance the absorption and bioavailability of isoflavone contents. Recent approaches were also released using nanotechnology, such as Metal-Organic Framework MIL-100(Fe), to deliver an effective and safe dose of genistein (Botet-Carreras et al. 2021). Capsules and tablets are the most common pharmaceutical dosage forms of genistein. Therefore, genistein efficacy and safety had been proven by a number of preclinical studies and considered one of the novel potentials for tumor management and prevention.

5.3.3 LUTEOLIN

Luteolin (3,4,5,7-tetrahydroxy flavone) is an abundantly available flavonoid in nature, particularly in fruits and vegetables such as celery, sweet bell peppers, and parsley (Saleem et al. 2021). Traditionally, luteolin-rich plants are used in China for the treatment of many diseases, including hypertension, inflammatory, and malignant disorders (Saleem et al. 2021). Hence, luteolin has distinct biological effects, including antioxidant, anti-inflammatory, anti-allergy, and anticancer (Imran et al. 2019). Luteolin is capable of mitigating cancer progression via affecting cell transformation, angiogenesis, invasion, and metastasis. Depending on the type of cancer, luteolin confers various mechanisms as reviewed by Imran et al. (2019), including (1) suppression of cell proliferation by inhibition of MAPK pathways, PI3K-Akt, and CDK2; (2) induction of apoptosis and inhibition of cell survival signaling associated with DNA damage, redox modulation and kinases suppression, through activation of DR5, caspase-8 and caspase-9, Fas, Bax, P53, JNK, inhibition of FASN, XIAP, Bcl-XL, PI3K-Akt, EGFR, NF-κB and MAPK pathways; (3) hampering angiogenesis by inhibition of VEGF, MMP-9, PI3k/Akt and NF-κB; and (4) inhibition of metastasis by suppression of PI3k/Akt, NF-κB, IL-6, and FAK. According to the above discussion, luteolin could exhibit a wide range of preventive and therapeutic activities against cancer cells.

Concerning the luteolin formulations, several methods were applied to promote its bio-availability, aqueous solubility, and bioactivities, such as folacin-modified nanoparticles, nanoparticles, nanostructured lipid carriers (NLCs), folic acid-modified reactive oxygen species (ROS)-responsive nanoparticles, nanospheres, liposomes, and lipid-based nanovesicles for topical delivery (Kazmi et al. 2021). It is available in the market in a capsule dosage form as a natural flavonoid product. According to the type of cancer, the effective dose is varied; for example, studies of breast cancer revealed that 10 mg/kg for 48 hours inhibits the cancer proliferation significantly (Imran et al. 2019). Among many natural compounds, luteolin has been highlighted as a promising chemopreventive and therapeutic agent due to its safety and efficacy against many tumors.

5.3.4 Resveratrol

Resveratrol (3,5,4-trihydroxystilbene) has three phenol rings connected by an ethylene bridge, a naturally occurring polyphenol (stilbenoid). There are two isomeric forms of resveratrol: *cis-* and *trans-*resveratrol, with *trans-*resveratrol being the more common. Resveratrol was discovered in large concentrations in the root of Japanese knotweed (*Polygonum cuspidatum*). Vine plants also produce resveratrol in high numbers in reaction to biotic infections (e.g., *Botrytis cinerea*), but it can also be formed in response to abiotic conditions. Other palatable plants that generate resveratrol include hops, peanuts, and a variety of berries (blackberries, blackcurrants, blueberries, mulberries, and cranberries) (Chun-Fu et al. 2013).

Resveratrol has been extensively studied for its anti-inflammatory and antioxidant capabilities and protective activity against metabolic disorders and cardiac diseases, as well as a variety of other biological features. Also, resveratrol has been linked to a reduction in age-related symptoms and the avoidance of early mortality in obese animals in several studies. Additionally, resveratrol is associated with deceleration or avoidance of cognitive deterioration, although there have been few clinical investigations into the effects of resveratrol on Alzheimer's disease (AD) (Ramírez-Garza et al. 2018).

Furthermore, resveratrol has been proven to have chemopreventive and chemotherapeutic effects on cancers *in vitro* and *in vivo* through several mechanisms, making it a promising anti-cancer drug. Resveratrol inhibits carcinogenesis at all three stages: initiation, promotion, and progression. Resveratrol has also been found to directly stimulate the apoptotic pathway through multiple pathways (Li et al. 2010). The ability of resveratrol to limit the activation of numerous carcinogens and/or accelerate their detoxification, to avoid oxidative damage to target cells, to diminish inflammatory responses, and to reduce cancer cell growth reflects its chemopreventive potential. Resveratrol's antioxidizing property for scavenging ROS and increasing the activities of some antioxidizing enzymes also indicates its chemoprotective benefits (Wang et al. 2018). Resveratrol has the ability to activate NF-κB (nuclear factor kappa B) and SIRTI, which are key regulators of the inflammatory response, as well as to block several key cytokines, including IL-1b, TNF-α, and IL-6, and oxidoreductases like CBR, AKR, and COXs. Furthermore, chemoprotection mediated by RES can be achieved by lowering the expression of EMMPRIN, a key regulator for the production of matrix metalloproteinase (MMP) to transport metal ions.

Furthermore, resveratrol triggers the mitochondrial (Smac/DIABLO), caspase-9, and caspase-3 enzymatic systems, upregulating death-induced cytokines and their receptors, as well as cyclin-dependent kinase inhibitors and tumor suppressor genes, causing cancer cells to undergo apoptosis. Resveratrol also inhibits invasion and metastasis by AMPK activation and inhibition of phosphoinositide 3-kinase (PI3K)/Akt, hedgehog (HH), hippo-YAP, PKC, EGFR kinase, NF-κB, activating protein-1 (AP-1) and HIF-1α (Rauf et al. 2018). Moreover, several studies have shown that resveratrol can affect immune cells directly and indirectly. Cancer cells treated with resveratrol upregulate stress proteins, such as ligands for the immune receptor NKG2D including MICA or ULBPs and death receptor 5 (DR5). The binding of these proteins by immune cells expressing the related receptor (NKG2D receptor) or ligand (TRAIL), result in cancer cell death (Trung and An 2018).

Despite the fact that *in vitro* studies have demonstrated that resveratrol has significant therapeutic potential, animal and clinical trials have shown few encouraging results due to oral resveratrol's extremely low absorption. As a result, alternative formulations and delivery systems have been achieved to avoid first-pass metabolism and increase resveratrol bioavailability, such as oral transmucosal delivery of resveratrol using ribose lozenges, which resulted in larger and faster blood concentrations of resveratrol. In another approach consisting of red grape cells (RGC) in which resveratrol with one hexose moiety was the major polyphenol, this approach had a high bioavailability and solubility in body fluids, as well as quick gastrointestinal absorption when compared to resveratrol alone. Resveratrol's glycosylated structure gives it increased stability and resistance to enzymatic metabolism (Talib et al. 2020).

5.3.5 ALLICIN

Allicin is a sulfenic acid thioester or allyl thiosulfinate. It belongs to the Liliaceae family and is mostly found in garlic (*Allium sativum*). Asians have traditionally used allicin as a traditional medicine to treat a variety of diseases. Allicin has been shown to have antibacterial, antiviral, antioxidant, anti-inflammatory, and tumor suppression properties, and can aid in prevention of heart disease (Borlinghaus et al. 2014).

Allicin has also been shown to have anticancer properties. According to Chen et al., allicin inhibited cholangiocarcinoma cell multiplication and invasion. Through upregulation of SHP-1 and inhibition of STAT3 activity, it promoted apoptosis and blocked cell migration. Furthermore, in a nude mouse model of cholangiocarcinoma, it inhibited tumor growth (Chen et al. 2018). In addition, allicin's effect on the radiosensitivity of colorectal cancer cells has been studied *in vivo*. The findings revealed that allicin, through inhibiting the NF-κB signaling pathway, improves the sensitivity of X-ray radiation in colorectal cancer (Huang et al. 2020). Allicin also inhibits melanoma cell development by upregulating cyclin D1 and lowering MMP-9 mRNA expression. Furthermore, allicin's antigrowth and antiproliferation properties are achieved by halting the cell cycle at the G2/M phase and inducing apoptosis, which inhibits the growth of malignant tumors. Allicin causes apoptosis through mitochondria-mediated apoptosis, which involves both caspase-dependent and caspase-independent pathways as well as the death receptor pathway. However, data has shown that allicin enhanced p53 expression in gastric cancer cells, particularly those containing the wild-type p53 gene, implying that allicin caused those cells to die via the p53 pathway (Chu et al. 2013).

Because of its hydrophobic nature, allicin is unstable and can easily penetrate cell membranes. Allinase, the enzyme that transforms alliin to allicin, is most active at pH 7. Many kinds of garlic supplements now have an enteric-coated formulation. Additionally, allicin's chemical stability was improved by combining it with an antibody to target a specific pancreatic cancer marker. In MIA PaCa-2 cells, this compound effectively triggered apoptosis in a way similar to the way chemotherapy destroys cancerous tumors, but in a much more potent form. Furthermore, allicin's stability was increased by encapsulating it in liposomes, which protected it from adverse conditions. Its noxious odor was also reduced as a result of this (Talib et al. 2020).

5.3.6 QUERCETIN

Quercetin (QUE; 3,5,7,30,40-pentahydroxyflavone) is a naturally occurring polyphenolic flavonoid, which is widely found in a variety of plants such as *Aesculus hippocastanum, Hypericum perforatum*, and *Ginkgo biloba*, and is also present in fruits and vegetables including green and red tea, coffee, onions, apples, broccoli, and berries. Quercetin has been shown in numerous studies to have antioxidant, anti-inflammatory, and anti-aging properties. As a result, quercetin has a powerful anticancer, anti-obesity, and antidiabetic action (Zou et al. 2021).

According to *in vivo* and *in vitro* studies, quercetin regulates and causes apoptosis in cancer cells and exhibits pro-apoptotic action by upregulating the p53 gene and decreasing the Bcl-2 protein. Furthermore, when Bcl-2 transcription is suppressed, the cell undergoes apoptosis, which may halt tumor development. In addition, quercetin has the ability to increase the expression of death receptor 5 (DR5), leading to activation of tumor necrosis factor–related apoptosis-inducing ligand (TRAIL) and, as a result, cancerous cells' apoptosis (Tang et al. 2020). Also, quercetin has been shown to reduce the expression of epidermal growth factor receptor (EGFR), a tyrosine kinase implicated in the formation of a wide range of solid cancers, resulting in cell growth inhibition and apoptosis induction. Moreover, quercetin inhibited cell growth by inducing cell cycle arrest, which was found in the G1 phase, and was attributed to the downregulation of cyclin B1 and cyclin-dependent kinase 1 (CDK1), essential components of G2/M cell cycle progression (Jeong et al. 2009).

Quercetin has low bioavailability as a result of its low water solubility, so nano-formulations have been created, including microemulsions, nanoparticles, liposomes, and solid lipid nanoparticles. Encapsulating quercetin in biodegradable monomethoxy poly-(ethylene glycol)-poly ("-caprolactone") micelles resulted in complete quercetin dispersion in water, as well as PEGylated liposomal quercetin, which has also been developed (Lipo-Que). *In vitro*, Lipo-Que inhibited cell growth and promoted apoptosis in cisplatin-resistant (A2780cp) and cisplatin-sensitive (A2780s) human ovarian cancer models *in vitro* (Talib et al. 2020).

5.3.7 EPIGALLOCATECHIN-3-GALLATE (EGCG)

The major catechin found in green tea is the (−)-epigallocatechin-3-gallate (EGCG), a polyphenolic compound which has several related catechins that are known to be responsible for the health benefits related to the consumption of green tea (Lai et al. 2020). Epidemiological studies suggest that drinking green tea may be significantly beneficial to health. This is supported by animal studies that support the consumption of high levels of EGCG such as in green tea and may have a significant effect on preventing tumors, heart disease, and other medical conditions. Studies on different types of cancer cell lines, including MCF-7, A549, and HeLa, have shown that the chemopreventive effect of EGCG is facilitated by the induction of apoptosis and cell cycle arrest, and the inhibition of angiogenesis, metastasis, and migration (Mukhtar and Ahmad 2000). Patterns of DNA methylation are recognized by the coordinated action of DNMTs and its associated factors, such as the polycomb proteins, in the presence of S-adenosylmethionine (SAM) that works as a methyl donor for the methyl group. When SAM is demethylated, it forms S-adenosylhomocysteine (SAH), which is a potent inhibitor of DNMT. EGCG has the ability to inhibit cancer-associated stages and decrease the effect on DNA methylation by blocking DNMTs; additionally, it possess strong free radical scavenging activity and works as an antioxidant. By inhibiting the DNMT, it may prevent the methylation of the newly synthesized DNA strand, which results in the reversal of the re-expression of the silenced genes and hypermethylation. The clinical studies propose that EGCG blocks the promotion of tumor growth via blocking receptors in the cancerous cells. Moreover, EGCG may enable direct binding to specific cancer developing carcinogens (Singh, Shankar, and Srivastava 2011).

5.3.8 Emodin

Emodin, also called (1,3,8-trihydroxy-6-methylanthraquinone), is a natural anthraquinone derivative. It is a popular ingredient of different Chinese herbs such as in the rhizome and root of *Rheum palmatum* (Polygonaceae), which is known for the treatment of inflammation, gallstones, osteomyelitis, and hepatitis and is a known vasorelaxant and diuretic. Furthermore, emodin has proved to possess a wide spectrum of pharmacological effects, such as antibacterial, antiviral, anti-allergic, antidiabetic, anti-osteoporotic, immunosuppressive, neuroprotective and hepato-protective effects (Semwal et al. 2021). A study showed that emodin also acts as an anticancer agent by modulating the expression of apoptosis-related genes to induce apoptosis in A549 cells and growth inhibition. The gene expression of FASL was upregulated, although the expression levels of MCL1, C-MYC, and CCND1 were downregulated. Novel functions of emodin have been reported, specifically that emodin improves the repair of cisplatin- and UV-induced DNA damage and might even promote nucleotide excision repair (NER) capabilities in human fibroblast cells (WI38) (Zhang et al. 2021). Another study showed that emodin is able to provoke cell cycle arrest. An MTT assay, electron microscopy, and flow cytometry were used to study the inhibitory effect of emodin on the human hepatoma cell line (SMMC-7721). The results showed that the proliferation of SMMC-7721 cells was inhibited in a concentration-dependent and time-dependent manner, that cells in G2/M phase increased significantly, and that the part of S-phase cells gradually declined (Zhang et al. 2015). Emodin/cisplatin co-treatment inhibited the growth of gallbladder carcinoma cells and human ovarian carcinoma *in vivo*. This mechanism might involve the downregulation of MRP1 expression and ABCG2 expression (Teng et al. 2021). Emodin has reversed the multidrug resistance in promyelocytic leukemia (HL-60/ADR cells). Moreover, it decreased the expression of MDR proteins including topo MRP1 and IIβ besides increasing the intracellular accumulation of daunorubicin (DNR) and adriamycin (ADR) (Talib et al. 2021).

5.3.9 Parthenolide

Parthenolide (a sesquiterpene lactone) is a bioactive chemical found mainly in *Tanacetum parthenium* (Asteraceae), often known as feverfew plant. Parthenolide is found mainly in plant shoots, or apical parts, such as flowers and leaves, as well as in trace amounts in the roots. Parthenolide has been found to have anti-inflammatory, antioxidant, antileishmanial, antifungal, and anticancer properties (Mathema et al. 2012). Earlier, parthenolide was used to treat migraine, fever, and rheumatoid arthritis, while in recent times, it was found that parthenolide has an anticancer effect in many types of tumors (Talib et al. 2020). Its nucleophilic methylene-γ-lactone ring and epoxide group allow for good interactions with biological sites and it is responsible for the cytotoxic action of parthenolide by interruption of DNA replication (Talib et al. 2020). A variety of anticancer and pro-apoptotic properties are the results of these interactions that are linked to its capacity to cause oxidative stress (Mathema et al. 2012). Many studies have reported that parthenolide induces apoptosis in a variety of cancer such as pancreatic cancer, lung cancer, cervical cancer, and lymphocytic leukemia (Talib and Al Kury 2018). Parthenolide was found to induce apoptosis by many mechanisms; one of these mechanisms is inhibiting the signaling pathways of NF-κB, STAT3, and MAPK (Talib and Al Kury 2018). Also, parthenolide can induce apoptosis by upregulation of proapoptotic proteins (e.g., Bax and Bim) and downregulation of anti-apoptotic protein (e.g., Bcl-2). Furthermore, parthenolide increases the intracellular reactive oxygen species (ROS), and it can also induce apoptosis by activation of caspases 3, 7, 8, and 9, which are important mediators of apoptosis (Talib and Al Kury 2018). In addition to the previously mentioned effects, parthenolide has a role in the inhibition of COX, angiogenesis inhibition, and induction of autophagy by the inhibition of PI3K/AKT signaling pathway (Talib and Al Kury 2018) (Jeyamohan et al. 2016). One of the most important properties of parthenolide is the ability to induce apoptosis in malignant cells while having no impact on normal cells (Mathema et al. 2012). Parthenolide has poor oral bioavailability derived from its hydrophobicity, which limits its clinical use as an oral anticancer drug; however, the derivatization of a more hydrophilic form of parthenolide has helped to overcome this limitation (Talib et al. 2020). Different delivery systems were used to improve the hydrophilicity and bioavailability of parthenolide. These systems include micelles, a carboxyl-functionalized nanographene (fGn) delivery system, and various types of liposome delivery system (Talib et al. 2020). There are no clinical studies that have been established to assess the anticancer activity of parthenolide on the Clinical Trials website (https://clinicaltrials.gov/).

5.3.10 Thymoquinone

Thymoquinone (TQ) is the main bioactive compound of *Nigella sativa* (black seed) and constitutes about 11.8% of the volatile oil of *Nigella sativa* seeds (Alobaedi, Talib, and Basheti 2017). Thymoquinone (2-isopropyl-5-methyl-1,4-benzoquinone) is a yellow crystalline chemical that was isolated using thin-layer chromatography on silica gel roughly five decades ago (Majdalawieh, Fayyad, and Nasrallah 2017). TQ has shown to have powerful antioxidant, anti-inflammatory, hypoglycemic, anticancer, cardio-, neuro-, nephro-, and hepatoprotective properties (Ballout and Gali-Muhtasib 2020). TQ has demonstrated promising *in vitro* and *in vivo* effects on a variety of cancer types, including breast, lung, prostate, colorectal, gastric, osteosarcoma, and bladder cancer (Ballout and Gali-Muhtasib 2020). The anticancer effect of TQ was observed through apoptosis induction, antiproliferative, antioxidant, and cytotoxic effects, and cell cycle arrest, in addition to effects on angiogenesis and metastasis (Alobaedi, Talib, and Basheti 2017; Majdalawieh, Fayyad, and Nasrallah 2017). TQ can induce apoptosis, which is one of the important mechanisms of cell death, by upregulating pro-apoptotic genes and proteins, such as Bax/Bak, and downregulating anti-apoptotic genes and proteins, such as Bcl-2 and Bcl-xL (Khan et al. 2017). Also, thymoquinone can induce apoptosis through the activation of the P53, PPARγ, and PI3K/AKT signaling pathways, and inhibition of the inhibitory signaling pathways of apoptosis such as NF-κB, STAT3, and PI3K/AKT (Majdalawieh, Fayyad, and Nasrallah 2017). It also has an antiproliferative activity, particularly when combined with doxorubicin, and 5-fluorouracil, which enhanced cytotoxicity in breast cancer in mice. The antioxidant activity of TQ has been explained by its effect on the reduction of CYP1A2 and CYP 3A4, and an increase of phase II enzyme, GST (Talib et al. 2020). Furthermore, many studies have demonstrated that TQ treatment induced G0/G1 cell-cycle arrest, which was associated with increases in the expression of the cyclin-dependent kinase inhibitor p16, and a decrease in cyclin D1 protein expression. Also, TQ induced G2/M cell-cycle arrest, which was correlated with an increase in the expression of the tumor suppressor protein p53 and a decrease in cyclin B1 protein (Talib et al. 2020). Furthermore, TQ has a role in cancer metastasis, as it was found that TQ prevents endothelial invasion, and cell migration in different cell lines (Khan et al. 2017). Although thymoquinone is safe, and effective at very low doses, hydrophobicity is the main challenge that faces its formulation and bioavailability. Many formulations have been developed to enhance thymoquinone bioavailability, such as thymoquinone-loaded liposomes, thymoquinone-encapsulated nanoparticles, and nanoparticulate formulation based on polyethylene glycol or PLGA in addition to chemical derivatives of thymoquinone like thymoquinone-4-palmitoylhydrazone

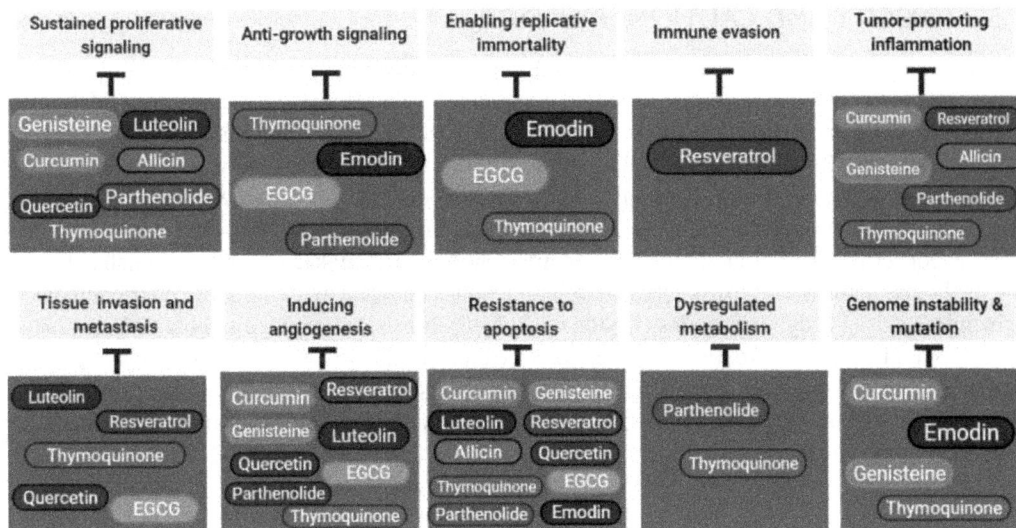

FIGURE 5.2 Effects of natural products on cancer hallmarks.

and thymoquinone-4-α-linolenoylhydrazone that show improvement in bioavailability (Talib et al. 2020). Although many studies have been conducted on thymoquinone, there were limited clinical studies on thymoquinone. Al-Amri and Bamosa observed no serious systemic toxicity in adult patients with solid tumors or hematological cancers treated with thymoquinone in a phase I study. It was also shown that the human body could tolerate up to 2600 mg of thymoquinone per day (Al-Amri and Bamosa 2009). Figure 5.2 summarizes cancer hallmarks with natural products targeting each hallmark.

5.4 OTHER FOODS, HERBS, SPICES, AND BOTANICALS USED IN CANCER MANAGEMENT

Medicinal plants, herbs, and spices are a rich source of highly potent bioactive compounds, which are used as traditional remedies and bioprecursors for drug development, particularly cancer chemotherapies (Roy, Ahuja, and Bharadvaja 2017; Bachrach 2012). Rosemary (*Rosmarinus officinalis*) and saffron (*Crocus sativus*) are spices used mainly for flavoring foods, however; they exhibited an antitumorigenesis effect via targeting cancer initiation and progression pathways (Zheng et al. 2016). Crocin and crocetin, the main constituents of saffron, have been reported to induce apoptosis and suppress angiogenesis in cancer cells (Zhou et al. 2020; Bakshi et al. 2010). On the other hand, rosemary extracts inhibited tumor cell proliferation and survival by targeting mTOR signaling, ERK, AKT, and AMPK expression (Jaglanian and Tsiani 2020; O'Neill et al. 2022). Ginger (*Zingiber officinale*) is another example of herbal medicine with anticancer potential. It reduced tumor cell growth, increased the level of p53, and mediated DNA damage (Nedungadi et al. 2021; Sarami et al. 2020). Lemon verbena (*Aloysia citrodora*) is one of the medicinal plants that gain a lot of attention for its biological activity, especially in cancer research. It suppressed tumor growth via various mechanisms of action in *in vitro* and *in vivo* studies (Salama et al. 2021; Rashid et al. 2022). All in all, most of the natural products that obtain anticarcinogenic activity are still under research and going through different experimental models; nevertheless, some of them are already used as adjuvant therapy in cancer treatment.

5.5 TOXICITY AND CAUTIONARY NOTES

Natural compounds from plants have been used in treating different kinds of diseases since ancient times, and also served as a source of single compound drugs. Herbal medicines are widely used around the world due to their health benefits and safety (Yeung, Gubili, and Mao 2018; Jermini et al. 2019). A variety of plants have indeed been used traditionally for therapeutic applications due to their general safety, but it is also crucial to know that some plants are extremely toxic and can even be deadly (Gardner and McGuffin 2013). Furthermore, adverse effects can occur due to different reasons concerning herbal medicine such as misidentification, intake overuse, and mislabeling of the medicinal herbs (Ekor 2013). Drug-herb interactions can occur with the same pharmacological principles as drug-drug interactions (Rodda et al. 2010). It is recommended to obtain herbal medicines from a registered herbalist to reduce toxicity incidences. Also, avoiding the consumption of herbal remedies along with drugs that have a narrow therapeutic window and keep monitoring herbal intake in case of pregnancy and breastfeeding mothers will help regarding herbal medicine toxicity (Fatima and Nayeem 2016).

5.6 CONCLUSION

Plant-derived natural products are promising sources for new anticancer therapies. Their high structural diversity, ability to target multiple pathways, and relatively low toxicity make these products an attractive target to discover new anticancer agents. Many natural products have proven their ability to inhibit cancer cells through interfering with multiple pathways in various cancer hallmarks. Some natural products reached the clinical use and may be considered as standard therapy in future. Further studies are needed to design a suitable experimental protocol to fully identify the anticancer potential of nature products and to clearly explain their mechanisms of action.

5.7 SUMMARY POINTS

- Cancer hallmarks summarize the main cellular and physiological alteration during the process of tumorigenesis.
- Plant-derived natural products showed high potential to target multiple cancer hallmarks.
- Apoptosis induction, angiogenesis inhibition, and cell cycle arrest are the most common mechanisms of natural products to target cancer cells.
- Some adverse effects and toxicity are associated with misidentification, overuse, and mislabeling of medicinal herbs. Drug-herb interactions are another source of toxicity.
- Plant-derived natural products are a promising source for new anticancer therapies. However, further studies are needed to reduce possible toxicity and to design a suitable experimental protocol to fully identify the anticancer potential of these natural products.

REFERENCES

Al-Amri, Ali M., and Abdullah O. Bamosa. 2009. "Phase I safety and clinical activity study of thymoquinone in patients with advanced refractory malignant disease." *E-Medical Journal* no. 10 (3):107–111.
Alobaedi, Omar H., Wamidh H. Talib, and Iman A. Basheti. 2017. "Antitumor effect of thymoquinone combined with resveratrol on mice transplanted with breast cancer." *Asian Pacific Journal of Tropical Medicine* no. 10 (4):400–408.
Bachrach, Zohara. 2012. "Contribution of selected medicinal plants for cancer prevention and therapy." *Acta Facultatis Medicae Naissensis* no. 29 (3).
Bakshi, Hamid, Smitha Sam, Roya Rozati, Phalisteen Sultan, Tajamul Islam, Babita Rathore, Zahoor Lone, Manik Sharma, Jagrati Triphati, and Ramesh Chand Saxena. 2010. "DNA fragmentation and cell cycle arrest: A hallmark of apoptosis induced by crocin from kashmiri saffron in a human pancreatic cancer cell line." *Asian Pac J Cancer Prev* no. 11 (3):675–679.

Ballout, Farah Rabih, and Hala Gali-Muhtasib. 2020. "Thymoquinone: A potential therapy against cancer stem cells." *Pharmacognosy Reviews* no. 14 (28).

Bensinger, Steven J., and Heather R. Christofk. 2012. "New aspects of the Warburg effect in cancer cell biology." *Seminars in Cell & Developmental Biology* no. 23 (4):352–361. doi:10.1016/j.semcdb.2012.02.003

Bergers, Gabriele, and Laura E. Benjamin. 2003. "Tumorigenesis and the angiogenic switch." *Nature Reviews Cancer* no. 3 (6):401–410.

Bodnar, Andrea G., Michel Ouellette, Maria Frolkis, Shawn E. Holt, Choy-Pik Chiu, Gregg B. Morin, Calvin B. Harley, Jerry W. Shay, Serge Lichtsteiner, and Woodring E. Wright. 1998. "Extension of life-span by introduction of telomerase into normal human cells." *Science* no. 279 (5349):349–352.

Borlinghaus, Jan, Frank Albrecht, Martin C. H. Gruhlke, Ifeanyi D. Nwachukwu, and Alan J. Slusarenko. 2014. "Allicin: Chemistry and biological properties." *Molecules* no. 19 (8):12591–12618.

Botet-Carreras, Adrià, Cristina Tamames-Tabar, Fabrice Salles, Sara Rojas, Edurne Imbuluzqueta, Hugo Lana, María José Blanco-Prieto, and Patricia Horcajada. 2021. "Improving the genistein oral bioavailability via its formulation into the metal–organic framework MIL-100 (Fe)." *Journal of Materials Chemistry B* no. 9 (9):2233–2239.

Chakraborty, Chiranjib, Ashish Ranjan Sharma, Garima Sharma, and Sang-Soo Lee. 2020. "The interplay among miRNAs, major Cytokines, and cancer-related inflammation." *Molecular Therapy–Nucleic Acids* no. 20:606–620. doi:10.1016/j.omtn.2020.04.002

Chakraborty, Sayan, Kizito Njah, and Wanjin Hong. 2020. "Agrin mediates angiogenesis in the tumor microenvironment." *Trends in Cancer* no. 6 (2):81–85. doi:10.1016/j.trecan.2019.12.002

Chen, Huinan, Biqiang Zhu, Lei Zhao, Yang Liu, Fuya Zhao, Jing Feng, Ye Jin, Jiayu Sun, Rui Geng, and Yunwei Wei. 2018. "Allicin inhibits proliferation and invasion in vitro and in vivo via SHP-1-mediated STAT3 signaling in cholangiocarcinoma." *Cellular Physiology and Biochemistry* no. 47 (2):641–653.

Chu, Yung-Lin, Chi-Tang Ho, Jing-Gung Chung, Rajasekaran Raghu, Yi-Chen Lo, and Lee-Yan Sheen. 2013. "Allicin induces anti-human liver cancer cells through the p53 gene modulating apoptosis and autophagy." *Journal of Agricultural and Food Chemistry* no. 61 (41):9839–9848.

Chun-Fu, WU, YANG Jing-Yu, WANG Fang, and WANG Xiao-Xiao. 2013. "Resveratrol: botanical origin, pharmacological activity and applications." *Chinese Journal of Natural Medicines* no. 11 (1):1–15.

Dang, Chi V., Jung-whan Kim, Ping Gao, and Jason Yustein. 2008. "The interplay between MYC and HIF in cancer." *Nature Reviews Cancer* no. 8 (1):51–56.

Efferth, Thomas, and Franz Oesch. 2021. "Repurposing of plant alkaloids for cancer therapy: Pharmacology and toxicology." *Seminars in Cancer Biology* no. 68:143–163.

Ekor, M. 2013. The growing use of herbal medicines: Issues relating to adverse reactions and challenges in monitoring safety. *Front. Neurol.* no. 4:1–10.

Fatima, Nudrat, and Naira Nayeem. 2016. "Toxic effects as a result of herbal medicine intake." In *Toxicology-New Aspects to This Scientific Conundrum*. London, UK: Tech Open, 193–207.

(FDA), US Food and Drug Administration. 2021. *Notice to US Food and Drug Administration of the Conclusion that the Intended Use of Curcumin is Generally Recognized as Safe* 2018 [cited November 28, 2021]. Available from chrome-extension://efaidnbmnnnibpcajpcglclefindmkaj/viewer.html?pdfurl=https%3A%2F%2F.

Ferguson, Lynnette R., Helen Chen, Andrew R. Collins, Marisa Connell, Giovanna Damia, Santanu Dasgupta, Meenakshi Malhotra, Alan K. Meeker, Amedeo Amedei, Amr Amin, S. Salman Ashraf, Katia Aquilano, Asfar S. Azmi, Dipita Bhakta, Alan Bilsland, Chandra S. Boosani, Sophie Chen, Maria Rosa Ciriolo, Hiromasa Fujii, Gunjan Guha, Dorota Halicka, William G. Helferich, W. Nicol Keith, Sulma I. Mohammed, Elena Niccolai, Xujuan Yang, Kanya Honoki, Virginia R. Parslow, Satya Prakash, Sarallah Rezazadeh, Rodney E. Shackelford, David Sidransky, Phuoc T. Tran, Eddy S. Yang, and Christopher A. Maxwell. 2015. "Genomic instability in human cancer: Molecular insights and opportunities for therapeutic attack and prevention through diet and nutrition." *Seminars in Cancer Biology* no. 35:S5–S24. doi:10.1016/j.semcancer.2015.03.005

Gardner, Zoë, and Michael McGuffin. 2013. *American Herbal Products Association's Botanical Safety Handbook.* Boca Raton and London: CRC Press.

Giordano, Antonio, and Giuseppina Tommonaro. 2019. "Curcumin and cancer." *Nutrients* no. 11 (10):2376.

Gupta, Subash C., Sridevi Patchva, and Bharat B. Aggarwal. 2013. "Therapeutic roles of curcumin: Lessons learned from clinical trials." *The American Association of Pharmaceutical Scientists* no. 15 (1):195–218.

Hanahan, Douglas, and Robert A. Weinberg. 2011. "Hallmarks of cancer: the next generation." *Cell* no. 144 (5):646–674.

Hassanpour, Seyed Hossein, and Mohammadamin Dehghani. 2017. "Review of cancer from perspective of molecular." *Journal of Cancer Research and Practice* no. 4 (4):127–129.

Hou, Jiajie, Michael Karin, and Beicheng Sun. 2021. "Targeting cancer-promoting inflammation–have anti-inflammatory therapies come of age?" *Nature Reviews Clinical Oncology*:1–19.

Huang, W. L., S. F. Wu, S. T. Xu, Y. C. Ma, R. Wang, and S. Jin. 2020. "Allicin enhances the radiosensitivity of colorectal cancer cells via inhibition of NF-κB signaling pathway." *Journal of Food Science* no. 85 (6):1924–1931. doi:10.1111/1750-3841.15156

Imran, Muhammad, Abdur Rauf, Tareq Abu-Izneid, Muhammad Nadeem, Mohammad Ali Shariati, Imtiaz Ali Khan, Ali Imran, Ilkay Erdogan Orhan, Muhammad Rizwan, and Muhammad Atif. 2019. "Luteolin, a flavonoid, as an anticancer agent: A review." *Biomedicine Pharmacotherapy* no. 112:108612.

Jaglanian, Alina, and Evangelia Tsiani. 2020. "Rosemary extract inhibits proliferation, survival, Akt, and mTOR signaling in triple-negative breast cancer cells." *International Journal of Molecular Sciences* no. 21 (3):810.

Jeong, Jae-Hoon, Jee Young An, Yong Tae Kwon, Juong G Rhee, and Yong J. Lee. 2009. "Effects of low dose quercetin: Cancer cell-specific inhibition of cell cycle progression." *Journal of Cellular Biochemistry* no. 106 (1):73–82.

Jermini, Mégane, Julie Dubois, Pierre-Yves Rodondi, Khalil Zaman, Thierry Buclin, Chantal Csajka, Angela Orcurto, and Laura E Rothuizen. 2019. "Complementary medicine use during cancer treatment and potential herb-drug interactions from a cross-sectional study in an academic centre." *Scientific Reports* no. 9 (1):1–11.

Jeyamohan, Sridharan, Rajesh Kannan Moorthy, Mahesh Kumar Kannan, and Antony Joseph Velanganni Arockiam. 2016. "Parthenolide induces apoptosis and autophagy through the suppression of PI3K/Akt signaling pathway in cervical cancer." *Biotechnology Letters* no. 38 (8):1251–1260.

Kazmi, Imran, Fahad A. Al-Abbasi, Muhammad Shahid Nadeem, Hisham N. Altayb, Sultan Alshehri, and Syed Sarim Imam. 2021. "Formulation, optimization and evaluation of luteolin-loaded topical nanoparticulate delivery system for the skin cancer." *Pharmaceutics* no. 13 (11):1749.

Khan, Md Asaduzzaman, Mousumi Tania, Shangyi Fu, and Junjiang Fu. 2017. "Thymoquinone, as an anticancer molecule: From basic research to clinical investigation." *Oncotarget* no. 8 (31):51907.

Lai, Wing-Fu, Mirza Muhammad Faran Ashraf Baig, Wing-Tak Wong, and Bao Ting Zhu. 2020. "Epigallocatechin-3-gallate in functional food development: From concept to reality." *Trends in Food Science and Technology* no. 102:271–279.

Li, Haitao, William Ka Kei Wu, Zongping Zheng, Chun Tao Che, Zhi Jie Li, Dan Dan Xu, Clover Ching Man Wong, Cai Guo Ye, Joseph Jao Yiu Sung, and Chi Hin Cho. 2010. "3, 3′, 4, 5, 5′-pentahydroxy-trans-stilbene, a resveratrol derivative, induces apoptosis in colorectal carcinoma cells via oxidative stress." *European Journal of Pharmacology* no. 637 (1–3):55–61.

Majdalawieh, Amin F., Muneera W. Fayyad, and Gheyath K. Nasrallah. 2017. "Anti-cancer properties and mechanisms of action of thymoquinone, the major active ingredient of *Nigella sativa*." *Critical Reviews in Food Science and Nutrition* no. 57 (18):3911–3928.

Majolo, Fernanda, Luciana Knabben de Oliveira Becker Delwing, Diorge Jônatas Marmitt, Ivan Cunha Bustamante-Filho, and Márcia Inês Goettert. 2019. "Medicinal plants and bioactive natural compounds for cancer treatment: Important advances for drug discovery." *Phytochemistry Letters* no. 31:196–207.

Martin, Tracey A., Lin Ye, Andrew J. Sanders, Jane Lane, and Wen G. Jiang. 2013. "Cancer invasion and metastasis: Molecular and cellular perspective." In *Madame Curie Bioscience Database [Internet]*. Austin, TX: Landes Bioscience.

Mathema, Vivek Bhakta, Young-Sang Koh, Balkrishna Chand Thakuri, and Mika Sillanpää. 2012. "Parthenolide, a sesquiterpene lactone, expresses multiple anti-cancer and anti-inflammatory activities." *Inflammation* no. 35 (2):560–565.

Mukhtar, Hasan, and Nihal Ahmad. 2000. "Tea polyphenols: Prevention of cancer and optimizing health." *The American Journal of Clinical Nutrition* no. 71 (6):1698S–1702S.

Nedungadi, Divya, Anupama Binoy, Vivek Vinod, Muralidharan Vanuopadath, Sudarslal Sadasivan Nair, Bipin G. Nair, and Nandita Mishra. 2021. "Ginger extract activates caspase independent paraptosis in cancer cells via ER stress, mitochondrial dysfunction, AIF translocation and DNA damage." *Nutrition and Cancer* no. 73 (1):147–159.

O'Neill, Eric J., Jessy Moore, Joon Song, and Evangelia Litsa Tsiani. 2022. "Inhibition of non–small cell lung cancer proliferation and survival by Rosemary extract is associated with activation of ERK and AMPK." *Life* no. 12 (1):52.

Orlikova, B., and M. Diederich. 2012. "Power from the garden: Plant compounds as inhibitors of the hallmarks of cancer." *Current Medicinal Chemistry* no. 19 (14):2061–2087.

PubChem. 2021. *Curcumin* 2021 [cited November 18, 2021]. Available from https://pubchem.ncbi.nlm.nih.gov/compound/Curcumin.

Ramírez-Garza, Sonia L., Emily P. Laveriano-Santos, María Marhuenda-Muñoz, Carolina E. Storniolo, Anna Tresserra-Rimbau, Anna Vallverdú-Queralt, and Rosa M. Lamuela-Raventós. 2018. "Health effects of resveratrol: Results from human intervention trials." *Nutrients* no. 10 (12):1892.

Rashid, Hasan M., Asma I. Mahmod, Fatma U. Afifi, and Wamidh H. Talib. 2022. "Antioxidant and antiproliferation activities of Lemon Verbena (*Aloysia citrodora*): An in vitro and in vivo study." *Plants* no. 11 (6). doi:10.3390/plants11060785

Rauf, Abdur, Muhammad Imran, Masood Sadiq Butt, Muhammad Nadeem, Dennis G. Peters, and Mohammad S. Mubarak. 2018. "Resveratrol as an anti-cancer agent: A review." *Critical Reviews in Food Science and Nutrition* no. 58 (9):1428–1447.

Rodda, Harish Chandra, Raj Kumar Molmoori, Sujatha Samala, Nagaraj Banala, and Veeresham Ciddi. 2010. "An insight into herb-drug interactions." *Intern. J. Pharma. Scien. Nanotech.* no. 2 (4).

Roy, Arpita, Shruti Ahuja, and Navneeta Bharadvaja. 2017. "A review on medicinal plants against cancer." *Journal of Plant Sciences and Agricultural Research* no. 2 (1):8–12.

Rusin, Marek, Artur Zajkowicz, and Dorota Butkiewicz. 2009. "Resveratrol induces senescence-like growth inhibition of U-2 OS cells associated with the instability of telomeric DNA and upregulation of BRCA1." *Mechanisms of Ageing and Development* no. 130 (8):528–537.

Sa, Gaurisankar, and Tanya Das. 2008. "Anti cancer effects of curcumin: Cycle of life and death." *Cell Division* no. 3 (1):1–14.

Salama, Yousef, Nidal Jaradat, Koichi Hattori, and Beate Heissig. 2021. "Aloysia citrodora essential oil inhibits melanoma cell growth and migration by targeting HB-EGF-EGFR signaling." *International Journal of Molecular Sciences* no. 22 (15):8151.

Saleem, Hammad, Sirajudheen Anwar, Ahmed Alafnan, and Nafees Ahemad. 2021. "Chapter 22 – Luteolin." In *A Centum of Valuable Plant Bioactives*, edited by Muhammad Mushtaq and Farooq Anwar, 509–523. Cambridge, MA: Academic Press.

Sarami, Soroush, Maryam Dadmanesh, Zuhair M. Hassan, and Khodayar Ghorban. 2020. "Study on the effect of ethanol ginger extract on cell viability and p53 level in breast and pancreatic cancer." *Archives of Pharmacy Practice* no. 1:115.

Semwal, Ruchi Badoni, Deepak Kumar Semwal, Sandra Combrinck, and Alvaro Viljoen. 2021. "Emodin – a natural anthraquinone derivative with diverse pharmacological activities." *Phytochemistry* no. 190:112854.

Singh, Brahma N., Sharmila Shankar, and Rakesh K. Srivastava. 2011. "Green tea catechin, epigallocatechin-3-gallate (EGCG): Mechanisms, perspectives and clinical applications." *Biochemical Pharmacology* no. 82 (12):1807–1821.

Stohs, Sidney J., Oliver Chen, Sidhartha D. Ray, Jin Ji, Luke R. Bucci, and Harry G. Preuss. 2020. "Highly bioavailable forms of curcumin and promising avenues for curcumin-based research and application: A review." *Molecules* no. 25 (6):1397.

Sung, Hyuna, Jacques Ferlay, Rebecca L. Siegel, Mathieu Laversanne, Isabelle Soerjomataram, Ahmedin Jemal, and Freddie Bray. 2021. "Global cancer statistics 2020: GLOBOCAN estimates of incidence and mortality worldwide for 36 cancers in 185 countries." *CA: A Cancer Journal for Clinicians* no. 71 (3):209–249. doi:10.3322/caac.21660

Talib, Wamidh H. 2018. "Melatonin and cancer hallmarks." *Molecules* no. 23 (3):518.

Talib, Wamidh H., and Lina T. Al Kury. 2018. "Parthenolide inhibits tumor-promoting effects of nicotine in lung cancer by inducing P53-dependent apoptosis and inhibiting VEGF expression." *Biomedicine and Pharmacotherapy* no. 107:1488–1495.

Talib, Wamidh H., Izzeddin Alsalahat, Safa Daoud, Reem Fawaz Abutayeh, and Asma Ismail Mahmod. 2020. "Plant-derived natural products in cancer research: Extraction, mechanism of action, and drug formulation." *Molecules* no. 25 (22):5319.

Talib, Wamidh H., Ahmad Riyad Alsayed, Muna Barakat, May Ibrahim Abu-Taha, and Asma Ismail Mahmod. 2021. "Targeting drug chemo-resistance in cancer using natural products." *Biomedicines* no. 9 (10):1353.

Tang, Si-Min, Xue-Ting Deng, Jian Zhou, Quan-Peng Li, Xian-Xiu Ge, and Lin Miao. 2020. "Pharmacological basis and new insights of quercetin action in respect to its anti-cancer effects." *Biomedicine & Pharmacotherapy* no. 121:109604.

Teng, Xue, Shu Ya Wang, Yuan Qi Shi, Xiao Fan Fan, Shuang Liu, Yue Xing, Yuan Yuan Guo, and Mei Dong. 2021. "The role of emodin on cisplatin resistance reversal of lung adenocarcinoma A549/DDP cell." *Anti-Cancer Drugs* no. 32 (9):939–949.

Trung, Ly Quoc, and Dao T. T. An. 2018. "Is resveratrol a cancer immunomodulatory molecule?" *Frontiers in Pharmacology* no. 9:1255.

Tuli, Hardeep Singh, Muobarak Jaber Tuorkey, Falak Thakral, Katrin Sak, Manoj Kumar, Anil Kumar Sharma, Uttam Sharma, Aklank Jain, Vaishali Aggarwal, and Anupam Bishayee. 2019. "Molecular mechanisms of action of genistein in cancer: Recent advances." *Frontiers in Pharmacology* no. 10:1336.

Wang, Haijun, Ke Zhang, Jia Liu, Jie Yang, Yidan Tian, Chen Yang, Yushan Li, Minglong Shao, Wei Su, and Na Song. 2021. "Curcumin regulates cancer progression: Focus on ncRNAs and molecular signaling pathways." *Frontiers in Oncology* no. 11:1202.

Wang, Hui, Tianyue Jiang, Wei Li, Na Gao, and Tao Zhang. 2018. "Resveratrol attenuates oxidative damage through activating mitophagy in an in vitro model of Alzheimer's disease." *Toxicology Letters* no. 282:100–108.

Wang, Ting-ye, and Jia-xu Chen. 2019. "Effects of curcumin on vessel formation insight into the pro-and anti-angiogenesis of curcumin." *Evidence-Based Complementary Alternative Medicine* no. 2019.

Yaswen, Paul, Karen L. MacKenzie, W. Nicol Keith, Patricia Hentosh, Francis Rodier, Jiyue Zhu, Gary L. Firestone, Ander Matheu, Amancio Carnero, Alan Bilsland, Tabetha Sundin, Kanya Honoki, Hiromasa Fujii, Alexandros G. Georgakilas, Amedeo Amedei, Amr Amin, Bill Helferich, Chandra S. Boosani, Gunjan Guha, Maria Rosa Ciriolo, Sophie Chen, Sulma I. Mohammed, Asfar S. Azmi, Dipita Bhakta, Dorota Halicka, Elena Niccolai, Katia Aquilano, S. Salman Ashraf, Somaira Nowsheen, and Xujuan Yang. 2015. "Therapeutic targeting of replicative immortality." *Seminars in Cancer Biology* no. 35:S104–S128. doi:10.1016/j.semcancer.2015.03.007

Yeung, K. Simon, Jyothirmai Gubili, and Jun J. Mao. 2018. "Herb-drug interactions in cancer care." *Oncology* no. 32 (10):516–520.

Zhang, Fang-Yuan, Run-Ze Li, Cong Xu, Xing-Xing Fan, Jia-Xin Li, Wei-Yu Meng, Xuan-Run Wang, Tu-Liang Liang, Xiao-Xiang Guan, and Hu-Dan Pan. 2021. "Emodin induces apoptosis and suppresses non–small-cell lung cancer growth via downregulation of sPLA2-IIa." *Phytomedicine* 153786.

Zhang, Xia, Yingping Chen, Ting Zhang, and Yaming Zhang. 2015. "Inhibitory effect of emodin on human hepatoma cell line SMMC-7721 and its mechanism." *African Health Sciences* no. 15 (1):97–100.

Zheng, Jie, Yue Zhou, Ya Li, Dong-Ping Xu, Sha Li, and Hua-Bin Li. 2016. "Spices for prevention and treatment of cancers." *Nutrients* no. 8 (8):495.

Zhou, Ye, Mingde Zang, Junyi Hou, Jiangli Wang, Yakai Huang, Xusheng Ding, and Yanong Wang. 2020. "Crocetin suppresses angiogenesis through inhibiting Sonic hedgehog signaling pathway in gastric cancer."

Zou, Haoyang, Haiqing Ye, Rajamanikkam Kamaraj, Tiehua Zhang, Jie Zhang, and Petr Pavek. 2021. "A review on pharmacological activities and synergistic effect of quercetin with small molecule agents." *Phytomedicine*:153736.

6 Fruit Extracts as Anticancer Agents

*Trien Trey Tang, Hayden Young Lee
and Yujiang Fang*

ABBREVIATIONS

BE   blueberry extract
CE   cranberry extract
KE   kiwi extract
OD   optical density
PCNA   proliferating cell nuclear antigen
RE   raspberry extract
XRT   radiation therapy

6.1 INTRODUCTION

Cancer chemotherapy is well-known to be an arduous treatment for patients due to its adverse side effects. While there is an array of chemotherapeutics available depending on the particular neoplasm, the toxicity associated with their administration often leads to multi-system damage, psychological deficits, medical emergencies, and death (Livshits, Rao, and Smith 2014). Thus, there is greater focus in the oncological community towards various medications with fewer or no associated adverse effects.

A promising option that fulfills this need is fruit extract of various plants that demonstrate favorable health outcomes following *in vitro* and clinical examination. In recent years, there is a growing body of literature that explored various fruit extracts' effects on cancer lines in the laboratory (Shu et al. 2021; Akhouri, Kumari, and Kumar 2020; Nozaki et al. 2016). While there are few clinical trials where patients receive fruit extract as part of cancer therapy, a particular study utilizing pomegranate extract revealed prostate cancer patients demonstrating favorable health results, such as longer neoplastic doubling time and fewer adverse effects than traditional chemotherapeutic alternatives (Paller, Pantuck, and Carducci 2017). If this is expanded to non-neoplastic disorders, then there are many more clinical trials that show fruit extract improve patient outcomes with similar absence or decrease of treatment toxicity (Upadya et al. 2019; Rao et al. 2016; Sangsefidi et al. 2021). Though this is an exciting field of study, more research should be introduced to further explore the efficacy and safety of utilizing this treatment modality.

To explore the mechanisms of fruits' demonstrated anticancer properties in such studies, the most notable bioactive molecules are discussed. Fruits contain polyphenols, a well-described category of nutrients shown to have anti-inflammatory properties by taking part in free radical reduction, potential cancer-apoptotic pathways, and dysplasia-reducing pathways (Ganesan and Xu 2017). There are thousands of polyphenols, but some are better examined in the literature to reduce cancer proliferation *in vitro*. For example, when resveratrol, a polyphenol found in a number of fruits, was administered in cancer lines directly, various pro-apoptotic proteins increased and anti-apoptotic proteins decreased (Galiniak, Aebishern, and Bartusik-Aebisher 2019).

DOI: 10.1201/9781003260028-7

This begs the question of how fruit extract can perform in more specific cancer therapies, particularly as a sensitizing agent that potentially enhances the effect of radiation on neoplasms. Radiation therapy is complex and involves different types of rays (e.g., electromagnetic, particulate), dosages, and fractions (Baskar et al. 2012). Further, cancer cells can be predisposed to greater injury in radiotherapy if exposed to an effective sensitizing agent, or radiosensitizer (Citrin 2019). The exploration of radiosensitizers as effective and safe treatment components in cancer therapy is an active field of research and ranges from substances like nanomaterials to biological matter – like fruit extract (Wang et al. 2018). The use of fruit as a radiosensitizer, specifically, remains largely uninvestigated. This opens the oncological field to research utilizing fruit as a nontoxic option in radiosensitivity and radiation studies, as fruit extract – as discussed earlier – has been well described to have anticancer properties valuable in efficacious treatments for patients.

This chapter therefore provides a discussion of certain fruit extracts as potential treatments in cancer therapy, both alone and as radiosensitizing agents.

6.2 BACKGROUND

It is common cultural knowledge that fruits are generally healthy. Even more, with the recent media attention to fruits in the form of "immunity shots" and "juice cleanse," the health benefits of fruits have been under increasing scrutiny. Such benefits known to the general public include antioxidizing, anti-obesity, anti-inflammatory, and pro-cardiovascular effects, with the idea that higher fruit consumption leads to a higher quality of life (Zeb 2020; Soerjomataram et al. 2010; Aune et al. 2017; Miller et al. 2017). Accordingly, the World Health Organization and the Food and Agriculture Organization of the United Nations recommend that adults consume at least five servings of fruits per day. This recommendation stems from hundreds of studies supporting that increased consumption of fruit is negatively correlated with obesity. Thus, fruit consumption indeed generally leads to better health outcomes, not just in regard to cancer.

A more enigmatic concept is that of radiotherapy, which is – not wrongly – often associated with severe health problems and drastic medical intervention to correct it. Unfortunately, as with chemotherapy, radiotherapy is associated with poorer quality of life due to lengthy durations of treatment, costs, hospital stays, and various acute and chronic side effects (Kawamura et al. 2020). On the other hand, radiotherapy alongside surgery has proven to be an efficacious intervention that eliminates many cancers in patients facing poor prognosis. Unknown to many is radiotherapy utilized in a palliative manner, reducing pain associated with certain tumors, such as in bone metastases, in patients with complex medical issues, and in end-of-life care (Arscott et al. 2020).

Associating these two ideas is a new topic and, even in the scientific community, is yet to be widely explored. In this chapter, we discuss four fruits that have been studied for their antiproliferative and pro-apoptotic agency.

6.3 ETIOLOGY AND *IN VITRO* STUDY

The complexity of cancer treatment can be divided into two aspects of cancer. First, each cancerous cell line has its own etiology, or manner of disease. Practically speaking, cervical cancer cell lines must be approached and treated differently than melanoma. Second, cancerous cells are essentially a derivative of neighboring healthy cells, and thus the strength of treatment is inversely correlated with the toxicity. Therefore, the difficulty is that current non-surgical modalities, such as chemotherapy and radiotherapy, are like a dull surgical knife because they often cause collateral damage. Thus, the key component of treatment is to identify and maneuver potential focalized regulators of cancer proliferation.

The success of cancer treatment was measured directly by the effect of intervention via fruit extract on both cancer cell survival and proliferation. To quantify cancer survival, studies utilize a clonal survival assay to measure response to treatment. In other words, this assay describes the extent of apoptosis, or controlled cell death, occurring in the tumor compared to a control that is not exposed to any intervention. Next, cancer cell proliferation is measured by a quick cell proliferation assay when exposed to fruit extract and compared to a control. This is quantified via proliferating cell nuclear antigen (PCNA) staining or optical density (OD). Ideal cancer treatments should lead to decreases in cancer cell survival and proliferation. These measurements summarize the antitumor effects of bioactive molecules from fruit extract.

To determine the specific mechanism of action on cancer persistence, cancer experiments often measure changes in concentration and expression of specific apoptotic and proliferative molecules. These compounds are markers that display tumor survival and proliferation from a molecular perspective and are frequently measured. The classification of apoptotic and proliferative is further divided into pro-apoptotic and anti-apoptotic, as well as pro-proliferative and antiproliferative, respectively. Fruit extracts serving as potential treatments for cancer would ideally have a pro-apoptotic and antiproliferative effect.

6.4   KIWI AND RASPBERRIES

In two separate *in vitro* studies, kiwi extract (KE) and raspberry extract (RE) showed significant antitumor effects on skin cancer and cervical cancer, respectively.

Kiwi fruit (*Actinidia* spp.) is a bright translucent green fruit with a contrasting dull brown hairy skin. It has well-documented mechanisms for improving gastrointestinal health, specifically in regard to bowel movement and the gut microbiome. Additionally, kiwi fruit has a high concentration of antioxidants, including vitamin C, vitamin E, and bioactive polyphenols, and thus is a potential treatment method for cancer cells (Richardson, Ansell, and Drummond 2018).

Raspberries (*Rubus* spp.) are dark reddish fruits that have increased in popularity due to various health benefits related to neurocognitive function in both children and adults, likely due to the antioxidative effect of various components (Bell and Williams 2021). These antioxidants include polyphenols, ellagitannin, and anthocyanins, groups of actively studied components associated with favorable health outcomes in patients. This composition suggests that raspberries may play a role in the reduction of cancer cell survival.

Via clonal survival assays and quick proliferative assays, survival and proliferation were measured for both cell lines after exposure to respective fruit extracts (Kou et al. 2021). Over a 72-hour period, human cell line melanoma CRL-11147 showed approximately 30% of total surviving colonies when treated with KE compared to the control (100%). PCNA staining and OD measurement revealed proliferation of 0.4 and 0.5 compared to the control (1.0) (Figure 6.1).

The cervical cancer cell line, HeLa, upon exposure to RE, showed 40% survival compared to the control (Sham et al. 2021). OD measurement revealed a proliferation of 0.6 compared to the control (Figure 6.2). Because different cancer cell lines are utilized, these measures cannot be adequate evidence to suggest KE is a more effective antitumor treatment. Yet, these studies serve to show the general effectiveness of fruit extract on *in vitro* cancer cells.

Further analysis of the KE effect on melanoma CRL-11147 revealed significant downregulation of pro-proliferative proteins cyclin E and CDK4. Table 6.1 notes the various molecules of interest that change in levels of expression in response to treatment throughout these studies. In any matter, cyclins and CDKs are well-studied molecules that together form a complex that regulates cell cycle progression. In cancer cells, these complexes are dysregulated and allow improper advancement through the cell cycle (Gao, Leone, and Wang 2020). There was also upregulation of pro-apoptotic molecule TRAIL R1 compared to the control. TRAIL R1 is a receptor that binds TRAIL. This

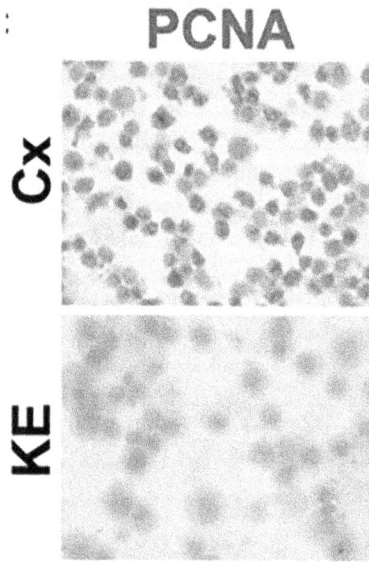

FIGURE 6.1   Kiwi treatment IHC. Cervical cancer cell survival before and after kiwi extract administration, measured by PCNA staining.

Source: From Kou et al. (2021), with permissions.

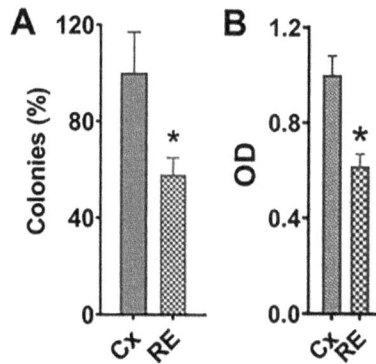

FIGURE 6.2   Results from raspberry treatment. Cervical cancer cell survival decreases after raspberry extract administration. OD = optical density.

Source: From Bai et al. (2021), permissions pending.

TABLE 6.1
Factor Chart

Fruit Extract	Cancer	Pro-Apoptotic Factor	Anti-Apoptotic factor	Antiproliferative Factor	Pro-Proliferative factor
Kiwi extract (KE)	Melanoma (CRL11147)	TRAILR1	–	–	Cyclin E, CDK4
Raspberry extract (RE)	Cervical (HeLa)	Fas	–	p53	–
Blueberry extract (BE)	Cervical (HeLa)	TRAIL	–	p21	Cyclin D, cyclin E
Cranberry extract (CE)	Glioblastoma (U87)	–	Survivin	P21, cyclin D	Cyclin B, CDK4

Note: Comparison of apoptotic and proliferative factors by cell line and fruit extract.

binding subsequently induces apoptosis. In essence, KE was effective in demonstrating both slowing of cancer cell division and increasing cell death.

HeLa cervical cancer cells, upon exposure to RE, displayed upregulation of antiproliferative molecule p53, which is a critical cyclin–CDK complex inhibitor that prevents improper cell cycle progression (Macaluso et al. 2005). There was also upregulation of the pro-apoptotic molecule Fas, an important receptor molecule in the extrinsic apoptotic pathway. This suggests that RE treatment, like that of KE, leads to marked disruption of cancer survival.

In summary, both KE and RE demonstrated a significant reduction in cell proliferation and increased apoptosis. It is important to note that the tests were performed *in vitro*, and thus the study does not encompass the total complexity of tumor growth (i.e., angiogenic factor of cancerous cells). Nevertheless, these findings show promising steps toward finding a safer alternative treatment that may work in conjunction with other treatment modalities.

6.5 RADIOSENSITIVITY

Perhaps the more attractive application of fruit extract in cancer treatment is in conjunction with radiotherapy. Currently, approximately 50% of all cancer patients receive radiation therapy alone or with other modalities (Baskar et al. 2012). The key benefit of radiation therapy is that it is a localized treatment using high-energy radiation to damage the DNA and other molecular structures of cancer cells compared to the systematic approach of traditional chemotherapy.

However, the degree of sensitivity of different cancer types to radiation therapy (XRT) is influenced by a multitude of factors including, the cell type, status of the patient, and stage of cancer (Wang 1999). The probability of successful XRT can be increased by using radiosensitizing chemicals. In preliminary studies, resveratrol, a polyphenolic compound found in grapes and other plant species, was found to have a radiosensitizing effect, meaning that XRT treatment showed greater effects when the cell line was saturated with fruit extracts. Similar results in other fruits with high polyphenolic compounds and sought to understand the underlying mechanisms.

6.6 BLUEBERRIES AND CRANBERRIES AS RADIOSENSITIZERS

In two separate studies, the effects of blueberry extract (BE) and cranberry extract (CE) on cancer were examined in conjunction with radiotherapy. The fruit extracts thus served as radiosensitizers.

To provide context, blueberries (*Vaccinium* spp.) are a widely consumed fruit that has been shown to help maintain healthy function of the nervous system, specifically in age-related cognitive deficits, and to improve learning in children (Tran and Tran 2021). In regards to anticancer effects, blueberries consist of various phenols that display antioxidant properties. Flavonoids, a group of phenolic compounds, include a potent antioxidant known as anthocyanin that is prevalent in blueberries. Anthocyanin has been shown to have antiproliferative and pro-apoptotic effects on cancer cells, making it a promising research candidate to study its effect on various tumor lines (Hazafa et al. 2020). Similarly, resveratrol is another compound found in blueberries that is shown to be an effective radiosensitizer for prostate cancer lines (Fang, DeMarco, and Nicholl 2012). With these compounds, blueberry extract overall may have an influential impact on cancer cell growth as a radiosensitizer for radiation.

In a similar fashion, cranberries (*Vaccinium macrocarpon*) are considered a healthy food that plays a role in prebiotic maintenance of gut and urinary tract microbiota and may help prevent urinary tract infections (Coleman and Ferreira 2020). Importantly, the antitumor effects of cranberries are notably found in flavonoids, such as myricetin and quercetin. These flavonoids have been shown to be effective radiosensitizers in more focused studies (Singh et al. 2009). Like blueberries, cranberry extract may be an effective radiosensitizer for radiotherapy.

Davidson et al. examined BE extract effect on cervical cancer cells in radiotherapy (Davidson et al. 2019). Bai et al. similarly quantified CE effect on glioblastoma cells in radiotherapy (Bai et al. 2021). In both studies, controls were produced, including a cancer line that was not exposed to radiotherapy or fruit extract, as well as a cell line that was only exposed to radiotherapy without fruit extract.

Clonal survival assays and quick cell proliferative assays were conducted for both cell lines with respective fruit extract with and without radiotherapy. The cervical cancer cells exposed to BE showed approximately 70% survival without radiotherapy and approximately 40% survival with radiotherapy compared to the control (100%) (Figure 6.3).

PCNA staining and OD measurement showed proliferation of 0.2 and 0.4, respectively, compared to the control (1.0) in the proliferative assay. Glioblastoma cells exposed to CE showed approximately 40% survival without radiotherapy and approximately 20% survival with radiotherapy compared to the control (Figure 6.4).

Only OD was measured in the proliferative assay, resulting in 0.4 compared to the control (Figure 6.5).

Much like KE and RE effects on melanoma cells and cervical cancer cells, the quantifications of CE and BE effects cannot be compared because of the different cancer cell lines in respective experiments, nor was it the aim of the studies. Thus, one cannot infer that CE is a more effective radiosensitizer than BE. The effectiveness of radiation therapy, however, does appear to be notably increased via exposure of cancer cells to these fruit extract radiosensitizers.

Each cell line was also examined for concentrations of apoptotic and proliferative markers in the individual studies. Again, Table 6.1 marks notable changes in these markers' expression according to the particular cancer and treatment. Cervical cancer cells exposed to BE and radiotherapy expressed significantly more pro-apoptotic molecule, TRAIL, and had significantly higher caspase-3 activity. Caspase-3 is a vital protease enzyme that executes cell apoptosis, such that increased caspase-3 denotes increased cancer cell death. There was also significantly less expression of pro-proliferative molecules cyclin D and cyclin E. Finally, there was significantly less

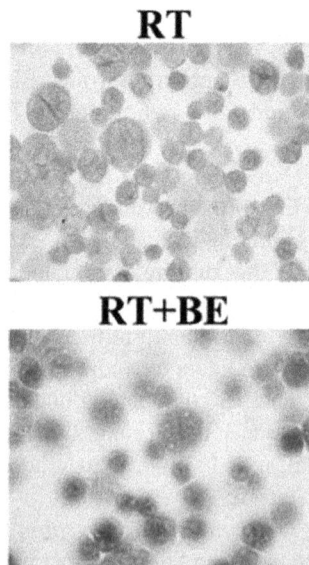

FIGURE 6.3 Blueberry immunohistochemistry. Cervical cancer cell survival reduction in radiotherapy (RT) versus radiotherapy with blueberry extract (RT + BE).

Source: From Davidson et al. (2019), with permissions.

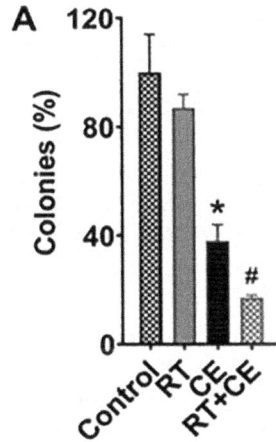

FIGURE 6.4 Cranberry immunohistochemistry. Colony survival decreased with radiotherapy (RT), cranberry extract (CE), and radiotherapy with cranberry extract (RT + CE).

Source: From Bai et al. (2021), permissions pending.

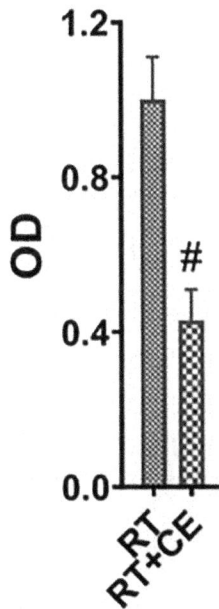

FIGURE 6.5 Cranberry optical density. Glioblastoma cell line decreases after the administration of radiotherapy (RT) and radiotherapy with cranberry extract (RT + CE).

Source: From Bai et al. (2021), permissions pending.

antiproliferative molecule p21, which suggests that BE does not necessarily have a singular effect on cervical cancer. Overall, the increase in pro-apoptotic and decrease in pro-proliferative molecules contribute to tumor death.

Based on the results of the aforementioned studies, CE should show a decrease in pro-proliferative factor, cyclin D, but actually increased this pro-proliferative factor. However, this is a common instance in oncology, where therapeutics often do not have consistent effect on the many complex cellular pathways regulating proliferation. As such, based on this molecule alone, the survival assay should show an increase in glioblastoma U87 colony size. However, there was a 60% decrease in the size of the U87 colony when treated with CE alone. This is supported by the decrease in expression of pro-proliferative markers cyclin B and CDK4, as well as a decrease in expression of survivin, an anti-apoptotic molecule, and an increase in p21, an antiproliferative marker. Survivin acts upstream from the extrinsic apoptotic pathway and regulates the interaction of other proteins with caspases (Wheatley and Altieri 2019). The results from studies suggest there are underlying mechanisms that must be considered for future studies.

6.7   CLOSING REMARKS

The discussed research on fruit as radiosensitizers for cancer therapy has yielded promising results. This begs the question of what other substances future studies should test in the field of radiation oncology.

These studies only tested the effects of four fruits, but there are many substances found in nature that yield anticancer properties, extending past fruits to various vegetables and seeds (Ni et al. 2021; Xu, Cao, and Chen 2015; Dandawate et al. 2016; Mohanraj and Sivasankar 2014). For simplicity, only a handful of such studies are referred, but the literature – specifically found on PubMed, an extensive database of clinical and biomedical journal articles – shows a large and growing interest in analyzing these substances for molecules demonstrating anticancer effects. Yet, the idea to test the extract of these botanical substances on cancer cell lines is novel idea and has ultimately few studies directly exploring their effects on tumors. As such, there is space in basic science and clinical research to investigate their direct impact on the wide array of existing neoplasms.

Further, the study of fruit extracts as sensitizers in radiotherapy is new and largely unexplored. The studies provided in this chapter are among a small handful of research articles today that test the cytotoxicity of fruit combined with radiation. Thus, not only is space open in the scientific community to continue work on the direct effect of fruits and vegetables on cancer viability, but there is much more work to be done discovering their potential role as radiosensitizers. This is expanded upon in section 6.8.

It should be noted that although the experiments conducted on blueberry, cranberry, kiwi, and raspberry extracts tested over 20 enzymes involved in critical proliferative and apoptotic pathways, the results of the experiments could have been swayed by untested or undetected molecules. To explain, these experiments are limited due to only examining proteins considered to be most important to cancer proliferation and apoptosis. There is a vast amount of proteins that signal proliferation and apoptosis that are not tested in these studies, including other cyclins, CDKs, interleukins, inflammatory factors, and many others. It is impossible for these few studies to grasp this massive scope, providing even more availability for future research to investigate these uninvestigated molecules.

Overall, the study of fruits in oncology is novel and yields high potential. Despite being a common part of daily life, fruits are not just a delicious snack; they provide an interesting and valuable avenue of research in modern cancer therapy and radiation medicine.

6.8   OTHER FOODS, HERBS, SPICES, AND BOTANICALS USED IN CANCER

As previously mentioned, fruit extract refers to only a section of possible natural substances available that can prove to be beneficial, nontoxic cancer therapeutics. To further discuss this, there are other botanicals that have shown promising effect *in vivo*. A particular example includes extract from *Corchorus olitorius* leaves having increased cytotoxicity of neoplasms from gastric, pancreatic, and melanoma cell lines (Tosoc et al. 2021). There are many other examples in the literature that investigate similar experiments and yield similar results (Reza et al. 2021; Nisa et al. 2017;

Pitchakarn et al. 2010). In the case of radiotherapy, there are much fewer studies that utilize non-fruit botanicals as radiosensitizers. This may be due to fewer researchers having adequate training or access to laboratory radiation equipment, more complexity in study methodologies, and simply the lack of awareness or interest in utilizing substances like extract from fruits, vegetables, and seeds in radiation oncology. However, as an example of efficacy, a study demonstrated extract from *Bouea macrophylla* seeds (and specific bioactive compounds within, such as the gallotannin, a polyphenol-originating compound) providing increased radiosensitivity of head and neck cancers, with marked increase in cell cycle arrests and radiation-induced cell death in response to ionizing radiation (Kantapan et al. 2021). As discussed in section 6.7, this field is not well explored. The scientific opportunity remains open to the testing of the many other medicinal plants found both in nature and domesticated origins.

6.9 TOXICITY AND CAUTIONARY NOTES

The vast majority of studies discussed investigating the effects of fruit extract on cancer lines, with and without radiotherapy, are *in vitro* or non-human *in vivo*. Regardless, the toxicity of traditional chemotherapeutics to patients demands caution be used in research for human clinical trials. Thus far, the few clinical trials available that utilize fruit extract in cancer therapy have demonstrated no obvious adverse effects related to treatment administration. It is duly important, however, that clinicians and biomedical researchers continue to exercise caution through usual consideration of patient medical history, predispositions, allergies, and other relevant factors.

Likewise, radiation therapy is a serious treatment that demands proper clinical judgement. Utilization of fruit extract as radiosensitizers is a promising field of research, but increased cytotoxicity of cancer cells in radiation as a result of sensitization may lead to collateral cellular damage to the patient. As such, continued study on the effect of fruit radiosensitization is needed prior to serious discussion of clinical application.

6.10 SUMMARY POINTS

- Radiotherapy has been shown to enhance the apoptosis of cancer lines with fruit extract during *in vitro* studies.
- Fruits contain antioxidants like polyphenols that may play a role in the reduction of cancer cell survival.
- Each fruit has different modes of action on each cancer line via varying effects on apoptotic and proliferative factors.
- Cervical cancers exposed to blueberry extract showed 40% survival in conjunction with radiotherapy.
- Colonies treated with cranberry extract showed a 60% decrease in size with a decrease in expression of pro-proliferative markers.
- A melanoma cancer line showed a 70% decrease in surviving colonies after treatment with kiwi extract.
- A cervical cancer line showed a 60% decrease in surviving colonies after treatment with raspberry extract.

REFERENCES

Akhouri, Vivek, Manorma Kumari, and Arun Kumar 2020. "Therapeutic effect of *Aegle marmelos* fruit extract against DMBA induced breast cancer in rats 2020." *Scientific Reports* 10, no. 1 (October): 18016. doi:10.1038/s41598-020-72935-2

Arscott, William Tristram, Jaclyn Emmett, Alireza Fotouhi Ghiam, and Joshua A. Jones 2020. "Palliative radiotherapy: Inpatients, outpatients, and the changing role of supportive care in radiation oncology." *Hematology/Oncology Clinics of North America* 34, no. 1 (February): 253–277. doi:10.1016/j. hoc.2019.09.009

Aune, Dagfinn, Edward Giovannucci, Paolo Boffetta, Lars T. Fadnes, NaNa Keum, Teresa Norat, Darren C. Greenwood, Elio Riboli, Lars J. Vatten, and Serena Tonstad 2017. "Fruit and vegetable intake and the risk of cardiovascular disease, total cancer and all-cause mortality – a systematic review and dose-response meta-analysis of prospective studies." *International Journal of Epidemiology* 46, no. 3 (June): 1029–1056. doi:10.1093/ije/dyw319

Bai, Qian, Zachary E. Hunzeker, Ziwen Zhu, Marco Lequio, Conner M. Willson, Huaping Xiao, Mark R. Wakefield, and Yujiang Fang 2021. "Cranberry extract is a potent radiosensitizer for glioblastoma." *Anticancer Research* 41, no. 7 (July): 3337–3341. doi:10.21873/anticanres.15121

Baskar, Rajamanickam, Kuo Ann Lee, Richard Yeo, and Kheng-Wei Yeoh 2012. "Cancer and radiation therapy: Current advances and future directions." *International Journal of Medical Sciences* 9, no. 3 (February): 193–199. doi:10.7150/ijms.3635

Bell, Lynne, and Claire M. Williams 2021. "Blueberry benefits to cognitive function across the lifespan." *International Journal of Food Sciences and Nutrition* 72, no. 5 (August): 650–652. doi:10.1080/096374 86.2020.1852192

Citrin, Deborah E. 2019. "Radiation modifiers." *Hematology/Oncology Clinics of North America* 33, no. 6 (December): 1041–1055. doi:10.1016/j.hoc.2019.08.004

Coleman, Christina M. and Daneel Ferreira 2020. "Oligosaccharides and complex carbohydrates: A new paradigm for cranberry bioactivity." *Molecules* 25, no. 4 (February): 881. doi:10.3390/molecules25040881

Dandawate, Prasad R., Dharmalingam Subramaniam, Subhash B. Padhye, and Shrikant Anant 2016. "Bitter melon: A panacea for inflammation and cancer." *Chinese Journal of Natural Medicines* 14, no. 2 (February): 81–100. doi:10.1016/S1875-5364(16)60002-X

Davidson, Kristoffer T., Ziwen Zhu, Qian Bai, Huaping Xiao, Mark R. Wakefield, and Yujiang Fang 2019. "Blueberry as a potential radiosensitizer for treating cervical cancer." *Pathology Oncology Research: POR* 25, no. 1 (January): 81–88. doi:10.1007/s12253-017-0319-y

Fang, Yujiang, Vincent G. DeMarco, and Michael B. Nicholl 2012. "Resveratrol enhances radiation sensitivity in prostate cancer by inhibiting cell proliferation and promoting cell senescence and apoptosis." *Cancer Science* 103, no. 6 (April): 1090–1098. doi:10.1111/j.1349-7006.2012.02272.x

Galiniak, Sabina, David Aebishern, and Doroto Bartusik-Aebisher 2019. "Health benefits of resveratrol administration." *Acta Biochimica Polonica* 66, no. 1 (February): 13–21. doi:10.18388/abp.2018_2749

Ganesan, Kumar, and Baojun Xu 2017. "Polyphenol-rich lentils and their health promoting effects." *International Journal of Molecular Sciences* 18, no. 11 (November): 2390. doi:10.3390/ijms18112390

Gao, Xueliang, Gustavo W. Leone, and Haizhen Wang 2020. "Cyclin D-CDK4/6 functions in cancer." *Advances in Cancer Research* 148 (April): 147–169. doi:10.1016/bs.acr.2020.02.002

Hazafa, Abu, Khalil-Ur- Rehman, Nazish Jahan, and Zara Jabeen 2020. "The role of polyphenol (flavonoids) compounds in the treatment of cancer cells." *Nutrition and Cancer* 72, no. 3 (July): 386–397. doi:10.10 80/01635581.2019.1637006

Kantapan, Jiraporn, Nathupakorn Dechsupa, Damrongsak Tippanya, Wannapha Nobnop and Imjai Chitapanarux 2021. "Gallotannin from *Bouea macrophylla* seed extract suppresses cancer stem-like cells and radiosensitizes head and neck cancer." *International Journal of Molecular Sciences* 22, no. 17 (August): 9253. doi:10.3390/ijms22179253

Kawamura, Hidemasa, Nobuteru Kubo, Hiro Sato, Yuhei Miyasaka, Hiroshi Matsui, Kazuto Ito, Kazuhiro Suzuki, and Tatsuya Ohno 2020. "Quality of life in prostate cancer patients receiving particle radiotherapy: A review of the literature." *International Journal of Urology: Official Journal of the Japanese Urological Association* 27, no. 1 (January): 24–29. doi:10.1111/iju.14102

Kou, Leon, Ziwen Zhu, Chase Redington, Qian Bai, Mark Wakefield, Marco Lequio, and Yujiang Fang 2021. "Potential use of kiwifruit for treatment of melanoma." *Medical Oncology* 38, no. 3 (February): 25. doi:10.21873/anticanres.15413

Livshits, Zhanna, Rama B. Rao., and Silas W. Smith. 2014. "An approach to chemotherapy-associated toxicity." *Emergency Medicine Clinics of North America* 32, no. 1 (February): 167–203. doi:10.1016/j.emc.2013.09.002

Macaluso, Marcella, Micaela Montanari, Caterina Cinti, and Antonio Giordano 2005. "Modulation of cell cycle components by epigenetic and genetic events." *Seminars in Oncology* 32, no. 5 (October): 452–457. doi:10.1053/j.seminoncol.2005.07.009

Miller, Victoria, Andrew Mente, Mahshid Dehghan, Sumathy Rangarajan, Xiaohe Zhang, Sumathi Swaminathan, Gilles Dagenais, et al. 2017. "Fruit, vegetable, and legume intake, and cardiovascular disease and deaths in 18 countries (PURE): A prospective cohort study." *Lancet* 390, no. 10107 (November): 2037–2049. doi:10.1016/S0140-6736(17)32253-5

Mohanraj, Remya, and Subha Sivasankar 2014. "Sweet potato (*Ipomoea batatas* [L.] Lam)–a valuable medicinal food: A review." *Journal of Medicinal Food* 17, no. 7 (July): 733–741. doi:10.1089/jmf.2013.2818

Ni, Chunlei, BaiLing Li, Yangyue Ding, Yue Wu, Qiuye Wang, Jiarong Wang, and Jianjun Cheng 2021. "Anti-cancer properties of Coix seed oil against HT-29 colon cells through regulation of the PI3K/AKT signaling pathway." *Foods (Basel, Switzerland)* 10, no. 11 (November): 2833. doi:10.3390/foods10112833

Nisa, Fatma Zuhrotun, Mary Astuti, Agnes Murdiati, and Sofia Mubarika Haryana 2017. "Anti-proliferation and apoptosis induction of aqueous leaf extract of *Carica papaya* L. on human breast cancer cells MCF-7." *Pakistan Journal of Biological Sciences: PJBS* 20, no. 1 (December): 36–41. doi:10.3923/pjbs.2017.36.41

Nozaki, Reo, Toru Kono, Hiroki Bochimoto, Tsuyoshi Watanabe, Kaori Oketani, Yuichi Sakamaki, Naoto Okubo, Koji Nakagawa, and Hiroshi Takeda 2016. "Zanthoxylum fruit extract from Japanese pepper promotes autophagic cell death in cancer cells." *Oncotarget* 7, no. 43 (October): 70437–70446. doi:10.18632/oncotarget.11926

Paller, C. J., A. Pantuck, and M. A. Carducci 2017. "A review of pomegranate in prostate cancer." *Prostate Cancer and Prostatic Diseases* 20, no. 3 (September): 270. doi:10.1038/pcan.2017.19

Pitchakarn, Pornsiri, Kumiko Ogawa, Shugo Suzuki, Satoru Takahashi, Makoto Asamoto, Teera Chewonarin, Pornngram Limtrakul, and Tomoyuki Shirai 2010. "*Momordica charantia* leaf extract suppresses rat prostate cancer progression in vitro and in vivo." *Cancer Science* 101, no. 10 (October): 2234–2240. doi:10.1111/j.1349-7006.2010.01669.x

Rao, Amanda, Elizabeth Steels, Warrick J. Inder, Suzanne Abraham, and Luis Vitetta 2016. "Testofen, a specialised *Trigonella foenum-graecum* seed extract reduces age-related symptoms of androgen decrease, increases testosterone levels and improves sexual function in healthy aging males in a double-blind randomised clinical study." *The Aging Male: The Official Journal of the International Society for the Study of the Aging Male* 19, no. 2 (June): 134–142. doi:10.3109/13685538.2015.1135323

Reza, A. S. M. Ali, Md Anwarul Haque, Joy Sarker, Mst Samima Nasrin, Md Mahbubur Rahman, Au Montakim Tareq, Zidan Khan, Mamunur Rashid, Md Golam Sadik, Toshifumi Tsukahara, and Ahm Khurshid Alam 2021. "Antiproliferative and antioxidant potentials of bioactive edible vegetable fraction of *Achyranthes ferruginea* Roxb. in cancer cell line." *Food Science & Nutrition* 9, no. 7 (June): 3777–3805. doi:10.1002/fsn3.2343

Richardson, David P., Juliet Ansell, and Lynley N. Drummond 2018. "The nutritional and health attributes of kiwifruit: A review." *European Journal of Nutrition* 57, no. 8 (December): 2659–2676. doi:10.1007/s00394-018-1627-z

Sangsefidi, Zohreh Sadat, Faezeh Yarhosseini, Mahdieh Hosseinzadeh, Alimohammad Ranjbar, Mohsen Akhondi-Meybodi, Hossein Fallahzadeh, and Hassan Mozaffari-Khosravi 2021. "The effect of (*Cornus mas* L.) fruit extract on liver function among patients with nonalcoholic fatty liver: A double-blind randomized clinical trial." *Phytotherapy Research: PTR* 35, no. 9 (September): 5259–5268. doi:10.1002/ptr.7199

Sham, Nelson, Chenglu Qin, Ziwen Zhu, Chase G. Redington, Huaping Xiao, Qian Bai, Mark R. Wakefield, Leon Kou, and Yujiang Fang 2021. "Raspberry extract with potential antitumor activity against cervical cancer." *Anticancer Research* 41, no. 7 (July): 3343–3348. doi:10.21873/anticanres.15122

Shu, Chih-Wen, Jing-Ru Weng, Hsueh-Wei Chang, Pei-Feng Liu, Jih-Jung Chen, Chien-Chi Peng, Jia-Wen Huang, Wei-Yu Lin, and Ching-Yu Yen 2021. "*Tribulus terrestris* fruit extract inhibits autophagic flux to diminish cell proliferation and metastatic characteristics of oral cancer cells." *Environmental Toxicology* 36, no. 6 (June): 1173–1180. doi:10.1002/tox.23116

Singh, Ajay P., Ted Wilson, Amanda J. Kalk, James Cheong, and Nicholi Vorsa 2009. "Isolation of specific cranberry flavonoids for biological activity assessment." *Food Chemistry* 116, no. 4 (October): 963–968. doi:10.1016/j.foodchem.2009.03.062

Soerjomataram, Isabelle, Dian Oomen, Valery Lemmens, Anke Oenema, Vassiliki, Benetou, Antonio Trichopoulou, Jan Willem Coebergh, Jan Barendregt, and Esther de Vries 2010. "Increased consumption of fruit and vegetables and future cancer incidence in selected European countries." *European Journal of Cancer* 46, no. 14 (September): 2563–2580. doi:10.1016/j.ejca.2010.07.026

Tosoc, John Paul Sese, Olga Macas Nuñeza, Thangirala Sudha, Noureldien H. E. Darwish, and Shaker A. Mousa 2021. "Anticancer effects of the *Corchorus olitorius* aqueous extract and its bioactive compounds on human cancer cell lines." *Molecules (Basel, Switzerland)* 26, no. 19 (October): 6033. doi:10.3390/molecules26196033

Tran, Phuong H. L., and Thao T. D. Tran 2021. "Blueberry supplementation in neuronal health and protective technologies for efficient delivery of blueberry anthocyanins." *Biomolecules* 11, no. 1 (January): 102. doi:10.3390/biom11010102

Upadya, Haridas, S. Prabhu, Avarinda Prasad, Deepa Subramanian, Swati Gupta, and Ajay Goel 2019. "A randomized, double blind, placebo controlled, multicenter clinical trial to assess the efficacy and safety of *Emblica officinalis* extract in patients with dyslipidemia." *BMC Complementary and Alternative Medicine* 19, no. 1 (January): 27. doi:10.1186/s12906-019-2430-y

Wang, C. C. 1999. *Clinical Radiation Oncology: Indications, Techniques, and Results*. Hoboken: J. Wiley & Sons.

Wang, Hao, Xaioyu Mu, Hua He, and Xiao-Dong Zhang 2018. "Cancer radiosensitizers." *Trends in Pharmacological Sciences* 39, no. 1 (December): 24–48. doi:10.1016/j.tips.2017.11.003

Wheatley, Sally P. and Dario C. Altieri 2019. "Survivin at a glance." *Journal of Cell Science* 132, no. 7 (April): jcs223826. doi:10.1242/jcs.223826

Xu, Lishan, Jingjing Cao, and Wenrong Chen 2015. "Structural characterization of a broccoli polysaccharide and evaluation of anti-cancer cell proliferation effects." *Carbohydrate Polymers* 126 (August): 179–184. doi:10.1016/j.carbpol.2015.03.011

Zeb, Alam 2020. "Concept, mechanism, and applications of phenolic antioxidants in foods." *Journal of Food Biochemistry* 44, no. 9 (September): e13394. doi:10.1111/jfbc.13394

Section II

Specific Agents, Items and Extracts

7 Amur Maackia (*Maackia amurensis*) Seed Lectin History and Potential Effect on Cancer Progression, Inflammation and Viral Infection

Tyler J. Hellmig, Eamonn J. Brace, Amanda Greenspan, Christopher Laugier, Abhay Aradhya, Sayan Basu, Saumil Parikh, Katarzyna Jachimowska, Xiaoxuan (Farrah) Wu, Yongquan Shen, Kelly L. Hamilton and Gary S. Goldberg

ABBREVIATIONS

ACE2	angiotensin-converting enzyme 2
ALL	acute lymphoblastic leukemia
Ang	angiotensin
CA-125	cancer antigen 125
CD43	leukosialin
ConA	concanavalin A
Gal	galactose
GalNAc	*N*-acetylgalactosamine
JAK-STAT	Janus kinase–signal transducer and activator of transcription
MAPK	mitogen-activated protein kinase
MASL	*Maackia Amurensis* seed lectin
ML1	mistletoe lectin
mTOR	mammalian target of rapamycin
Muc1	mucin
Muc16	mucin 16
NF-κB	nuclear factor kappa B
Nrp1	neuropilin-1
NSCLC	non–small cell lung cancer (NSCLC)
OSCC	oral squamous cell carcinoma
PDPN	podoplanin
PNA	peanut agglutinin
RAAS	renin–angiotensin–aldosterone system
TF antigen	Thomsen-Friedenreich antigen
TGFβ	transforming growth factor beta
VEGF	vascular endothelial growth factor

DOI: 10.1201/9781003260028-9

7.1 INTRODUCTION AND *MAACKIA AMURENSIS* HISTORY

Maackia amurensis (also called Amur maackia) is a legume tree native to the Amur River region in northeastern China, Korea, and Russia. It was named in honor of the 19th-century naturalist Richard Otto (or Karlovic) Maack noted for his exploration of the Amur River valleys along the Siberian and Chinese borders (Ruprecht, 1856). It is grown today as a hardy ornamental tree in many areas of the world.

M. amurensis has a long history as a medicinal plant. It was documented in the ancient Chinese book *Er Ya* (尔雅), which was compiled as early as 1100 BC by Dan Ji, then edited and complemented by Confucius and his students no later than 200 BC. The *Er Ya* contains commentaries on art, nature, and living creatures (Pu, 1987). It describes three kinds of Huai (槐). The most common was called Guo Huai (国槐), with slim and light green leaves, and is currently known as *Sophora japonica* (Tang and Eisenbrand, 1992). Shou Gong Huai (守宫槐), with leaves closing at daytime and opening at night, has not been identified in recent literature. Finally, Huai Huai (怀槐), with big dark green leaves, has been identified as *M. amurensis* (Andrews, 1997; Ruprecht, 1856).

Almost 1000 years after the *Er Ya*, *M. amurensis* usage was recorded in the Chinese medicine encyclopedia *Bencao Tujing* (本草图经), which was written by Song Su in AD 1061. The *Bencao Tujing* describes up to 780 plants, animals, and minerals used in Chinese medicine, with 103 of them updated as new discoveries at that time (Cai, 1991). The *Bencao Tujing* describes a decoction prepared from the bark of *M. amurensis* to be used to treat hematochezia, which often results from colon cancer (Barnert and Messmann, 2009).

The *Bencao Gangmu* (本草纲目), or "Compendium of Materia Medica" published by Shizhen Li in 1596, also describes *M. amurensis* as a medicinal plant (see Figure 7.1). It prescribes a decoction

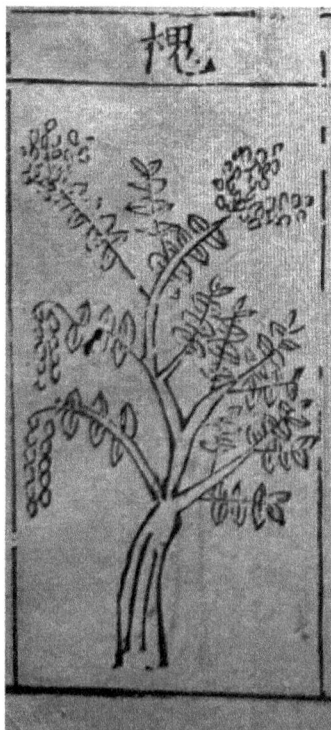

FIGURE 7.1 *Maackia amurensis* image from *Bencao Gangmu*.

to treat gastrointestinal bleeding complicated by cancers (Li, 1593). This solution is currently prescribed to be orally administered once a day to treat cancer, deep wounds, chronic ulcers, arthritis, cholecystitis, and other diseases (Sciences, 1955). Thus, *M. amurensis* has been utilized in traditional Chinese medicine for over 2000 years. In addition to China, *M. amurensis* extracts have been used to treat cancer and inflammation in Korea and Russia for many centuries (Fedoreev et al., 2010; Liu, 1997; Sun et al., 2008).

M. amurensis extracts contain a variety of compounds including flavonoids, alkaloids, polyphenols, and stilbenes (Fedoreev et al., 2010; Liu, 1997; Sun et al., 2008). However, *M. amurensis* lectin is an extremely abundant protein in the bark and seed extracts, and exhibits significant potential to inhibit viral infection, inflammation, and cancer progression (Carpintero-Fernandez et al., 2020; Hamilton et al., 2021; Honma et al., 2017; Kapoor et al., 2008; Ochoa-Alvarez et al., 2012; Sheehan et al., 2021).

7.2 LECTINS

Lectins are naturally occurring proteins. The word "lectin" is derived from the Latin word *legere*, which means "to select." Lectins are ubiquitous and found in virtually all organisms. They can be found throughout the cell, including the nucleus, cytoplasm, cell membranes, and can be secreted extracellularly (De Coninck and Van Damme, 2021). Mammalian lectins, often called "galectins," play important roles in numerous biological events, including defense against infections, immunity, intercellular interactions, signal transduction, cell migration, and cancer (Sharon and Lis, 2004). This chapter focuses on plant lectins, particularly *M. amurensis* seed lectin (MASL).

Lectins bind reversibly, but with high specificity and affinity, to sugar moieties on glycolipids and glycoproteins (De Coninck and Van Damme, 2021). These targets include mannose, galactose, *N*-acetylglucosamine, and sialic acids. Examples of a few lectins including peanut agglutinin (PNA), jacalin, concanavalin A (ConA), ricin, mistletoe lectin (ML1), and MASL along with their carbohydrate binding affinities are shown in Table 7.1.

Lectins generally do not generally possess intrinsic enzymatic activity (De Coninck and Van Damme, 2021). However, lectins exist as potentially bioactive ingredients in virtually all of our daily foods. These dietary lectins can exert effects since, unlike most proteins including antibodies, they can survive digestion to mediate systemic effects. For example, 100 g of raw peanuts can contain over 150 mg of peanut agglutinin (PNA). The concentration of bioactive PNA was found to be 50 nM in the blood of human subjects 1 hour after consuming 200 g of peanuts (Wang et al., 1998). These data demonstrate how plant lectins can resist gastrointestinal proteolysis to enter the circulatory system as bioactive food components. PNA is produced by *Arachis hypogaea* as a tetramer formed by identical 27.5 kD subunits which combine to produce a lectin of 110 kD. PNA has affinity

TABLE 7.1
Examples of Plant Lectins and Binding Moieties

Lectin	Source	Target Binding Domain
Maackia amurensis **seed lectin (MASL)**	Amur maackia	α-2,3 and α-2,6 sialic acids
Ricin	*Ricinus communis* (castor beans)	N-acetylgalactosamine and β-1,4 galactose
Mistletoe lectin	*Viscum album*	O-linked α-2,3 sialic acids
Jacalin-related lectins (JRL)	*Artocarpus heterophyllus* (jackfruit)	Galβ1–3GalNAc
Peanut agglutinin (PNA)	*Arachis hypogaea*	Galβ1–3GalNAc
Concanavalin A (Con A)	*Canavalia ensiformis* (jack bean seeds)	N-linked hexasaccharides, methyl mannosides, and methylglucosides

for O-linked glycoproteins including the Thomsen-Friedenreich antigen (TF antigen). The TF antigen is a disaccharide formed by O-glycosylation of galactosyl (β-1,3) *N*-acetylgalactosamine onto serine and threonine residues. This immunoreactive glycoantigen is rarely found in healthy cells but is frequently expressed by cancer cells, particularly endothelial carcinomas. PNA selectively binds to the Galβ1–3GalNAc core of the TF antigen (Cao et al., 1996). The binding specificity of PNA is similar to Jacalin-related lectins, as shown in Table 7.1.

Jacalins are a family of lectins isolated from the seeds of *Artocarpus heterophyllus*, more commonly known as jackfruit. Jacalin have a tetrameric structure with a molecular weight of 66 kD. Jacalin binds to O-linked Galβ1–3GalNAc residues of the TF antigen similar to, but with a higher affinity than, PNA. However, in contrast to PNA, jacalin can bind to sialylated forms of the TF antigen. This produces more carbohydrate interactions with especially strong electrostatic bonds and stability. The high affinity of jacalin for the TF antigen has been used in several applications. For example, it can be used to detect gastric and colorectal cancers (Hoffmann et al., 2020).

Concanavalin A (ConA) is a legume lectin extracted from jack beans (*Canavalia ensiformis*). ConA binds strongly to non-reducing terminal α-d-mannosyl and α-d-glucosyl groups in a manner dependent on calcium and manganese divalent cations. ConA can inhibit the growth of a number of cancer cell types (Li et al., 2011). For example, ConA can induce mitochondrial membrane collapse and caspase-dependent apoptosis in human melanoma cells (Liu et al., 2009).

Ricin is derived from the seeds of the castor bean plant (*Ricinus communis*). This lectin was first described as a highly toxic hemagglutinin in the 1880s (Lord et al., 1994). Like many lectins, ricin is a glycoprotein made up of A and B chains. The B chain binds to galactose (Gal) and *N*-acetylgalactosamine (GalNAc) in order to direct cell binding, uptake, and intracellular trafficking (Vance et al., 2020). The A chain is highly toxic since it contains a type 2 ribosome inactivating protein (RIP) domain. This RIP domain removes an adenine residue from the 28S ribosome RNA loop, which inactivates protein synthesis and leads to apoptosis. Foreign agents used a microscopic ricin pellet packed into the tip of an umbrella to assassinate the Bulgarian journalist Georgi Markov in a crowded London subway station in 1978. This "umbrella murder" lends a nefarious reputation to ricin that attests to the strong biological potential of plant lectins (Audi et al., 2005).

Mistletoe lectin binds to O-linked glycans containing α-2,3-sialic acid. Three mistletoe lectin isoforms have been described: ML1, ML2, and ML3. Mistletoe lectins possess a cytotoxic A chain and galactose binding B chains connected to each other by disulfide bonds. Like ricin, the mistletoe lectin A chain contains a cytotoxic type 2 RIP domain that inhibits protein synthesis at the ribosomal level (Poiroux et al., 2017). ML1 has been found to have immunomodulatory properties with the potential to inhibit tumor cell growth and metastasis. Indeed, ML1 is currently used to treat melanoma in Europe (Augustin et al., 2005) and is being studied in clinical trials aimed at pancreatic cancer (NCT02948309).

MASL is the major focus of this chapter. MASL consists of a tetramer formed by two 32 kD and two 37 kD subunits. These subunits have identical amino acid sequences, as shown in Figure 7.2. The primary sequence contains a C-terminal cysteine residue that enables them to form a disulfide bridge

```
1    sdelsftinn fvpneadllf qgeasvsstg vlqltrveng qpqqysvgra lyaapvriwd
61   nttgsvasfs tsftfvvkap nptitsdgla fflappdsqi psgrvskylg lfnnsnsdss
121  nqivavefdt yfghsydpwd pnyrhigidv ngiesiktvq wdwinggvaf atitylapnk
181  tliaslvyps nqtsfivaas vdlkeilpew vrvgfsaatg yptqvethdv lswsftstle
241  ancdaaten
```

FIGURE 7.2   Primary amino acid sequence of MASL.

and dimerize with each other (Ochoa-Alvarez et al., 2012). MASL is heavily glycosylated and has a strong affinity to glycans containing α-2,3-sialic acid moieties like ML1 (Kawaguchi et al., 1974; Yamamoto et al., 1997). However, unlike ML1, MASL does not contain a RIP domain. Rather, MASL contains an L-type lectin domain that is not inherently cytotoxic (Cummings and Etzler, 2009).

7.3 MASL TARGETS

Lectins target a variety of receptors that contain glycosylation sites needed to direct functions including cell adhesion, growth, and motility. In particular, MASL binds to α-2,3 sialic acid residues on extracellular receptors (Carpintero-Fernandez et al., 2020; Imberty et al., 2000; Ochoa-Alvarez et al., 2012). Therefore, identifying receptors that contain α-2,3 sialic acid residues should yield insights into how MASL might affect cell behavior. Some examples of these receptors include mucin 1 (Muc1), mucin 16 (Muc16), leukosialin (CD43), angiotensin-converting enzyme 2 (ACE2), and podoplanin (PDPN).

The Muc1 receptor is expressed on epithelial cells. It is upregulated in epithelial cancers including carcinomas of the lung, liver, breast, pancreas, and ovaries. In general, Muc1 appears to affect Janus kinase–signal transducer and activator of transcription (JAK-STAT) signaling to regulate inflammation, and increase mitogen activated protein kinase (MAPK) and vascular endothelial growth factor (VEGF) signaling that drives malignant neovascularization. Muc1 also regulates mammalian target of rapamycin (mTOR) and neuropilin-1 (Nrp1) activity in order to promote tumor progression (Chen et al., 2021).

The Muc16 receptor is expressed on epithelial cells where it serves as a mucosal barrier protein. However, Muc16 also serves as a clinically relevant biomarker called cancer antigen 125 (CA-125). Indeed, CA-125 is regarded as a biomarker for ovarian carcinoma and gastrointestinal tumors including pancreatic ductal adenocarcinoma, esophageal adenocarcinoma, gastric adenocarcinoma, and colorectal adenocarcinoma (Aithal et al., 2018; Chen et al., 2021).

The leukosialin (CD43) receptor is typically expressed by T lymphocytes, monocytes, granulocytes, and some B lymphocytes (de Laurentiis et al., 2011). The receptor is decorated with approximately 80 O-linked glycans, particularly α-2,3 sialic acids, that play a key role in its ability to affect T cell development, activation, and survival (Clark and Baum, 2012). Abnormal expression of this receptor has also been found in various lymphomas including MALTomas, T cell lymphomas, and B-cell lymphoblastic lymphoma (Arends et al., 1999).

The ACE2 receptor is a monocarboxypeptidase type I transmembrane glycoprotein. This receptor is expressed in various tissues including lung alveolar epithelial, heart, kidney, and gastrointestinal cells. ACE2 functions in the renin-angiotensin-aldosterone system (RAAS), which regulates blood volume and systemic vascular pressure. More specifically, ACE2 converts angiotensin (Ang) I to Ang (1–9) and Ang II to Ang (1–7) (Wiese et al., 2021). Ang (1–7) opposes vasoconstriction and proliferation to inhibit vascular cellular growth and inflammation (Simoes e Silva et al., 2013). In addition to its role in the RAAS system, ACE2 is also the entry receptor for SARS-CoV viruses, including SARS-CoV-2 which is responsible for COVID-19. The SARS viral spike protein targets the human ACE2 receptor to initiate infection. The viral spike and ACE2 proteins are highly glycosylated with sialic acid modifications, specifically α-2,3 and α-2,6 O-linked sialic acid residues. These modifications on the ACE2 cell receptor are needed for viral-host interactions and infection. MASL targets the ACE2 receptor, decreases ACE2 expression and glycosylation, suppresses binding of the SARS-CoV-2 spike protein, and decreases expression of inflammatory mediators that lead to acute respiratory distress syndrome (ARDS), as described below (Sheehan et al., 2021).

The podoplanin (PDPN) receptor mediates signaling events that direct a wide array of processes including circulatory system and organ development, inflammation, tumorigenesis, and viral infection. PDPN serves as an influenza virus receptor, and PDPN interactions with endogenous ligands and binding partners promote inflammation and cancer progression. The PDPN extracellular domain is heavily glycosylated with α-2,3 sialic acids (Krishnan et al., 2019, 2018; Quintanilla et al., 2019; Suzuki et al., 2022). Consequently, MASL can target the PDPN receptor to inhibit arthritis and cancer progression, as described below.

7.4 MASL AND CANCER

PDPN has emerged as a biologically relevant cancer biomarker and chemotherapeutic target. Increased PDPN expression is found in a variety of cancers, particularly in transformed cells that override contact normalization to break away from their microenvironment in order to realize their malignant and metastatic potential (Krishnan et al., 2019; Sheehan et al., 2022; Suzuki et al., 2022). Oncogenic kinase activity induces PDPN expression, which increases Rho GTPase activity to promote tumor cell invasion. RhoA, Rac1, and Cdc42 GTPases regulate cell protrusion, retraction, and polarity to direct cell migration (Acton et al., 2014; Ochoa-Alvarez et al., 2015; Shen et al., 2010; Wicki et al., 2006). MASL has been shown to target PDPN and inhibit Cdc42 activity required to establish cell polarity and directional cell migration. Consequentially, MASL can effectively inhibit tumor cell motility, including melanoma and oral squamous cell carcinoma (OSCC) cell migration at nanomolar concentrations (Hamilton et al., 2021; Krishnan et al., 2019; Ochoa-Alvarez et al., 2015; Ochoa-Alvarez et al., 2012; Retzbach et al., 2018).

In addition to inhibiting tumor cell motility, MASL can also inhibit tumor cell growth and viability. MASL has been reported to induce apoptosis of childhood acute lymphoblastic leukemic (ALL) cells (Kapoor et al., 2008). MASL can also enhance paclitaxel toxicity, induce BAX activity, and suppress Bcl-XL activity in order to activate caspases and cause apoptosis of non–small cell lung cancer (NSCLC) cells (Chhetra Lalli et al., 2019; Lalli et al., 2015; Mehta et al., 2013). However, MASL can kill colonic adenocarcinoma cells with and without caspase activity (Parshenkov and Hennet, 2022). MASL can also enhance doxorubicin and 5-fluorouracil toxicity, and trigger a mitochondrial permeability transition pore (MPTP) to kill human oral squamous cell carcinoma (OSCC) cells by caspase independent non-apoptotic necrosis (Ochoa-Alvarez et al., 2015).

In addition to affecting GTPase and cytotoxic activities that decrease tumor cell motility and viability, MASL also modulates oncogenic cascades including the Wnt-Bctn, TGFβ-SMAD, and JAK-STAT signaling pathways. These are scenarios shown schematically in Figure 7.3.

The Wnt-Bctn pathway has been linked to many cancers and is the driving force behind cancers resulting from adenomatous polyposis coli (APC) mutations (Klaus and Birchmeier, 2008). MASL inhibits the expression of at least 50 genes induced by Wnt-Bctn signaling including Wnt10a, Fzd2, and Sox2 (Hamilton et al., 2021). The Wnt10a ligand has been associated with cancers including renal cell, esophageal squamous cell, and colon carcinomas (Hsu et al., 2012; Kirikoshi et al., 2001; Nie et al., 2020). Wnt ligands bind to the Fzd2 receptor to activate oncogenic gene expression. These genes include the Sox2 transcription factor, which induces reversal of differentiated cells to stem cells and is implicated in a number of cancers including ovarian carcinoma, mammary carcinoma, and glioblastoma multiforme (Kinney et al., 2020; Schaefer and Lengerke, 2020).

TGFβ signaling phosphorylates SMADs, which translocate to the nucleus and induce expression of genes that can promote cancer progression (Tewari et al., 2022). These effectors can promote

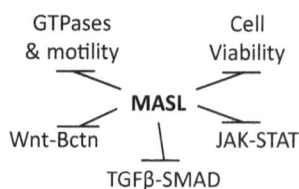

FIGURE 7.3 MASL can suppress oncogenic signaling cascades and increase apoptotic and necrotic pathways to inhibit cancer progression as indicated.

stromal cell recruitment and increase tumor spread (Motoyama et al., 2008; Yokoyama et al., 2017). MASL has been shown to decrease expression of the several members of this pathway including the Tgfbr3 receptor kinase, Smad5 and Smad6, and downstream effectors including Bmp4 and Bmp7 in OSCC cells (Hamilton et al., 2021).

A variety of factors, often cytokines, target their cognate receptors to activate JAK kinases. Activated JAKs phosphorylate STATs, which then enter the nucleus to induce expression of genes that can promote cell growth and motility. JAK-STAT signaling is implicated in a number of cancers including leukemias and lymphomas (Bousoik and Montazeri Aliabadi, 2018; Gadina et al., 2019). MASL modulates the expression of over 150 genes associated in the JAK-STAT pathway. For example, MASL increases the expression of the Kruppel-like factor Klf6 tumor suppressor in OSCC cells (Hamilton et al., 2021). Interestingly, Klf6 has been reported to inhibit OSCC cell migration and invasion (Hsu et al., 2017). Decreased Klf6 expression has also been found in prostate and colorectal cancers (Narla et al., 2001; Reeves et al., 2004). In addition to inducing the expression of tumor suppressor genes, MASL also decreases expression of tumor promoters associated with the JAK-STAT pathway. These include the Jak2 kinase, as well as Stat1 and Stat2 signal transducers which have been implicated in a number of malignancies including colorectal and skin cancers (O'Shea et al., 2015; Thomas et al., 2015).

Taken together, MASL inhibits oncogenic TGFβ-SMAD, JAK-STAT, and Wnt-Bctn signaling pathways, while also triggering caspase independent cell death and decreasing cell motility in a variety of cancers. MASL is a clear candidate for inclusion in the pharmacopeia of natural products with anticancer potential. Indeed, MASL is currently the focus of a human clinical trial aimed at oral cancer (NTC04188665). However, MASL shows potential to inhibit a variety of other cancers, as indicated by results shown in Figure 7.4.

7.5 MASL AND INFLAMMATION

Protein glycosylation modifications are associated with a variety of inflammatory diseases. In particular, alterations α-2,6 and α-2,3 sialic acids on chondrocytes are associated with arthritic progression and cartilage damage (Toegel et al., 2010; Wang et al., 2021). Endogenous lectins (galectins) target these glycoprotein carbohydrate motifs to affect extracellular matrix production, migration, growth, and inflammation. For example, galectins with affinity to α-2,3 sialic acid motifs presented by receptors on chondrocytes promote arthritic joint and bone destruction (Leppanen et al., 2005; Toegel et al., 2016).

Glycoprotein receptor activation stimulates the NF-κB pathway to induce inflammation that leads to arthritic conditions. This NF-κB activation induces cytokine production, particularly TNF-α and interleukins (e.g., IL-6 and IL-17), which initiate JAK-STAT and Src kinase signaling pathways that cause cartilage destruction (Akeson and Malemud, 2017; Lawrence, 2009; Toegel et al., 2016). PDPN has been identified as a receptor that galectins target to initiate this process, and is, therefore, an enticing therapeutic target (Carpintero-Fernandez et al., 2020; Ekwall et al., 2011; Krishnan et al., 2019; Takakubo et al., 2017). MASL can target PDPN to affect oncogenic signaling cascades, as described above. MASL can also target PDPN on chondrocytes and to decrease inflammatory signaling cascades, as shown in Figure 7.5 (Carpintero-Fernandez et al., 2020). One-hour treatment with 400 nM MASL significantly inhibits NF-κB nuclear translocation in arthritic human chondrocytes, and decreases IL-6 expression by twofold compared to parallel control cells. Accordingly, weekly oral MASL administration (40 mg/kg) effectively reduced cartilage extracellular matrix degradation in LPS-induced arthritic mice compared to placebo controls (Carpintero-Fernandez et al., 2020).

In addition to its involvement in arthritis, PDPN also plays a role in psoriasis. Erythematous skin plaques are a hallmark feature of psoriasis and psoriatic arthritis. In normal skin, PDPN is involved in the structure and function of sebaceous glands and hair follicles, but is not found in other areas of the epidermis. In contrast, robust PDPN expression is found in skin plaques of psoriasis lesions. Several factors can induce PDPN expression in keratinocytes including TGFβ along with IFNγ, IL-6, and IL-22 induced by JAK-STAT signaling (Honma et al., 2012). MASL has been shown to

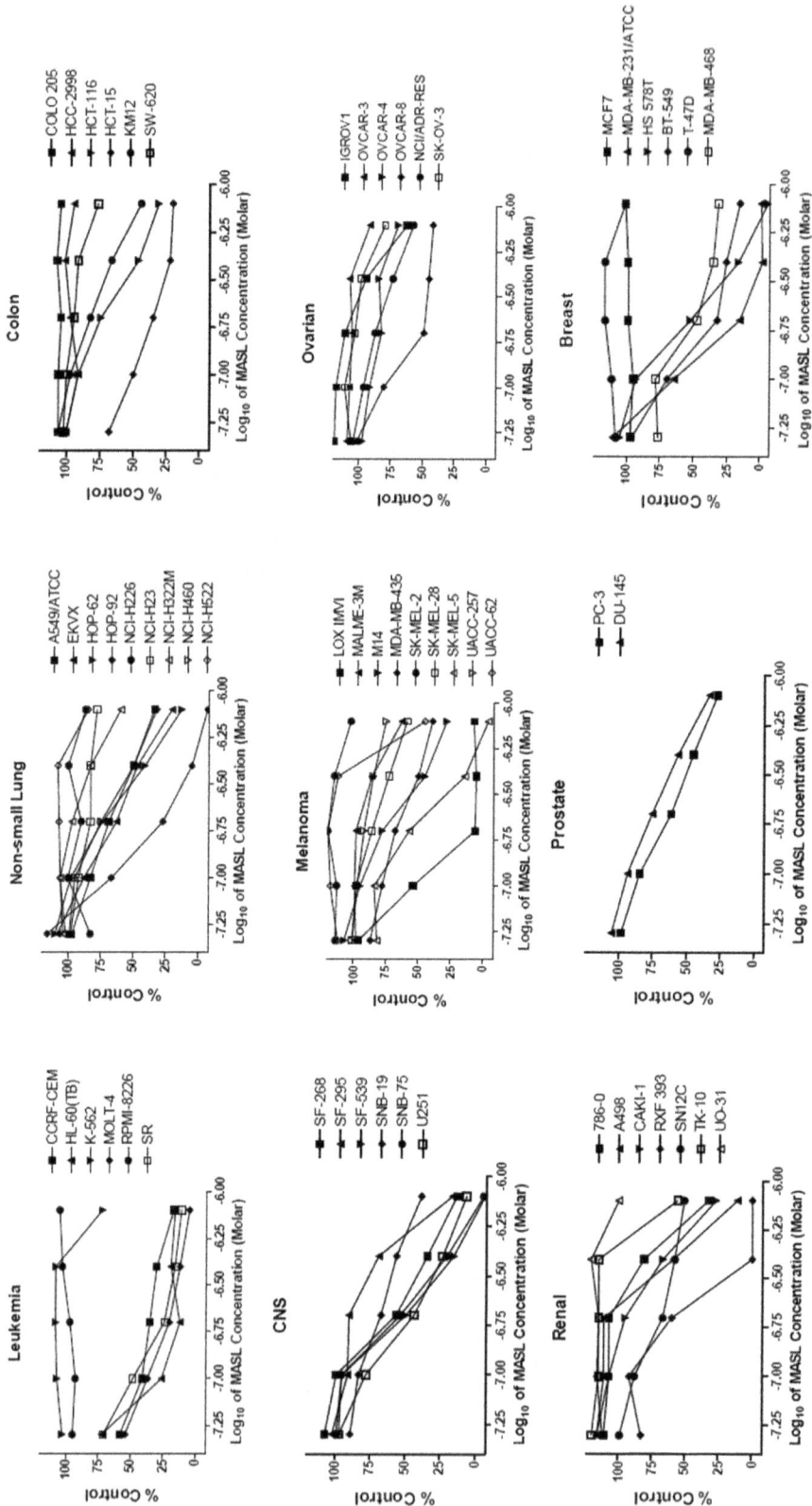

FIGURE 7.4 Effects of MASL on the NCI 60 cell line panel performed by the Developmental Therapeutics Program at the NCI. Cells were plated, grown for 24 hours, and then treated with indicated concentrations of MASL for 48 hours before evaluation by sulforhodamine B assay.

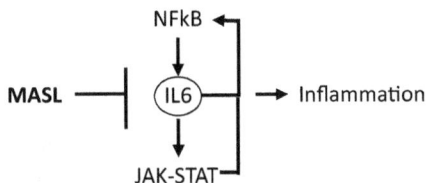

FIGURE 7.5   MASL inhibits NF-κB, interleukin, and JAK-STAT signaling cascades that cause arthritis and acute inflammatory syndromes.

suppress IL-22–induced keratinocyte hyperproliferation in reconstituted epidermis in cell culture (Honma et al., 2017).

In addition to arthritis, NF-κB, JAK-STAT, and IL-6 signaling events are also implicated in ARDS caused by inflammatory processes resulting from COVID-19 infection. During this process, IL-6 stimulates JAK-STAT signaling, which further increases IL-6 and NF-κB activity. NF-κB then further stimulates IL-6 production in a positive feedback mechanism referred to as the IL-6 amplifier, which induces the expression of additional cytokines such as IL-27 and TNF-α, and causes unbridled inflammation resulting in ARDS (Hirano and Murakami, 2020; Murakami et al., 2019). MASL can inhibit this inflammatory process, as shown in Figure 7.5. MASL has been shown to reduce NF-κB, IL-6, and JAK-STAT signaling in oral epithelial cells in a dose-dependent manner. Along with decreasing inflammatory signaling events, MASL treatment also increased the expression of anti-inflammatory proteins including HMOX1 and IL-36RN in these cells (Sheehan et al., 2021).

7.6   MASL ANTIVIRAL ACTIVITY

Viral and host receptor proteins are heavily glycosylated with motifs required for infection (Mitchell et al., 2017; Nabi-Afjadi et al., 2022). Lectins can target these motifs in order to inhibit viral-host interactions and subsequent infection. For example, bacterial cyanovirin-N and microvirin lectins bind to α-(1–2)-mannose moieties on the HIV viral GP120 envelope glycoprotein to prevent its interaction with the CD4 receptor needed for T-cell infection. In another example, *Galanthus nivalis* (snowdrop) agglutinin targets carbohydrates on envelope proteins to inhibit infection of viruses including SARS-CoV. Griffithsin lectin from red algae targets carbohydrate recognition domains on glycoproteins including the SARS-CoV spike protein to inhibit infection by viruses including HIV, hepatitis C virus (HCV), and the SARS-CoV coronavirus. Indeed, Griffithsin is being investigated as an antiviral agent in ongoing human clinical trials (Lee, 2019; Mitchell et al., 2017; Nabi-Afjadi et al., 2022).

Like Griffithsin, MASL can also associate with glycoproteins that mediate coronavirus infection. MASL targets sialic acid motifs that are presented by the SARS-CoV S1 spike protein and its host ACE2 receptor (Gong et al., 2021). In particular, MASL associates with the ACE2 receptor and decreases SARS-CoV-2 spike protein binding on human oral epithelial cells, as shown in Figure 7.6. In addition, MASL decreases ACE2 expression and sialic acid glycosylation in these cells. Consequentially, MASL also inhibits SARS-CoV-2 cytotoxic infection in a monkey kidney cell model system (Sheehan et al., 2021).

Results from recent studies indicate that MASL can also inhibit (BTV) infection. BTV is an orbivirus that uses its VP2 outer spike protein to infect host cells in domestic animals. VP2 has high affinity towards α-2,3 and α-2,6 sialic acid glycans on host receptors that mediate viral infection. *M. amurensis* lectin can, therefore, target these receptor motifs to inhibit BTV infection and virus propagation in susceptible sheep cells (Wu and Roy, 2022).

Like BTV, influenza virus also targets α-2,3 sialic acid residues on host cell receptors. Thus, potential influenza viral receptors include PDPN with is heavily glycosylated with sialic acids as described above. Interestingly, influenza infection induces PDPN expression in lung epithelial cells (Hofer et al., 2015). MASL has been shown to target PDPN and decreases its expression in human

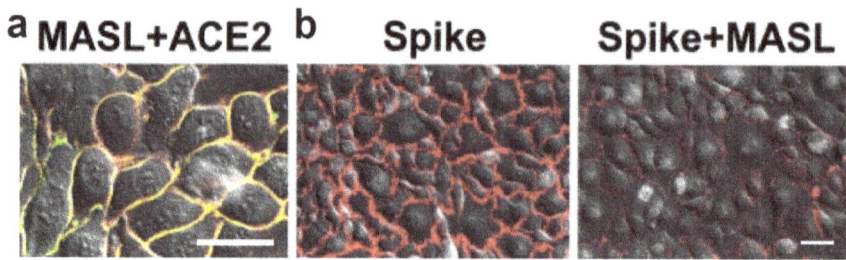

FIGURE 7.6 MASL associates with ACE2 and inhibits SARS-CoV-2 spike protein binding to human oral epithelial cells. (A) Human OSCC cells were incubated with Alexa 647 labeled ACE2 monoclonal antibody (green) and Alexa 595–labeled MASL (red) and examined by live cell confocal microscopy to visualize MASL-ACE2 colocalization (yellow). (B) Cells were incubated with Alexa 555–labeled SARS-CoV-2 spike protein (red) with and without MASL and visualized by confocal microscopy as indicated (bar = 50 μm).

oral epithelial cells (Hamilton et al., 2021; Krishnan et al., 2019; Ochoa-Alvarez et al., 2015; Ochoa-Alvarez et al., 2012). Taken together, these data suggest that MASL may target α-2,3 sialic acid receptors exemplified by PDPN to limit influenza viral pathogenicity.

7.7 CONCLUSION

MASL has an extensive history as a coincidental component in traditional medicines. It has earned its place in our collective pharmacopeia. It can target sialic acid motifs on specific receptors that drive cancer progression, inflammation, and viral infection. As such, MASL shows potential to treat a variety of afflictions including cancer, arthritis, and COVID-19.

7.8 SUMMARY POINTS

- MASL targets sialic acid motifs presented by extracellular receptors that drive cancer progression, inflammation, and viral infection.
- MASL can inhibit oncogenic TGFβ-SMAD, JAK-STAT, and Wnt-Bctn signaling pathways.
- MASL can trigger caspase independent death of malignant cells.
- MASL can inhibit inflammatory signaling cascades and progression of arthritis, psoriasis, and possibly acute respiratory disease.
- MASL can target receptors to inhibit SARS-CoV-2, bluetongue, and potentially influenza virus infection.

TABLE 7.2
Receptors with α-2–3 Sialic Acid Motifs

Receptor	Abbreviation
Podoplanin	PDPN
Mucin-1	Muc1
Mucin-16	Muc16 (CA-125)
Angiotensin converting enzyme-2	ACE-2
Leukosialin	CD43

REFERENCES

Acton, S.E., A.J. Farrugia, J.L. Astarita, D. Mourao-Sa, R.P. Jenkins, E. Nye, S. Hooper, J. van Blijswijk, N.C. Rogers, K.J. Snelgrove, I. Rosewell, L.F. Moita, G. Stamp, S.J. Turley, E. Sahai, and C. Reis e Sousa. 2014. Dendritic cells control fibroblastic reticular network tension and lymph node expansion. *Nature.* 514:498–502.

Aithal, A., S. Rauth, P. Kshirsagar, A. Shah, I. Lakshmanan, W.M. Junker, M. Jain, M.P. Ponnusamy, and S.K. Batra. 2018. MUC16 as a novel target for cancer therapy. *Expert Opin Ther Targets.* 22:675–686.

Akeson, G., and C.J. Malemud. 2017. A role for soluble IL-6 receptor in osteoarthritis. *J Funct Morphol Kinesiol.* 2.

Andrews, S. 1997. Trees of the year: *Cladrastis* and *Maackia.* United Kingdom.

Arends, J.E., F.J. Bot, I.A. Gisbertz, and H.C. Schouten. 1999. Expression of CD10, CD75 and CD43 in MALT lymphoma and their usefulness in discriminating MALT lymphoma from follicular lymphoma and chronic gastritis. *Histopathology.* 35:209–215.

Audi, J., M. Belson, M. Patel, J. Schier, and J. Osterloh. 2005. Ricin poisoning: A comprehensive review. *JAMA.* 294:2342–2351.

Augustin, M., P.R. Bock, J. Hanisch, M. Karasmann, and B. Schneider. 2005. Safety and efficacy of the long-term adjuvant treatment of primary intermediate- to high-risk malignant melanoma (UICC/AJCC stage II and III) with a standardized fermented European mistletoe (*Viscum album* L.) extract. Results from a multicenter, comparative, epidemiological cohort study in Germany and Switzerland. *Arzneimittelforschung.* 55:38–49.

Barnert, J., and H. Messmann. 2009. Diagnosis and management of lower gastrointestinal bleeding. *Nature Reviews: Gastroenterology & Hepatology.* 6:637–646.

Bousoik, E., and H. Montazeri Aliabadi. 2018. "Do we know Jack" about JAK? A closer look at JAK/STAT signaling pathway. *Front Oncol.* 8:287.

Cai, J. 1991. 承先启后的《图经本草》(Maps of Materia). *Jilin Journal of Chinese Traditional Medicine.* 3:1–4.

Cao, Y., P. Stosiek, G.F. Springer, and U. Karsten. 1996. Thomsen-Friedenreich–related carbohydrate antigens in normal adult human tissues: a systematic and comparative study. *Histochemistry and Cell Biology.* 106:197–207.

Carpintero-Fernandez, P., M. Varela-Eirin, A. Lacetera, R. Gago-Fuentes, E. Fonseca, S. Martin-Santamaria, and M.D. Mayan. 2020. New therapeutic strategies for osteoarthritis by targeting sialic acid receptors. *Biomolecules.* 10.

Chen, W., Z. Zhang, S. Zhang, P. Zhu, J.K. Ko, and K.K. Yung. 2021. MUC1: Structure, function, and clinic application in epithelial cancers. *Int J Mol Sci.* 22.

Chhetra Lalli, R., K. Kaur, A. Chakraborti, R. Srinivasan, and S. Ghosh. 2019. *Maackia amurensis* agglutinin induces apoptosis in cultured drug resistant human non–small cell lung cancer cells. *Glycoconjugate Journal.* 36:473–485.

Clark, M.C., and L.G. Baum. 2012. T cells modulate glycans on CD43 and CD45 during development and activation, signal regulation, and survival. *Ann N Y Acad Sci.* 1253:58–67.

Cummings, R.D., and M.E. Etzler. 2009. R-type Lectins. In Essentials of Glycobiology. nd, A. Varki, R.D. Cummings, J.D. Esko, H.H. Freeze, P. Stanley, C.R. Bertozzi, G.W. Hart, and M.E. Etzler, editors, Cold Spring Harbor, New York.

De Coninck, T., and E.J.M. Van Damme. 2021. Review: The multiple roles of plant lectins. *Plant Sci.* 313:111096.

de Laurentiis, A., M. Gaspari, C. Palmieri, C. Falcone, E. Iaccino, G. Fiume, O. Massa, M. Masullo, F.M. Tuccillo, L. Roveda, U. Prati, O. Fierro, I. Cozzolino, G. Troncone, P. Tassone, G. Scala, and I. Quinto. 2011. Mass spectrometry-based identification of the tumor antigen UN1 as the transmembrane CD43 sialoglycoprotein. *Molecular & Cellular Proteomics: MCP.* 10:M111 007898.

Ekwall, A.K., T. Eisler, C. Anderberg, C. Jin, N. Karlsson, M. Brisslert, and M.I. Bokarewa. 2011. The tumor-associated glycoprotein podoplanin is expressed in fibroblast-like synoviocytes of the hyperplastic synovial lining layer in rheumatoid arthritis. *Arthritis Res. Ther.* 13:R40.

Fedoreev, S.A., N.I. Kulish, L.I. Glebko, T.V. Pokushalova, M.V. Veselova, A.S. Saratikov, A.I. Vengerovskii, and V.S. Chuchalin. 2010. Maksar: A preparation based on Amur maackia. *Pharmaceutical Chemistry Journal.* 38:605–610.

Gadina, M., M.T. Le, D.M. Schwartz, O. Silvennoinen, S. Nakayamada, K. Yamaoka, and J.J. O'Shea. 2019. Janus kinases to jakinibs: From basic insights to clinical practice. *Rheumatology.* 58:i4–i16.

Gong, Y., S. Qin, L. Dai, and Z. Tian. 2021. The glycosylation in SARS-CoV-2 and its receptor ACE2. *Signal Transduct Target Ther.* 6:396.

Hamilton, K.L., S.A. Sheehan, E.P. Retzbach, C.A. Timmerman, G.B. Gianneschi, P.J. Tempera, P. Balachandran, and G.S. Goldberg. 2021. Effects of *Maackia amurensis* seed lectin (MASL) on oral squamous cell carcinoma (OSCC) gene expression and transcriptional signaling pathways. *Journal of Cancer Research and Clinical Oncology.* 147:445–457.

Hirano, T., and M. Murakami. 2020. COVID-19: A new virus, but a familiar receptor and cytokine release syndrome. *Immunity.* 52:731–733.

Hofer, C.C., P.S. Woods, and I.C. Davis. 2015. Infection of mice with influenza A/WSN/33 (H1N1) virus alters alveolar type II cell phenotype. *American Journal of Physiology: Lung Cellular and Molecular Physiology.* 308:L628–L638.

Hoffmann, M., M.R. Hayes, J. Pietruszka, and L. Elling. 2020. Synthesis of the Thomsen-Friedenreich–antigen (TF-antigen) and binding of Galectin-3 to TF-antigen presenting neo-glycoproteins. *Glycoconjugate Journal.* 37:457–470.

Honma, M., M. Minami-Hori, H. Takahashi, and H. Iizuka. 2012. Podoplanin expression in wound and hyperproliferative psoriatic epidermis: Regulation by TGF-beta and STAT-3 activating cytokines, IFN-gamma, IL-6, and IL-22. *J. Dermatol. Sci.* 65:134–140.

Honma, M., T. Shibuya, M. Fujii, S. Iinuma, N. Saito, M. Kishibe, and A. Ishida-Yamamoto. 2017. *Maackia amurensis* seed lectin can suppress IL-22 induced hyperproliferative reconstituted epidermis. *Journal of Dermatalogical Science.* 86:E46.

Hsu, L.S., R.H. Huang, H.W. Lai, H.T. Hsu, W.W. Sung, M.J. Hsieh, C.Y. Wu, Y.M. Lin, M.K. Chen, Y.S. Lo, and C.J. Chen. 2017. KLF6 inhibited oral cancer migration and invasion via downregulation of mesenchymal markers and inhibition of MMP-9 activities. *Int J Med Sci.* 14:530–535.

Hsu, R.J., J.Y. Ho, T.L. Cha, D.S. Yu, C.L. Wu, W.P. Huang, P. Chu, Y.H. Chen, J.T. Chen, and C.P. Yu. 2012. WNT10A plays an oncogenic role in renal cell carcinoma by activating WNT/beta-catenin pathway. *PloS One.* 7:e47649.

Imberty, A., C. Gautier, J. Lescar, S. Perez, L. Wyns, and R. Loris. 2000. An unusual carbohydrate binding site revealed by the structures of two *Maackia amurensis* lectins complexed with sialic acid–containing oligosaccharides. *J. Biol. Chem.* 275:17541–17548.

Kapoor, S., R. Marwaha, S. Majumdar, and S. Ghosh. 2008. Apoptosis induction by *Maackia amurensis* agglutinin in childhood acute lymphoblastic leukemic cells. *Leuk. Res.* 32:559–567.

Kawaguchi, T., I. Matsumoto, and T. Osawa. 1974. Studies on hemagglutinins from *Maackia amurensis* seeds. *J. Biol. Chem.* 249:2786–2792.

Kinney, B.A., A. Al Anber, R.H. Row, Y.J. Tseng, M.D. Weidmann, H. Knaut, and B.L. Martin. 2020. Sox2 and Canonical Wnt signaling interact to activate a developmental checkpoint coordinating morphogenesis with mesoderm fate acquisition. *Cell Reports.* 33:108311.

Kirikoshi, H., S. Inoue, H. Sekihara, and M. Katoh. 2001. Expression of WNT10A in human cancer. *International Journal of Oncology.* 19:997–1001.

Klaus, A., and W. Birchmeier. 2008. Wnt signalling and its impact on development and cancer. *Nature Reviews. Cancer.* 8:387–398.

Krishnan, H., W.T. Miller, F.J. Blanco, and G.S. Goldberg. 2019. Src and podoplanin forge a path to destruction. *Drug Discov Today.* 24:241–249.

Krishnan, H., J. Rayes, T. Miyashita, G. Ishii, E.P. Retzbach, S.A. Sheehan, A. Takemoto, Y.W. Chang, K. Yoneda, J. Asai, L. Jensen, L. Chalise, A. Natsume, and G.S. Goldberg. 2018. Podoplanin: An emerging cancer biomarker and therapeutic target. *Cancer Science.* 109:1292–1299.

Lalli, R.C., K. Kaur, S. Dadsena, A. Chakraborti, R. Srinivasan, and S. Ghosh. 2015. *Maackia amurensis* agglutinin enhances paclitaxel induced cytotoxicity in cultured non–small cell lung cancer cells. *Biochimie.* 115:93–107.

Lawrence, T. 2009. The nuclear factor NF-kappaB pathway in inflammation. *Cold Spring Harb Perspect Biol.* 1:a001651.

Lee, C. 2019. Griffithsin, a highly potent broad-spectrum antiviral lectin from red algae: From discovery to clinical application. *Mar Drugs.* 17.

Leppanen, A., S. Stowell, O. Blixt, and R.D. Cummings. 2005. Dimeric galectin-1 binds with high affinity to alpha2,3-sialylated and non-sialylated terminal N-acetyllactosamine units on surface-bound extended glycans. *The Journal of Biological Chemistry.* 280:5549–5562.

Li, S. 1593. *Bencao Gangmu* (A Materia Medica, Arranged according to Drug Descriptions and Technical Aspects) Ming Dynasty, China.

Li, W.W., J.Y. Yu, H.L. Xu, and J.K. Bao. 2011. Concanavalin A: A potential anti-neoplastic agent targeting apoptosis, autophagy and anti-angiogenesis for cancer therapeutics. *Biochemical and Biophysical Research Communications.* 414:282–286.

Liu, B., M.W. Min, and J.K. Bao. 2009. Induction of apoptosis by Concanavalin A and its molecular mechanisms in cancer cells. *Autophagy.* 5:432–433.

Liu, W. 1997. 植物多糖抗肿瘤活性研究进展 (A new medicinal plant resource – *Maackia amurensis*). *Chinese Wild Plant Resource.* 5:22–25.

Lord, J.M., L.M. Roberts, and J.D. Robertus. 1994. Ricin: Structure, mode of action, and some current applications. *FASEB Journal: Official Publication of the Federation of American Societies for Experimental Biology.* 8:201–208.

Mehta, S., R. Chhetra, R. Srinivasan, S.C. Sharma, D. Behera, and S. Ghosh. 2013. Potential importance of *Maackia amurensis* agglutinin in non–small cell lung cancer. *Biol Chem.* 394:889–900.

Mitchell, C.A., K. Ramessar, and B.R. O'Keefe. 2017. Antiviral lectins: Selective inhibitors of viral entry. *Antiviral Res.* 142:37–54.

Motoyama, K., F. Tanaka, Y. Kosaka, K. Mimori, H. Uetake, H. Inoue, K. Sugihara, and M. Mori. 2008. Clinical significance of BMP7 in human colorectal cancer. *Annals of Surgical Oncology.* 15:1530–1537.

Murakami, M., D. Kamimura, and T. Hirano. 2019. Pleiotropy and specificity: Insights from the interleukin 6 family of cytokines. *Immunity.* 50:812–831.

Nabi-Afjadi, M., M. Heydari, H. Zalpoor, I. Arman, A. Sadoughi, P. Sahami, and S. Aghazadeh. 2022. Lectins and lectibodies: Potential promising antiviral agents. *Cell Mol Biol Lett.* 27:37.

Narla, G., K.E. Heath, H.L. Reeves, D. Li, L.E. Giono, A.C. Kimmelman, M.J. Glucksman, J. Narla, F.J. Eng, A.M. Chan, A.C. Ferrari, J.A. Martignetti, and S.L. Friedman. 2001. KLF6, a candidate tumor suppressor gene mutated in prostate cancer. *Science.* 294:2563–2566.

Nie, X., H. Liu, L. Liu, Y.D. Wang, and W.D. Chen. 2020. Emerging roles of Wnt Ligands in human colorectal cancer. *Front Oncol.* 10:1341.

Ochoa-Alvarez, J.A., H. Krishnan, J.G. Pastorino, E. Nevel, D. Kephart, J.J. Lee, E.P. Retzbach, Y. Shen, M. Fatahzadeh, S. Baredes, E. Kalyoussef, M. Honma, M.E. Adelson, M.K. Kaneko, Y. Kato, M.A. Young, L. Deluca-Rapone, A.J. Shienbaum, K. Yin, L.D. Jensen, and G.S. Goldberg. 2015. Antibody and lectin target podoplanin to inhibit oral squamous carcinoma cell migration and viability by distinct mechanisms. *Oncotarget.* 6:9045–9060.

Ochoa-Alvarez, J.A., H. Krishnan, Y. Shen, N.K. Acharya, M. Han, D.E. McNulty, H. Hasegawa, T. Hyodo, T. Senga, J.G. Geng, M. Kosciuk, S.S. Shin, J.S. Goydos, D. Temiakov, R.G. Nagele, and G.S. Goldberg. 2012. Plant lectin can target receptors containing sialic acid, exemplified by podoplanin, to inhibit transformed cell growth and migration. *PLoS One.* 7:e41845.

O'Shea, J.J., D.M. Schwartz, A.V. Villarino, M. Gadina, I.B. McInnes, and A. Laurence. 2015. The JAK-STAT pathway: Impact on human disease and therapeutic intervention. *Annu Rev Med.* 66:311–328.

Parshenkov, A., and T. Hennet. 2022. Glycosylation-dependent induction of programmed cell death in murine adenocarcinoma cells. *Frontiers in Immunology.* 13:797759.

Poiroux, G., A. Barre, E.J.M. van Damme, H. Benoist, and P. Rouge. 2017. Plant lectins targeting O-Glycans at the cell surface as tools for cancer diagnosis, prognosis and therapy. *Int J Mol Sci.* 18.

Pu, Z. 1987. History of Chinese Linguistics. Shanghai Ancient Books Publishing House, Shanghai. 69–85 pp.

Quintanilla, M., L. Montero-Montero, J. Renart, and E. Martin-Villar. 2019. Podoplanin in inflammation and cancer. *Int J Mol Sci.* 20.

Reeves, H.L., G. Narla, O. Ogunbiyi, A.I. Haq, A. Katz, S. Benzeno, E. Hod, N. Harpaz, S. Goldberg, S. Tal-Kremer, F.J. Eng, M.J. Arthur, J.A. Martignetti, and S.L. Friedman. 2004. Kruppel-like factor 6 (KLF6) is a tumor-suppressor gene frequently inactivated in colorectal cancer. *Gastroenterology.* 126:1090–1103.

Retzbach, E.P., S.A. Sheehan, E.M. Nevel, A. Batra, T. Phi, A.T.P. Nguyen, Y. Kato, S. Baredes, M. Fatahzadeh, A.J. Shienbaum, and G.S. Goldberg. 2018. Podoplanin emerges as a functionally relevant oral cancer biomarker and therapeutic target. *Oral Oncology.* 78:126–136.

Ruprecht, F.J. 1856. *Maackia amurensis. Bull. Cl. Phys.-Math. Acad. Imp. Sci. Saint-Petersburg.* 15:143.

Schaefer, T., and C. Lengerke. 2020. SOX2 protein biochemistry in stemness, reprogramming, and cancer: The PI3K/AKT/SOX2 axis and beyond. *Oncogene.* 39:278–292.

Sciences, C.A.O. 1955. Illustrated Manual of China Main Plants- the Family Leguminosae. Science Press, Beijing.

Sharon, N., and H. Lis. 2004. History of lectins: From hemagglutinins to biological recognition molecules. *Glycobiology.* 14:53R–62R.

Sheehan, S.A., K.L. Hamilton, E.P. Retzbach, P. Balachandran, H. Krishnan, M. Leone, M. Lopez-Gonzalez, S. Suryavanshi, P. Kumar, R. Russo, and G.S. Goldberg. 2021. Evidence that *Maackia amurensis* seed lectin (MASL) exerts pleiotropic actions on oral squamous cells with potential to inhibit SARS-CoV-2 infection and COVID-19 disease progression. *Exp Cell Res.* 403:112594.

Sheehan, S.A., E.P. Retzbach, Y. Shen, H. Krishnan, and G.S. Goldberg. 2022. Heterocellular N-cadherin junctions enable nontransformed cells to inhibit the growth of adjacent transformed cells. *Cell Commun Signal.* 20:19.

Shen, Y., C.S. Chen, H. Ichikawa, and G.S. Goldberg. 2010. SRC induces podoplanin expression to promote cell migration. *J. Biol. Chem.* 285:9649–9656.

Simoes e Silva, A.C., K.D. Silveira, A.J. Ferreira, and M.M. Teixeira. 2013. ACE2, angiotensin-(1–7) and Mas receptor axis in inflammation and fibrosis. *Br J Pharmacol.* 169:477–492.

Sun, W., Q. Guo, and Y. Liu. 2008. 民间药怀槐的化学成分和药理作用研究进展 (The folk medicine Huai Huai chemical composition and pharmacological research). *Chinese Journal of Ethnomedicine and Ethnopharmacy*:35–38.

Suzuki, H., M.K. Kaneko, and Y. Kato. 2022. Roles of podoplanin in malignant progression of tumor. *Cells.* 11.

Takakubo, Y., H. Oki, Y. Naganuma, K. Saski, A. Sasaki, Y. Tamaki, Y. Suran, T. Konta, and M. Takagi. 2017. Distribution of podoplanin in synovial tissues in rheumatoid arthritis patients using biologic or conventional disease-modifying anti-rheumatic drugs. *Current Rheumatology Reviews.* 13:72–78.

Tang, W., and G. Eisenbrand. 1992. Sophora japonica L. *In* Chinese Drugs of Plant Origin: Chemistry, Pharmacology, and Use in Traditional and Modern Medicine. Springer Berlin Heidelberg, Berlin, Heidelberg. 945–955.

Tewari, D., A. Priya, A. Bishayee, and A. Bishayee. 2022. Targeting transforming growth factor-beta signalling for cancer prevention and intervention: Recent advances in developing small molecules of natural origin. *Clin Transl Med.* 12:e795.

Thomas, S.J., J.A. Snowden, M.P. Zeidler, and S.J. Danson. 2015. The role of JAK/STAT signalling in the pathogenesis, prognosis and treatment of solid tumors. *British Journal of Cancer.* 113:365–371.

Toegel, S., M. Pabst, S.Q. Wu, J. Grass, M.B. Goldring, C. Chiari, A. Kolb, F. Altmann, H. Viernstein, and F.M. Unger. 2010. Phenotype-related differential alpha-2,6- or alpha-2,3-sialylation of glycoprotein N-glycans in human chondrocytes. *Osteoarthritis and Cartilage/OARS, Osteoarthritis Research Society.* 18:240–248.

Toegel, S., D. Weinmann, S. Andre, S.M. Walzer, M. Bilban, S. Schmidt, C. Chiari, R. Windhager, C. Krall, I.M. Bennani-Baiti, and H.J. Gabius. 2016. Galectin-1 couples glycobiology to inflammation in osteoarthritis through the activation of an NF-kappaB-regulated gene network. *Journal of Immunology.* 196:1910–1921.

Vance, D.J., A.Y. Poon, and N.J. Mantis. 2020. Sites of vulnerability on ricin B chain revealed through epitope mapping of toxin-neutralizing monoclonal antibodies. *PloS One.* 15:e0236538.

Wang, Q., L.G. Yu, B.J. Campbell, J.D. Milton, and J.M. Rhodes. 1998. Identification of intact peanut lectin in peripheral venous blood. *Lancet.* 352:1831–1832.

Wang, Y., A. Khan, A. Antonopoulos, L. Bouche, C.D. Buckley, A. Filer, K. Raza, K.P. Li, B. Tolusso, E. Gremese, M. Kurowska-Stolarska, S. Alivernini, A. Dell, S.M. Haslam, and M.A. Pineda. 2021. Loss of alpha2–6 sialylation promotes the transformation of synovial fibroblasts into a pro-inflammatory phenotype in arthritis. *Nat Commun.* 12:2343.

Wicki, A., F. Lehembre, N. Wick, B. Hantusch, D. Kerjaschki, and G. Christofori. 2006. Tumor invasion in the absence of epithelial-mesenchymal transition: Podoplanin-mediated remodeling of the actin cytoskeleton. *Cancer Cell.* 9:261–272.

Wiese, O., A.E. Zemlin, and T.S. Pillay. 2021. Molecules in pathogenesis: Angiotensin converting enzyme 2 (ACE2). *Journal of Clinical Pathology.* 74:285–290.

Wu, W., and P. Roy. 2022. Sialic acid binding sites in VP2 of Bluetongue virus and their use during virus entry. *Journal of Virology.* 96:e0167721.

Yamamoto, K., Y. Konami, and T. Irimura. 1997. Sialic acid-binding motif of *Maackia amurensis* lectins. *J. Biochem.* 121:756–761.

Yokoyama, Y., T. Watanabe, Y. Tamura, Y. Hashizume, K. Miyazono, and S. Ehata. 2017. Autocrine BMP-4 signaling is a therapeutic target in colorectal cancer. *Cancer Res.* 77:4026–4038.

8 Apricot (*Prunus armeniaca* L.) Kernels and Usage in Cancer Studies

Teodora Todorova

ABBREVIATIONS

ABCF2	ATP-binding cassette, subfamily F, member 2
Bax	BCL2-associated X, apoptosis regulator
Bcl-2	B-cell lymphoma 2
EXO1	exonuclease 1
FRAP1	FK506 binding protein 12-rapamycin-associated protein 1
LC-ESI/MS	liquid chromatography–electrospray ionization/mass spectrometry
MRE11A	MRE11 meiotic recombination 11 homolog A
TOP1	topoisomerase 1
Ty1	transposon of yeast, family 1

8.1 INTRODUCTION

The apricot (*Prunus armeniaca* L.) is one of the members of the Rosaceae family. It is cultivated in regions with well-determined seasons. The apricot is used in traditional medicine to cure skin problems, vaginal infections, infertility, eye inflammation, and other disorders (Yiğit et al., 2009). Most of the parts that are used are fruits: raw or dried, and kernels. The wide application is often related to the various constituents in the apricot fruit such as carbohydrates, vitamins C and K, β-carotene, niacin, thiamine, organic acids, phenols, volatile compounds, esters, and terpenoids (Michalcová et al., 2016), while the bitter apricot kernel extract is known to contain flavonoids, polyphenols, glycosides, vitamins, and metal ions (Qin et al., 2019). Therefore, apricot-based extracts have been used in the pharmaceutical industry for years as an ingredient in different pharmaceuticals with anti-inflammatory, antimicrobial, or regenerative properties.

In alternative medicine, the bitter apricot kernels are prescribed as a remedy for respiratory disorders and skin diseases (Qin et al., 2019; Geng et al., 2016). Data exist that this extract possesses antihyperlipidemic, anti-inflammatory, anticancer, antioxidant, antimicrobial, anti-asthmatic, analgesic, and atherosclerotic effects, among others (Qin et al., 2019; Chang et al., 2006; Do et al., 2006; Korekar et al., 2011).

Apricot kernels, depending on the cultivar, contain various amounts of amygdalin as a major cyanogenic glycoside (EFSA CONTAM Panel, 2016; Michalcová et al., 2016). Data already exist that amygdalin is commonly used in alternative medicine as a remedy for migraine, hypertonia, chronic inflammation, asthma, bronchitis, emphysema, leprosy, diabetes, colorectal cancer, and vitiligo (Halenár et al., 2021; Zhou et al., 2012; Yan et al., 2006; Chang et al., 2005).

8.2 BACKGROUND

The apricot (*P. armeniaca* L.), a member of the Rosaceae family, and bitter apricot kernels are known in traditional medicine as remedies for respiratory disorders, skin diseases (Qin et al., 2019; Geng et al., 2016), hemorrhages, infertility, eye inflammation, spasm and vaginal infections (Yiğit

DOI: 10.1201/9781003260028-10

et al., 2009), and memory loss (Vahedi-Mazdabadi et al., 2020). Their application as a cardio-, reno-, and hepatoprotective, antiparasitic, antitussive, anti-aging, anticancer, anti-atherosclerotic, anti-anginal, and an antioxidant agent is also reported (Erdogan-Orhan & Kartal, 2011; Gupta et al., 2018). There is evidence that this extract has antihyperlipidemic, anti-inflammatory, antimicrobial, anti-asthmatic, analgesic, and other beneficial properties (Qin et al., 2019; Chang et al., 2006; Do et al., 2006; Korekar et al., 2011).

This wide application is often related to the various constituents in the apricot fruit and bitter apricot kernel extract such as carbohydrates, vitamins (A, C, and K), β-carotene, niacin, thiamine, organic acids, flavonoids, polyphenols, volatile compounds, esters, terpenoids, iron, potassium, calcium, phosphorous, glycosides, essential trace minerals, and fiber (Michalcová et al., 2016; Wani et al., 2017, Qin et al., 2019). Therefore, the extract has been used in the pharmaceutical industry for years as an ingredient in different pharmaceuticals with anti-inflammatory, antimicrobial, or regenerative properties. In Iranian traditional medicine, apricot is recommended for the treatment of dementia (Vahedi-Mazdabadi et al., 2020).

Practitioners prescribed apricot-based products such as kernels and amygdalin as a remedy for different medical conditions, including cancer. Amygdalin is not approved by the National Cancer Institute or the US Food and Drug Administration (FDA) because of potential toxicity but it has been applied in the anticancer therapies in northern Europe and Mexico (Todorova et al., 2017).

8.3 ORIGIN AND DISTRIBUTION

The apricot (*P. armeniaca* L.) is cultivated in regions with favorable environmental conditions (Yiğit et al., 2009; Gupta et al., 2018). It is believed that the apricot originated in China and it has been cultivated since 2000 BC (Crisosto & Kader, 1999; Faust et al., 1998; Ali et al., 2015). Recently, around 69 countries are considered the main apricot producers (FAOSTAT, 2020). The number one producer is Turkey (Uzundumlu et al., 2021).

8.4 PHYTOCHEMICALS PRESENTED

Bitter apricot kernel extract contains various biologically active substances such as flavonoids, polyphenols, glycosides, vitamins, metal ions, carbohydrates, organic acids, volatile compounds, esters, and terpenoids (Michalcová et al., 2016; Wani et al., 2017; Qin et al., 2019).

Phytochemical characterization performed by liquid chromatography–electrospray ionization/mass spectrometry (LC-ESI/MS) revealed the presence of 35 phenolic compounds (Qin et al., 2019). The most abundant were salicylic and gentisic acids followed by caffeic acid, ferulic acid, vanillic acid, and m-coumaric acid.

A total of 14 anthocyanins were identified in the methanol extracts of apricot kernel skins (Qin et al., 2019).

Dimitrov et al. (2021) confirmed the presence of at least 50 compounds already reported in other studies and apricot varieties (Qin et al., 2019; Rai et al., 2016; Erdogan-Orhan & Kartal, 2011).

Amygdalin has been found as the major cyanogenic glycoside in apricot kernels (EFSA CONTAM Panel, 2016; Michalcová et al., 2016). Stoewsand et al. (1975) reported variations depending on the cultivar. The wild apricot kernels had been found to contain 200 mg/100 g, whereas domestic bitter apricot cultivars contain relatively low levels: 11.7 mg/100 g. The amygdalin quantity in an extract prepared from a Bulgarian cultivar was determined to be 57.8 μg/mL (Dimitrov et al., 2021). The presence of three more glycosides – linamarin, deidaclin, and prulaurasin along with amygdalin – has been reported for the first time in the same research.

8.5 ANTICANCER ACTIVITY

Many studies have provided information concerning the potential anticancer activity of apricot and the main glycoside, amygdalin (Table 8.1).

One of the first known successful applications of amygdalin was in Russia in 1845 (Moss, 1996). In the late 1970s and early 1980s, amygdalin was reported to selectively kill cancer cells in the tumor without systemic toxicity and to effectively relieve pain in cancer patients (Zhou et al., 2012). Rats and mice were transplanted with various rodent tumors, such as osteogenic sarcoma, melanoma, carcinosarcoma, lung cancer, and leukemia. Amygdalin with or without the enzyme β-glycosidase was administered to animals by intraperitoneal injection.

None of the administered doses of amygdalin affected the studied solid tumors or leukemias. No statistically significant increase in animal survival was observed in any of the treatment groups (Laster & Schabel, 1975).

Other studies have shown positive results. Amygdalin has been shown to enhance its antitumor activity in combination with vitamin A in mice with mammary adenocarcinomas. It was injected intramuscularly, vitamin A was taken orally through a feeding tube, and enzymes were injected into and around tumor masses. No anticancer activity was observed with amygdalin alone (Manner et al., 1978).

The ability of amygdalin alone and in combination with β-glycosidase to inhibit growth and induce apoptosis in HepG2 cells was studied. All samples had an effect on HepG2 proliferation and responded in a dose- and time-dependent manner. The anti-HepG2 activity of amygdalin was weak, but its β-glycosidase-activated activity was enhanced (Zhou et al., 2012).

White blood cells and prostate cancer cell samples were used to study the potential of amygdalin to stimulate the immune system. Amygdalin greatly increases the ability of patients' white blood cells to adhere to their own prostate cancer cells, suggesting an increase in the immune system's potential for amygdalin (Bhatti et al., 1981).

The ability of amygdalin and β-glycosidase to indirectly sensitize hypoxic cells (oxygen-starved cells) at the center of the tumor to the lethal effects of gamma radiation has been studied. Cells in

TABLE 8.1
Various Antitumor Activities of Apricot and Amygdalin

Product	Type of Cancer	References
Amygdalin	Prostate cancer	Chang et al., 2006; Makarević et al., 2016
Raw Chinese apricot and peach kernels extracts; amygdalin	Colorectal cancer	Park et al., 2005; Cassiem & de Kock, 2019; Dimitrov et al., 2021; Todorova et al., 2017
Amygdalin; hydrophobic substances from Japanese apricot	Breast cancer	Nakagawa et al., 2007; Lee & Moon, 2016; Moradipoodeh et al., 2019; Abboud et al., 2019; Albogami & Alnefaie, 2021
Amygdalin	Cervical cancer	Choi et al., 2005; Chen et al., 2013
Bitter and sweet apricot extracts	Pancreatic cancer	Aamazadeh et al., 2020, 2022
A substance extracted from the Japanese apricot; apricot kernels; amygdalin	Hepatocellular carcinoma	Okada et al., 2007; Dimitrov et al., 2021; Todorova et al., 2017
Amygdalin	Oral cancer	Sireesha et al., 2019
Amygdalin	Bladder cancer	Makarević et al., 2014a, 2014b
Amygdalin	Renal cell carcinoma	Juengel et al., 2016
Amygdalin	Chronic myeloid leukemia	Park et al., 2006
Amygdalin	Non–small cell lung cancer	Qian et al., 2015

the periphery of the tumor are not deprived of oxygen and are more sensitive to gamma radiation. Probably cells inside the tumor take in less cyanide than cells located on the periphery of the tumor. Amygdalin and β-glycosidase have been shown to act as indirect radiation sensitizers of hypoxic tumor cells (Biaglow & Durand, 1978).

Cultured human blood cancer cells were treated with amygdalin alone or in combination with an antibody that was chemically attached to β-glycosidase. The target of this antibody is the glycoprotein MUC 1. The results show that amygdalin alone does not kill cancer blood cells effectively, but its ability to kill cells in the presence of the antibody-enzyme complex was 36 times higher (Syrigos et al., 1998).

Park et al. (2005) reported that amygdalin inhibits genes associated with the cell cycle in SNU-C4 human colorectal cancer cells such as exonuclease 1 (EXO1), ATP-binding cassette, subfamily F, member 2 (ABCF2), MRE11 meiotic recombination 11 homolog A (MRE11A) topoisomerase 1 (TOP1) and FK506 binding protein 12-rapamycin-associated protein 1 (FRAP1). A decrease in mRNA levels of these genes after amygdalin treatment was obtained.

Amygdalin induces cell death in a dose-dependent manner and shows significant cytotoxicity in human chronic myeloid leukemia K562 cells. cDNA microarray showed that amygdalin regulates genes belonging to the cell cycle in K562 cells. It damages DNA and thus stops the S-phase by modulating such regulatory genes (Park et al., 2006).

Another research shows that amygdalin reduces proliferative potential by lowering the mitochondrial activity of cervical cancer cells, accumulating G1-phase cells, and leading to their death (Jarocha & Majka, 2011).

Treatment of human prostate cancer cells DU145 and LNCaP with high concentrations of amygdalin induces apoptotic cell death. Amygdalin inhibits the expression of Bcl-2, an anti-apoptotic protein, increases the expression of Bax, a proapoptotic protein, and increases the enzyme activity of caspase 3 in a dose-dependent manner (Chang et al., 2006).

In another study, the viability of the human HeLa cancer line was significantly inhibited by amygdalin. Amygdalin-treated HeLa cells develop typical apoptotic changes by suppressing Bcl2 expression and increasing Bax expression (Chen et al., 2013).

To date, the FDA has not approved the use of amygdalin for the treatment of cancer due to insufficient clinical evidence of its efficacy and potential toxicity. Despite the failure of clinical trials to show the anticancer effects of amygdalin in the United States and Europe, it continues to be produced and used as an anticancer therapy in Northern Europe and Mexico (Chang et al., 2006).

8.6   MECHANISM OF ACTION

The selective action of amygdalin in healthy and cancer cells is explained by the fact that everywhere in the human body, except in cancer cells, there is an enzyme called rhodanese, and only in cancer cells in very large quantities is the enzyme β-glycosidase. When administered, amygdalin is destroyed by the enzyme rhodanese. It breaks down hydrogen cyanide and benzaldehyde into two products, thiocyanate and benzoic acid, which are good for healthy cells.

Upon contact of amygdalin with cancer cells in which β-glycosidase is present, a chemical reaction occurs, with hydrogen cyanide and benzaldehyde synergistically combining to form a toxin that destroys them. The whole process is known as selective toxicity, as only cancer cells become specific targets for amygdalin and are destroyed (Enculescu, 2009).

One of the possible mechanisms of action of amygdalin is related to the regulation of Bax and Bcl-2 expression (Chang et al., 2006).

Based on the research reported by Dimitrov et al. (2021), the tumor cell line HepG2 was more sensitive to apricot kernels than HT-29, which is in accordance with our previous study on the action of amygdalin (Todorova et al., 2017) as well as with another study where HepG2 was found to be more sensitive to apricot kernels than MCF-7 and HCT-116 cell lines (Gomaa, 2013).

The amygdalin mode of action is summarized in Figure 8.1.

An important step in anticancer research of plant-based natural products is to evaluate their potential toxicity. Data provided in Todorova et al. (2017) reveals that amygdalin in small doses up to 100 µg/mL does not induce point mutation, mitotic crossing over, and mitotic gene conversion. As discussed in this work, tumorigenesis is related to several molecular events such as point mutations, small deletions or inversions, mitotic recombination, or chromosome loss. The results obtained provide evidence for the inability of amygdalin itself to provoke events related to tumorigenesis (Todorova et al., 2017).

Further experiments provided evidence that apricot kernels' extract possesses antimutagenic activity primarily by activation of the error-prone recombinational repair as a main DNA damage repair pathway (Dimitrov et al., 2021). The action of apricot kernels' extract does not differ significantly depending on the mutagen studied.

Data concerning the mitigation of mitotic gene conversion induced by MMS (Dimitrov et al., 2021) and bleomycin (unpublished data) provide evidence for well-expressed antirecombinogenic activity which is not dose dependent (Figure 8.2).

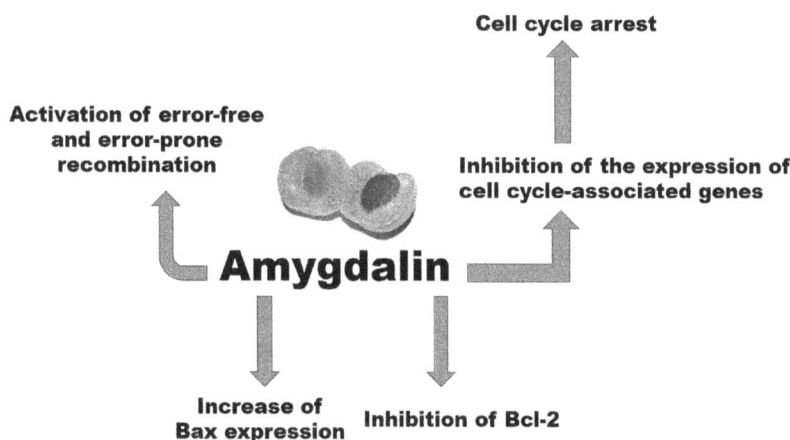

FIGURE 8.1 Summarized mechanism of action of amygdalin on a molecular level.

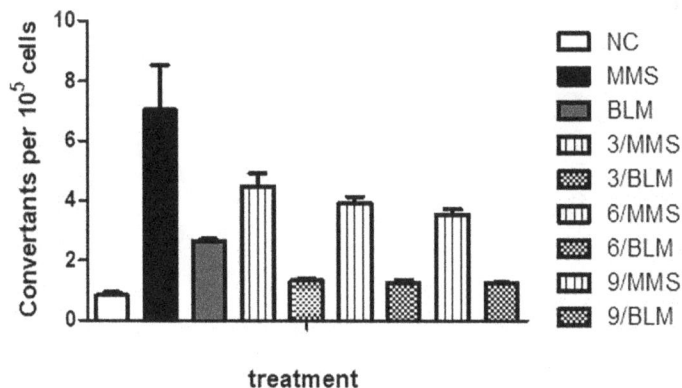

FIGURE 8.2 Potential antirecombinogenic activity, measured as "a number of convertants per 10^5 cells." BLM = bleomycin; 3/BLM, 6/BLM, 9/BLM = pretreatment with 3, 6, 9 µg/mL apricot kernels' extract and subsequent treatment with bleomycin; MMS = methyl methanesulfonate; 3/MMS, 6/MMS, 9/MMS = pretreatment with 3, 6, 9 µg/mL apricot kernels' extract and subsequent treatment with MMS; NC = negative control. Where no error bars are evident, they are equal to or less than the values.

The same was obtained for the other genetic marker: mitotic crossing-over (Figure 8.3). Interestingly, bleomycin was not found to be a strong mitotic crossing-over inducer.

The best-expressed protective activity of apricot kernels (Figure 8.4) was reported based on the reduction of the number of reverse mutation events – a marker used for error-prone recombination (Dimitrov et al., 2021).

Amygdalin prevented mutations caused by methyl methanesulfonate (Todorova et al., 2017) and radiomimetics (unpublished data) by activating both error-free and error-prone recombination events.

The mechanism of anticarcinogenic action was studied based on the potential inhibition of Ty1 retrotransposition in *Saccharomyces cerevisiae* (Figure 8.5). Data reported provided information that amygdalin mitigates the action of the standard carcinogen chromium (Cr^{VI}) as well as the action of bleomycin in terms of cell survival and Ty1 transposition rates.

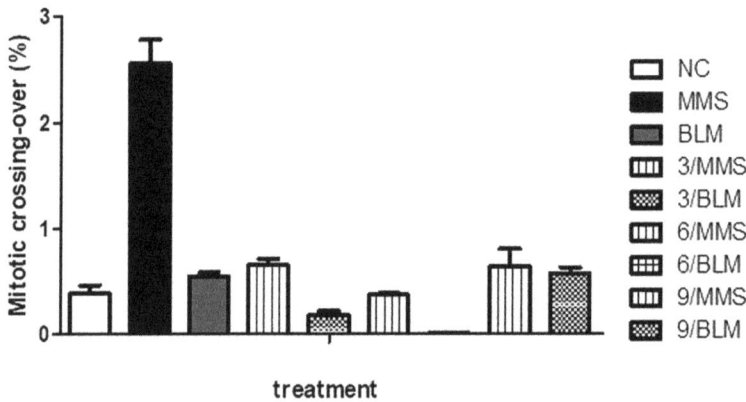

FIGURE 8.3 Potential antirecombinogenic activity, measured as "percent of mitotic crossing-over." BLM = bleomycin; 3/BLM, 6/BLM, 9/BLM = pretreatment with 3, 6, 9 µg/mL apricot kernels' extract and subsequent treatment with bleomycin; MMS = methyl methanesulfonate; 3/MMS, 6/MMS, 9/MMS = pretreatment with 3, 6, 9 µg/mL apricot kernels' extract and subsequent treatment with MMS; NC = negative control. Where no error bars are evident, they are equal to or less than the values.

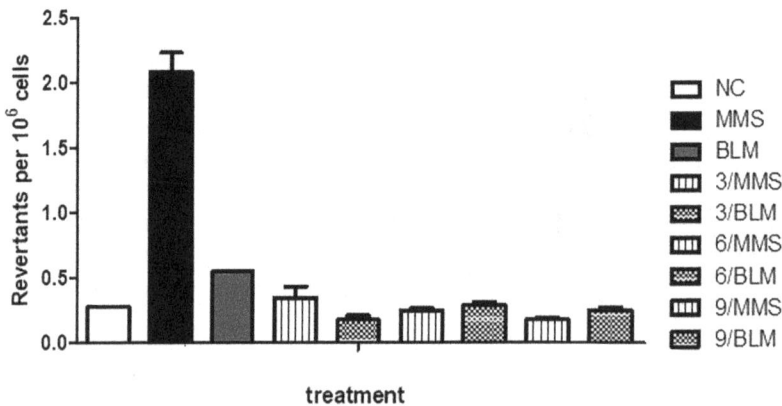

FIGURE 8.4 Potential antimutagenic activity, measured as "a number of revertants per 10^6 cells." BLM = bleomycin; 3/BLM, 6/BLM, 9/BLM = pretreatment with 3, 6, 9 µg/mL apricot kernels' extract and subsequent treatment with bleomycin; MMS = methyl methanesulfonate; 3/MMS, 6/MMS, 9/MMS = pretreatment with 3, 6, 9 µg/mL apricot kernels' extract and subsequent treatment with MMS; NC = negative control. Where no error bars are evident, they are equal to or less than the values.

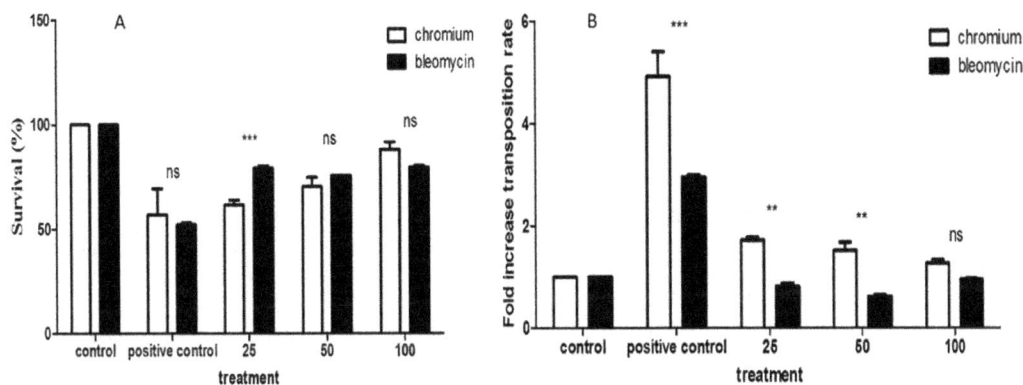

FIGURE 8.5 Effect of pretreatment with 25, 50, and 100 µg/mL and subsequent treatment with hexavalent chromium or bleomycin: (A) survival rate and (B) fold increase transposition rate.

8.7 OTHER FOODS, HERBS, SPICES, AND BOTANICALS USED IN CANCER

Herbal medicine practices have been known as an integral feature in local healthcare for many years with around 80% of Asian and African populations relying on them (Oyenihi et al., 2021). About 49% of the FDA-approved anticancer drugs were based on natural products or derivatives (Newman & Cragg, 2012). There is enormous research on anticancer phytochemicals and medicinal plants in the last decades (Dutta et al., 2019), which unfortunately does not correspond with the number of new plant-derived drugs (Oyenihi et al., 2021). By now, results provide evidence concerning the anticancer potential of quercetin, silymarin, resveratrol, melatonin, taurine, curcumin, and so forth (discussed in Dutta et al., 2019; Singh et al., 2020).

Even so, many data point out that the herbal preparations or extracts possess better expressed anticancer activity than single phytochemical compounds which should be taken into consideration when performing in-depth scientific research for their use and patient safety (Oyenihi et al., 2021).

8.8 TOXICITY AND CAUTIONARY NOTES

Contradictory data exist concerning the effect of amygdalin on organisms (reviewed in He et al., 2020). It has been reported that ingestion of amygdalin preparations and bitter apricot kernels results in acute cyanide toxicity in humans. The acute lethal oral dose of hydrogen cyanide (HCN) is 0.5–3.5 mg/kg body weight and the toxicity threshold for cyanide in whole blood is 0.5 mg/L (approximately 20 µM) (EFSA CONTAM Panel, 2016). Unrestrained consumption of kernels may cause various adverse reactions such as diarrhea, vomiting, abdominal pain, and in extreme cases death (Jaszczak-Wilke et al., 2021). It should be taken into consideration that amygdalin is not approved by the FDA because of potential toxicity. More data is needed concerning the potential range of doses that may provide anticancer activity without posing a health risk.

8.9 SUMMARY POINTS

- This chapter focuses on the anticancer potential of apricot (*P. armeniaca* L.).
- *P. armeniaca* L. is cultivated in regions with favorable environmental conditions.
- The apricot originated in China.
- One of the first known successful applications of amygdalin was in Russia in 1845.
- Amygdalin affects the mitochondrial activity of cancer cells.
- Amygdalin inhibits the expression of Bcl-2.
- Apricot kernels' extract possesses antimutagenic activity primarily by activation of the error-prone recombinational repair as a main DNA damage repair pathway.

REFERENCES

Aamazadeh, F., Barar, J., Rahbar Saadat, Y., & Ostadrahimi, A. (2022). In vitro evaluation of cytotoxic and apoptotic activities of ethanolic extract of sweet apricot kernel on PANC-1 pancreatic cancer cells. *Nutrition & Food Science*, *52*(1), 12–25.

Aamazadeh, F., Ostadrahimi, A., Rahbar Saadat, Y., & Barar, J. (2020). Bitter apricot ethanolic extract induces apoptosis through increasing expression of Bax/Bcl-2 ratio and caspase-3 in PANC-1 pancreatic cancer cells. *Molecular Biology Reports*, *47*(3), 1895–1904.

Abboud, M. M., Al Awaida, W., Alkhateeb, H. H., & Abu-Ayyad, A. N. (2019). Antitumor action of amygdalin on human breast cancer cells by selective sensitization to oxidative stress. *Nutrition and Cancer*, *71*(3), 483–490.

Albogami, S., & Alnefaie, A. (2021). Role of amygdalin in blocking DNA replication in breast cancer in vitro. *Current Pharmaceutical Biotechnology*, *22*(12), 1612–1627.

Ali, S., Masud, T., Abbasi, K. S., Mahmood, T., & Hussai, A. (2015). Apricot: Nutritional potentials and health benefits-a review. *Annals. Food Science and Technology*, *16*, 175–189.

Bhatti, R. A., Ablin, R. J., & Guinan, P. D. (1981). Tumor-associated directed immunity in prostatic cancer: Effect of amygdalin. *IRCS Medical Science research Biochemistry*, *9*(1), 19.

Biaglow, J. E., & Durand, R. E. (1978). The enhanced radiation response of an in vitro tumor model by cyanide released from hydrolysed amygdalin. *International Journal of Radiation Biology & Related Studies in Physics, Chemistry & Medicine*, *33*(4), 397–401.

Cassiem, W., & de Kock, M. (2019). The anti-proliferative effect of apricot and peach kernel extracts on human colon cancer cells in vitro. *BMC Complementary and Alternative Medicine*, *19*(1), 1–12.

Chang, H. K., Shin, M. S., Yang, H. Y., Lee, J. W., Kim, Y. S., Lee, M. H, Kim, J., Kim, K. H., & Kim, C. J. (2006). Amygdalin induces apoptosis through regulation of Bax and Bcl-2 expressions in human DU145 and LNCaP prostate cancer cells. *Biological and Pharmaceutical Bulletin*, *29*(8), 1597–1602.

Chang, H. K., Yang, H. Y., Lee, T. H., Shin, M. C., Lee, M. H., Shin, M. S., . . . & Cho, S. (2005). Armeniacae semen extract suppresses lipopolysaccharide-induced expressions of cycloosygenase-2 and inducible nitric oxide synthase in mouse BV2 microglial cells. *Biological and Pharmaceutical Bulletin*, *28*(3), 449–454.

Chen, Y., Ma, J., Wang, F., Hu, J., Cui, A., Wei, C., . . . & Li, F. (2013). Amygdalin induces apoptosis in human cervical cancer cell line HeLa cells. *Immunopharmacology and Immunotoxicology*, *35*(1), 43–51.

Choi, S. P., Song, Y. K., Kim, K. J., & Lim, H. H. (2005). Amygdalin extract from Armeniacae semen induces apoptosis through Bax-dependent caspase-3 activation in human cervical cancer cell line ME-180. *The Journal of Korean Medicine*, *26*(4), 130–142.

Crisosto, C. H., & Kader, A. A. (1999). Apricots postharvest quality maintenance guidelines. *Department of pomology university of California*.

Dimitrov, M., Iliev, I., Bardarov, K., Georgieva, D., & Todorova, T. (2021). Phytochemical characterization and biological activity of apricot kernels' extract in yeast-cell based tests and hepatocellular and colorectal carcinoma cell lines. *Journal of Ethnopharmacology*, *279*, 114333.

Do, J. S., Hwang, J. K., Seo, H. J., Woo, W. H., & Nam, S. Y. (2006). Antiasthmatic activity and selective inhibition of type 2 helper T cell response by aqueous extract of semen armeniacae amarum. *Immunopharmacology and Immunotoxicology*, *28*(2), 213–225.

Dutta, S., Mahalanobish, S., Saha, S., Ghosh, S., & Sil, P. C. (2019). Natural products: An upcoming therapeutic approach to cancer. *Food and Chemical Toxicology*, *128*, 240–255.

EFSA Contam Panel. (2016). EFSA panel on contaminants in the food chain, scientific opinion on the acute health risks related to the presence of cyanogenic glycosides in raw apricot kernels and products derived from raw apricot kernels. *EFSA Journal*, *14*(4), 4424. doi:10.2903/j.efsa.2016.4424

Enculescu, M. (2009). Vitamin B17/Laetrile/Amygdalin (a review) bulletin UASVM. *Animal Science and Biotechnologies*, *66*(1–2).

Erdogan-Orhan, I., & Kartal, M. (2011). Insights into research on phytochemistry and biological activities of *Prunus armeniaca* L. (apricot). *Food Research International*, *44*(5), 1238–1243. doi:10.1016/j. foodres.2010.11.014

FAOSTAT. (2020). Fruit production in the world. Available from: www.fao.org/faostat/en/#data/qc. [Last accessed on 2020 Feb 29]

Faust, M., Suranyi, D., & Nyujto, F. (1998). Origin and dissemination of apricot. *Horticultural Reviews-Westport then New York*, *22*, 225–260.

Geng, H., Yu, X., Lu, A., Cao, H., Zhou, B., Zhou, L., & Zhao, Z. (2016). Extraction, chemical composition, and antifungal activity of essential oil of bitter almond. *International Journal of Molecular Sciences, 17*(9), 1421.

Gomaa, E. Z. (2013). In vitro antioxidant, antimicrobial, and antitumor activities of bitter almond and sweet apricot (*Prunus armeniaca* L.) kernels. *Food Science and Biotechnology, 22*(2), 455–463.

Gupta, S., Chhajed, M., Arora, S., Thakur, G., & Gupta, R. (2018). Medicinal value of apricot: A review. *Indian Journal of Pharmaceutical Sciences, 80*(5), 790–794.

Jarocha, D., & Majka, M. (2011). Influence of amygdalin on biology of cervical carcinoma cells. In *Abstracts of the 2nd Congress of Biochemistry and Cell Biology*. Krakow, p. 280.

Jaszczak-Wilke, E., Polkowska, Ż., Koprowski, M., Owsianik, K., Mitchell, A. E., & Bałczewski, P. (2021). Amygdalin: Toxicity, anticancer activity and analytical procedures for its determination in plant seeds. *Molecules (Basel, Switzerland), 26*(8), 2253. doi:10.3390/molecules26082253

Juengel, E., Thomas, A., Rutz, J., et al. (2016) Amygdalin inhibits the growth of renal cell carcinoma cells in vitro. *International Journal of Molecular Medicine, 37*(2), 526–532.

Halenár, M., Medveďová, M., Maruniaková, N., Packová, D., & Kolesárová, A. (2021). Dose-response of porcine ovarian granulosa cells to amygdalin treatment combined with deoxynivalenol. *Journal of Microbiology, Biotechnology and Food Sciences, 2021,* 77–79.

He, X. Y., Wu, L. J., Wang, W. X., Xie, P. J., Chen, Y. H., & Wang, F. (2020). Amygdalin-A pharmacological and toxicological review. *Journal of Ethnopharmacology, 254,* 112717.

Korekar, G., Stobdan, T., Arora, R., Yadav, A., & Singh, S. B. (2011). Antioxidant capacity and phenolics content of apricot (*Prunus armeniaca* L.) kernel as a function of genotype. *Plant Foods for Human Nutrition, 66*(4), 376–383.

Laster, W. R., Jr., & Schabel, F. M., Jr. (1975). Experimental studies of the antitumor activity of amygdalin alone and in combination with beta-glucosidase. *Cancer Chemotherapy Reports, 59*(5), 951–965.

Lee, H. M., & Moon, A. (2016). Amygdalin regulates apoptosis and adhesion in Hs578T triple-negative breast cancer cells. *Biomolecules & Therapeutics, 24*(1), 62–66. doi:10.4062/biomolther.2015.172

Makarević, J., Rutz, J., Juengel, E., Kaulfuss, S., Reiter, M., Tsaur, I., . . . & Blaheta, R. A. (2014a). Amygdalin blocks bladder cancer cell growth in vitro by diminishing cyclin A and cdk2. *PLoS One, 9*(8), e105590.

Makarević, J., Rutz, J., Juengel, E., Kaulfuss, S., Tsaur, I., Nelson, K., . . . & Blaheta, R. A. (2014b). Amygdalin influences bladder cancer cell adhesion and invasion in vitro. *PLoS One, 9*(10), e110244.

Makarević, J., Tsaur, I., Juengel, E., Borgmann, H., Nelson, K., Thomas, C., . . . & Blaheta, R. A. (2016). Amygdalin delays cell cycle progression and blocks growth of prostate cancer cells in vitro. *Life Sciences, 147,* 137–142.

Manner, H. W., Disanti, S. J., & Maggio, M. I. (1978). Amygdalin, vitamin A and enzyme induced regression of murine mammary adenocarcinomas. *Journal of Manipulative and Physiological Therapeutics, 1*(4), 246–248.

Michalcová, K., Halenár, M., Tušimová, E., Kováčik, A., Chrastinová, Ľ., Ondruška, Ľ., . . . & Kolesárová, A. (2016). Blood plasma levels of anterior pituitary hormones of rabbits after apricot seed exposure in vivo. *Journal of Central European Agriculture, 17*(4), 1241–1252.

Moradipoodeh, B., Jamalan, M., Zeinali, M., Fereidoonnezhad, M., & Mohammadzadeh, G. (2019). In vitro and in silico anticancer activity of amygdalin on the SK-BR-3 human breast cancer cell line. *Molecular Biology Reports, 46,* 6361–6370. doi:10.1007/s11033-019-05080-3

Moss, R. W. (1996). The cancer industry: The classic exposé on the cancer establishment. In *The Cancer Industry: The Classic Exposé on the Cancer Establishment*. Brooklyn, NY: First Equinox Press, 450 p.

Nakagawa, A., Sawada, T., Okada, T., Ohsawa, T., Adachi, M., & Kubota, K. (2007). New antineoplastic agent, MK615, from UME (a Variety of) Japanese apricot inhibits growth of breast cancer cells in vitro. *The Breast Journal, 13*(1), 44–49.

Newman, D. J., & Cragg, G. M. (2012). Natural products as sources of new drugs over the 30 years from 1981 to 2010. *Journal of Natural Products, 75*(3), 311–335.

Okada, T., Sawada, T., Osawa, T., Adachi, M., & Kubota, K. (2007). A novel anti-cancer substance, MK615, from ume, a variety of Japanese apricot, inhibits growth of hepatocellular carcinoma cells by suppressing Aurora A kinase activity. *Hepato-Gastroenterology, 54*(78), 1770–1774.

Oyenihi, O. R., Oyenihi, A. B., Erhabor, J. O., Matsabisa, M. G., & Oguntibeju, O. O. (2021). Unravelling the anticancer mechanisms of traditional herbal medicines with metabolomics. *Molecules, 26*(21), 6541.

Park, H. J., Baik, H. W., Lee, S. K., Yoon, S. H., Zheng, L. T., Yim, S. V., . . . & Chung, J. H. (2006). Amygdalin modulates cell cycle regulator genes in human chronic myeloid leukemia cells. *Molecular & Cellular Toxicology, 2*(3), 159–165.

Park, H. J., Yoon, S. H., Han, L. S., Zheng, L. T., Jung, K. H., Uhm, Y. K., . . . & Hong, S. P. (2005). Amygdalin inhibits genes related to cell cycle in SNU-C4 human colon cancer cells. *World Journal of Gastroenterology: WJG, 11*(33), 5156.

Qian, L., Xie, B., Wang, Y., & Qian, J. (2015). Amygdalin-mediated inhibition of non–small cell lung cancer cell invasion in vitro. *International Journal of Clinical and Experimental Pathology, 8*(5), 5363.

Qin, F., Yao, L., Lu, C., Li, C., Zhou, Y., Su, C., . . . & Shen, Y. (2019). Phenolic composition, antioxidant and antibacterial properties, and in vitro anti-HepG2 cell activities of wild apricot (*Armeniaca sibirica* L. Lam) kernel skins. *Food and Chemical Toxicology, 129*, 354–364.

Rai, I., Bachheti, R. K., Saini, C. K., Joshi, A., & Satyan, R. S. (2016). A review on phytochemical, biological screening and importance of Wild Apricot (*Prunus armeniaca* L.). *Oriental Pharmacy and Experimental Medicine, 16*(1), 1–15.

Singh, N., Kushwaha, P., Gupta, A., & Prakash, O. (2020). Recent advances of novel therapeutic agents from botanicals for prevention and therapy of breast cancer: An updated review. *Current Cancer Therapy Reviews, 16*(1), 5–18.

Sireesha, D., Reddy, B. S., Reginald, B. A., Samatha, M., & Kamal, F. (2019). Effect of amygdalin on oral cancer cell line: An in vitro study. *Journal of Oral and Maxillofacial Pathology: JOMFP, 23*(1), 104.

Stoewsand, G. S., Anderson, J. L., & Lamb, R. C. (1975). Cyanide content of apricot kernels. *Journal of Food Science, 40*(5), 1107–1120.

Syrigos, K. N., Rowlinson-Busza, G., & Epenetos, A. A. (1998). In vitro cytotoxicity following specific activation of amygdalin by beta-glucosidase conjugated to a bladder cancer associated monoclonal antibody. *International Journal of Cancer, 78*(6), 712–719.

Todorova, A., Pesheva, M., Iliev, I., Bardarov, K., & Todorova, T. (2017). Antimutagenic, antirecombinogenic, and antitumor effect of amygdalin in a yeast cell – based test and mammalian cell lines. *Journal of Medicinal Food, 20*(4), 360–366.

Uzundumlu, A. S., Karabacak, T., & Ali, A. (2021). Apricot production forecast of the leading countries in the period of 2018–2025. *Emirates Journal of Food and Agriculture*, 682–690.

Vahedi-Mazdabadi, Y., Karimpour-Razkenari, E., Akbarzadeh, T., Lotfian, H., Toushih, M., Roshanravan, N., . . . & Ostadrahimi, A. (2020). Anti-cholinesterase and neuroprotective activities of sweet and bitter apricot kernels (*Prunus armeniaca* L.). *Iranian Journal of Pharmaceutical Research: IJPR, 19*(4), 216.

Wani, S. M., Hussain, P. R., Masoodi, F. A., Ahmad, M., Wani, T. A., Gani, A., . . . & Suradkar, P. (2017). Evaluation of the composition of bioactive compounds and antioxidant activity in fourteen apricot varieties of North India. *Journal of Agricultural Science, 9*(5), 66–82.

Yan, J., Tong, S., Li, J., & Lou, J. (2006). Preparative isolation and purification of amygdalin from *Prunus armeniaca* L. with high recovery by high-speed countercurrent chromatography. *Journal of Liquid Chromatography & Related Technologies, 29*(9), 1271–1279.

Yiğit, D., Yiğit, N., & Mavi, A. (2009). Antioxidant and antimicrobial activities of bitter and sweet apricot (*Prunus armeniaca* L.) kernels. *Brazilian Journal of Medical and Biological Research, 42*(4), 346–352.

Zhou, C., Qian, L., Ma, H., Yu, X., Zhang, Y., Qu, W., . . . & Xia, W. (2012). Enhancement of amygdalin activated with β-D-glucosidase on HepG2 cells proliferation and apoptosis. *Carbohydrate Polymers, 90*(1), 516–523.

9 Barberry (*Berberis vulgaris*) *Composition and Use of Extracts in Cancer Studies*

*Farnaz Shahdadian, Mohammad Bagherniya,
Gholamreza Askari, Prashant Kesharwani,
Rajkumar Rajendram and Amirhossein Sahebkar*

ABBREVIATIONS

ACC	acetyl-CoA carboxylase
AEG-1	astrocyte elevated gene-1 protein
AFP	acetylaminofluorene
ALP	alkaline phosphatase
AMPK	AMP-activated protein kinase
APAF-1	apoptotic protease activating factor 1
BAX	BCL2 associated X
BCL-2	B-cell lymphoma-2
BCL-XL	B-cell lymphoma extra-large
BH	berberine hydrochloride
BIM	Bcl-2-like protein 11
CDKs	cyclin-dependent kinases
COX2	cyclooxygenase-2
DAXX	death-domain-associated protein
DHFR	dihydrofolate reductase
ECM	extracellular matrix
EGFR-ERK	epidermal growth factor receptor activated/extracellular signal–regulated kinase
ER	endoplasmic reticulum
FAK	focal adhesion kinase
FN	fibronectin
GBM	glioblastoma multiforme
GGT	gamma glutamyl transferase
GST	glutathione S-transferase
HCC	hepatocellular carcinoma
HIF	hypoxia-inducible factor
IFN-β	interferon beta
IGF-1	insulin-like growth factor
IGFBPs	IGF-binding proteins
IL-6	interleukin-6
JNK	c-Jun N-terminal kinase
LDL-C	low-density lipoprotein cholesterol
MAPK	mitogen-activated protein kinase
MEK/ERK	mitogen-activating protein kinase/extracellular receptor kinase
MMP	matrix metalloproteinase

DOI: 10.1201/9781003260028-11

MTDH	metadherin
mTOR	mammalian target of rapamycin
NF-κB	nuclear factor kappa B
p-mTOR	phosphorylated mammalian target of rapamycin
PCD II	programmed cell death type II
PGE2	prostaglandin E2
PI3K/Akt	phosphatidil-inositol-3-kinase/Akt
PPAR-γ	expression levels of peroxisome proliferator-activated receptor gamma
PUMA	p53 upregulated modulator of apoptosis
RCT	randomized clinical trials
RIAISs	radiation-induced acute intestinal symptoms
RILI	radiation-induced lung injury
ROS	reactive oxygen species
sICAM-1	soluble intercellular adhesion molecular-1
TBP	TATA binding protein
TGF-β1	transforming growth factor beta-1
TNF-α	tumor necrosis factor alpha
TS	thymidylate synthase
u-PA	urokinase type plasminogen activator
VASP	vasodilator stimulated phosphoprotein
VEGF	vascular endothelial growth factor

9.1   *BERBERIS VULGARIS*

B. vulgaris (barberry) is a member of the Berberidaceae family (Arayne, Sultana, and Bahadur 2007). It is believed that *B. vulgaris* originated in Eastern Asia before the Paleocene Epoch (Li, Kvaček, et al. 2010). It is cultivated in southern Europe, the northeastern United States and the Middle East (Mokhber-Dezfuli et al. 2014; Kim, Kim, and Landrum 2004). It is particularly common in the northeastern cities of Iran (Fatehi et al. 2005). It is a thorny, bushy plant, approximately 1–3 m tall, with yellow to brown bark and ovoid leaves; *B. vulgaris* bears pendulous yellow flowers that eventually turn to oblong red berries with a sour taste (Shamsa, Ahmadiani, and Khosrokhavar 1999). The dried fruit of this plant is used as a food additive, and beverages, including juice, syrup, and concentrates can be produced from the fresh fruit. Anthocyanin, which is found in the fruit, is used as a natural coloring agent in the food industry (Alemardan et al. 2013).

9.2   CHEMICAL AND NUTRITIONAL COMPONENTS OF *B. VULGARIS*

Various compounds have been isolated from different parts of this plant (i.e., root, bark, fruit, shoots, flowers, and leaves). These include isoquinoline alkaloids (acanthine, bargustanine, berbamine, berberrubine, berberine, beriambine, bervulcine, columbamine, jatrorrhizine, lambertine, magnoflorine, palmatine, and thaliemidine), coumarin (aesculetin), vitamins (ascorbic acid and vitamin K), phenylpropanoid (caffeic acid and chlorogenic acid), carotenoids, flavonoids (chrysanthemin, delphinidin-3-o-beta-d-glucosido, pelargonin, and petunidin-3-o-beta-d-glucoside), carbohydrate (glucan, pectin, polysaccharide, sucrose, and xylan), and flavonol (hyperoside and quercetin) (Imanshahidi and Hosseinzadeh 2008; Zarei et al. 2015). Several organic acids, including citric acid, chelidonic acid, malic acid, pectinic, tannin, resin, and mucilagic acid have also been identified in the roots (Zarei et al. 2012; Fatehi et al. 2005).

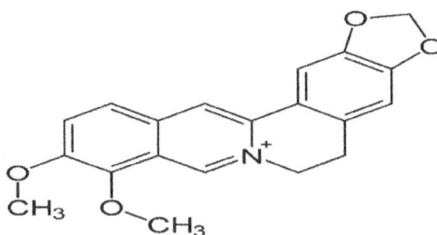

FIGURE 9.1 Chemical structure of berberine.

One of the most important isoquinoline alkaloids in barberry is berberine. This protoberberine compound (Figure 9.1) is found in the root, bark, and fruit of *B. vulgaris* (Mazzini, Bellucci, and Mondelli 2003).

9.3 HEALTH AND PHARMACEUTICAL APPLICATION OF *B. VULGARIS* AND BERBERINE

B. vulgaris has recently attracted attention as an herbal medicine and is being used for the prevention and treatment of a wide range of diseases (Imenshahidi and Hosseinzadeh 2019; Mohammadi et al. 2014; Sobhani et al. 2021). Several double-blind randomized clinical trials suggest that *B. vulgaris* effectively reduces serum glucose, glycosylated hemoglobin (HbA_{1c}), triglycerides, total cholesterol, low-density lipoprotein cholesterol (LDL-C), and apo B (Shidfar et al. 2012; Awasthi et al. 2015; Di Pierro et al. 2017). It also improves the oxidant-antioxidant balance, reducing the serum concentration of high-sensitivity C-reactive protein and interleukin-6 (Giuseppe et al. 2017; Mohammadi et al. 2014).

Several clinical benefits have been attributed to berberine. These include antimicrobial, anti-inflammatory, hypotensive, and anticancer properties (Dash, Kumar, and Pareek 2020; Kumar et al. 2020; Tew et al. 2020; Cicero and Tartagni 2012; Lopes et al. 2020; Wang et al. 2020; Ayati et al. 2017; Bagheriya et al. 2018; Hesari et al. 2018; Sahebkar and Watts 2017; Ziasarabi, Sahebkar, and Ghasemi 2021). It has important applications in the prevention and treatment of diseases of the cardiovascular, endocrine, immune, renal, and gastrointestinal systems, as well as polycystic ovary syndrome and Alzheimer disease (Kalmarzi et al. 2019). There is also significant interest in the use of *B. vulgaris* and berberine to treat many types of cancer (Sakaguchi et al. 2020; Mortazavi et al. 2020; Loo et al. 2020) (Figure 9.2).

9.4 *B. VULGARIS,* BERBERINE, AND CANCER STUDIES

Cancer is a leading cause of morbidity and mortality worldwide (Bray et al. 2021). There are several therapeutic options for the treatment of cancer, including chemotherapy, radiotherapy, and surgery (partial or total removal of a tumor). Yet, outcomes remain unsatisfactory in view of the side effects of the currently available treatments and their limited ability to cure cancer if complete resection is not possible (Samadi et al. 2020; Sheahan 2014).

However, novel therapies for cancer have been developed from recent advances in the understanding of the molecular mechanisms in the pathogenesis of malignancy. These include immunotherapy and gene therapy (Samadi et al. 2020).

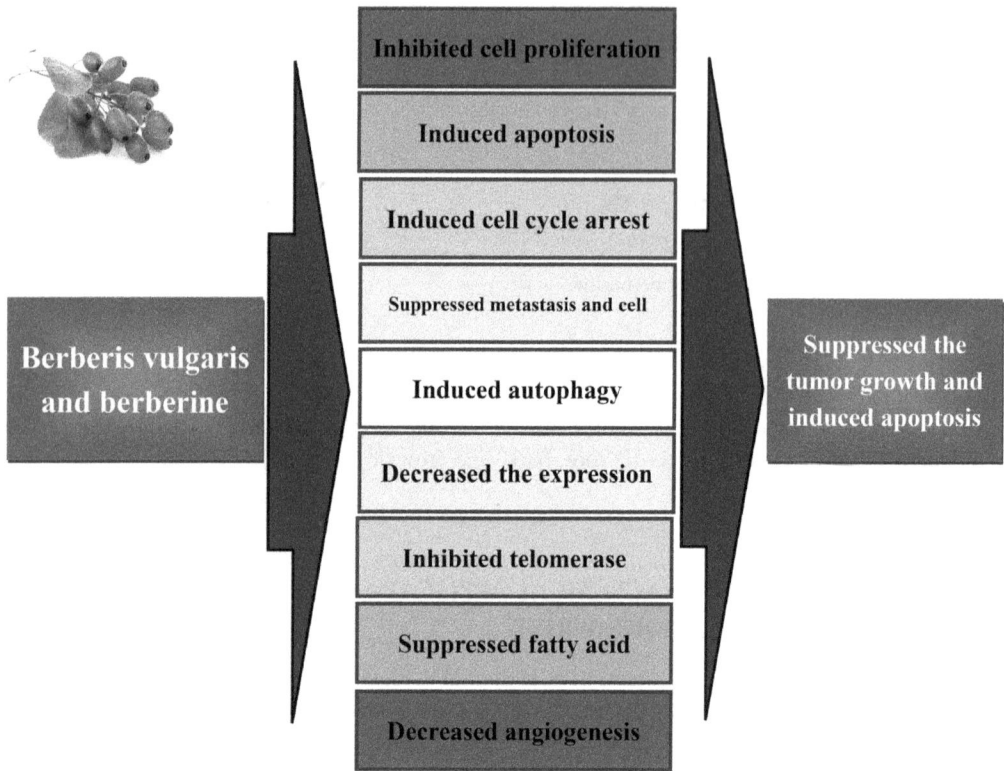

FIGURE 9.2   Schematic summary of the anticancer mechanisms of *Berberis vulgaris* and berberine.

Besides the standard therapies, plant-derived medicine has attracted a great deal of attention as a potential treatment for cancer (Samadi et al. 2020). One of the most important plants in cancer studies is *B. vulgaris* and its natural phytochemicals. This chapter describes the studies which have investigated their use to treat cancer.

9.5   *B. VULGARIS* AND CANCER STUDIES IN EXPERIMENTAL AND MOLECULAR STUDIES

The cytotoxic and anticancer properties of *B. vulgaris* and berberine have been shown in several experimental and molecular studies (Table 9.1). Berberine, by inhibiting the proliferation and synthesis of fatty acids, plays an important role in the suppression of the growth of tumor cells. This may be applicable as a novel approach to the treatment of cancer (Gu et al. 2020). Hoshyar et al. (Hoshyar, Mahboob, and Zarban 2016) investigated the cytotoxic effect of *B. vulgaris* and its extract on human breast carcinoma cells. This study suggested that *B. vulgaris* exerted its anticancer effect through antioxidant, antiproliferative, antimigratory, and apoptotic effects (Hoshyar, Mahboob, and Zarban 2016). So, a new therapeutic approach for breast cancer could include *B. vulgaris* (Hoshyar, Mahboob, and Zarban 2016).

Another study investigated the therapeutic effect of berberine on glioblastoma multiforme (Wang et al. 2016). Berberine significantly decreased the growth of cancer cells by induction of autophagy via increasing levels of 5′ adenosine monophosphate (AMP)-activated protein kinase (AMPK) and suppressing the expression of phosphorylated-mammalian target of rapamycin

TABLE 9.1
Experimental and Molecular Studies of the Pharmacological Applications of *Berberis vulgaris* and Berberine in the Treatment of Various Types of Cancer

Reference	Study Design	Type of Cancer/Cell Line	Treatment	Dose	Duration	Results
(Gu et al. 2020)	*In vitro* study	Human colon cancer cell line (HCT116), cervical cancer cell line (HeLa)	Berberine	2.5–10 μmol/L	0–60 hours	Inhibited proliferation and growth of tumor
(Hoshyar, Mahboob, and Zarban 2016)	*In vitro* study	Human breast cancer (MCF-7)	Alcoholic extract of *Berberis*	1.5 and 3 mg/mL	48 hours	Induced apoptosis
(Wang et al. 2016)	*In vitro/in vivo* study	Glioblastoma multiforme (GBM)	Berberine	–	24–48 hours	Induced autophagy by increasing AMPK and suppressing p-mTOR
(Li et al. 2014)	*In vitro* study	Nasopharyngeal carcinoma (CNE-1 cells)	Berberine hydrochloride	2.5, 5, 10, 20 and 40 μg/mL	0–48 hours	Reduced cell viability and proliferation, inhibited cell invasion and migration, and increased cell apoptosis
(Zhang et al. 2012)	*In vivo* study	Murine sarcoma S180	Berberine	30 mg/kg, (IV)	–	Decreased tumor weight and volume
(Choi et al. 2009)	*In vitro* study	Human prostate cancer (LNCaP cells, PC-3 cells)	Berberine	0, 5, 10, 20, 50, and 100 μM	0–48 hours	Inhibited cancerous cell proliferation and cell growth in a concentration- and time-dependent manner and induced the apoptotic proteins and apoptotic cell death
(Motaleb et al. 2008)	Experimental (rat)	Hepatocellular carcinoma (HCC)	*B. vulgaris* fruit extract	25, 50 or 100 mg/kg	11 weeks	Decreased the liver enzymes activities, including GST, GGT, and ALP, and inhibition the gene expression of AFP during hepatocarcinogenesis
(Hanachi, Othman, and Motaleb 2008)	Experimental (rat)	HCC	*B. vulgaris* aqueous extract	25, 50 or 100 mg/kg	11 weeks	Increased the TUNEL-positive apoptotic cells and induction of apoptosis
(Orfila et al. 2000)	*In vitro* study	Cell lines of uterus, ovary, larynx carcinoma	Berberine	–	–	Cytotoxic activity against different types of cell lines

Abbreviations: AFP = alpha-fetoprotein; ALP = alkaline phosphatase; AMPK = 5′ adenosine monophosphate (AMP)-activated protein kinase; GGT = gamma glutamyltransferase; GGT = glutathione S-transferase; p-mTOR = phosphorylated-mammalian target of rapamycin; TUNEL = terminal deoxynucleotidyl transferase deoxyuridine triphosphate nick end labeling.

(p-mTOR) (Wang et al. 2016). A study by Li et al. evaluated the effect of berberine hydrochloride (BH) on the apoptosis, invasion, proliferation, and migration of CNE-1 nasopharyngeal carcinoma cells (Li et al. 2014). The results suggested that decreased expression of Twist reduced the viability, proliferation, migration, and invasion of these malignant cells. The ability of BH to increase caspase-3 activity induced apoptosis in malignant cells (Li et al. 2014). Zhang et al. also concluded that berberine, a natural compound, could be a valuable antitumor agent in clinical practice (Zhang et al. 2012).

Another *in vitro* study investigated the effect of berberine on human prostate cancer cells (Choi et al. 2009). The results suggested that berberine reduced the weight, volume, and growth of tumors as well as the proliferation of cancer cells (Choi et al. 2009). Berberine, by increasing the expression of apoptotic proteins, including Bax and caspase-3, had an important role in tumor treatment (Choi et al. 2009). Motaleb et al. investigated the effect of an extract from the fruit of *B. vulgaris* in rats with liver cancer. In this model it was demonstrated that *B. vulgaris* may have a chemopreventive effect against hepatocarcinogenesis (Motaleb et al. 2008).

An extract of *B. vulgaris* also had a dose-dependent effect on the treatment of cancer by induction of apoptosis (Hanachi, Othman, and Motaleb 2008). The cytotoxic activity of berberine has been evaluated *in vitro*. Berberine had cytotoxic effect against different types of cell lines, including HeLa (uterus carcinoma), SVKO3 (ovary carcinoma), Hep-2 (larynx carcinoma), primary cultures from mouse embryos, and human fibroblast cells (Orfila et al. 2000).

9.6 RANDOMIZED CLINICAL TRIALS OF *B. VULGARIS* IN CANCER

The anticancer effect of *B. vulgaris* and berberine has been assessed in a small number of human clinical studies (Table 9.2). The RCT by Pirouzpanah et al. evaluated the effect of *B. vulgaris* juice on plasma concentration of IGF-binding proteins (IGFBPs), insulin-like growth

TABLE 9.2

The Randomized Clinical Trial Studies of the Pharmacological Applications of *Berberis vulgaris* and Berberine in Various Types of Cancer

Reference	Study Design	Type of Cancer	Treatment	Sample Size/ Trial Group	Dose/Duration	Results
(Pirouzpanah et al. 2019)	Double blind, RCT	Benign breast disease	*B. vulgaris* juice	85/44	*B. vulgaris* juice, 480 mL/day for 8 weeks	Decreased the expression of PPAR, VEGF, and HIF and prevented breast tumorigenesis
(Asemani et al. 2018)	Parallel, triple blind, RCT	Benign breast disease	*B. vulgaris* juice	85/44	*B. vulgaris* juice, 480 mL/day for 8 weeks	Decreased glycemic profiles and inhibited tumor growth
(Li, Wang, et al. 2010)	Double blind, RCT	Cervical cancer	Berberine	42/21	300 mg three times daily for 6 months	Decreased the complication of radiation in abdominal or pelvic areas, including RIAISs
(Liu et al. 2008)	Double blind, RCT	Lung cancer	Berberine	90/42	20 mg kg^{-1} once a day for 6 months	Reduced the radiation-induced lung injury in patients with lung cancer

Abbreviations: HIF = hypoxia-inducible factor; PPAR = peroxisome proliferator-activated receptor; RCT = randomized controlled trial; RIAIS = radiation-induced acute intestinal symptom; VEGF = vascular endothelial growth factor.

factor (IGF-1), and expression of peroxisome proliferator-activated receptor gamma (PPAR-γ), vascular endothelial growth factor (VEGF) and hypoxia-inducible factors (HIF) in women with benign breast disease. *B. vulgaris* juice decreased plasma levels of IGF-1, the IGF-1/IGFBP-1 ratio, and the expression of PPAR, VEGF, and HIF (Pirouzpanah et al. 2019). These tumorigenic factors are associated with the growth of cancer cells and promote malignant change (Pirouzpanah et al. 2019). Asemani et al. investigated the effect of *B. vulgaris* juice on glycemic profiles in women with benign breast disease (Asemani et al. 2018). *B. vulgaris* juice had beneficial effects on functions related to insulin signaling that are associated with tumorigenesis (Asemani et al. 2018).

A double-blind RCT evaluated the effect of berberine on the severity of radiation-induced acute intestinal symptoms (RIAISs). This is a common complication of radiotherapy to the abdomen or pelvis. Berberine (300 mg three times a day) in patients with cervical cancer reduced the severity of RIAISs due to pelvic or abdominal radiotherapy (Li, Wang, et al. 2010). It also had an effective role in cancer treatment process and reduction of complications (Li, Wang, et al. 2010). Liu et al. conducted a double blind RCT of the effect of berberine on radiation-induced lung injury (RILI) in patients with lung cancer. Berberine reduced RILI and improved pulmonary function in lung cancer. It exerted this effect by reducing soluble intercellular adhesion molecular-1 (sICAM-1) and transforming growth factor beta-1 (TGF-β1) (Liu et al. 2008).

9.7 ANTICANCER MECHANISMS AND MOLECULAR PATHWAYS OF *B. VULGARIS* AND BERBERINE

This section comprehensively explains the anticancer mechanisms of *B. vulgaris* and berberine. These include antiproliferative and apoptotic activities, arrest of the cell cycle, and inhibiting cell invasion and migration. These effects involve several molecular pathways in different types of cancer.

9.7.1 INHIBITED CELL PROLIFERATION AND INDUCED APOPTOSIS

Abnormal cell proliferation and blockage of apoptosis are mechanisms related to tumorigenesis and progression of cancer. Berberine inhibits cell proliferation. Berberine exerts this effect through several pathways. Berberine upregulates p53 expression, which is an important tumor suppressor protein. It plays a beneficial role in cell cycle arrest, regulation of proliferation, cell growth, and induction of apoptosis, and subsequently induces nuclear stress that results in inhibition of cell proliferation and death of cells (Sakaguchi et al. 2020). Berberine downregulates metadherin (MTDH) or astrocyte elevated gene-1 protein (AEG-1). These oncogenic factors are strongly expressed in several types of cancer (Sun, Wang, and Tong 2019).

Apoptosis (programmed cell death) controls the molecular sequences that contribute to cell death. Suppression of apoptosis is tumorigenic. Berberine, a pro-apoptotic agent, stimulates cell death via both the extrinsic and intrinsic pathways of apoptosis (Samadi et al. 2020). In the extrinsic (cytoplasmic) pathway, berberine stimulates the expression of Fas receptor. This a surface death receptor that contributes to programmed cell death, when Fas binds Fas ligand (FasL). Stimulation of Fas subsequently activates caspase-8 and caspase-3, which are involved in induction of apoptosis (Zapata et al. 2001).

However, berberine induces the production of reactive oxygen species (ROS). The higher production of ROS increases intracellular calcium through the endoplasmic reticulum (ER). This stimulates of caspase-12 (induction of apoptosis) and suppresses the expression of B-cell lymphoma-2 (BCL-2) family proteins that act as anti-apoptotic protein.

In addition, the production of ROS increases the activity of p38 mitogen-activated protein kinase (MAPK) and c-Jun N-terminal kinase (JNK). This subsequently increases p53 and p53 upregulated modulator of apoptosis (PUMA) that enhance the levels of BCL2 associated X (BAX) and Bcl-2-like protein 11 (BIM), which contribute to apoptosis. In the intrinsic pathway, berberine increases cytochrome c and apoptotic protease activating factor 1 (APAF-1) and suppresses the expression of BCL-2 and B-cell lymphoma extra-large (BCL-XL) proteins (anti-apoptotic agents) through mitochondrial membrane potential (Samadi et al. 2020; Fulda and Debatin 2006; Hockenbery et al. 1990).

9.7.2 Induced Cell Cycle Arrest

Previous studies suggested that berberine, the most important isoquinoline alkaloid of barberry, might have a useful effect on cell cycle arrest. Two important types of regulatory molecules are related to the control of cell cycle process. These are the cyclins and cyclin-dependent kinases (CDKs). Berberine increases the expression of proteins Cip/p21 and Kip/p27 and decreases the expression of cyclins D1, D2, and E and cyclin-dependent kinases Cdk2, Cdk4, and Cdk6. This arrests the cell cycle at the G_0/G_1 phase and contributes to the decline in the population of cells in the S and G_2/M phases (Li et al. 2017). In addition, berberine through the activation of miR-23a, plays an important role in increasing the expression of inhibitors of the cell cycle, including p53 and p21 (a potent cyclin-dependent kinase inhibitor) that results in cell cycle arrest (Zheng et al. 2014).

9.7.3 Suppressed Metastasis and Cell Invasion

Local invasion and metastasis are important characteristics of malignant that increase the risk of mortality. The extracellular matrix (ECM) acts as a mechanical barrier against movement of the cell. Matrix metalloproteinases (MMPs) could degrade the ECM, facilitating metastasis and cell invasion. In addition, MMP contributes to tumor progression and MMP-3. This form of MMP regulates angiogenesis, cell invasion, and metastasis (Yilmaz, Christofori, and Lehembre 2007).

The effect of berberine on the inhibition of cell invasion and metastasis has been investigated. The mechanisms by which berberine suppresses cell invasion and metastasis are as follows.

First, berberine inhibits the expression of MMP-3 (decrease both mRNA and protein) by regulating negative extracellular signal–regulated kinase (ERK) activation. ERK is an important signaling cassette that has roles in different types of cellular process, including cell differentiation, adhesion, proliferation, migration, and survival (Ho et al. 2009; Samadi et al. 2020).

Second, berberine reduces the levels of MMP-2 and MMP-9 by downregulating transforming growth factor beta-1 (TGF-β1) and ephrin-B2, which suppress cell migration and growth (Ho et al. 2009; Samadi et al. 2020). Third, nuclear factor kappa B (NF-κB) is a ubiquitous transcription factor that reduces cell apoptosis and metastasis. Berberine inhibits the toll-like receptor 9 (TLR9)-myeloid differentiation factor 88 (MyD88)–nuclear factor kappa-B (NF-κB) pathway related to metastasis (Ho et al. 2009; Samadi et al. 2020; Zhu et al. 2022). Fourth, the expression of vasodilator stimulated phosphoprotein (VASP) and fibronectin (FN) is an indicator in metastatic and poor prognosis cancer. Berberine binds to VASP and alters its secondary structure. Berberine also down regulates FN expression (Jeong et al. 2018; Su et al. 2016). Fifth, by the suppression of the focal adhesion kinase (FAK), urokinase type plasminogen activator (u-PA), IκB kinase (IKK) through the inhibition of the ERK/MAPK and NF-κB pathways, berberine plays a role in decreasing cell invasion and migration (Ho et al. 2009; Samadi et al. 2020). These actions suppress cell invasion and metastasis and subsequently improve progression toward apoptosis.

9.7.4 Induced Autophagy

Autophagy is involved in programmed cell death type II (PCD II) and suppression of tumors (Hsieh, Athar, and Chaudry 2009). Berberine may have a role in the induction of autophagy. Stimulation of P38 mitogen-activated protein kinase (MAPK) and suppression of Akt signaling by berberine could inhibit the mTOR signaling pathway. mTOR is a serine/threonine protein kinase that acts as an important regulator of cell growth, cell proliferation, and synthesis of the proteins. In addition, berberine play an important role in activation of Beclin-1. mTOR-signaling pathway inhibition and Beclin-1 activation are involved in autophagy (Wang et al. 2010). In addition, a study on the glioblastoma (GBM) cells demonstrated that berberine contributes to autophagy by increasing the AMP-activated protein kinase (AMPK) levels and suppressing the levels of phosphorylated mammalian target of rapamycin (p-mTOR) (Wang et al. 2016).

9.7.5 Decreased the Expression of Hypoxia-Inducible Factors (HIFs) and Angiogenesis

HIF is a tumorigenic factor that enhances growth of tumor and metastasis. *B. vulgaris* juice and its isoquinoline alkaloid, berberine, decrease levels of HIF through different mechanisms. *B. vulgaris* juice decreases IGF-1, increases IGFBP-1, and subsequently reduces the IGF-1/IGFBP-1 ratio that alters the phosphatidil-inositol-3-kinase/Akt (PI3K/Akt) pathway and mitogen activating protein kinase/extracellular receptor kinase (MEK/ERK). This process decreases the expression of HIF-1α and subsequently downregulates the expression of vascular endothelial growth factor (VEGF) and angiogenesis (Pirouzpanah et al. 2019).

9.7.6 Suppressed Fatty Acid Synthesis and Declined Extracellular Vesicles Biogenesis

De novo synthesis of fatty acids enhances tumor cells to proliferate and grow. A rate-limiting enzyme in the first step of fatty acid synthesis is acetyl-CoA carboxylase (ACC). AMP-activated protein kinase (AMPK) controls the activation of ACC. Berberine, by stimulating AMPK, inhibits the activation of ACC. This suppresses fatty acid synthesis and decreases the biogenesis of extracellular vesicles. So, berberine could be a new therapeutic agent against cancer (Gu et al. 2020).

9.8 TELOMERASE INHIBITION

Telomerase, also known as a terminal transferase, is a ribonucleoprotein enzyme that is responsible for adding a species-dependent telomere repeat sequence to the 3′ end of telomeres. Suppression of telomerase leads to inhibition of proliferation and apoptosis in cancerous cells. As the tendency of berberine to bind with G-quadruplex DNA structures is high, berberine plays an important role in downregulating telomerase activity and exerts its apoptotic effect in tumor cells (Rocca et al. 2015).

9.9 THE ANTI-INFLAMMATORY EFFECT OF *B. VULGARIS* AND BERBERINE

The anti-inflammatory properties of berberine suppress cell proliferation. Berberine suppresses the expression of the cyclooxygenase-2 (COX_2) and decreases the production of prostaglandin E_2 (PGE_2) by inhibition of AP-1 binding or the AP-1 promoter site. Berberine could also increase the expression of antitumor cytokines, including interferon-β (IFN-β) and tumor necrosis factor alpha (TNF-α). Furthermore, berberine inhibits the production of interleukin-6 (IL-6) suppressing the inflammatory response driven by epidermal growth factor receptor activated/extracellular signal–regulated kinase (EGFR-ERK) signaling (Song, Hao, and Fan 2020).

9.10 OTHER MOLECULAR ANTICANCER MECHANISMS OF *B. VULGARIS* AND BERBERINE

Berberine plays an important role in breaking double-stranded deoxyribonucleic acid (DNA) and changing the conformation of DNA. It then inhibits the transcription of genes via block of the relation of TATA binding protein (TBP) with the TATA box in the promoters of genes. So, berberine could suppress the replication of DNA. In addition, berberine could bind to the death-domain-associated protein (DAXX) and downregulate the expression of DAXX.

The decreased expression of DAXX activates p53, subsequently leading to apoptosis. Furthermore, two enzymes that regulate the folate cycle, thymidylate synthase (TS) and dihydrofolate reductase (DHFR), are necessary in the biosynthesis of DNA and cell growth. Previous data suggest that berberine could suppress the expression of TS and DHFR. Thus its antiproliferative effect may block the growth of malignant cells, especially in cells resistant to cisplatin (Guamán Ortiz et al. 2014).

9.11 OTHER FOODS, HERBS, SPICES, AND BOTANICALS USED IN CANCER

Previous surveys indicated that about 50% of cancer patients use herbs, spices, and botanicals as alternative and complementary medicine for prevention and treatment of different types of cancer (Boon and Wong 2004). In addition, herbs and spices have an important role in prevention of normal tissue injury, tumor recurrence, and metastasis. Furthermore, the use of herbs and botanicals in cancer patients is associated with reduction of radiotherapy and chemotherapy side effects, as well as depression, fatigue, insomnia, nausea, and vomiting (Zulfiker et al. 2017; Liu et al. 2019). Natural herbs and spices have a helpful role in prevention and treatment of various types of cancer through several mechanisms, including prevention of invasion and metastasis, activation of anticancer immunity, promotion of cancer cell apoptosis, synergistic enhancement of the efficacy of radiotherapy and chemotherapy, and inhibition of cancer cell growth. Garlic (*Allium sativum*) and its bioactive components, including allicin, diallyl disulfide, and allyl isothiocyanate, have a beneficial role in prevention and treatment of cancer. In addition, considered as an herb, ginger (*Zingiber officinale*) could significantly decrease the duration and severity of nausea and vomiting, which are side effects of chemotherapy. This property of ginger might be related to its bioactive components such as zingiberone, ingerol, paradol, zingiberene, shagoal, and curcumin. The bioactive content of green tea, including epigallocatechin gallate, epigallocatechin, catechin, theophylline, gallic acid, and theanine, plays a beneficial role in both prevention and treatment of cancers. In addition, some spices, including cinnamon, pepper (black and red), saffron, thyme, and turmeric could decrease the incidence of different types of cancers and might play a role in treatment of cancers. Other effective herbs, spices, botanicals, and foods used in cancer treatment are basil, cardamom, caraway, cloves, coriander, cumin, dill, fennel, licorice, mustard, marjoram, nutmeg, oregano, paprika, parsley, peppermint, rosemary, sage, tarragon, reishi, ginseng, tomato, and onion. Incidence and promotion of cancers are related to oxidative stress, inflammation, imbalance in the microbiome, and tumorigenesis. Thus by modification of microbiota, antioxidant, antitumorigenesis activity, and suppression of carcinogenic pathways, many herbs and spices could protect humans against cancer (Boon and Wong 2004; Kaefer and Milner 2008; Liu et al. 2019).

9.12   TOXICITY AND CAUTIONARY NOTES

A survey assessed the safety of oral usage of barberry in an *in vivo* study. The results showed that oral usage of barberry did not have any significant adverse effect on organs in laboratory animals and found no significant hepatotoxicity and hematotoxicity (Sarhadynejad et al. 2016). However, other surveys revealed that *B. vulgaris* and berberine might be involved in ulceration and upset of the gastrointestinal system, phototoxicity, immunotoxicity, cardiotoxicity, jaundice, and neurotoxicity in a dose-response manner and related to the route and duration of *B. vulgaris* and berberine use. In addition, *B. vulgaris* and berberine should be applied with caution in pregnant women, neonates, and persons with G6PD deficiency. Furthermore, because of the inhibitory effect of berberine on CYP enzymes, co-administration of drugs that metabolized with these enzymes with berberine should be be carried out with caution (Rad, Rameshrad, and Hosseinzadeh 2017). To clarify the effective dose and duration of *B. vulgaris* and berberine on cancer prevention and treatment, more studies with accurate design in animals and human are warranted.

9.13   CONCLUSION

B. vulgaris and its isoquinoline alkaloid, berberine, has attracted attention in herbal medicine. Its potential to prevent and treat various types of cancer has been studied. *B. vulgaris* and berberine act through multiple mechanisms, including inhibition of cell proliferation, apoptosis, cell cycle arrest, suppression of metastasis and cell invasion, autophagy, decreased HIF expression and angiogenesis, suppression of fatty acid synthesis and reduced extracellular vesicles biogenesis, and various molecular pathways that have an important role in treatment of cancer.

Thus, *B. vulgaris* and its isoquinoline alkaloid, berberine, could be trialed as novel therapeutic agents in cancer studies. The effect of different forms of *B. vulgaris* and berberine on the development and treatment of various types of cancer has been investigated in several molecular and experimental studies. However, very few clinical studies have assessed the anticancer effect of *B. vulgaris*. There is a paucity of clinical data on the optimum dose and duration, anticancer efficacy, and potential side effect profile in humans. This should be studied further. Research should also be carried out to clarify causality, shed a light on the underlying pathogenesis, and identify the effective dose and side effects in human studies.

9.14   SUMMARY POINTS

- This chapter focuses on the use of *B. vulgaris* and berberine for the treatment of cancer.
- On account of antioxidant, cardioprotective, anti-inflammatory, and hypoglycemic properties, *B. vulgaris* and berberine have attracted attention in herbal medicine and are used for the prevention and treatment of a wide range of diseases.
- Various compounds including isoquinoline alkaloids, coumarin, vitamins, phenylpropanoid, carotenoids, flavonoids, carbohydrate, and flavonol have been isolated from different parts of this plant.
- One of the most important isoquinoline alkaloids in barberry is berberine. This protoberberine compound is found in the root, bark, and fruit of *B. vulgaris*.
- Besides the standard therapies, plant-derived medicine has attracted a great deal of attention as a potential treatment for cancer, and one of the most important plants in cancer studies is *B. vulgaris* and its natural phytochemicals.
- Berberine, by inhibiting the proliferation and synthesis of fatty acids, plays an important role in the suppression of the growth of tumor cells.
- The anticancer mechanisms of *B. vulgaris* and berberine include antiproliferative and apoptotic activities, inhibiting cell invasion and migration and arrest of the cell cycle.

- *B. vulgaris* and berberine should be applied with caution in pregnant women, neonates, and persons with G6PD deficiency.
- Because of the inhibitory effect of berberine on CYP enzymes, co-administration of drugs that metabolized with these enzymes with berberine should be carried out with caution.

REFERENCES

Alemardan, Ali, Wahab Asadi, Mehdi Rezaei, Leila Tabrizi, and Siavash Mohammadi. 2013. "Cultivation of Iranian seedless barberry (*Berberis integerrima* 'Bidaneh'): A medicinal shrub." *Industrial Crops and Products* 50:276–287.

Arayne, M. Saeed, Najma Sultana, and Saima Sher Bahadur. 2007. "The berberis story: *Berberis vulgaris* in therapeutics." *Pakistan Journal of Pharmaceutical Sciences* 20 (1):83–92.

Asemani, S., V. Montazeri, B. Baradaran, M. A. Tabatabiefar, and S. Pirouzpanah. 2018. "The Effects of *Berberis vulgaris* juice on insulin indices in women with benign breast disease: A randomized controlled clinical trial." *Iran J Pharm Res* 17 (Suppl):110–121.

Awasthi, Harshika, Rajendra Nath, Kauser Usman, Dayanandan Mani, Sanjay Khattri, Anuradha Nischal, Manju Singh, and Kamal Kumar Sawlani. 2015. "Effects of a standardized Ayurvedic formulation on diabetes control in newly diagnosed Type-2 diabetics; a randomized active controlled clinical study." *Complementary Therapies in Medicine* 23 (4):555–561.

Ayati, S. H., B. Fazeli, A. A. Momtazi-borojeni, A. F. G. Cicero, M. Pirro, and A. Sahebkar. 2017. "Regulatory effects of berberine on microRNome in Cancer and other conditions." *Critical Reviews in Oncology/Hematology* 116:147–158. doi:10.1016/j.critrevonc.2017.05.008

Bagherniya, M., V. Nobili, C. N. Blesso, and A. Sahebkar. 2018. "Medicinal plants and bioactive natural compounds in the treatment of non–alcoholic fatty liver disease: A clinical review." *Pharmacological Research* 130:213–240. doi:10.1016/j.phrs.2017.12.020

Boon, Heather, and Jacqueline Wong. 2004. "Botanical medicine and cancer: A review of the safety and efficacy." *Expert Opinion on Pharmacotherapy* 5 (12):2485–2501.

Bray, Freddie, Mathieu Laversanne, Elisabete Weiderpass, and Isabelle Soerjomataram. 2021. "The ever-increasing importance of cancer as a leading cause of premature death worldwide." *Cancer* 127 (16):3029–3030.

Choi, Myoung Suk, Ju Hoon Oh, Sun Mi Kim, Hai Young Jung, Hwan Soo Yoo, Yong Moon Lee, Dong Cheul Moon, Sang Bae Han, and Jin Tae Hong. 2009. "Berberine inhibits p53-dependent cell growth through induction of apoptosis of prostate cancer cells." *International Journal of Oncology* 34 (5):1221–1230.

Cicero, Arrigo F. G., and Elisa Tartagni. 2012. "Antidiabetic properties of berberine: From cellular pharmacology to clinical effects." *Hospital Practice* 40 (2):56–63.

Dash, Sonali, Manish Kumar, and Nidhi Pareek. 2020. "Enhanced antibacterial potential of berberine via synergism with chitosan nanoparticles." *Materials Today: Proceedings* 31:640–645.

Di Pierro, Francesco, Pietro Putignano, Tarcisio Ferrara, Carmela Raiola, Giuliana Rapacioli, and Nicola Villanova. 2017. "Retrospective analysis of the effects of a highly standardized mixture of *Berberis aristata, Silybum marianum*, and monacolins K and KA in patients with dyslipidemia." *Clinical Pharmacology: Advances and Applications* 9:1.

Fatehi, Mohammad, Tarek M. Saleh, Zahra Fatehi-Hassanabad, Khadige Farrokhfal, Mostafa Jafarzadeh, and Samaneh Davodi. 2005. "A pharmacological study on *Berberis vulgaris* fruit extract." *Journal of Ethnopharmacology* 102 (1):46–52.

Fulda, S., and K. M. Debatin. 2006. "Extrinsic versus intrinsic apoptosis pathways in anticancer chemotherapy." *Oncogene* 25 (34):4798–4811. doi:10.1038/sj.onc.1209608

Giuseppe, Derosa, D'Angelo Angela, Romano Davide, and Maffioli Pamela. 2017. "Effects of a combination of *Berberis aristata, Silybum marianum* and monacolin on lipid profile in subjects at low cardiovascular risk; a double-blind, randomized, placebo-controlled trial." *International Journal of Molecular Sciences* 18 (2):343.

Gu, Songgang, Xuhong Song, Rufei Xie, Cong Ouyang, Lingzhu Xie, Qidong Li, Ting Su, Man Xu, Tian Xu, Dongyang Huang, and Bin Liang. 2020. "Berberine inhibits cancer cells growth by suppressing fatty acid synthesis and biogenesis of extracellular vesicles." *Life Sciences* 257:118122. doi:10.1016/j.lfs.2020.118122

Guamán Ortiz, Luis Miguel, Paolo Lombardi, Micol Tillhon, and Anna Ivana Scovassi. 2014. "Berberine, an epiphany against cancer." *Molecules* 19 (8):12349–12367.

Hanachi, P., F. Othman, and G.R. Motaleb. 2008. "Effect of *Berberis vulgaris* aqueous extract on the apoptosis, sodium and potassium in hepatocarcinogenic rats." *Iranian Journal of Basic Medical Sciences* 11 (2 (38)).

Hesari, A., F. Ghasemi, A. F. G. Cicero, M. Mohajeri, O. Rezaei, S. M. G. Hayat, and A. Sahebkar. 2018. "Berberine: A potential adjunct for the treatment of gastrointestinal cancers?" *Journal of Cellular Biochemistry* 119 (12):9655–9663. doi:10.1002/jcb.27392

Ho, Yung-Tsuan, Chi-Cheng Lu, Jai-Sing Yang, Jo-Hua Chiang, Tsai-Chung Li, Siu-Wan Ip, Te-Chun Hsia, Ching-Lung Liao, Jaung-Geng Lin, and W. Gibson Wood. 2009. "Berberine induced apoptosis via promoting the expression of caspase-8,-9 and-3, apoptosis-inducing factor and endonuclease G in SCC-4 human tongue squamous carcinoma cancer cells." *Anticancer Research* 29 (10):4063–4070.

Hockenbery, D., G. Nuñez, C. Milliman, R. D. Schreiber, and S. J. Korsmeyer. 1990. "Bcl-2 is an inner mitochondrial membrane protein that blocks programmed cell death." *Nature* 348 (6299):334–336. doi:10.1038/348334a0

Hoshyar, R., Z. Mahboob, and A. Zarban. 2016. "The antioxidant and chemical properties of *Berberis vulgaris* and its cytotoxic effect on human breast carcinoma cells." *Cytotechnology* 68 (4):1207–1213. doi:10.1007/s10616-015-9880-y

Hsieh, Ya-Ching, Mohammad Athar, and Irshad H Chaudry. 2009. "When apoptosis meets autophagy: Deciding cell fate after trauma and sepsis." *Trends in Molecular Medicine* 15 (3):129–138.

Imanshahidi, M., and H. Hosseinzadeh. 2008. "Pharmacological and therapeutic effects of *Berberis vulgaris* and its active constituent, berberine." *Phytother Res* 22 (8):999–1012. doi:10.1002/ptr.2399

Imenshahidi, Mohsen, and Hossein Hosseinzadeh. 2019. "Berberine and barberry (*Berberis vulgaris*): A clinical review." *Phytotherapy Research* 33 (3):504–523.

Jeong, Yisun, Daeun You, Hyun-Gu Kang, Jonghan Yu, Seok Won Kim, Seok Jin Nam, Jeong Eon Lee, and Sangmin Kim. 2018. "Berberine suppresses fibronectin expression through inhibition of c-Jun phosphorylation in breast cancer cells." *Journal of Breast Cancer* 21 (1):21–27.

Kaefer, Christine M., and John A. Milner. 2008. "The role of herbs and spices in cancer prevention." *The Journal of Nutritional Biochemistry* 19 (6):347–361.

Kalmarzi, Rasool Nasiri, Seyyed Nima Naleini, Damoon Ashtary-Larky, Ilaria Peluso, Leila Jouybari, Alireza Rafi, Fereshteh Ghorat, Nishteman Heidari, Faezeh Sharifian, and Jalal Mardaneh. 2019. "Anti-inflammatory and immunomodulatory effects of barberry (*Berberis vulgaris*) and its main compounds." *Oxidative Medicine and Cellular Longevity* 2019.

Kim, Young-Dong, Sung-Hee Kim, and Leslie R. Landrum. 2004. "Taxonomic and phytogeographic implications from ITS phylogeny in *Berberis* (Berberidaceae)." *Journal of Plant Research* 117 (3):175–182.

Kumar, Ravi, Mansi Awasthi, Anamika Sharma, Yogendra Padwad, and Rohit Sharma. 2020. "Berberine induces dose-dependent quiescence and apoptosis in A549 cancer cells by modulating cell cyclins and inflammation independent of mTOR pathway." *Life Sciences* 244:117346.

Li, Cai-Hong, Dong-Fang Wu, Hang Ding, Yang Zhao, Ke-Yuan Zhou, and De-Feng Xu. 2014. "Berberine hydrochloride impact on physiological processes and modulation of twist levels in nasopharyngeal carcinoma CNE-1 cells." *Asian Pacific Journal of Cancer Prevention* 15 (4):1851–1857.

Li, Guang-hui, Dong-lin Wang, Yi-de Hu, Ping Pu, De-zhi Li, Wei-dong Wang, Bo Zhu, Ping Hao, Jun Wang, Xian-qiong Xu, Jiu-qing Wan, Yi-bing Zhou, and Zheng-tang Chen. 2010. "Berberine inhibits acute radiation intestinal syndrome in human with abdomen radiotherapy." *Medical Oncology* 27 (3):919–925. doi:10.1007/s12032-009-9307-8

Li, Liang, Xingchun Wang, Rampersad Sharvan, Jingyang Gao, and Shen Qu. 2017. "Berberine could inhibit thyroid carcinoma cells by inducing mitochondrial apoptosis, G0/G1 cell cycle arrest and suppressing migration via PI3K-AKT and MAPK signaling pathways." *Biomedicine & Pharmacotherapy* 95:1225–1231.

Li, Ye-Liang, Zlatko Kvaček, David K Ferguson, Yu-Fei Wang, Cheng-Sen Li, Jian Yang, Tsun-Shen Ying, Albert G Ablaev, and Hai-Ming Liu. 2010. "The fossil record of *Berberis* (Berberidaceae) from the Palaeocene of NE China and interpretations of the evolution and phytogeography of the genus." *Review of Palaeobotany and Palynology* 160 (1–2):10–31.

Liu, Wei, Binbin Yang, Lu Yang, Jasmine Kaur, Calvin Jessop, Rushdi Fadhil, David Good, Guoying Ni, Xiaosong Liu, and Tamim Mosaiab. 2019. "Therapeutic effects of ten commonly used Chinese herbs and their bioactive compounds on cancers." *Evidence-Based Complementary and Alternative Medicine* 2019.

Liu, Yunfang, Huiming Yu, Cheng Zhang, Yufeng Cheng, Likuan Hu, Xiaohui Meng, and Yuxia Zhao. 2008. "Protective effects of berberine on radiation-induced lung injury via intercellular adhesion molecular-1 and transforming growth factor-beta-1 in patients with lung cancer." *European Journal of Cancer* 44 (16):2425–2432.

Loo, Yan Shan, Thiagarajan Madheswaran, Ramkumar Rajendran, and Rajendran J. C. Bose. 2020. "Encapsulation of berberine into liquid crystalline nanoparticles to enhance its solubility and anticancer activity in MCF7 human breast cancer cells." *Journal of Drug Delivery Science and Technology* 57:101756.

Lopes, Tairine Zara, Fabio Rogerio de Moraes, Antonio Claudio Tedesco, Raghuvir Krishnaswamy Arni, Paula Rahal, and Marilia Freitas Calmon. 2020. "Berberine associated photodynamic therapy promotes autophagy and apoptosis via ROS generation in renal carcinoma cells." *Biomedicine & Pharmacotherapy* 123:109794.

Mazzini, Stefania, Maria Cristina Bellucci, and Rosanna Mondelli. 2003. "Mode of binding of the cytotoxic alkaloid berberine with the double helix oligonucleotide d (AAGAATTCTT) 2." *Bioorganic & Medicinal Chemistry* 11 (4):505–514.

Mohammadi, A., A. Sahebkar, T. Kermani, M. Zhilaee, S. Tavallaie, and M. G. Mobarhan. 2014. "Barberry administration and pro-oxidant – antioxidant balance in patients with metabolic syndrome." *Iranian Red Crescent Medical Journal* 16 (12). doi:10.5812/ircmj.16786

Mokhber-Dezfuli, Najmeh, Soodabeh Saeidnia, Ahmad Reza Gohari, and Mahdieh Kurepaz-Mahmoodabadi. 2014. "Phytochemistry and pharmacology of *Berberis* species." *Pharmacognosy Reviews* 8 (15):8.

Mortazavi, Hamed, Banafsheh Nikfar, Seyed-Alireza Esmaeili, Fatemeh Rafieenia, Ehsan Saburi, Shahla Chaichian, Mohammad Ali Heidari Gorji, and Amir Abbas Momtazi-Borojeni. 2020. "Potential cytotoxic and anti-metastatic effects of berberine on gynaecological cancers with drug-associated resistance." *European Journal of Medicinal Chemistry* 187:111951.

Motaleb, G., P. Hanachi, O. Fauziah, and R. Asmah. 2008. "Effect of *Berberis vulgaris* fruit extract on alpha-fetoprotein gene expression and chemical carcinogen metabolizing enzymes activities in hepatocarcinogenesis rats." *International Journal of Cancer Management (Iranian Journal of Cancer Prevention)* 1 (1).

Orfila, Luz, María Rodríguez, Trina Colman, Masahisa Hasegawa, Elizabeth Merentes, and Francisco Arvelo. 2000. "Structural modification of berberine alkaloids in relation to cytotoxic activity in vitro." *Journal of Ethnopharmacology* 71 (3):449–456. doi:10.1016/S0378-8741(00)00177-X

Pirouzpanah, S., S. Asemani, A. Shayanfar, B. Baradaran, and V. Montazeri. 2019. "The effects of *Berberis vulgaris* consumption on plasma levels of IGF-1, IGFBPs, PPAR-γ and the expression of angiogenic genes in women with benign breast disease: a randomized controlled clinical trial." *BMC Complement Altern Med* 19 (1):324. doi:10.1186/s12906-019-2715-1

Rad, Seyede Zohre Kamrani, Maryam Rameshrad, and Hossein Hosseinzadeh. 2017. "Toxicology effects of *Berberis vulgaris* (barberry) and its active constituent, berberine: A review." *Iranian Journal of Basic Medical Sciences* 20 (5):516.

Rocca, Roberta, Federica Moraca, Giosuè Costa, Stefano Alcaro, Simona Distinto, Elias Maccioni, Francesco Ortuso, Anna Artese, and Lucia Parrotta. 2015. "Structure-based virtual screening of novel natural alkaloid derivatives as potential binders of h-telo and c-myc DNA G-quadruplex conformations." *Molecules* 20 (1):206–223.

Sahebkar, A., and G. F. Watts. 2017. "Mode of action of berberine on lipid metabolism: A new-old phytochemical with clinical applications?" *Current Opinion in Lipidology* 28 (3):282–283. doi:10.1097/MOL.0000000000000409

Sakaguchi, Minoru, Daiki Kitaguchi, Shiho Morinami, Yuki Kurashiki, Haruna Hashida, Saki Miyata, Maki Yamaguchi, Miyu Sakai, Natsuko Murata, and Satoshi Tanaka. 2020. "Berberine-induced nucleolar stress response in a human breast cancer cell line." *Biochemical and Biophysical Research Communications* 528 (1):227–233.

Samadi, Parisa, Parisa Sarvarian, Elham Gholipour, Karim Shams Asenjan, Leili Aghebati-Maleki, Roza Motavalli, Mohammad Hojjat-Farsangi, and Mehdi Yousefi. 2020. "Berberine: A novel therapeutic strategy for cancer." *IUBMB Life* 72 (10):2065–2079.

Sarhadynejad, Zarrin, Fariba Sharififar, Abbas Pardakhty, Mohammad-Hadi Nematollahi, Saeedeh Sattaie-Mokhtari, and Ali Mandegary. 2016. "Pharmacological safety evaluation of a traditional herbal medicine 'Zereshk-e-Saghir' and assessment of its hepatoprotective effects on carbon tetrachloride induced hepatic damage in rats." *Journal of Ethnopharmacology* 190:387–395.

Shamsa, F., A. Ahmadiani, and R. Khosrokhavar. 1999. "Antihistaminic and anticholinergic activity of barberry fruit (*Berberis vulgaris*) in the guinea-pig ileum." *Journal of Ethnopharmacology* 64 (2):161–166.

Sheahan, Patrick. 2014. "Management of advanced laryngeal cancer." *Rambam Maimonides Medical Journal* 5 (2):e0015. doi:10.5041/RMMJ.10149

Shidfar, Farzad, Shima Seyyed Ebrahimi, Sharieh Hosseini, Iraj Heydari, Shahrzad Shidfar, and Giti Hajhassani. 2012. "The effects of *Berberis vulgaris* fruit extract on serum lipoproteins, apoB, apoA-I, homocysteine, glycemic control and total antioxidant capacity in type 2 diabetic patients." *Iranian Journal of Pharmaceutical Research: IJPR* 11 (2):643.

Sobhani, Z., M. Akaberi, M. S. Amiri, M. Ramezani, S. A. Emami, and A. Sahebkar. 2021. "Medicinal species of the genus berberis: A review of their traditional and ethnomedicinal uses, phytochemistry and pharmacology." *Advances in Experimental Medicine and Biology* 1308:547–577. doi:10.1007/978-3-030-64872-5_27

Song, Danyang, Jianyu Hao, and Daiming Fan. 2020. "Biological properties and clinical applications of berberine." *Frontiers of Medicine* 14 (5):564–582.

Su, Ke, Pengchao Hu, Xiaolan Wang, Changchun Kuang, Qingmin Xiang, Fang Yang, Jin Xiang, Shan Zhu, Lei Wei, and Jingwei Zhang. 2016. "Tumor suppressor berberine binds VASP to inhibit cell migration in basal-like breast cancer." *Oncotarget* 7 (29):45849.

Sun, Yong, Wentao Wang, and Yuwen Tong. 2019. "Berberine inhibits proliferative ability of breast cancer cells by reducing metadherin." *Medical Science Monitor: International Medical Journal of Experimental and Clinical Research* 25:9058.

Tew, Xin Nee, Natalie Jia Xin Lau, Dinesh Kumar Chellappan, Thiagarajan Madheswaran, Farrukh Zeeshan, Murtaza M. Tambuwala, Alaa A. A. Aljabali, Sri Renukadevi Balusamy, Haribalan Perumalsamy, and Gaurav Gupta. 2020. "Immunological axis of berberine in managing inflammation underlying chronic respiratory inflammatory diseases." *Chemico-Biological Interactions* 317:108947.

Wang, Jiwei, Qichao Qi, Zichao Feng, Xin Zhang, Bin Huang, Anjing Chen, Lars Prestegarden, Xingang Li, and Jian Wang. 2016. "Berberine induces autophagy in glioblastoma by targeting the AMPK/mTOR/ULK1-pathway." *Oncotarget* 7 (41):66944–66958. doi:10.18632/oncotarget.11396

Wang, Ning, Yibin Feng, Meifen Zhu, Chi-Man Tsang, Kwan Man, Yao Tong, and Sai-Wah Tsao. 2010. "Berberine induces autophagic cell death and mitochondrial apoptosis in liver cancer cells: the cellular mechanism." *Journal of Cellular Biochemistry* 111 (6):1426–1436.

Wang, Zhi-Cheng, Jing Wang, Huang Chen, Jie Tang, Ai-Wu Bian, Ting Liu, Li-Fang Yu, Zhengfang Yi, and Fan Yang. 2020. "Synthesis and anticancer activity of novel 9, 13-disubstituted berberine derivatives." *Bioorganic & Medicinal Chemistry Letters* 30 (2):126821.

Yilmaz, Mahmut, Gerhard Christofori, and Francois Lehembre. 2007. "Distinct mechanisms of tumor invasion and metastasis." *Trends in Molecular Medicine* 13 (12):535–541.

Zapata, J. M., K. Pawlowski, E. Haas, C. F. Ware, A. Godzik, and J. C. Reed. 2001. "A diverse family of proteins containing tumor necrosis factor receptor-associated factor domains." *J Biol Chem* 276 (26):24242–24252. doi:10.1074/jbc.M100354200

Zarei, Ali, Saeed Changizi-Ashtiyani, Soheila Taheri, and Majid Ramezani. 2015. "A quick overview on some aspects of endocrinological and therapeutic effects of *Berberis vulgaris* L." *Avicenna Journal of Phytomedicine* 5 (6):485.

Zarei, Ali, Mehrdad Shariati, Shahnaz Shekar Forosh, Saeid Ashtiyani, and Fateme Rasekh. 2012. "The effect of *Physalis alkekengi* extract on the physiologic function of organ tissues: A mini-review." *Journal of Arak University of Medical Sciences* 15 (7):94–104.

Zhang, Lei, Jingjing Li, Fei Ma, Shining Yao, Naisan Li, Jing Wang, Yongbin Wang, Xiuzhen Wang, and Qizheng Yao. 2012. "Synthesis and cytotoxicity evaluation of 13-n-alkyl berberine and palmatine analogues as anticancer agents." *Molecules* 17 (10):11294–11302.

Zheng, Fang, Qin Tang, JingJing Wu, ShunYu Zhao, ZhanYang Liang, Liuning Li, WanYin Wu, and Swei Hann. 2014. "p38α MAPK-mediated induction and interaction of FOXO3a and p53 contribute to the inhibited-growth and induced-apoptosis of human lung adenocarcinoma cells by berberine." *Journal of Experimental & Clinical Cancer Research* 33 (1):1–12.

Zhu, Yi, Na Xie, Yilu Chai, Yisen Nie, Ke Liu, Yufei Liu, Yang Yang, Jinsong Su, and Chuantao Zhang. 2022. "Apoptosis Induction, a sharp edge of berberine to exert anti-cancer effects, focus on breast, lung, and liver cancer." *Frontiers in Pharmacology* 13.

Ziasarabi, P., A. Sahebkar, and F. Ghasemi. 2021. "Evaluation of the effects of nanomicellar curcumin, ber-
     berine, and their combination with 5-fluorouracil on breast cancer cells." *Advances in Experimental
     Medicine and Biology* 1328:21–35. doi:10.1007/978-3-030-73234-9_3
Zulfiker, Abu Hasanat Md, Saeed M. Hashimi, David A. Good, I. Darren Grice, and Ming Q. Wei. 2017. "Cane
     toad skin extract – induced upregulation and increased interaction of serotonin 2A and D2 receptors via
     Gq/11 signaling pathway in CLU213 cells." *Journal of Cellular Biochemistry* 118 (5):979–993.

10 Chuanxinlian/Kalmegh (*Andrographis paniculata* (Burm.f.) Nees)

Discoveries in Esophageal, Gastric and Colorectal Cancer Studies

Clara Bik-San Lau and Grace Gar-Lee Yue

ABBREVIATIONS

AKT1	RAC-alpha serine/threonine-protein kinase 1
AP	*Andrographis paniculata*
BMP4	bone morphogenetic protein 4
CAM	complementary and alternative medicine
CXCR4	C-X-C chemokine receptor type 4
EGFR	epidermal growth factor receptor
HER2	human epidermal growth factor receptor 2
NF-κB	nuclear factor kappa B
PBMCs	peripheral blood mononuclear cells
STAT3	signal transducer and activator of transcription 3
TRAIL	tumor necrosis factor–related apoptosis-inducing ligand

10.1 INTRODUCTION

Andrographis paniculata (Burm. f.) Nees. belongs to the Acanthaceae family. This annual plant is commonly regarded as "king of the bitters." The plant is known as *Chuanxinlian* in China, *Kalmegh* in India, *fathalaichon* in Thailand, *Hempedu bumi* in Malaysia, and *green chiretta* in the United States (Medicinal Plant Names Services, Royal Botanic Gardens, Kew). This plant is in fact native to India and Sri Lanka, and cultivated or naturalized in Cambodia, Indonesia, Laos, Malaysia, Myanmar, Thailand, Vietnam, and China (Hossain et al. 2014; Hu et al. 2011).

As a traditional Indian medicinal plant, the whole plant of *A. paniculata* (AP) (Figure 10.1A) is used for treating snakebite and insect sting, dyspepsia, influenza, malaria, and respiratory infections (Chopra 1980). The aerial part has been recorded for treatment of common cold, hypertension, diabetes, cancer, malaria, snakebite, and urinary tract infection (World Health Organization 2002; Saxena et al. 1998). The dried leaves of AP have been reported as an alternative for treating uncomplicated acute upper respiratory tract infection (Poolsup et al. 2004), as well as colic pain, loss of appetite, irregular stools, hepatitis, tuberculosis, mouth ulcers, and diarrhea (Saxena et al. 1998). Besides, AP roots have been used for febrifuge, stomachic and as an antimalarial (Chopra 1980; Dua et al. 2004). In traditional Chinese medicine, the *Andrographis* herb (Figure 10.1B) refers to the dried aerial part of AP, collected in early autumn (when foliage branches grow luxuriantly) and then dried under the sun (Chinese Pharmacopoeia Commission 2015). Among the different traditional medicine systems, AP plant parts can be used alone in decoction, juice, powder, or infusion form, or

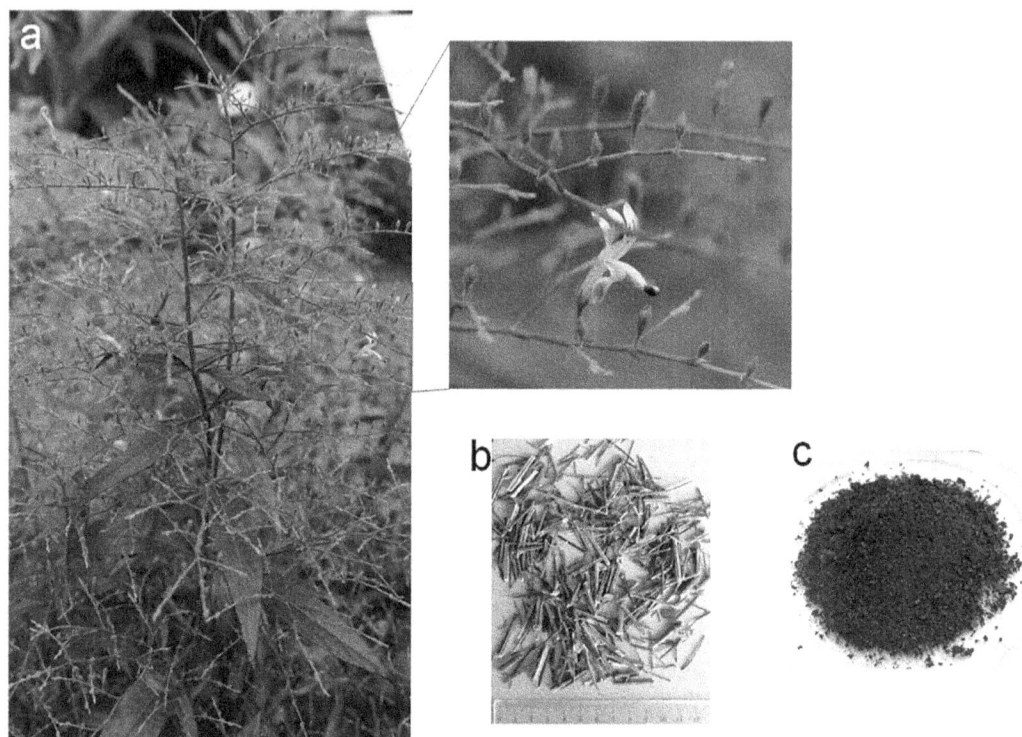

FIGURE 10.1 Photos showing (a) the growing plant of *Andrographis paniculata*, (b) *Andrographis* herb, and (c) *A. paniculata* dried aqueous extract.

Source: Photos taken by Grace G. L. Yue.

in combination with other herbs for various pharmacological activities (Hossain et al. 2021; Kumar et al. 2021).

10.1.1 BACKGROUND

A. paniculata is a well-known medicinal plant that has been used for centuries in subtropical Asia. In Ayurvedic medicine, Kalmegh, which can be found from Himachal Pradesh to Assam and Mizoram and all over southern India, is regarded as hepatoprotective, cholinergic, antispasmodic, stomachic, anthelmintic, alterative, blood purifier, and febrifuge. It is also used for treatment of cold and upper respiratory tract infections. This herb has also been mentioned in around 26 different polyherbal formulations in Ayurveda as a remedy for treating various disorders (Kumar et al. 2004). In Southeast Asia, such as in Thailand and Malaysia, AP is used as a relief for the symptoms of common cold and sore throat and is regarded as a hepatoprotective medicinal plant (Kumar et al. 2021). In China, the plant can be found in different provinces including Anhui, Fujian, Guangdong, Guangxi, Hainan, Hubei, Hunan, Jiangsu, Jiangxi, Yunnan, and Zhejiang (Hu et al. 2011). The medicinal use of AP has been formally recorded since the 1930s in the Chinese medicinal literature *Herbal Collection in Lingnan* 《岭南采药录》. As recorded in Chinese Pharmacopoeia since the 1970s, the actions of AP are for clearing heat, remove toxin, cooling blood, and disperse swelling. AP is prescribed in common cold with fever, swollen sore throat, mouth and tongue sores, whooping cough, cough in consumptive disease, diarrhea and dysentery, heat strangury with difficulty and pain, swelling abscess, sores and ulcers, and bites of insects, worms and snakes (Chinese Pharmacopoeia Commission 2015, 2020). AP is also found as ingredients in Chinese medicine preparations listed in Chinese Pharmacopoeia and *Chinese Medicine Prescription*《中药成方制剂》. For example, Chuanxinlian Pian 穿心莲片, which is made of ethanolic extract of AP, is used for common cold and sore throat (Chinese Pharmacopoeia Commission 2015, 2020). Xiyanping injection 喜炎平注射液, whose major component is andrographolide sulfonate, is a Chinese patent medicine approved for treatment of bronchitis in China (Zheng et al. 2020). Another Chinese medicine preparation containing AP, Xiaoyan Lidan tablets 消炎利胆片, are frequently used for syndromes of the liver and gallbladder, cholecystitis, and cholangitis (Yang et al. 2016). AP is also commonly used as an ingredient in folk remedies as recorded in the herbal medicine literature *Handbook of Commonly Used Chinese Herbal Medicine*《常用中草药手册》, *Fujian Zhongcaoyao*《福建中草药》, *Jiangxi Caoyao*《江西草药》, and *Guangxi Zhongcaoyao*《广西中草药》. The indications of these formulas include antimalarial, cold and fever, bronchitis, tuberculosis, pneumonia, cholecystitis, and hypertension.

Regarding phytochemistry, various constituents are found to be present in different parts of the AP plant (Kumar et al. 2021; Rastogi et al. 1990). For example, 14-deoxyandrographolide was found at the highest level in leaves at transfer stage, while andrographolide was found at the highest level in leaves at both the vegetative and seed-forming stages (Pholphana et al. 2013). Besides, the presence of andrographolide and dehydroandrographolide were reported in leaves and stems of AP, but not in roots as demonstrated in an HPTLC fingerprint analysis (Shao et al. 2014). The principal component analysis also showed the difference of constituents in roots against those from leaves and stems (Shao et al. 2014), while the rare noriridoids, andrographidoids A–E, and xanthones along with a known iridoid curvifloruside F were isolated from the roots of AP (Dua et al. 2004).

Modern pharmacological studies on AP have focused mainly on its efficacies for respiratory and digestive diseases. Among the ongoing clinical trials registered in https://ClinicalTrials.gov, the majorities are related to respiratory infection, bronchitis, and multiple sclerosis. In these human clinical trials and meta-analyses, results suggest that AP preparations might be effective in treating upper respiratory symptoms associated with cold and flu and in reducing the severity of cough and sore throat (Kumar et al. 2021; Saxena et al. 2010). Other clinical studies also demonstrated the efficacy of AP for rheumatoid arthritis (Burgos et al. 2009) and ulcerative colitis (Tang et al. 2011). In recent years, tremendous attention has been paid to the efficacy of AP in upper respiratory tract infections, including COVID-19 management, which is a recent hot topic globally.

On the other hand, the anticancer activities of AP extract and its major components, particularly andrographolide, have also attracted scientists' attention in the past two decades. Hence, this emerging therapeutic effect of AP, its anticancer effect, will be introduced and thoroughly discussed in this chapter, with special focus on esophageal, gastric, and colorectal cancer. Since only water and ethanol are edible solvents, this chapter will only include those studies using aqueous and ethanolic extracts of AP.

10.2 EFFICACY OF AP EXTRACTS IN ESOPHAGEAL CANCER

10.2.1 CLINICAL STUDIES

A clinical trial in esophageal cancer patients treated with Chinese herbal formula Xiaoliuxing 消瘤行 containing AP, *Chrysanthemum indicum* (Yejuhua), *Scutellaria barbata* (Banzhilian), and *Patrinia scabiosifolia* (Baijiangcao) for 6 months could increase the rate of complete response when compared with untreated control group (Bi et al. 2008). In addition, our recently completed clinical study (ClinicalTrials.gov Identifier: NCT04196075) aimed at validating the adjuvant effect of AP on palliative management of patients with advanced or metastatic esophageal cancer. In this study, 30 patients with locally advanced or metastatic squamous esophageal cancer were recruited and prescribed AP concentrated granules (hot water extract) manufactured under GMP standards for 4 months. The recruited patients were consulted by both Western physicians and Chinese medicine practitioner, and follow-up clinical assessments were conducted at certain intervals. At the end of the clinical trial, patients who managed to complete the entire AP treatment were shown to have better overall survival and quality of life when compared with those patients who received partial AP treatment (Chiu et al. 2023).

10.2.2 Animal Studies

Our previous animal studies revealed that AP aqueous extract (Figure 10.1C) could suppress the human esophageal xenograft growth and metastasis in nude mice (Li et al. 2017; Yue et al. 2015). Mice were intraperitoneally inoculated with human esophageal cancer cells EC109 and were orally administered AP aqueous extract for 21 days. The tumor weight and metastasis in lungs and livers were significantly reduced after AP treatment (Yue et al. 2015), while in the carcinogen-induced esophageal tumorigenesis mouse model, decreased dysplasia level in esophageal tissues could be observed after AP treatment (Yue et al. 2019). Besides, the immunomodulatory activities, such as decreased regulatory T cells population and cytokine production, of AP aqueous extract treatment were firstly demonstrated in this esophageal tumorigenesis model. The clinically relevant mouse model for cancer research, the patient-derived xenograft model, has also been set up in our laboratory to illustrate the efficacy of AP aqueous extract on the growth of patient-derived esophageal xenografts (Yue et al. 2019). Furthermore, we have recently shown that the inhibitory effect of AP aqueous extract on liver metastasis might partially depend on the changes of commensal gut microbiota by AP (Cheung et al. 2020).

10.2.3 Mechanistic Studies in Cancer Cells

Our previous cell-based studies showed that AP aqueous extract could suppress the proliferation of esophageal squamous carcinoma cells EC109 and KYSE520, as well as the migration of vascular and lymphatic endothelial cells (HMEC-1 and LEC) (Yue et al. 2015). Our results also showed that AP inhibited cell motility and reversed anoikis resistance in EC109 cells (Yue et al. 2015). In addition, AP aqueous extract and its absorbed components in Caco-2 cells could downregulate the expression of tetraspanin 8 (*TM4SF3*) in EC109 cells (Li et al. 2017; Yue et al. 2015). Furthermore, these absorbed components reduced the expressions of NF-κB, HER2, and CXCR4 in EC109 cells. In order to elucidate the underlying mechanism of action, transcriptome analysis has been performed in AP aqueous extract–treated EC109 cells. Results revealed that multiple genes related to proliferation, apoptosis, intercellular adhesion, metastatic processes, and drug resistance, such as WNT, TGF-β, MAPK, and ErbB signaling pathways, were regulated by AP treatment; meanwhile, the expressions of BMP4, SMAD7, WNT4, and AXIN2 genes were apparently downregulated in EC109 cells after AP treatment (Li et al. 2018). Nevertheless, by using the network pharmacology as a tool, the molecular basis of AP in esophageal cancer treatment was further elucidated in our recent *in vitro* study (Cheung et al. 2022). Results showed that cellular molecules such as epidermal growth factor receptor (EGFR), signal transducer and activator of transcription 3 (STAT3), and RAC-alpha serine/threonine-protein kinase 1 (AKT1) were identified as the predicted targets of AP in esophageal cancer treatment. This prediction has been validated in EC109 cells treated with AP aqueous extract so that more scientific evidence is available to support the efficacy of AP aqueous extract in esophageal cancer (Cheung et al. 2022).

10.3 EFFICACY OF AP EXTRACTS IN GASTRIC CANCER

Up till now, no clinical study of AP extract in gastric cancer has been reported.

10.3.1 Animal Studies

Treatment with 80% hydroalcoholic extract of AP for 14 days significantly decreased the activities of glutathione S-transferase, DT-diaphorase, and superoxide dismutase in the forestomach of butyl-ated hydroxyanisole-treated mice (Singh et al. 2001). These findings indicate the chemopreventive potential of AP extract against chemotoxicity. A later study also demonstrated the ulcer-preventing effect of AP hydroalcoholic extract in mice, whose gastric ulcers were induced by ethanol, aspirin, and pylorus ligation. The effect of AP extract might partly relate to the regulation of $H^+/K^+ATPase$ activity and/or mucin-preserving effects (Panneerselvam and Arumugam 2011).

10.3.2 Mechanistic Studies in Cancer Cells

Andrographis EP80 (an *Andrographis* extract standardized to 80% andrographolide content) was shown to inhibit proliferation, reduce colony formation, and enhance apoptotic activity in gastric cancer cell lines MKN74 and NUGC4 (Ma et al. 2021). The AP extract also altered the expression levels of ferroptosis-associated genes, such as heme oxygenase-1 (HMOX1), glutamate-cysteine ligase catalytic (GCLC), and glutamate-cysteine ligase modifier (GCLM) (Ma et al. 2021).

10.4 EFFICACY OF AP EXTRACTS IN COLORECTAL CANCER

So far, there is no clinical study of AP extract on colorectal cancer. Nonetheless, a clinical study was planned in 2013, in which the efficacy and safety of andrographolides combined with capecitabine in treatment of elderly patients with locally advanced or recurrent or metastasis inoperable colorectal cancer would be determined. However, due to the low accrual rate, the trial was terminated as of March 9, 2022 (https://clinicaltrials.gov/ct2/show/NCT01993472).

10.4.1 Animal Studies

The AP ethanolic extract was shown to exert the chemoprotective effects in the azoxymethane-induced aberrant crypt foci (ACF) rat model. The number of ACF of the AP-treated rats was significantly reduced (Al-Henhena et al. 2014). Another study using the dimethylbenzanthracene (DMBA)-induced cancer rat model demonstrated that AP ethanolic extract treatment for 5 weeks attenuated the hyperplasia in lung parenchymal and colonic epithelial tissues, indicating the inhibitory effect of AP ethanolic extract on the development of cancer at the hyperplasia stage by reducing telomerase activity (Budiatin et al. 2021). Furthermore, a standardized *Andrographis* extract (Andrographis EP80) was shown to suppress the human colon HCT116 xenografts growth and activate ferroptosis-related genes in tumor xenografts (Shimura et al. 2021). A recent study also showed that a mixture of AP ethanolic extract and Indian barberry bark and root methanolic extract (containing berberine) exerted its synergistic amplified anticancer effects in human colon RKO tumor–bearing mice (Zhao et al. 2022).

10.4.2 Mechanistic Studies in Cancer Cells

The antiproliferative activities of AP extracts in colon cancer cells have been studied since 2008. The AP ethanolic extract exhibited moderate cytotoxic activity in colon 205 cell line (Geethangili et al. 2008). Recent studies on the standardized *Andrographis* extract (Andrographis EP80) demonstrated that the extract exerted the anticancer effect by activating ferroptosis and downregulating the β-catenin/Wnt-signaling pathways (Sharma et al. 2020). The antitumor activity of this extract could also be enhanced by combination with oligomeric proanthocyanidins (flavonoids present in grape seed extract) (Shimura et al. 2021).

Apart from the aforementioned, the efficacies of AP extracts in other types of cancer have been summarized in Table 10.1.

TABLE 10.1

Efficacy of AP Extracts in Other Types of Cancer

Types of AP Extracts	Activities	References
Aqueous extract	The hepatoprotective property of AP is for delaying the hepatic tumorigenic condition induced by hexachlorocyclohexane	Trivedi and Rawal 1998
Ethanol extract	IC_{50} value for both neuroblastoma IMR-32 and colon HT-29 cell lines at 200 µg/mL	Kumar et al. 2004
Ethanol extract	Induced cell cycle arrest and affected an intrinsic mitochondria-dependent pathway of apoptosis by regulating the expression of some pro-apoptotic markers in leukemia HL-60 cells	Cheung et al. 2005
Ethanol extract	Inhibited the tumor growth in thymoma cells-carrying mice by stimulating cytotoxic T lymphocyte production via the enhanced secretion of IL-2 and IFN-c by T cells	Sheeja and Kuttan 2007
Ethanol extract	Moderate cytotoxic activity against Jurkat (human lymphocytic cancer), PC-3 (human prostate cancer) and colon 205 (human colon cancer) cells	Geethangili et al. 2008
Ethanol extract	Enhance cell-mediated immune response in metastatic melanoma tumor-bearing mice	Sheeja and Kuttan 2010
Water extract of mature leaf stage; ethanolic extract of first true leaf stage	Cytotoxic effects in liver (HepG2 and SK-Hep1) and bile duct (HuCCA-1 and RMCCA-1) cancer cells	Suriyo et al. 2014

10.5 OTHER PHARMACOLOGICAL ACTIVITIES OF AP EXTRACTS THAT ARE RELATED TO CANCER

10.5.1 IMMUNOMODULATION

The immunomodulatory activities of AP were reported in early 1990s that AP ethanolic extract and purified diterpene andrographolides induced significant stimulation of antibody and delayed-type hypersensitivity response to sheep red blood cells in mice (Puri et al. 1993). AP ethanolic extract was shown to downregulate proinflammatory cytokine production in tumor-bearing mice (Sheeja and Kuttan 2010). Furthermore, andrographolide has been reported to enhance proliferation and cytokine productions of peripheral blood lymphocytes (Panossian et al. 2002), and a mixture of andrographolides was also shown to enhance immune function and to reverse the immunosuppression induced by cyclophosphamide *in vivo* (Naik and Hule 2009). Besides, HMPL-004 (AP extract) was shown to inhibit chronic colitis progression in a T cell–driven model of colitis, in which the extract treatment could alter early T cell proliferation, differentiation, and T_H1/T_H17 responses (Michelsen et al. 2013). AP ethanolic extract was also shown to inhibit TNF-α-induced ICAM-1 expression via attenuation of activation of the IKK/IκB/NF-κB pathway, which in turn plays a role in the anti-inflammatory effect of AP (Lin et al. 2019).

In a recent clinical trial, a standardized *A. paniculata* extract (KalmCold) consumption for 30 days was shown to increase T cells, T helper cells, and significantly increase IFN-γ, IL-4, and decrease IL-2 in healthy adults (Rajanna et al. 2021). There was no treatment-related adverse effects following SAPE intake for 30 days. Furthermore, a recent network analysis identified five targets (IL-6, VEGFA, PTGST2, TNF-α, and MMP-9) responsible for AP anti-inflammatory effects, while further validation is pending (Zhu et al. 2021).

On the other hand, our previous studies demonstrated the immunomodulatory activities of AP aqueous extract (which has seldom been reported), that AP aqueous extract could increase the proliferation and TNF-α and IFN-γ productions in PBMCs (Yue et al. 2019), while in the immunocompetent mice with esophageal tumorigenesis, the regulatory T cells population in lymph nodes and production of IL-10 and IL-12 in spleen lymphocytes were all reduced in AP aqueous extract–treated mice (Yue et al. 2019).

10.5.2 Anti-Angiogenesis

The *in vivo* anti-angiogenic effects of AP ethanolic extract and andrographolide have been demonstrated in the study by Sheeja et al. (2007). The melanoma cell line–induced capillary formation on the ventral skin surface of C57BL/6 mice was significantly inhibited by AP ethanolic extract treatment (Sheeja et al. 2007). The inhibitory effects were through regulating production of various pro- and anti-angiogenic factors such as nitric oxide, VEGF, IL-2, and TIMP-1. In fact, our *in vitro* study also showed that AP aqueous extract inhibited the migration of human microvascular endothelial cells HMEC-1 (Yue et al. 2015).

10.6　POTENTIAL ACTIVE INGREDIENTS IN AP AND THEIR ANTICANCER ACTIVITIES

The plant AP contains the active phytochemicals in the aerial parts (leaves and stems), such as diterpenoids and 2′-oxygenated flavonoids, including andrographolide, neoandrographolide, dehydroandrographolide, 14-deoxyandrographolide, 14-deoxy-11, 12-didehydroandrographolide, isoandrographolide, 14-deoxyandrographolide-19-β-D-glucoside, and homoandrographolide (Kumar et al. 2021). In fact, the four diterpenoids andrographolide, neoandrographolide, dehydroandrographolide and 14-deoxyandrographolide (Figure 10.2) are the chemical markers for AP, according to Chinese Pharmacopoeia 2020.

Our previous *in vitro* absorption study using human colon Caco-2 cell monolayer showed that seven known chemical constituents were identified in the basolateral side of the monolayer after

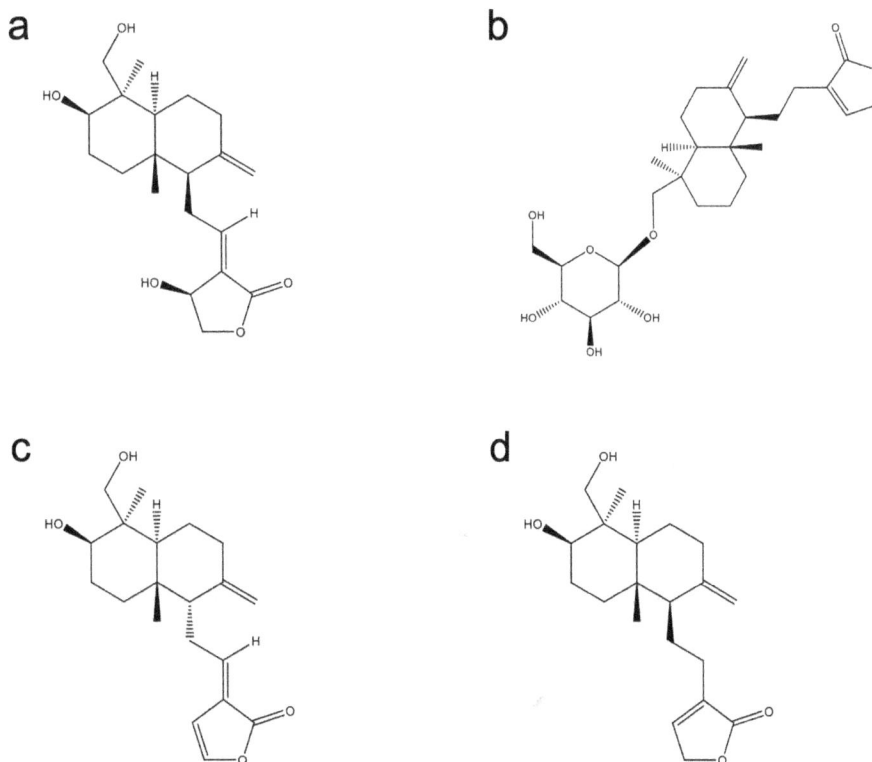

FIGURE 10.2　Chemical structures of (a) andrographolide, (b) neoandrographolide, (c) dehydroandrographolide, and (d) 14-deoxyandrographolide.

addition of 400–6400 µg/mL of AP aqueous extract on the apical side of the monolayer, namely andrographolide, andropanoside, dehydroandrographolide, deoxyandrographolide, neoandrographolide, 5-hydroxy-7,8-dimethoxyflavone, and 5-hydroxy-7,8-dimethoxyflavanone (Li et al. 2017). These absorbable AP aqueous extract components, which could pass through the human intestinal Caco-2 cell monolayer, were shown to regulate the mRNA and protein expression of metastasis-related factors in esophageal cancer EC-109 cells (Li et al. 2017).

Our recent network pharmacology study also revealed 22 potential active AP compounds against esophageal cancer, including anti-inflammatory compounds panicolin and moslosooflavone (5-hydroxy-7,8-dimethoxyflavone), as well as cytotoxic compound deoxyandrographiside. These compounds were proven to be present in the AP aqueous extract and their modulation on the metastasis-related gene expressions were also shown in EC109 cells (Cheung et al. 2022).

It is interesting to note that andrographolide becomes the rising star of multi-targeted molecules which may act on various signaling pathways, such as JNK, Stat3, PI3K/Akt, modulate expression of death receptor, tumor necrosis factor-related apoptosis-inducing ligand (TRAIL) ligand, and tumor suppressors, which lead to inhibition in inflammation, angiogenesis, and metastasis. Apart from andrographolide, other components of AP have been screened for their cytotoxicities in cancer cells (Kumar et al. 2021; Malik et al. 2021). A few of these compounds, which have been studied in detail, are listed in Table 10.2.

TABLE 10.2
Potential Active Components of AP with Underlying Anticancer Mechanistic Studies

Cancer Types	Cell Lines	Activities	References
Esophageal cancer	ECA109	Andrographolide increased cleaved-caspase 3 and Bax; decreased Bcl-2 and NF-κB	Wang et al. 2016b
	Ec9706	Andrographolide downregulated Bcl-2 gene expression and increased the activities of caspase-3 and caspase-9, which lead to apoptosis	Dai et al. 2009
Gastric cancer	SGC7901 and AGS	Andrographolide activated the expression of p53 protein and gene and downregulated the levels of Mdm-2 (negative regulator of p53)	Gao et al. 2021
	AGS-EBV	Andrographolide induced cell cytotoxicity and apoptosis	Malat et al. 2021
	Adenocarcinoma cell BGC823 Mucinous adenocarcinoma MGC803	Andrographolide blocked E-selectin expression and hence adhesion of cancer cells	Jiang et al. 2007
Colorectal cancer	HCT116 HCT116/5-FUR	Andrographolide upregulated expression of Bax	Wang et al. 2016a
	T84 and COLO 205	Andrographolide induced ROS; suppressed level of cyclins B1/D1 and phosphorylation of Akt and mTOR	Banerjee et al. 2017
	CT26 and HT29	Andrographolide reduced MMP2 activity and attenuated ERK signaling pathway	Chao et al. 2010
	Lovo	Andrographolide induced cell cycle G1/S phase arrest, and increased p53, p21, and p16 expressions	Shi et al. 2008
	HCT116	Andrographolide enhanced TRAIL-induced apoptosis	Zhou et al. 2008
	SW620	Dehydroandrographolide as a novel TMEM16A inhibitor exerted its anticancer activity partly through a TMEM16A-dependent mechanism	Sui et al. 2015

10.7 TOXICITY AND CAUTIONARY NOTES

10.7.1 Toxicity Evaluation on *Andrographis* Extracts/Andrographolide

According to a systematic review and meta-analysis on the safety of AP, which included ten randomized controlled trials (RCTs) and three intensive monitoring studies, the incidence of serious adverse effects was very rare with the pooled incidence (95% CI) from RCTs of 0.02 per 1000 patients (0.0–0.5) (Worakunphanich et al. 2021). The findings indicated that AP is generally safe, though patients using AP are advised to be closely monitored for any adverse effects (Worakunphanich et al. 2021). So far, no detailed unwanted plant-drug (chemotherapeutics) interactions can be found for AP. On the other hand, a systematic review and meta-analysis on the adverse effects of herbal preparations of AP stated that the reported adverse drug reactions of nine AP herbal preparations in ten studies were mainly mild to moderate gastrointestinal, skin, and subcutaneous tissue disorders (Shang et al. 2022). Hence, herbal preparations of AP are essentially safe. However, it is important to note that adverse effects of andrographolide derivative injections (andrographolide sulfonate, potassium sodium dehydroandrographolide succinate, and potassium dehydroandrographolide succinate) could be fatal or anaphylactic shock could happen in patients. Therefore, the use of these injections must be with caution (Shang et al. 2022).

On the other hand, few preclinical toxicity evaluation studies have been conducted previously. Mice that received oral extracts of AP (10 g/kg body weight) once a day for 7 days were shown to be vital and none of the mice died (Tian et al. 2022). The oral acute toxicity of ethanolic extract LD_{50} was >17 g/kg, and the use of extract up to 1000 mg/kg for 60 days did not produce subchronic testicular toxicity effect in male rats (Burgos et al. 1997). In recent studies, a single oral administration of the standardized AP first true leaf ethanolic extract 5000 mg/kg did not cause significant acute toxicological effects (Worasuttayangkurn et al. 2019), while another 85% ethanolic AP extract at 10 g/kg also did not induce abnormal consequences (Tian et al. 2022). The repeated-dose toxicity tests also demonstrated that repeated intragastric administration of 85% ethanolic AP extract (1 g/kg) for 8 weeks in rats did not lead to any obvious toxic effects (Tian et al. 2022).

10.8 BENEFICIAL HERB-DRUG INTERACTION

Instead of unwanted herb-drug interaction, the combination of *Andrographis* extracts/constituents with chemotherapeutics may result in beneficial antiproliferative or antitumor effects. For example, in our human esophageal xenograft-bearing mouse model, we demonstrated that mice received 3-week treatment with AP aqueous extract plus chemotherapeutics (cisplatin and 5-fluorouracil) exhibited better antitumor efficacy when compared with AP extract or chemotherapeutics alone (Li et al. 2017). These two regimens inhibited the growth of intraperitoneal EC109 tumor nodules synergistically (with combination index <0.7) (Li et al. 2017). In addition, the decrease in platelet count and hemoglobin concentration observed in the chemotherapeutics-treated mice was slightly improved in the combined treatment. In another study, the antitumor effect of *Andrographis* extract (Andrographis EP80) was also shown to be more effective when used in combination with 5-fluorouracil (5-FU) in the colon cancer HCT116 xenograft model (Sharma et al. 2020). The combined treatment further enhanced the dysregulation on the expressions of ferroptosis-related genes (e.g., HMOX1, GCLC, GCLM) and Wnt-signaling pathways (Sharma et al. 2020). Furthermore, in another study using HCT116 cells which are 5-FU resistant, andrographolide was shown to significantly re-sensitize HCT116/5-FUR cells to cytotoxicity of 5-FU by elevating the apoptosis level of HCT116/5-FUR cells with highly increased level of Bax (Wang et al. 2016a).

10.9　FUTURE PROSPECTIVE-ADJUVANT USE OF AP IN CANCER TREATMENT

A. paniculata has long been used as an herbal medicine in Chinese, Ayurveda, and other traditional medicine systems. Apart from its promising efficacies in respiratory tract infections and its anti-inflammatory properties, this herb and its major constituents have gained attention for in-depth investigation and further development as anticancer agents in recent years.

Herbal medicine is a form of complementary and alternative medicine (CAM), and most herbal medicines are used in conjunction with Western conventional therapy rather than as a replacement. Previous studies demonstrated that between 11% and 95% of oncology patients use CAMs (Davis et al. 2012; Enioutina et al. 2017). CAMs are popular in cancer patients since they can help to cope with both physical and emotional impact of their disease and treatment. Herbal medicine consumption can be beneficial to cancer patients or survivors because they will play important roles in modulating immune system and relieve discomfort from conventional therapies such as chemotherapies and/or radiotherapy. In several clinical trials, herbal medicines were reported to have favorable therapeutic effects in improving quality of life among cancer patients (Chung et al. 2015).

In view of the clinical and preclinical studies of AP and its major constituents in treating esopha-geal, gastric, and colorectal cancer summarized in this chapter, there should be great potential for developing this herb as an adjuvant agent for management of such types of cancer. Since we have demonstrated that the potencies of reverse anoikis resistance by andrographolide (Yue et al. 2015) or downregulation of metastasis-related gene expression by panicolin and moslosooflavone (Cheung et al. 2022) were not as high as AP aqueous extract, we strongly believe that AP aqueous extract as a whole, rather than any single active component, is worth further development as an adjuvant for cancer treatment.

10.10　SUMMARY POINTS

- *A. paniculata* is a medicinal plant in both Ayurvedic medicine and traditional Chinese medicine.
- Potential anticancer activities of AP extract in esophageal, gastric, and colorectal cancer.
- AP contains active phytochemicals such as diterpenoids and flavonoids, with its well-known component andrographolide.
- With mild gastrointestinal side effects, AP extract is generally safe to be used.
- Potential beneficial effects can be obtained from the combination of AP and chemotherapeutics.
- AP aqueous extract has great potential to be developed as an adjuvant for cancer treatment.

REFERENCES

Al-Henhena, N., R. P. Ying, S. Ismail, W. Najm, S. A. Khalifa, H. El-Seedi, et al. 2014. Chemopreventive effi-cacy of *Andrographis paniculata* on azoxymethane-induced aberrant colon crypt foci *in vivo*. PLoS One 9 (11):e111118.

Banerjee, A., V. Banerjee, S. Czinn, and T. Blanchard. 2017. Increased reactive oxygen species lev-els cause ER stress and cytotoxicity in andrographolide treated colon cancer cells. Oncotarget 8 (16):26142–26153.

Bi, X., X. L. Song, and J. Z. Zhang. 2008. Efficacy of formula "Xiaoliuxing" for advanced esophageal cancer. Zhong Cheng Yao 30 (9):1266–1268.

Budiatin, A. S., I. B. Sagitaras, I. P. Nurhayati, N. Khairah, K. Nisak, I. Susilo, et al. 2021. Attenuation of hyperplasia in lung parenchymal and colonic epithelial cells in DMBA-induced cancer by administering *Andrographis paniculata* Nees extract using animal model. J Basic Clin Physiol Pharmacol 32 (4):497–504.

Burgos, R. A., E. E. Caballero, N. S. Sanchez, R. A. Schroeder, G. K. Wikman, and J. L. Hancke. 1997. Testicular toxicity assessment of *Andrographis paniculata* dried extract in rats. J Ethnopharmacol 58 (3):219–224.

Burgos, R. A., J. L. Hancke, J. C. Bertoglio, V. Aguirre, S. Arriagada, M. Calvo, et al. 2009. Efficacy of an *Andrographis paniculata* composition for the relief of rheumatoid arthritis symptoms: A prospective randomized placebo-controlled trial. Clin Rheumatol 28 (8):931–946.

Chao, H. P., C. D. Kuo, J. H. Chiu, and S. L. Fu. 2010. Andrographolide exhibits anti-invasive activity against colon cancer cells via inhibition of MMP2 activity. Planta Med 76 (16):1827–1833.

Cheung, H. Y., S. H. Cheung, J. Li, C. S. Cheung, W. P. Lai, W. F. Fong, et al. 2005. Andrographolide isolated from *Andrographis paniculata* induces cell cycle arrest and mitochondrial-mediated apoptosis in human leukemic HL-60 cells. Planta Med 71 (12):1106–1111.

Cheung, M. K., G. G. L. Yue, A. J. Gomes, E. C. Wong, J. K. Lee, F. H. Kwok, et al. 2022. Network pharmacology reveals potential functional components and underlying molecular mechanisms of *Andrographis paniculata* in esophageal cancer treatment. Phytother Res 36 (4):1748–1760.

Cheung, M. K., G. G. L. Yue, K. Y. Tsui, A. J. Gomes, H. S. Kwan, P. W. Y. Chiu, et al. 2020. Discovery of an interplay between the gut microbiota and esophageal squamous cell carcinoma in mice. Am J Cancer Res 10 (8):2409–2427.

Chinese Pharmacopoeia Commission. 2015, 2020. Pharmacopoeia of the People's Republic of China, Vol. 2015, 2020. Beijing: China Medical Science Press.

Chiu, P. W. Y., G. G. L. Yue, M. K. Cheung, H. C. Yip, S. K. Chu, M. Y. Yung, et al. 2023. The effect of *Andrographis paniculata* water extract on palliative management of metastatic esophageal squamous cell carcinoma – A phase II clinical trial. Phytother Res doi: 10.1002/ptr.7815.

Chopra, R. N. 1980. Glossary of Indian Medicinal Plants. New Delhi: Council for Scientific and Industrial Research.

Chung, V. C., X. Wu, E. P. Hui, E. T. Ziea, B. F. Ng, R. S. Ho, et al. 2015. Effectiveness of Chinese herbal medicine for cancer palliative care: Overview of systematic reviews with meta-analyses. Sci Rep 5:18111.

Dai, G. F., J. Zhao, Q. D. Wang, S. J. Mao, W. Xia, and H. M. Liu. 2009. Studies on the apoptosis induction mechanism of andrographolide in human esophageal cancer Ec9706 cells. Chinese Pharmacological Bulletin 25 (2):173–176.

Davis, E. L., B. Oh, P. N. Butow, B. A. Mullan, and S. Clarke. 2012. Cancer patient disclosure and patient-doctor communication of complementary and alternative medicine use: A systematic review. Oncologist 17 (11):1475–1481.

Dua, V. K., V. P. Ojha, R. Roy, B. C. Joshi, N. Valecha, C. U. Devi, et al. 2004. Anti-malarial activity of some xanthones isolated from the roots of *Andrographis paniculata*. J Ethnopharmacol 95 (2–3):247–251.

Enioutina, E. Y., E. R. Salis, K. M. Job, M. I. Gubarev, L. V. Krepkova, and C. M. Sherwin. 2017. Herbal medicines: Challenges in the modern world. Part 5. Status and current directions of complementary and alternative herbal medicine worldwide. Expert Rev Clin Pharmacol 10 (3):327–338.

Gao, H., H. Li, W. Liu, S. K. Mishra, and C. Li. 2021. Andrographolide induces apoptosis in gastric cancer cells through reactivation of p53 and inhibition of Mdm-2. Dokl Biochem Biophys 500 (1):393–401.

Geethangili, M., Y. K. Rao, S. H. Fang, and Y. M. Tzeng. 2008. Cytotoxic constituents from *Andrographis paniculata* induce cell cycle arrest in jurkat cells. Phytother Res 22 (10):1336–1341.

Hossain, M. S., Z. Urbi, A. Sule, and K. M. Hafizur Rahman. 2014. *Andrographis paniculata* (Burm. f.) Wall. ex Nees: A review of ethnobotany, phytochemistry, and pharmacology. Sci World J 2014:274905.

Hossain, S., Z. Urbi, H. Karuniawati, R. B. Mohiuddin, A. Moh Qrimida, A. M. M. Allzrag, et al. 2021. *Andrographis paniculata* (Burm. f.) Wall. ex Nees: An updated review of phytochemistry, antimicrobial pharmacology, and clinical safety and efficacy. Life (Basel) 11 (4):348.

Hu, J., Y. Deng, and F. D. Thomas. 2011. Andographis Wallich ex Nees in Wallich, Pl. Asiat. Rar. 3: 77, 116. 1832. Flora of China 19:473–474.

Jiang, C. G., J. B. Li, F. R. Liu, T. Wu, M. Yu, and H. M. Xu. 2007. Andrographolide inhibits the adhesion of gastric cancer cells to endothelial cells by blocking E-selectin expression. Anticancer Res 27 (4B):2439–2447.

Kumar, R. A., K. Sridevi, N. V. Kumar, S. Nanduri, and S. Rajagopal. 2004. Anticancer and immunostimulatory compounds from *Andrographis paniculata*. J Ethnopharmacol 92 (2–3):291–295.

Kumar, S., B. Singh, and V. Bajpai. 2021. *Andrographis paniculata* (Burm.f.) Nees: Traditional uses, phytochemistry, pharmacological properties and quality control/quality assurance. J Ethnopharmacol 275:114054.

Li, L., G. G. L. Yue, J. K. Lee, E. C. Wong, K. P. Fung, J. Yu, et al. 2017. The adjuvant value of *Andrographis paniculata* in metastatic esophageal cancer treatment: From preclinical perspectives. Sci Rep 7 (1):854.

Li, L., G. G. L. Yue, J. K. Lee, E. C. Wong, K. P. Fung, J. Yu, et al. 2018. Gene expression profiling reveals the plausible mechanisms underlying the antitumor and antimetastasis effects of *Andrographis paniculata* in esophageal cancer. Phytother Res 32 (7):1388–1396.

Lin, H. C., C. C. Li, Y. C. Yang, T. H. Chiu, K. L. Liu, C. K. Lii, et al. 2019. *Andrographis paniculata* diterpenoids and ethanolic extract inhibit TNFalpha-induced ICAM-1 expression in EA.hy926 cells. Phytomedicine 52:157–167.

Ma, R., T. Shimura, C. Yin, Y. Okugawa, T. Kitajima, Y. Koike, et al. 2021. Antitumor effects of *Andrographis* via ferroptosis-associated genes in gastric cancer. Oncol Lett 22 (1):523.

Malat, P., T. Ekalaksananan, C. Heawchaiyaphum, S. Suebsasana, S. Roytrakul, Y. Yingchutrakul, et al. 2021. Andrographolide inhibits lytic reactivation of Epstein-Barr virus by modulating transcription factors in gastric cancer. Microorganisms 9 (12):2561.

Malik, Z., R. Parveen, B. Parveen, S. Zahiruddin, M. Aasif Khan, A. Khan, et al. 2021. Anticancer potential of andrographolide from *Andrographis paniculata* (Burm.f.) Nees and its mechanisms of action. J Ethnopharmacol 272:113936.

Michelsen, K. S., M. H. Wong, B. Ko, L. S. Thomas, D. Dhall, and S. R. Targan. 2013. HMPL-004 (*Andrographis paniculata* extract) prevents development of murine colitis by inhibiting T-cell proliferation and TH1/TH17 responses. Inflamm Bowel Dis 19 (1):151–164.

Naik, S. R., and A. Hule. 2009. Evaluation of immunomodulatory activity of an extract of andrographolides from *Andrographis paniculata*. Planta Med 75 (8):785–791.

Panneerselvam, S., and G. Arumugam. 2011. A biochemical study on the gastroprotective effect of hydroalcoholic extract of *Andrographis paniculata* in rats. Indian J Pharmacol 43 (4):402–408.

Panossian, A., T. Davtyan, N. Gukassyan, G. Gukasova, G. Mamikonyan, E. Gabrielian, et al. 2002. Effect of andrographolide and Kan Jang – fixed combination of extract SHA-10 and extract SHE-3 – on proliferation of human lymphocytes, production of cytokines and immune activation markers in the whole blood cells culture. Phytomedicine 9 (7):598–605.

Pholphana, N., N. Rangkadilok, J. Saehun, S. Ritruechai, and J. Satayavivad. 2013. Changes in the contents of four active diterpenoids at different growth stages in *Andrographis paniculata* (Burm.f.) Nees (Chuanxinlian). Chin Med 8 (1):2.

Poolsup, N., C. Suthisisang, S. Prathanturarug, A. Asawamekin, and U. Chanchareon. 2004. *Andrographis paniculata* in the symptomatic treatment of uncomplicated upper respiratory tract infection: Systematic review of randomized controlled trials. J Clin Pharm Ther 29 (1):37–45.

Puri, A., R. Saxena, R. P. Saxena, K. C. Saxena, V. Srivastava, and J. S. Tandon. 1993. Immunostimulant agents from *Andrographis paniculata*. J Nat Prod 56 (7):995–999.

Rajanna, M., B. Bharathi, B. R. Shivakumar, M. Deepak, D. Prashanth, D. Prabakaran, et al. 2021. Immunomodulatory effects of *Andrographis paniculata* extract in healthy adults: An open-label study. J Ayurveda Integr Med 12 (3):529–534.

Rastogi, R. P., B. N. Mehrotra, S. Sinha, P. Pant, and R. Seth. 1990. Compendium of Indian Medicinal Plants, Vol. 1990–1994. New Delhi: Central Drug Research Institute and Publications & Information Directorate.

Saxena, R. C., R. Singh, P. Kumar, S. C. Yadav, M. P. Negi, V. S. Saxena, et al. 2010. A randomized double blind placebo controlled clinical evaluation of extract of *Andrographis paniculata* (KalmCold) in patients with uncomplicated upper respiratory tract infection. Phytomedicine 17 (3–4):178–185.

Saxena, S., D. C. Jain, R. S. Bhakuni, and R. P. Sharma. 1998. Chemistry and pharmacology of *Andrographis* species. Indian Drugs 35:458–467.

Shang, Y. X., C. Shen, T. Stub, S. J. Zhu, S. Y. Qiao, Y. Q. Li, et al. 2022. Adverse effects of andrographolide derivative medications compared to the safe use of herbal preparations of *Andrographis paniculata*: Results of a systematic review and meta-analysis of clinical studies. Front Pharmacol 13:773282.

Shao, Y. H., J. G. Wang, X. P. Lai, X. W. Wu, and P. Ding. 2014. HPTLC fingerprint analysis of andrographolides from *Andrographis paniculata*. Zhong Yao Cai 37 (2):219–223.

Sharma, P., T. Shimura, J. K. Banwait, and A. Goel. 2020. Andrographis-mediated chemosensitization through activation of ferroptosis and suppression of beta-catenin/Wnt-signaling pathways in colorectal cancer. Carcinogenesis 41 (10):1385–1394.

Sheeja, K., C. Guruvayoorappan, and G. Kuttan. 2007. Antiangiogenic activity of *Andrographis paniculata* extract and andrographolide. Int Immunopharmacol 7 (2):211–221.

Sheeja, K., and G. Kuttan. 2007. Activation of cytotoxic T lymphocyte responses and attenuation of tumor growth *in vivo* by *Andrographis paniculata* extract and andrographolide. Immunopharmacol Immunotoxicol 29 (1):81–93.

Sheeja, K., and G. Kuttan. 2010. *Andrographis paniculata* downregulates proinflammatory cytokine production and augments cell mediated immune response in metastatic tumor-bearing mice. Asian Pac J Cancer Prev 11 (3):723–729.

Shi, M. D., H. H. Lin, Y. C. Lee, J. K. Chao, R. A. Lin, and J. H. Chen. 2008. Inhibition of cell-cycle progression in human colorectal carcinoma Lovo cells by andrographolide. Chem Biol Interact 174 (3):201–210.

Shimura, T., P. Sharma, G. G. Sharma, J. K. Banwait, and A. Goel. 2021. Enhanced anti-cancer activity of andrographis with oligomeric proanthocyanidins through activation of metabolic and ferroptosis pathways in colorectal cancer. Sci Rep 11 (1):7548.

Singh, R. P., S. Banerjee, and A. R. Rao. 2001. Modulatory influence of *Andrographis paniculata* on mouse hepatic and extrahepatic carcinogen metabolizing enzymes and antioxidant status. Phytother Res 15 (5):382–390.

Sui, Y., F. Wu, J. Lv, H. Li, X. Li, Z. Du, et al. 2015. Identification of the novel TMEM16A inhibitor dehydroandrographolide and its anticancer activity on SW620 cells. PLoS One 10 (12):e0144715.

Suriyo, T., N. Pholphana, N. Rangkadilok, A. Thiantanawat, P. Watcharasit, and J. Satayavivad. 2014. *Andrographis paniculata* extracts and major constituent diterpenoids inhibit growth of intrahepatic cholangiocarcinoma cells by inducing cell cycle arrest and apoptosis. Planta Med 80 (7):533–543.

Tang, T., S. R. Targan, Z. S. Li, C. Xu, V. S. Byers, and W. J. Sandborn. 2011. Randomised clinical trial: Herbal extract HMPL-004 in active ulcerative colitis: A double-blind comparison with sustained release mesalazine. Aliment Pharmacol Ther 33 (2):194–202.

Tian, J., C. Li, J. Meng, L. Wang, Y. Tong, Y. Zhao, et al. 2022. Pharmacological effects and safety of *Andrographis paniculata* (Burm.f.) Nees. J Food Sci 87 (3):1319–1330.

Trivedi, N., and U. M. Rawal. 1998. Effect of aqueous extract of *Andrographis paniculata* on liver tumor. Indian J Pharmacol 30 (5):318–322.

Wang, W., W. Guo, L. Li, Z. Fu, L. Liu, J. Gao, et al. 2016a. Andrographolide reversed 5-FU resistance in human colorectal cancer by elevating BAX expression. Biochem Pharmacol 121:8–17.

Wang, Z. M., Y. H. Kang, X. Yang, J. F. Wang, Q. Zhang, B. X. Yang, et al. 2016b. Andrographolide radiosensitizes human esophageal cancer cell line ECA109 to radiation *in vitro*. Dis Esophagus 29 (1):54–61.

Worakunphanich, W., M. Thavorncharoensap, S. Youngkong, K. Thadanipon, and A. Thakkinstian. 2021. Safety of *Andrographis paniculata*: A systematic review and meta-analysis. Pharmacoepidemiol Drug Saf 30 (6):727–739.

Worasuttayangkurn, L., W. Nakareangrit, J. Kwangjai, P. Sritangos, N. Pholphana, P. Watcharasit, et al. 2019. Acute oral toxicity evaluation of *Andrographis paniculata*-standardized first true leaf ethanolic extract. Toxicol Rep 6:426–430.

World Health Organization. 2002. Herba andrographidis. In WHO Monographs on Selected Medicinal Plants, 12–25. Geneva: World Health Organization.

Yang, N., A. Xiong, R. Wang, L. Yang, and Z. Wang. 2016. Quality evaluation of traditional Chinese medicine compounds in Xiaoyan Lidan tablets: Fingerprint and quantitative analysis using UPLC-MS. Molecules 21 (2):83.

Yue, G. G. L., J. K. Lee, L. Li, K. M. Chan, E. C. Wong, J. Y. Chan, et al. 2015. *Andrographis paniculata* elicits anti-invasion activities by suppressing TM4SF3 gene expression and by anoikis-sensitization in esophageal cancer cells. Am J Cancer Res 5 (12):3570–3587.

Yue, G. G. L., L. Li, J. K. Lee, H. F. Kwok, E. C. Wong, M. Li, et al. 2019. Multiple modulatory activities of *Andrographis paniculata* on immune responses and xenograft growth in esophageal cancer preclinical models. Phytomedicine 60:152886.

Zhao, Y., S. Roy, C. Wang, and A. Goel. 2022. A combined treatment with berberine and *Andrographis* exhibits enhanced anti-cancer activity through suppression of DNA replication in colorectal cancer. Pharmaceuticals (Basel) 15 (3):262.

Zheng, R., L. Tao, J. S. W. Kwong, C. Zhong, C. Li, S. Chen, et al. 2020. Risk factors associated with the severity of adverse drug reactions by Xiyanping injection: A propensity score-matched analysis. J Ethnopharmacol 250:112424.

Zhou, J., G. D. Lu, C. S. Ong, C. N. Ong, and H. M. Shen. 2008. Andrographolide sensitizes cancer cells to TRAIL-induced apoptosis via p53-mediated death receptor 4 up-regulation. Mol Cancer Ther 7 (7):2170–2180.

Zhu, N., J. Hou, and N. Yang. 2021. Network pharmacology integrated with experimental validation revealed the anti-inflammatory effects of *Andrographis paniculata*. Sci Rep 11 (1):9752.

11 Crisp-Leaved Fleabane (*Pulicaria undulata*) *Molecular Actions and Pathways in Tumor Cells*

*Mohamed-Elamir F. Hegazy,
Heba K. Nabih and Thomas Efferth*

ABBREVIATIONS

AKT–mTOR	AKT–mammalian target of rapamycin
CDK	cyclin dependent kinase
EO	essential oil
ERK	extracellular signal–regulated protein kinase
HO-1	heme oxygenase-1
iNOS	inducible NO synthase
Keap1	Kelch-like ECH-associated protein 1
NF-κB	nuclear factor kappa B
NQO	quinine oxidoreductase
NRF2	nuclear erythroid 2-cognate factor 2
PARP	poly-ADP-ribose polymerase
PI3K/Akt	phosphoinositide 3-kinase and AKT
PLC	phospholipase C
PU	*Pulicaria undulata*
ROS	reactive oxygen species
VEGF	vascular endothelial growth factor
VEGF-B	vascular endothelial growth factor B
VEGFR-2	vascular endothelial growth factor receptor 2

11.1 INTRODUCTION

Pulicaria undulata (PU) is one of the most significant plant species in the genus *Pulicaria*, which is part of the Asteraceae family and has around 100 herbaceous plant species (Xu et al. 2015). *Pulicaria* species are extensively dispersed in Asia, Africa, and Europe. Because of their historic uses all around the world, these plants are regarded as highly significant medicinal herbs (Hegazy et al. 2012; Elshamy et al. 2018; Assaeed et al. 2020; Al-Maqtari et al. 2020).

Pulicaria plants are well-known for their therapeutic properties. Several *Pulicaria* species have been often used by Arabian nomads and herbalists to treat inflammation, diabetes, and gastrointestinal ailments (Liu et al. 2010; Kumar et al. 2012; Emam et al. 2019). In this area of the world, the plants are also used as tonics, food preservatives, in fragrances, and in salads. They are also used in various other dishes. There are additional records of anti-ulcer, antibacterial, antioxidant, and anticancer bioactivities of *Pulicaria* species (Vanhaelen et al. 1991; Al-Hajj et al. 2017).

DOI: 10.1201/9781003260028-13

P. undulata (L.) (syn. *P. crispa* (Forssk.) Benth et Hook) is an Egyptian desert plant that has been described as a highly useful traditional herb for the treatment of diabetes, abscesses, heart and skin problems, and chills (Hammiche and Maiza 2006). This plant was utilized in Egypt as an anti-inflammatory herbal beverage as well as an insect repellent (Hegazy et al. 2012).

Antioxidant (Hussein et al. 2017; Mohammed et al. 2020; Mustafa et al. 2020), neuroprotective (Issa et al. 2020), anti-ulcer (Fahmi et al. 2019), anti-acetylcholinesterase (Mustafa et al. 2020), anticancer (Abdallah et al. 2019), and antiglucosidase inhibitory activities (Rasool et al. 2013) have all been identified for distinct extracts and components of this plant.

One of the reasons for the plant's widespread usage in herbal teas, fragrances, and as insect repellents is its volatile components. Many papers have been published on the chemical characterization of essential oils (EOs) of various *P. undulata* ecospecies from various countries, including Sudan (Mohamed et al. 2020), Iran (Javadinamin and Asgarpanah 2014), Algeria (Boumaraf et al. 2016), Yemen (Ali et al. 2012), and Egypt (Ahmed and Ibrahim 2017). However, it was evident from the comparison of these ecospecies that their EOs differed in quality and quantity. This led to the conclusion that the production of natural metabolites in the plant kingdom, including EOs, is influenced by environmental and climatic factors as well as genetic variability (Nematollahi et al. 2006; Javadinamin and Asgarpanah 2014; Dekinash et al. 2019; Hassan et al. 2021).

The volatile oil compositions of *P. undulata* from various geographic regions (Rav et al. 2011; Ali et al. 2012; Boumaraf et al. 2016; McNeil et al. 2018; Emam et al. 2019; Mohamed et al. 2020) have been thoroughly examined. Among the principal volatile elements of the plants' essential oil are carvotanacetone, carvacrol, borneol, linalool, and camphor. There were notable differences in EO concentration, oil yields, and oil components from *P. undulata* growing in geographically various sites (Rav et al. 2011; McNeil et al. 2018). In addition to isoflavone glycosides, the flavonoid class of chemicals, primarily of kaempferol and quercetin glycosidic origin, has been detected in *P. undulata* (Kumar et al. 2012).

The presence of saponins, steroids, triterpenes, coumarins, and tannins, among other secondary metabolites, has been described (Mohamed et al. 2020). Local herbalists and nomads in northern Sudan have traditionally used *P. undulata* as a medicine for epilepsy, influenza, the common cold, gastrointestinal problems, backache, inflamed joints, and other inflammations (Hussein et al. 2017).

11.2 BACKGROUND

P. undulata contains a number of bioactive chemical constituents, such as sesquiterpene lactones (Hegazy et al. 2012; Hegazy et al. 2020; Assaeed et al. 2020), flavonoids, and phenolics (Hussein et al. 2017; Elshamy et al. 2018), terpenes (Abdallah et al. 2019), and steroids (Elhady et al. 2021). These potent bioactive compounds could be applied as valuable promising materials for the manufacturing of novel drugs against infections (Helal et al. 2019; Khan et al. 2021; Mohammed et al. 2021) and other diseases such as cancer (Elhady et al. 2021; Hegazy et al. 2020; Abdallah et al. 2019; Emam et al. 2019; Hegazy et al. 2018; Ahmed et al. 2018).

Cancer is the most common disease with increasing incidence, mortality, and morbidity (Kopustinskiene et al. 2020). There are many types of cancer, such as breast, colon, liver, leukemia, prostate, and pancreas carcinoma which are treated with surgery, chemotherapy, and radiotherapy with only moderate or weak success. Cancer cells may poorly respond to antitumor therapies because of the development of multidrug resistance phenomena and metastatic behavior (Choudhari et al. 2020; Wang et al. 2019).

Cancer is a complicated disorder with numerous diverse interrelated biochemical signaling pathways. To achieve an improvement for the successful of treatment against cancer, targeting these oncogenic signaling pathways should be initiated (Hanahan and Weinber 2011) using novel bioactive compounds from natural sources to avoid the severe and partly life-threatening side effects of chemically synthesized drugs (Law et al. 2020; Khazir et al. 2014).

Accordingly, we shed light in the present chapter on the molecular mechanisms of action of *P. undulata* along with the cancer-related pathways that may be critical for tumor cell survival and that might be targeted by *P. undulata*.

11.3   BIOACTIVITY OF *P. UNDULATA* AGAINST CANCER PROLIFERATION PATHWAYS

It was estimated that the methylene chloride:methanol (1:1) total extract of *P. undulata* could enhance the generation of reactive oxygen species (ROS) in a range from 80.7% to 100% in human leukemia cells (Hegazy et al. 2018). The upregulation of ROS production is one mechanism by most chemotherapies, flavonoids (Kma and Baruah 2021), and extracts of *P. undulata* that can lead to apoptosis through the induction of DNA damage, release of cytochrome c, and activation of caspases (Koundouros and Poulogiannis 2018; Emam et al. 2019). DNA damage is characterized by formation of specific foci containing activated H2A.X (γH2A.X) that induce cell cycle arrest through activation of checkpoint proteins, p53 (TP53) and the cyclin dependent kinase (CDK) inhibitor p21 (CDKN1A) (Passos et al. 2010).

Additionally, we isolated the major sequiterpene lactone metabolite, 2α-hydroxyalantolactone (PU-1), which exerted activity against sensitive and multidrug-resistant human cancer cells (Hegazy et al. 2020). This cytotoxic action of PU-1 in cancer cells was initiated through inhibition of the phosphoinositide 3-kinase and AKT (PI3K/Akt) pathway, induction of DNA damage, cell cycle arrest, and apoptosis. Moreover, PU-1 and other methylene chloride:methanol (1:1) *P. undulata* extracts such as Ivalin had anti-inflammatory effects in RAW264 macrophage cells. This prevention of inflammation-associated carcinogenesis was propagated through reduction of inducible NO synthase (iNOS) and nuclear factor kappa B (NF-κB) (Hegazy et al. 2012).

11.4   *P. UNDULATA'S* ANTI-ANGIOGENIC ACTIVITY

In one recent study, six anti-angiogenic and antiproliferative compounds were isolated from *P. undulata*, *i.e.*, xanthoxyline, stigmasterol, oleanolic acid, salvigenin, rhamnetin, and dihydroquercetin-40-methyl ether (Elhady et al. 2021). These compounds significantly reduced tumor weight and vascular endothelial growth factor (VEGF) signaling through the decrease of vascular endothelial growth factor B (VEGF-B) and vascular endothelial growth factor receptor 2 (VEGFR-2) levels in breast and Ehrlich's ascites carcinomas. Sequentially, the reduction in receptor tyrosine kinase VEGFR-2 level led to the inactivation of the mediated signaling pathways, including the phospholipase C (PLC)/extracellular signal–regulated protein kinase (ERK1/2) pathway as well as PI3K and its downstream molecule serine/threonine protein kinase B, known as AKT-mammalian target of rapamycin (PI3K–AKT–mTOR) pathway (Roskoski 2008). Accordingly, the suppression of PI3K/Akt pathway resulted in the induction of apoptosis, inhibition of mTORC1-dependent cell growth, hindering in metabolism of cancerous cells and their metastatic potential, and cell cycle arrest (Koundouros and Poulogiannis 2018).

11.5   ROLE OF *P. UNDULATA* IN OXIDATIVE STRESS

The Kelch-like ECH-associated protein 1 (Keap1)–nuclear erythroid 2-cognate factor 2 (NRF2) pathway is one cascade that is regulated by PI3K/Akt signaling. The transcription factor NRF2 represents a main mediator of ROS detoxification through its nuclear translocation, and inducing the expression of several phase II enzymes that are involved in the antioxidation process, including glutathione S-transferases, UDP-glucuronosyl transferases, NAD(P)H/quinine oxidoreductase (NQO), and heme oxygenase-1 (HO-1) (Kashyap et al. 2016; Koundouros and Poulogiannis 2018). Thus, upon inhibition of the PI3K/Akt pathway by the isolated active compounds of *P. undulata*,

NRF2 reduced its antioxidant transcription activity in cancerous cells leading to a loss of protection against excessive oxidative stress and cell survival (De Nicola et al. 2011; Sporn and Liby 2012).

11.6 *P. UNDULATA'S* EFFECT ON AUTOPHAGY

Increasing ROS activities can also induce the autophagy pathway via promotion of the autophagy mediator protein, Beclin-1 (Hegazy et al. 2018) by enhancing its dissociation from its bounded anti-apoptotic Bcl-2 protein. Thereafter, Beclin-1 is subjected to cleavage by caspases, and the cleaved products can bind to the mitochondrial membrane leading to activation of apoptosis process. Interestingly, mTORC2 – regulated by the PI3K axis – was directly involved in the regulation of most autophagic proteins. This provides evidence that the PI3K/Akt pathway is critical for the regulation of autophagy through its ability to integrate signals from the cellular environment and other signaling pathways such as the Ras/Raf/MEK/ERK and MAPK/JNK pathways to regulate the fate of autophagic response. The regulation of autophagy status within the cell is orchestrated by the cellular ROS levels. In the presence of high ROS levels, the PI3K β catalytic subunit is activated to promote autophagy, while under moderate levels of ROS, the PI3K α catalytic subunit inhibits autophagy via activation of Akt (inhibition of autophagy, and apoptosis) and NRF2 (decreases ROS level) to inhibit autophagy response (Kma and Baruah 2022).

Interestingly, the tumor suppressor p21 that initiates cell cycle arrest to allow DNA repair or facilitate apoptosis if DNA damage is severe and cannot be repaired – contributes to the regulation of NRF2 according to the cellular ROS levels. At low ROS levels, p21 activates the NRF2-dependent antioxidant response to protect cells against oxidative stress inducing damage, while at moderate levels of cellular ROS, p21 enhances cell cycle arrest to allow DNA repair. At high levels of oxidative stress, p21 blocks NRF2, the downstream pro-survival responses are inhibited, and the process of apoptosis is activated (Villeneuve et al. 2009).

11.7 ANTITUMOR BIOACTIVITY OF *P. UNDULATA'S* SECONDARY METABOLITE QUERCETIN

One of the most common secondary metabolites in *P. undulata* is quercetin (3,3′,4′,5,7-pentahydroxyflavone). Quercetin possesses many pharmacologic activities, such as antioxidant, antidiabetic, anti-inflammatory, and antiproliferative effects. Quercetin exerted anticancer properties against a broad range of cell lines from different cancer types by affecting several signaling pathways in different cancers (Kashyap et al. 2016; Vafadar et al. 2020).

Quercetin plays an important role as initiator of apoptosis by inducing caspase-3, and caspase-9, releasing cytochrome c, suppressing Bcl-xL and Bcl-2 anti-apoptotic proteins, upregulating Bax and other proapoptotic proteins, and cleaving poly-ADP-ribose polymerase (PARP) (Aalinkeel et al. 2008; Kim and Jang 2009). Hegazy et al. (2018) and Emam et al. (2019) reported similar results for the total *P. undulata* extract in different cancerous cell lines. Moreover, quercetin inhibited major survival signals, such as PI3K/AKT and ERKs (Kashyap et al. 2016) as also reported by Elhady et al. (2021) for six anti-angiogenic and antiproliferative compounds isolated from *P. undulata* and major metabolite PU-1 (Hegazy et al., 2020). Besides, quercetin promoted the p53-dependent apoptotic pathway via increasing the expression level of microRNA-34a in hepatocellular carcinoma (Lou et al. 2015), similar to the results obtained by Emam et al. (2019) for the total *P. undulata* extract in HepG2 cells.

Quercetin mediated the G1, S, and G2/M phase cell cycle arrest as a consequence of upregulation of p21 in multiple cancerous cell lines (Jeong et al. 2009), as also indicated by Hegazy et al. (2020) for PU-1. This flavonol also inhibited different steps of angiogenesis including proliferation, migration, and tube formation. This inhibition process was initiated through suppressing many signaling pathways such as VEGF receptor-2 (VEGF-R2)-regulated AKT/mTOR/P70S6K, ERK, STAT3 (regulator of matrix metalloproteinases, and VEGF), MAPK, PI3K/AKT, NF-κB, and hypoxia-inducible factor (HIF)-1α, a protein known to reduce the production and secretion of VEGF (Kashyap et al. 2016).

Surprisingly, various studies reported the protective effect of quercetin against the oxidative stress by activation of NRF2 translocation into nucleus to estimate the expression of several phase II enzymes (Kashyap et al. 2016).

11.8 CONCLUSION

There is a critical and increasing requirement to search for alternative anticancer therapies that are safer than current chemotherapies to avoid and to minimize the undesired side effects of current standard treatments. Natural plant sources represent an effective reservoir to identify agents with low toxicity. This favors plants along with their bioactive metabolites as promising candidates for novel anticancer medications. Exploring the molecular mechanisms and the mode of their action to different signaling pathways of cancer will aid the better understanding of cancer biology that will facilitate the design of novel, safe, and effective anticancer drugs.

The current chapter focuses on the cellular signaling pathways that are governed by the active secondary metabolites isolated from *P. undulata* in the treatment of tumor cells. We conclude that *P. undulata* may be a safe source that is rich in many bioactive phytochemical compounds that inhibit various carcinogenic pathways by increasing oxidative stress, DNA damage response, cell cycle arrest, autophagy, and apoptosis. Additionally, *P. undulata* can prevent cancer progression through inhibition of angiogenesis and the PI3K/AKT pathway (Figure 11.1). Collectively, *P.*

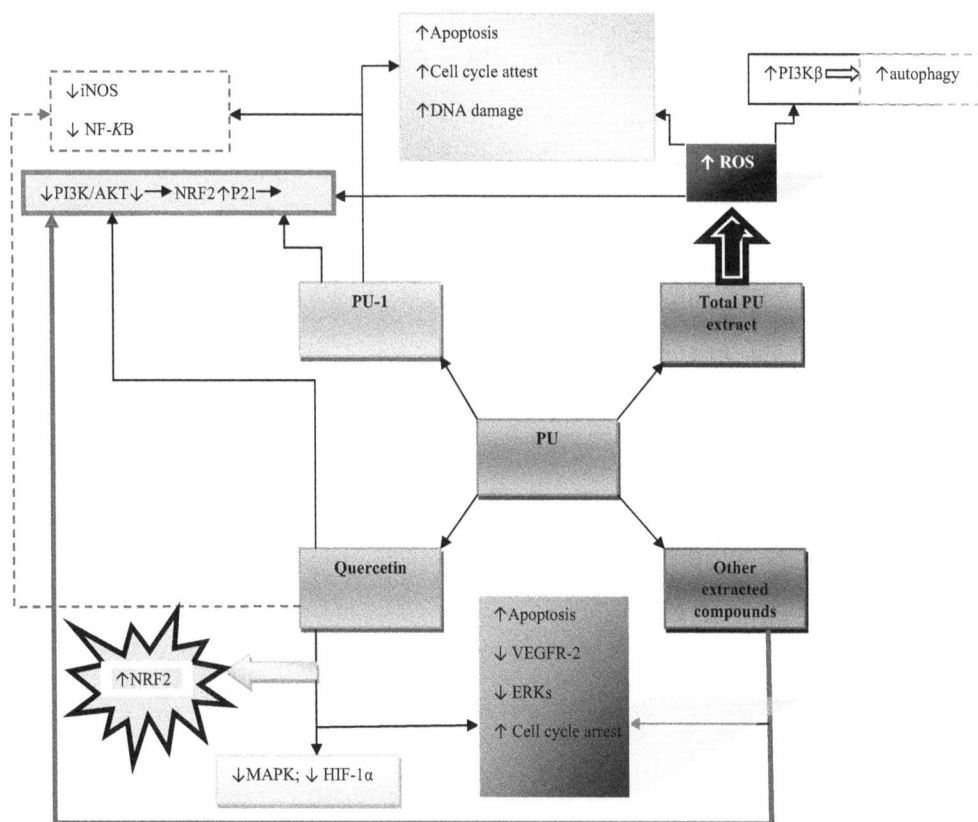

FIGURE 11.1 Molecular mechanism interactions of the bioactive compounds isolated from PU. ERK = extracellular signal–regulated protein kinase; HIF-1α = hypoxia-inducible factor; iNOS = inducible NO synthase; MAPK = mitogen-activated protein kinase; NF-κB = nuclear factor kappa B; NRF2 = nuclear erythroid 2-cognate factor 2; PI3K/Akt = phosphoinositide 3-kinase and AKT; PU = *Pulicaria undulata*; ROS = reactive oxygen species; VEGFR-2 = vascular endothelial growth factor receptor 2.

undulata and its secondary metabolites are promising novel anticancer drug candidates with various favorable properties that could add value in the field of drug discovery through further *in vitro* and *in vivo* studies.

11.9 SUMMARY POINTS

- This chapter focuses on the bioactivity of secondary metabolites isolated from *P. undulata* against tumor cells.
- *P. undulata* is a natural, safe source that is rich in many bioactive phytochemical compounds that can inhibit various carcinogenic pathways.
- *P. undulata* has an antitumor activity by increasing oxidative stress, DNA damage response, cell cycle arrest, autophagy, and apoptosis.
- *P. undulata* prevents cancer progression through inhibition of angiogenesis and the PI3K/AKT pathway.
- *P. undulata* could be used as an alternative anticancer therapy to avoid and to minimize the undesired side effects of the current traditional treatments.

REFERENCES

Aalinkeel, R., Bindukumar, B., Reynolds, J.L., Sykes, D.E., Mahajan, S.D., Chada, K.C. and S. A. Schwartz. 2008. The dietary bioflavonoid, quercetin, selectively induces apoptosis of prostate cancer cells by downregulating the expression of heat shock protein 90. Prostate, 68, 1773–1789.

Abdallah, H.M., Mohamed, G.A., Ibrahim, S.R.M., Asfour, H.Z. and M.T. Khayat. 2019. Undulaterpene A: A new triterpene fatty acid ester from *Pulicaria undulata*. Pharmacogn. Mag., 15, 671.

Ahmed, M.M., Samih, I.E., Giovanni, C., Massimo, B., Luana, Q., Giulio, L., Daniela, B., Sauro, V. and M. Filippo. 2018. Chemical composition and biological activities of the essential oil from *Pulicaria undulata* (L.) C. A. Mey. Growing wild in Egypt. Nat. Prod. Res., 34, 2358–2362. doi:10.1080/14786419.2018.1534107

Ahmed, S. and M. Ibrahim. 2017. Chemical investigation and antimicrobial activity of *Francoeuria crispa* (Forssk) grown wild in Egypt. J. Mater. Environ. Sci., 9, 1–6.

Al-Hajj, N.Q.M., Algabr, M.N., Omar, K.A. and H. Wang. 2017. Anticancer, antimicrobial and antioxidant activities of the essential oils of some aromatic medicinal plants (Pulicariainuloides-Asteraceae). J. Food Nutr. Res., 5, 490–495.

Ali, N.A.A., Sharopov, F.S., Alhaj, M., Hill, G.M., Porzel, A., Arnold, N., Setzer, W.N., Schmidt, J. and L. Wessjohann. 2012. Chemical composition and biological activity of essential oil from *Pulicaria undulata* from Yemen. Nat. Prod. Comm., 7, 1934578X1200700238

Al-Maqtari, Q.A., Mahdi, A.A., Al-Ansi, W., Mohammed, J.K., Wei, M. and W. Yao. 2020. Evaluation of bioactive compounds and antibacterial activity of *Pulicaria jaubertii* extract obtained by supercritical and conventional methods. J. Food Meas. Charact., 15, 449–456.

Assaeed, A., Elshamy, A., El Gendy, A.E.-N., Dar, B., Al-Rowaily, S. and A. Abd-ElGawad. 2020. Sesquiterpenes-rich essential oil from above ground parts of *Pulicaria somalensis* exhibited antioxidant activity and allelopathic effect on weeds. Agronomy, 10, 399.

Boumaraf, M., Mekkiou, R., Benyahia, S., Chalchat, J.-C., Chalard, P., Benayache, F. and S. Benayache. 2016. Essential oil composition of *Pulicaria undulata* (L.) DC. (Asteraceae) growing in Algeria. Int. J. Pharmacogn. Phytochem. Res., 8, 746–749.

Choudhari, A.S., Mandave, P.C., Deshpande, M., Ranjekar, P. and O. Prakash. 2020. Phytochemicals in cancer treatment: From preclinical studies to clinical practice. Front. Pharmacol., 10, 1614. doi:10.3389/fphar.2019.01614

Dekinash, M.F., Abou-Hashem, M.M., Beltagy, A.M. and F.K. El-Fiky. 2019. GC/MS profiling, in-vitro cytotoxic and antioxidant potential of the essential oil of *Pulicaria crispa* (Forssk) growing in Egypt. Int. J. Pharmacogn. Chin. Med., 3, 000175.

De Nicola, G.M., Karreth, F.A., Humpton, T.J., Gopinathan, A., Wei, C., Frese, K., Mangal, D., Yu, K.H., Yeo, C.J., Calhoun, E.S., Scrimieri, F., Winter, J.M., Hruban, R.H., Iacobuzio-Donahue, C., Kern, S.E., Blair, I.A. and D.A. Tuveson. 2011. Oncogene-induced Nrf2 transcription promotes ROS detoxification and tumorigenesis. Nature, 475(7354), 106–109.

Elhady, S.S., Abdelhameed, R.F.A., Zekry, S.H., Ibrahim, A.K., Habib, E.S., Darwish, K.M., Hazem, R.M., Mohammad, K.A., Hassanean, H.A. and S.A. Ahmed. 2021. VEGFR-mediated cytotoxic activity of *Pulicaria undulata* isolated metabolites: A biological evaluation and in silico study. Life, 11, 759.

Elshamy, A.I., Mohamed, T.A., Marzouk, M.M., Hussien, T.A., Umeyama, A., Hegazy, M.E.F. and T. Efferth. 2018. Phytochemical constituents and chemo systematic significance of *Pulicaria jaubertii* E. Gamal-Eldin (Asteraceae). Phytochem. Lett., 24, 105–109.

Emam, M.A., Khattab, H.I. and M.G. Hegazy. 2019. Assessment of anticancer activity of *Pulicaria undulata* on hepatocellular carcinoma HepG2 cell line. Tumor Biol., 1–10.

Fahmi, A.A., Abdur-Rahman, M., Naser, A.F.A., Hamed, M.A., Abd-Alla, H.I., Shalaby, N.M. and M.I. Nasr. 2019. Chemical composition and protective role of *Pulicaria undulata* (L.) CA Mey. subsp. *undulata* against gastric ulcer induced by ethanol in rats. Heliyon, 5, e01359.

Hammiche, V. and K. Maiza. 2006. Traditional medicine in Central Sahara: Pharmacopoeia of Tassili N'ajjer. J. Ethnopharmacol., 105, 358–367.

Hanahan, D. and R.A. Weinber. 2011. Hallmarks of cancer: The next generation. Cell. 144(5), 646–674.

Hassan, E.M., El Gendy, A.E.-N.G., Abd-ElGawad, A.M., Elshamy, A.I., Farag, M.A., Alamery, S.F. and E.A. Omer. 2021. Comparative chemical profiles of the essential oils from different varieties of *Psidium guajava* L. Molecules, 26, 119.

Hegazy, M.-E.F., Abdelfatah, S., Hamed, A.R., Mohamed, T.A., Elshemy, A.A., Saleh, I.A., Reda, E.H., Abdel-Azim, N.S., Shams, K.A., Sakr, M., Sugimoto, Y., Paré, P.W. and T. Efferth. 2018. Cytotoxicity of 40 Egyptian plant extracts targeting mechanisms of drug-resistant cancer cells. Phytomedicine, S0944711318305889.

Hegazy, M.-E.F., Dawood, M., Mahmoud, N., Elbadawi, M., Sugimoto, Y., Klauck, S.M., Mohamed, N. and T. Efferth. 2020. 2α-hydroxyalantolactone from *Pulicaria undulata*: Activity against multidrug-resistant tumor cells and modes of action. Phytomedicine, 81, 153409.

Hegazy, M.-E.F., Matsuda, H., Nakamura, S., Yabe, M., Matsumoto, T. and M. Yoshikawa. 2012. Sesquiterpenes from an Egyptian Herbal Medicine, *Pulicaria undulate*, with inhibitory effects on nitric oxide production in RAW264.7 macrophage cells. Chem. Pharm. Bull., 60(3), 363–370.

Helal, N.M., Ibrahim, N.A. and H. Khattab. 2019. Phytochemical analysis and antifungal bioactivity of *Pulicaria undulata* (L.) methanolic extract and essential oil. Egypt. J. Bot., 59(3), 827–844.

Hussein, S.R., Marzouk, M.M., Soltan, M.M., Ahmed, E.K., Said, M.M. and A. R. Hamed. 2017. Phenolic constituents of *Pulicaria undulata* (L.) C.A. Mey. subsp. *undulata* (Asteraceae): Antioxidant protective effects and chemo systematic significances. J. Food Drug Anal., 25, 333–339.

Issa, M.Y., Ezzat, M.I., Sayed, R.H., Elbaz, E.M., Omar, F.A. and E. Mohsen. 2020. Neuroprotective effects of *Pulicaria undulata* essential oil in rotenone model of Parkinson's disease in rats: Insights into its anti-inflammatory and anti-oxidant effects. S. Afr. J. Bot., 132, 289–298.

Javadinamin, A. and J. Asgarpanah. 2014. Essential oil composition of *Francoeuria undulata* (L.) Lack. growing wild in Iran. J. Essent. Oil Bear. Plants, 17, 875–879.

Jeong, J.H., An, J.Y., Kwon, Y.T., Rhee, J.G. and Y.J. Lee. 2009. Effects of low dose quercetin: Cancer cell-specific inhibition of cell cycle progression. J Cell Biochem., 106, 73–82.

Kashyap, D., Mittal, S., Sak, K., Singhal, P. and H.S. Tuli. 2016. Molecular mechanisms of action of quercetin in cancer: Recent advances. Tumor Biol. 37, 12927–12939.

Khan, T.A., Al Nasr, I.S., Mujawah, A.H. and W.S. Koko. 2021. Assessment of *Euphorbia retusa* and *Pulicaria undulata* activity against *Leishmania major* and *Toxoplasma gondii*. Tropical Biomedicine, 38(1), 135–141.

Khazir, J., Riley, D., Pilcher, L., De Maayer, P. and B. Mir. 2014. Anticancer agents from diverse natural sources. Nat. Prod. Commun., 9, 1655–1669.

Kim, G. and H. Jang. 2009. Jang protective mechanism of quercetin and rutin using glutathione metabolism on H_2O_2-induced oxidative stress in HepG2 cells. Ann. NY Acad. Sci., 1171, 530–537.

Kma, L. and T.J. Baruah. 2022. The interplay of ROS and the PI3K/Akt pathway in autophagy regulation. Biotechnol. Appl. Biochem. 69, 248–264.

Kopustinskiene, D.M., Jakstas, V., Savickas, A. and J. Bernatoniene. 2020. Flavonoids as anticancer agents. Nutrients, 12, 457.

Koundouros, N. and G. Poulogiannis. 2018. Phosphoinositide 3-Kinase/Akt signaling and redox metabolism in cancer. Front. Oncol., 8, 160.

Kumar, S., Saini, M., Kumar, V., Prakash, O., Arya, R., Rana, M. and D. Kumar. 2012. Traditional medicinal plants curing diabetes: A promise for today and tomorrow. Asian J. Trad. Med., 7, 178–188.

Law, J.W.-F., Law, L.N.-S., Letchumanan, V., Tan, L.T.-H., Wong, S.H., Chan, K.-G., Ab Mutalib, N.-S. and L.-H. Lee. 2020. Anticancer drug discovery from microbial sources: The unique mangrove streptomycetes. Molecules, 25, 5365.

Liu, L., Yang, J. and Y. Shi. 2010. Phytochemicals and biological activities of *Pulicaria* species. Chem. Biodiver., 7, 327–349.

Lou, G., Liu, Y., Wu, S., Xue, J., Yang, F., Fu, H., Zheng, M. and Z. Chen. 2015. The p53/miR-34a/SIRT1 positive feedback loop in quercetin-induced apoptosis. Cell Physiol Biochem., 35, 2192–202.

McNeil, M.J., Porter, R.B.R., Rainford, L., Dunbar, O., Francis, S., Laurieri, N. and R. Delgoda. 2018. Chemical composition and biological activities of the essential oil from *Cleome rutidosperma* DC. Fitoterapia, 129, 191–197.

Mohamed, E.A.A., Muddathir, A.M. and M.A. Osman. 2020. Antimicrobial activity, phytochemical screening of crude extracts, and essential oils constituents of two *Pulicaria* spp. growing in Sudan. Sci. Rep., 10, 1–8.

Mohammed, A.B., Yagi, S., Tzanova, T., Schohn, H., Abdelgadir, H., Stefanucci, A., Mollica, A., Mahomoodally, M.F., Adlan, T.A. and G. Zengin. 2020. Chemical profile, antiproliferative, antioxidant and enzyme inhibition activities of *Ocimum basilicum* L. and *Pulicaria undulata* (L.) CA Mey. grown in Sudan. S. Afr. J. Bot., 132, 403–409.

Mohammed, H.A., Al-Omar, M.S., Khan, R.A., Mohammed, S.A.A., Qureshi, K.A., Abbas, M.M., Al Rugaie, O., Abd-Elmoniem, E., Ahmad, A.M. and Y.I. Kandil. 2021. Chemical profile, antioxidant, antimicrobial, and anticancer activities of the water-ethanol extract of *Pulicaria undulata* growing in the Oasis of Central Saudi Arabian Desert. Plants, 10, 1811.

Mustafa, A.M., Eldahmy, S.I., Caprioli, G., Bramucci, M., Quassinti, L., Lupidi, G., Beghelli, D., Vittori, S. and F. Maggi. 2020. Chemical composition and biological activities of the essential oil from *Pulicaria undulata* (L.) CA Mey. Growing wild in Egypt. Nat. Prod. Res., 34, 2358–2362.

Nematollahi, F., Rustaiyan, A., Larijani, K., Nadimi, M. and S. Masoudi. 2006. Essential oil composition of *Artemisia biennisz* Willd. and *Pulicaria undulata* (L.) CA Mey., two compositae herbs growing wild in Iran. J. Essent. Oil Res., 18, 339–341.

Passos, F.J., Nelson, G., Wang, C., Richter, T., Simillion, C., Proctor, C.J., Miwa, S., Olijslagers, S., Hallinan, J., Wipat, A., Saretzki, G., Karl, L.R., Tom, K. and V.-Z. Thomas. 2010. Feedback between p21 and reactive oxygen production is necessary for cell senescence. Mol. Syst. Biol., 6, 347.

Rasool, N., Rashid, M.A., Khan, S.S., Ali, Z., Zubair, M., Ahmad, V.U., Khan, S.N., Choudhary, M.I. and R.B. Tareen. 2013. Novel α-glucosidase activator from *Pulicaria undulata*. Nat. Prod. Commun., 8, 757–759.

Rav, M., Valizadeh, J., Noroozifar, M. and M. Khorasani-Motlagh. 2011. Screening of chemical composition of essential oil, mineral elements and antioxidant activity in *Pulicaria undulata* (L.) CA Mey from Iran. J. Med. Plants Res., 5, 2035–2040.

Roskoski, R. 2008. VEGF receptor protein-tyrosine kinases: Structure and regulation. Biochem. Biophys. Res. Commun., 375, 287–291.

Sporn, M.B. and K.T. Liby. 2012. NRF2 and cancer: The good, the bad and the importance of context. Nat. Rev. Cancer, 12, 564–5671. doi:10.1038/nrc3278

Vafadar, A., Shabaninejad, Z., Movahedpour, A., Fallahi, F., Taghavipour, M., Ghasemi, Y., Akbari, M., Shafiee, A., Hajighadimi, S., Moradizarmehri, S., Razi, E., Savardashtaki, A. and H. Mirzaei. 2020. Quercetin and cancer: New insights into its therapeutic effects on ovarian cancer cells. Cell Biosci., 10, 32.

Vanhaelen, M., Lejoly, J., Hanocq, M. and L. Molle. 1991. Climatic and geographical aspects of medicinal plant constituents. In The Medicinal Plant Industry; Routledge Press: London, UK; pp. 59–75.

Villeneuve, N.F., Sun, Z., Chen, W. and D.D. Zhang. 2009. Nrf2 and p21 regulate the fine balance between life and death by controlling ROS levels. Cell Cycle, 8, 20, 3255–3256.

Wang, X., Zhang, H. and X. Chen. 2019. Drug resistance and combating drug resistance in cancer. Cancer Drug Resist., 2, 141–160.

Xu, T., Gherib, M., Bekhechi, C., Atik-Bekkara, F., Casabianca, H., Tomi, F., Casanova, J. and A. Bighelli. 2015. Thymyl esters derivatives and a new natural product modhephanone from *Pulicaria mauritanica* Coss. (Asteraceae) root oil. Flavour Fragr. J., 30(1), 83–90.

12 Felty Germander (*Teucrium polium* L.) Usage in the Middle East and Biological Basis of Its Effects and Special Focus on Cancers

Vahap Murat Kutluay and Neziha Yagmur Diker

ABBREVIATIONS

α2MG	alpha-2 macroglobulin
A375.S2	human malignant melanoma cell
A431	human epidermoid carcinoma cell
A549	human lung carcinoma cell
Aβ	amyloid beta
AFP	alpha fetoprotein
ALP	alkaline phosphatase
ALT	alanine aminotransaminase
AST	aspartate transaminase
BT20	human breast adenocarcinoma cell
CACO-2	human colorectal adenocarcinoma cell
CBG	corticosteroid-binding globulin
CYP3A	cytochrome P450, family 3, subfamily A
DU145	human prostate cancer cell
eNOS	endothelial nitric oxide synthase
EJ	human endometrial adenocarcinoma cell
FGF-2	fibroblast growth factor 2
FoxO1	forkhead box O1
GGT	gamma glutamyltransferase
GLUT-1	glucose transporter 1
HCY	homocysteine
HeLa	human cervical cancer cell
HRT18	human rectal adenocarcinoma cell
HT29	human colorectal adenocarcinoma cell
HUVECs	human umbilical vein endothelial cell
IGF-1	insulin-like growth factor 1
IL-1β	interleukin-1 beta
JNK	c-Jun N-terminal kinase
KB	human epithelial carcinoma cell
MatLyLu	rat prostate carcinoma cell
MCF-7	human breast adenocarcinoma cell

DOI: 10.1201/9781003260028-14

MDA	malondialdehyde
MTT	3-[4,5-dimethythiazol-2-yl]-2,5 diphenyl tetrazolium bromide
PC12	rat adrenal medullary tumor cell
PC3	human prostate adenocarcinoma cell
Pdx1	pancreas/duodenum homeobox protein 1
ROS	reactive oxygen species
Saos-2	human osteogenic sarcoma cell
Sirt3	NAD-dependent deacetylase sirtuin-3, mitochondrial
Sk-mel-3	human malignant melanoma cell
SW480	human colorectal carcinoma cell
T47D	human ductal epithelial breast tumor cell
TNF-α	tumor necrosis factor alpha
TP	*Teucrium polium* L.
VCAM-1	vascular cell adhesion protein 1
VEGF	vascular endothelial growth factor
VERO	African green monkey kidney epithelial cell
Walker 256/B	rat malignant breast cancer cell
WM1361A	human melanoma cell
WST-1	2-[4-iodophenyl]-3-[4-nitrophenyl]-5-[2,4-disulphophenyl]-2H tetrazolium sodium salt

12.1   INTRODUCTION

The *Teucrium* genus includes about 300 species worldwide and belongs to the Lamiaceae family. Phytochemical investigations on the genus have shown that the herb contains secondary metabolites such as terpenoids, steroids, flavonoids, iridoids, clerodanes, and phenylethanoid glycosides (Sadeghi et al. 2021). Neo-clerodane diterpenoids can be accepted chemotaxonomic markers for this genus. As like other members of the Lamiaceae family and *Teucrium* genus, *Teucrium polium* L. (TP) is also rich in essential oil. Essential oil has been investigated for its chemical composition, and the main components are reported as sesquiterpene hydrocarbons (germacrene D and β-caryophyllene) and monoterpene hydrocarbons (α- and β-pinene) (Candela et al. 2021). TP is an herbaceous plant and flowering time is between June and August. The plant is found mainly in the Mediterranean region and Middle East and various areas of the world such as Asia, Europe, and North Africa. Aerial parts of TP are rich in essential oil and polyphenols (Rahmouni et al. 2021). This plant has been used widely mainly in the Middle East as a traditional medicine to treat various diseases.

12.2   BACKGROUND

T. polium, a member of Lamiaceae family, is widely distributed in the Mediterranean region and Middle East (Figure 12.1). The botanical characteristics of *T. polium* are given in Table 12.1 (Ekim 1982).

The aerial parts are used in folk medicine and are widely consumed as an infusion and decoction in the Mediterranean region and Middle East. The plant is known with various local names through different countries. Even though the local names differ, the traditional use of the plant is similar and mostly center upon gastrointestinal diseases, diabetes, and liver diseases such as jaundice (Table 12.2).

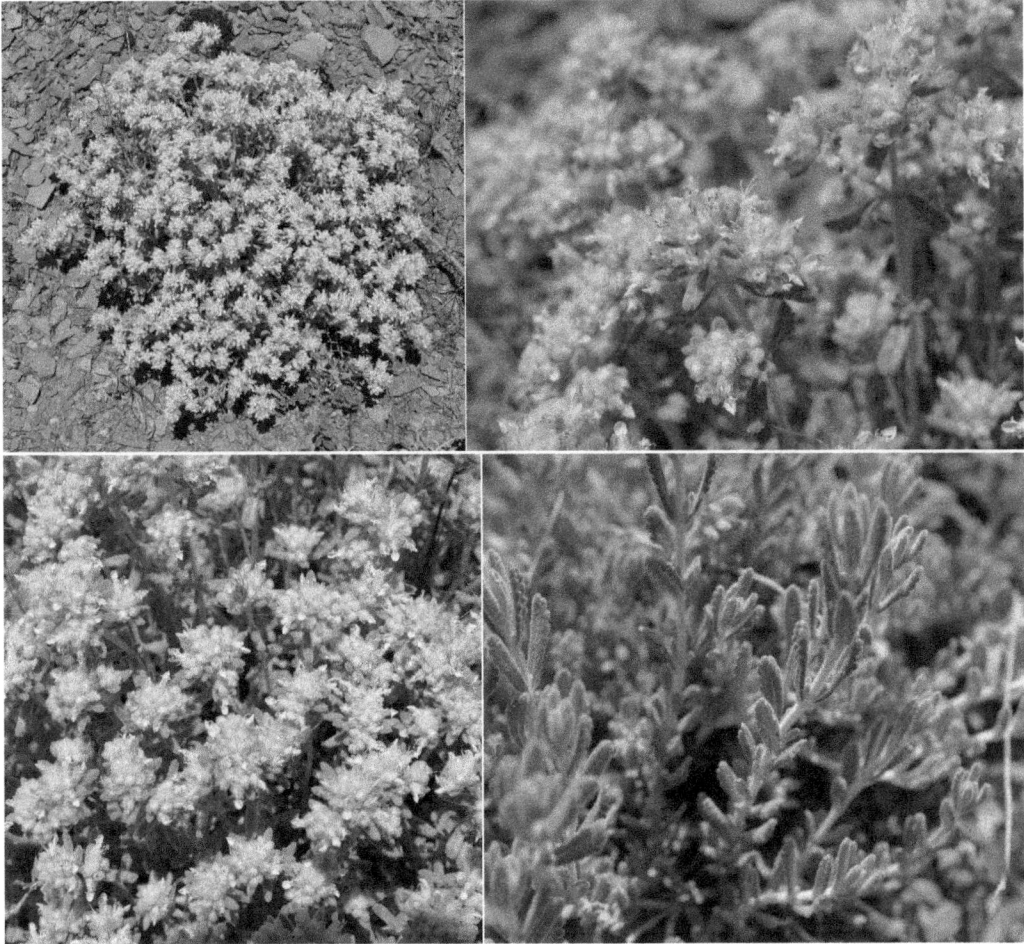

FIGURE 12.1   *Teucrium polium* L.

TP is known as *Gurisa* and *Jaadeh* in Syria and used for the treatment of diabetes, cancer, spasm, and stomach hyperacidity in Aleppo (Alachkar et al. 2011). In Saudi Arabia, the local name of the plant is *Jaad*, and it is traditionally used to treat liver diseases, inflammatory disorders, stomach and intestinal troubles, and rheumatism (Al-Asmari et al. 2014). Similar traditional use of TP in Palestine were reported, as it is used to treat digestive system, prostate, and skin disorders (Ali-Shtayeh et al. 2000). In addition, the leaves of the plant are used for stomachache, especially for children in Israel (Dafni et al. 1984).

It is widely used for stomach and colic spasm, inflammation, anorexia, jaundice, kidney stones, and as an antispasmodic and antidiabetic in Jordan, where the local name is *Jeada* (Alzweiri et al. 2011). Similarly it is called *Ja'ada* or *Ba'itran*, and *Lisan-al-'asfour* in Lebanon. When prepared as decoctions, it used for its effects in hyperglycemia, abdominal pain, vulnerary, goiter, and kidney stones. In addition, the plant's infusion treats hyperthermia, liver disease, and stomachic. Different from these, it is used for the treatment of malaria and jaundice as a poultice. In a steam bath, it is used for its cardiotonic and spasmolytic effects (El Beyrouthy et al. 2013). In Iran, TP has been

TABLE 12.1

Botanical Characteristics of *Teucrium polium* L.

Characteristic	*T. polium*
Habitus	Prostrate to erect
Stem	10–40 cm long
	With white, gray (sometimes golden) lanuginose-tomentose or crisped indumentum
	Internodes shorter or longer than leaves
Leaves	Oblong to narrowly obovate or linear, obtuse
	Crenate to the base or middle, flat or revolute-margined
	Usually tomentose
Flowers	Very shortly pedicellate
	Borne in heads (capitula)
Bracts	Linear-spathulate
	Crenate or entire
	Shorter to slightly longer than calyces
Calyx	3–5 mm
	Tubular-obconical
	Usually densely lanuginose or adpressed-canescent
	Divided to 1/4–1/3 into subequal
	Obtuse teeth
Corolla	Whitish
	Proximal lobes occasionally glabrous
Fruit	Nutlets, 2 mm
Locations	Dry places, *Quercus* scrub, rocky slopes, steppe, dunes, field margins, etc.
Altitude	Sea level to 2050 m

TABLE 12.2

Examples for Local Names of *Teucrium polium* L. in the Middle East

Country	Local Name
Iran	*Maryam-nokhodi*
Lebanon	*Ja'ada*
	Ba'itran
	Lisan-al-'asfour
Saudi Arabia	*Jaad*
Syria	*Gurisa*
	Jaadeh
Jordan	*Jeada*
Turkey	*Acıyavşan*
	Tüylü kısamahmut

widely used as folk medicine and the local name is *Maryam-nokhodi*. Aerial parts are internally used for pregnancy pains, flatulence, analgesic, liver disorders, jaundice, abortifacient, and coughing (Naghibi et al. 2005).

The plant, known as *Acıyavşan* or *Tüylü kısamahmut* in Turkey, is traditionally used for stomachache, hemorrhoids, common colds, abdominal pains, antipyretic, and sunstroke (Tuzlacı 2016). It is also reported to be used in fungal diseases (Altanlar et al. 2006).

The ethnobotanical use of *T. polium* in different regions are listed in more detail in Table 12.3.

TABLE 12.3

The Ethnobotanical Use of *Teucrium polium* L.

Used as/in the Treatment of	Plant Part(s)	Preparation	Additional Information about Utilization	Reference
Abortifacient	Aerial parts	Infusion	Not specified	Naghibi et al. 2005
Analgesic	Aerial parts	Infusion	Not specified For pregnancy pains	Naghibi et al. 2005
Anorexia	Aerial parts	Infusion	Not specified	Alzweiri et al. 2011
Anticancer	Aerial parts	Infusion	Crushed and prepared as tea	Alachkar et al. 2011;
Antidiabetic	Aerial parts	Infusion	Crushed and prepared as tea Not specified	Alachkar et al. 2011; Alzweiri et al. 2011
		Decoction	One tablespoon in 250 mL (10 min) for hypoglycemia	El Beyrouthy et al. 2013
Anti-inflammatory	Aerial parts	Not specified Infusion	Not specified	Al-Asmari et al. 2014 Alzweiri et al. 2011
Antimalarial	Aerial parts	Poultice	Not specified	El Beyrouthy et al. 2013
Antipyretic	Leaves Aerial parts	Infusion	Not specified	El Beyrouthy et al. 2013 Tuzlacı 2016
Antirheumatic	Aerial parts	Not specified	Not specified	Al-Asmari et al. 2014
Antispasmodic	Aerial parts	Infusion	Crushed and prepared as tea For stomach and colic spasm	Alachkar et al. 2011 Alzweiri et al. 2011
Cardiotonic	Aerial parts	Steam bath	Not specified	El Beyrouthy et al. 2013
Common colds, cough	Aerial parts	Infusion	Not specified	Naghibi et al. 2005; Tuzlacı 2016
Goiter	Aerial parts	Decoction	One tablespoon in 250 mL (10 min)	El Beyrouthy et al. 2013
Hemorrhoids	Aerial parts	Infusion	Not specified	Tuzlacı 2016
Intestinal troubles	Aerial parts	Not specified	Not specified	Al-Asmari et al. 2014; Ali-Shtayeh et al. 2000
		Infusion	For flatulence For abdominal pain	Naghibi et al. 2005 Tuzlacı 2016
		Decoction	One tablespoon in 250 mL (10 min) for abdominal pain	El Beyrouthy et al. 2013
Kidney stones	Aerial parts	Infusion	Not specified	Alzweiri et al. 2011
		Decoction	One tablespoon in 250 mL (10 min)	El Beyrouthy et al. 2013
Liver disorders	Aerial parts	Not specified	Not specified	Al-Asmari et al. 2014
		Infusion	For jaundice	Alzweiri et al. 2011; Naghibi et al. 2005
			Not specified	Naghibi et al. 2005
		Poultice	For jaundice	El Beyrouthy et al. 2013
	Leaves	Infusion	Not specified	El Beyrouthy et al. 2013
Prostate	Aerial parts	Not specified	Not specified	Ali-Shtayeh et al. 2000
Skin disorders	Aerial parts	Not specified	Not specified	Ali-Shtayeh et al. 2000
Stomachic	Aerial parts	Infusion	Crushed and prepared as tea for stomach hyperacidity	Alachkar et al. 2011
			Not specified	Al-Asmari et al. 2014
			For stomachache	Tuzlacı 2016
		Steam bath	Not specified	El Beyrouthy et al. 2013
	Leaves	Infusion	Prepared as tea for stomachache in children	Dafni et al. 1984
			Not specified	El Beyrouthy et al. 2013
Sunstroke	Aerial parts	Infusion	Not specified	Tuzlacı 2016

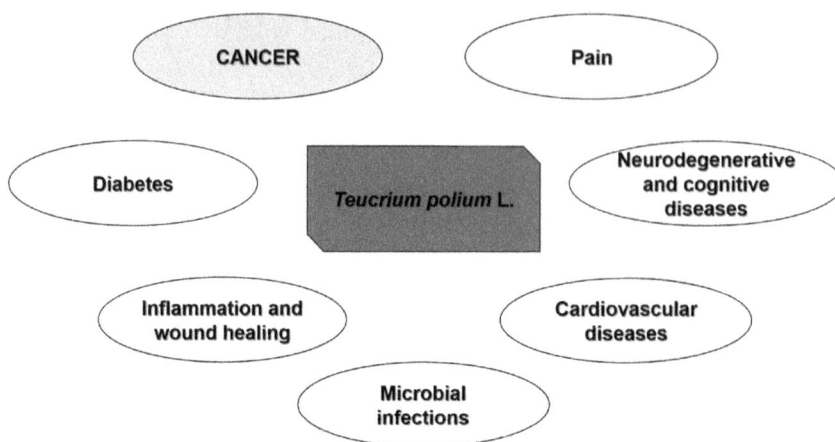

FIGURE 12.2　The main health problems tested against *Teucrium polium* L. for its biological effects.

12.3　EFFECTS OF *T. POLIUM* L. IN HEALTH PROBLEMS

Studies performed on *T. polium* are represented under subtitles by classifying them according to diseases (Figure 12.2).

12.3.1　PAIN

T. polium is used as a folk medicine in Iran to treat visceral pain (Zendehdel et al. 2011). TP, belonging to the Lamiaceae family, is a source of essential oil, like other members of the family. Abdollahi et al. has evaluated the antinociceptive activity of the aerial parts of the plant and tried to identify the source of the biological activity. For this purpose, researchers tested essential oil, extract, and essential oil free extract separately in a visceral pain model in mice. Though all samples decreased the number of abdominal writhings, findings showed that mainly essential oil is responsible for the analgesic effects of the plant, but even essential oil free extract decreased the number of writhing in mice (Abdollahi et al. 2003). Similarly, Zendehdal et al. tested hydroethanolic extract of TP in a writhing test model in mice and reported antinociceptive effect (Zendehdel et al. 2011).

A placebo controlled clinical study was performed in Iran to evaluate the effects of TP in primary dysmenorrhea. Seventy women aged between 20 and 30 years were screened. For a period of two cycles, 35 women took TP powder and other participants were treated with mefenamic acid. The severity of pain that participants suffered decreased significantly. Results of TP were compared with mefenamic acid, and it was reported that TP showed similar effect with handling pain in dysmenorrhea. There were no adverse effects reported in this study (Abadian et al. 2016).

12.3.2　NEURODEGENERATIVE AND COGNITIVE DISEASES

Alzheimer disease is a neurodegenerative disease that researchers are studying to find an effective treatment. Plants used in folk medicine were searched for their effects in neurodegenerative diseases. TP, one of those plants, was reported to be used for its memory enhancing effects in Anatolia (Orhan and Aslan 2009). A 75% ethanolic extract of aerial parts of TP showed a dose-dependent memory-enhancing effect evaluated by passive avoidance test in mice. Orhan and Aslan also reported the acetylcholine esterase inhibitory activity of TP with an IC_{50} value of 0.55 mg/mL (Orhan and Aslan 2009). Bendjabeur et al. reported that essential oil showed higher inhibitory acetylcholine esterase and butyrylcholinesterase activities than ethanol extract (Bendjabeur et al. 2018). Another target in drug discovery research is amyloid β (Aβ) protein that forms insoluble aggregates in Alzheimer disease. Aβ(25–35)-induced rats were used by different studies to evaluate the effects of TP administration on hippocampal neurons (Ghasemi et al. 2019; Simonyan et al. 2019). Ghasemi et al. reported that 75% ethanolic extract of aerial parts (3 mg/kg dose for rats) increased neuronal count in the hippocampus and showed memory enhancing effect (Ghasemi et al. 2019). Learning and memory can be affected in situations related to estrogen deficiency. Ovarian hormones are related to hippocampus and needed for memory. In a study performed in ovariectomized rats, TP was found to help neuronal survival and reduce neurodegenerative effects seen in the hippocampus (Simonyan and Chavushyan 2016). TP was also shown to reverse the effects of Aβ(25–35) in rats by reducing posttetanic potentiation and depression (Simonyan et al. 2019).

In an *in vivo* study, the anticonvulsive effect of aqueous extract and various fractions obtained from aerial parts of TP were tested. Results showed that flavonoid-rich aqueous extract and *n*-butanol fraction increased the onset time of seizure behavior in pentylenetetrazole-treated mice (Khoshnood-Mansoorkhani et al. 2010).

TP also reported to show a preventive effect on cognitive impairment resulting from diabetes mellitus. Diabetic rats treated with aqueous extract of TP with doses of 200 and 400 mg/kg had beneficial effects in learning and memory (Hasanein and Shahidi 2012).

12.3.3 CARDIOVASCULAR DISEASES

In Iran, TP has been used as a traditional medicine for a long time for heart failure (Niazmand et al. 2011). A study conducted by Niazmand et al. focused on the effects of aerial parts of the plant on blood pressure, intraventricular pressure, and heart rate in rabbits. It was reported that the extract showed positive inotropic effect and hypotensive effect but did not show an effect on heart rate (Niazmand et al. 2011). In another study performed in isolated rat thoracic aorta, TP showed vasorelaxant activity via both endothelium dependent and independent mechanisms through calcium influx inhibition in vascular smooth muscle cells (Niazmand et al. 2017).

Endothelium dysfunction has an important role in vascular problems. Diabetes may also cause atherosclerotic vascular complications (Khodadadi et al. 2018). Atherosclerosis, a major cause of coronary artery disease, is one of the major health problems in the world. Khodadadi et al. reported that TP showed vasorelaxation in rat aortic rings and increased eNOS expression and decreased VCAM-1 expression (Khodadadi et al. 2018). In another study, methanolic extract and polysaccharide extract obtained from TP aerial parts were found to increase the coagulation time and showed antiplatelet activity (Nor et al. 2019).

12.3.4 MICROBIAL INFECTIONS

Essential oils are well-known and frequently used for their antimicrobial activities. The antimicrobial activity studies on TP have been focused on both essential oil and plant extract. Essential oils have getting attention for their use in food industries against foodborne pathogens for preservation of food and health. Benali et al. tested the antibacterial effect of TP essential oil against gram-positive (*Listeria innocua* CECT 4030, *Staphylococcus aureus* CECT 976, and *Bacillus subtilis* DSM 6633) and gram-negative (*Proteus mirabilis*, *Escherichia coli* K12, and *Pseudomonas aeruginosa* CECT 118) bacteria. The essential oil showed antibacterial effect against all the bacteria tested (Benali et al. 2021). Moreover, essential oil derived from TP collected from northern Anatolia was reported to possess antimicrobial activity against *Pseudomonas aeruginosa* and methicillin-resistant *S. aureus* (Sevindik et al. 2016).

Ethanol extract obtained from the aerial parts of TP was reported to have antilisterial activity against the gram-positive bacteria *Listeria monocytogenes* in the agar diffusion method with a minimum inhibitory concentration of 50 µg/mL (Altanlar et al. 2006).

Methanol extract of TP was found to have antibacterial activity against *Acinetobacter baumannii*. In the same study, Alreshidi et al. also tested the antiviral activity of the methanolic extract against coxsackievirus B-3 and herpes simplex virus type 2 but reported that the extract was not active against the tested viruses (Alreshidi et al. 2020).

A mouthwash containing TP was tested in a double-blind clinical trial with 22 volunteer dental students. *Streptococcus mutans* is a pathogen that could threaten dental health and, in some cases, it can result in teeth loss. In this study, volunteers were divided into two groups using mouthwash with or without TP. The number of *S. mutans* significantly decreased in the group that used mouthwash containing TP (Tusi et al. 2020).

Another major health problem worldwide is leishmaniasis. Essential oil of TP was tested against *Leishmania major* and *L. infantum* promastigotes. Essential oil showed inhibitory activity on *L. major* and *L. infantum* with IC_{50} values of 0.09 and 0.15 µg/mL, respectively (Essid et al. 2015).

12.3.5 INFLAMMATION AND WOUND HEALING

A wound is tissue damage in skin where the healing process includes various processes such as inflammation. Mehrabani et al. reported the anti-ulcer effects of 80% ethanol extract of the TP plant in indomethacin-induced gastric ulcer model in rats. TP administration showed reduction in the ulcer indices over 90% after 4 weeks (Mehrabani et al. 2009).

An 80% ethanolic extract of the aerial parts of TP was tested for its wound healing effects in diabetic rats. A 10% TP ointment application showed wound healing activity comparable to phenytoin (Huseini et al. 2020). In another study, excisional wound healing in a diabetic mouse model was used to test the effects of TP. Mouse were topically treated with TP alone and as a mixture with aloe vera. The 10% TP ointment and mixture (5%+5%) both accelerated wound healing process and upregulated VEGF, IGF-1, GLUT-1, and FGF-2 expressions and decreased inflammatory cytokines IL-1β, MDA, and TNF-α (Gharaboghaz et al. 2020).

12.3.6 DIABETES

TP has been used traditionally for its antidiabetic effects. In an *in vivo* study, the extract prepared from TP aerial parts and metformin were given to the streptozotocin-induced diabetic rats for 6 weeks as gavage. Doses of 100, 200, and 400 mg/kg were chosen for the extract. The results showed that TP significantly reduced serum glucose level at all tested doses comparable to metformin, where 100 mg/kg found to show the higher hypoglycemic effect than metformin (Khodadadi et al. 2018). Tabatabaie and Yazdanparast similarly showed the hypoglycemic effect of TP extract in streptozotocin-induced diabetic rats. Aerial parts of the plant were extracted with 70% ethanol and used in *in vivo* experiments. After 42 days of treatment with TP, the negative impacts on both blood glucose and lipid levels were found to be ameliorated (Tabatabaie and Yazdanparast 2017). It was reported that β-cell mass and insulin secretion were regulated via FoxO1 and Pdx1 proteins and JNK pathway (Tabatabaie and Yazdanparast 2017).

In a sucrose-induced insulin resistance male rat model, the serum glucose level was decreased by the treatment ethanolic extract of TP leaves with dose of 50 mg/kg, 100 mg/kg, and 200 mg/ kg. In the same study, insulin, leptin, and triglyceride levels were decreased with extract treatment (Mousavi et al. 2012).

12.3.7 CANCER

Studies on the effects of TP in cancers mainly focus on *in vitro* cytotoxicity screening and its mechanism of action. A375.S2, A549, BT20, CACO-2, DU145 HRT18, HT29, MatLyLu, MCF-7, PC12, PC3, T47D, VERO, Walker 256/B, and WM1361A cells were used in different studies, and results are discussed below (Table 12.4).

TABLE 12.4

Cytotoxic Activity Results of Different *Teucrium polium* L. Extracts Tested *In Vitro* on Various Cell Lines

Extract	Cell Line	Result	References
Methanol extract of *T. polium* aerial parts	A375.S2	At 100 µg/mL concentration cell viability of 61%	(Abu-rish et al. 2016)
Ethanol extract of *T. polium* leaves	A549	IC_{50} value of 90 µg/mL	(Nematollahi-Mahani et al. 2007)
Ethanol extract of *T. polium* leaves	BT20	IC_{50} value of 106 µg/mL	(Nematollahi-Mahani et al. 2007)
Aqueous extract of *T. polium* aerial parts	DU145	100 µg/mL of extract blocked cell invasion and migration abilities and inhibited cell proliferation	(Kandouz et al. 2010)
Essential oil of *T. polium*	HT29	IC_{50} value of 67 µg/mL	(Hashem-Dabaghian et al. 2020)
Methanol extract of *T. polium*	HT29	IC_{50} value of 3 µg/mL	(Khodaei et al. 2018)
Methanol extract of *T. polium* aerial parts	MatLyLu	At 200 µg/mL cell viability% decreased under 50%	(Noumi et al. 2020)
Ethanol extract of *T. polium* leaves	MCF-7	IC_{50} value of 140 µg/mL	(Nematollahi-Mahani et al. 2007)
Ethanol extract of *T. polium* leaves	PC12	IC_{50} value of 120 µg/mL	(Nematollahi-Mahani et al. 2007)
Aqueous extract of *T. polium* aerial parts	PC3	100 µg/mL of extract blocked cell invasion and migration abilities and inhibited cell proliferation	(Kandouz et al. 2010)
Methanol extract of *T. polium* aerial parts	VERO	IC_{50} value of 209 µg/mL	(Alreshidi et al. 2020)
Methanol extract of *T. polium* aerial parts	Walker 256/B	At 200 µg/mL cell viability% decreased under 50%	(Noumi et al. 2020)

In a study by Alreshidi et al., cytotoxic activity of TP methanolic extract against VERO cells was tested using MTT method. Cells were treated with various concentrations of extract for 72 hours to determine cytotoxicity. As a result, the IC_{50} value was found as 209 µg/mL (Alreshidi et al. 2020).

Another *in vitro* study that aimed to screen antiproliferative activity against six cancer cell lines was performed by Abu-rish et al. At a concentration of 100 µg/mL for TP extract, no cytotoxicity was found against MCF-7, T47D, CACO-2, and WM1361A cells together with a very low cytotoxicity was found against HRT18 (rectum adenocarcinoma) cells. The cell viability value of 61% for A375.S2 cells was the lowest value in all tested cells (Abu-rish et al. 2016). Another cytotoxicity screening on A549, MCF-7, BT20, and PC12 cell lines were examined for ethanolic extract of TP leaves. Extract concentrations of 50, 100, 150, and 200 µg/mL were added to the cells and incubated for 48 hours to measure the cell proliferation using WST-1 method. IC_{50} values were found as 90, 120, 106, and 140 µg/mL for A549, PC12, BT20, and MCF-7 cells, respectively. In addition, TP was found to reduce colony formation in all the cell lines tested (Nematollahi-Mahani et al. 2007).

Essential oil of TP was also tested using MTT method. HT29 cells were incubated with different concentrations (0, 10, 25, 50, 75, 100, 150 µg/mL) of essential oil for 48 hours. The IC_{50} value for essential oil was found as 66.867 ± 1.37 µg/mL on HT-29 cells and induced apoptosis.

10-Epi-γ-eudesmol, spathulenol, elemol, α-pinene, and β-caryophyllene were reported as the main constituents of essential oil (Hashem-Dabaghian et al. 2020). In a study by Khodaei et al., this time methanolic extract was applied to HT-29 cells. The IC_{50} value was reported as 3 µg/mL for the extract. TP made an increase in ROS production and Sirt3 activity (Khodaei et al. 2018).

MatLyLu and Walker 256/B cancer cells were used to evaluate cytotoxicity of methanolic extract of TP aerial parts with a concentration range of 0–200 µg/mL. At 200 µg/mL for both cells, viability% decreased under 50% (Noumi et al. 2020).

A detailed study to assess the effects of TP on prostate cancer cell lines was performed by Kandouz et al. Aqueous extract of TP was tested for antiproliferative activity, cell cycle analysis, cell invasion assay, cell wounding assay, and immunofluorescence analysis on PC3 and DU145 cells. Kandouz et al. found that 1–4 days of incubation of PC3 and DU145 cells with TP extract resulted in the inhibition of cell proliferation, induction of apoptosis, and decrease in the number of cells at the G0–G1 fraction in cell cycle analysis. In prostate cancer cells, invasion and motility is an important process to reveal the effect on cell invasion PC3 and DU145 cells were incubated with 100 µg/mL of extract for 24 and 48 hours. The results showed that extract when compared to untreated cells cell invasion and migration was blocked. Moreover, Kandouz et al. reported that TP showed inhibition in signaling pathways that regulates E-cadherin/catenin complex (Kandouz et al. 2010).

Hepatocellular carcinoma is one of the cancer types that cause mortality worldwide. Movahedi et al. examined the protective effects of TP in liver cells in carcinogenic rats. After 28 weeks of treatment with TP decoction, biochemical markers such as ALT, AST, AFP, GGT, ALP, HCY, TNF-α, α2MG, and CBG were found to be regulated by the extract when compared to the control group. Movahedi et al. also reported a decrease in liver lesion score and increase in glucocorticoid activity with the treatment of TP (Movahedi et al. 2014).

Beside its effects alone, TP was tested together as a mixture with vincristine, vinblastine, and doxorubicin separately to evaluate its role as a chemosensitizer agent. Skmel-3, Saos-2, SW480, MCF-7, KB, EJ, and A431 cell lines were used in the study, and cytotoxicity and colony formation were assessed. Methanol extract of TP together with chemotherapeutic agent showed high cytotoxicity and inhibited colony formation through synergistic effect. In addition *T. polium* reduced cytotoxicity of vincristine and vinblastine against human fibroblasts (Rajabalian 2008).

In one of the most recent studies, Sheikhbahaei et al. reported that TP enhances the anti-angiogenic effect of Tranilast on HUVECs. Tranilast is a drug used for its antifibrotic effects and also has been studied for anti-angiogenic activity. Results of the study indicated that the combination showed significant anti-angiogenic effect (Sheikhbahaei et al. 2021).

12.4 OTHER FOODS, HERBS, SPICES, AND BOTANICALS USED IN CANCER

Ethnobotanical studies and related reviews indicate several plants used for the treatment of cancer traditionally in the Middle East (Abu-Darwish and Efferth 2018; Ben-Arye et al. 2012). Among a long list of plants used traditionally, various species from the *Arum, Artemisia*, and *Urtica* genera and *Calotropis procera, Citrullus colocynthis, Nigella sativa, Pulicaria crispa*, and *Withania somnifera* were reported to be used more often, according to a literature survey performed by Abu-Darwish and Efferth (2018).

In addition to the plants used traditionally, there have been *in vitro* studies performed on other members of *Teucrium* genus. In a study examined to investigate the effects of methanolic extract of *T. persicum* on PC-3, SW480, and T47D cell lines, *T. persicum* potently showed an inhibition on cell viability of the tested cells and induced apoptosis (Tafrihi et al. 2014). *T. mascatense* methanol extract was reported to show antiproliferative activity against MCF-7 and HeLa cells (Panicker et al. 2019). Another study on methanol, ethyl acetate, and acetone extracts of *T. chamaedrys* indicated that it induced apoptosis and modulated drug resistance in colorectal cancer cells (Milutinovic et al. 2019).

12.5 TOXICITY AND CAUTIONARY NOTES

T. polium has been reported to show several side effects such as hepatitis, vomiting, changes in kidney function, and allergic responses (Moeini and Tavakkoli 2020). Hepatotoxicity is generated by affecting CYP3A metabolism because the plant includes furano neoclerodane diterpenoids, especially teucrin A and teuchamaedryn. In France and Greece, several cases of acute liver failure causa of the *Teucrium* species have been reported in consequence of long-term (3–18 weeks) consumption of tea, and most cases had been observed in middle-aged women (Chitturi and Farrell 2008). In Turkey, this plant has been used to treat infantile colic in children, and liver dysfunction for infants was reported (Sezer and Bozaykut 2012). Despite toxic effects, *T. polium* has been contradictorily used in treating jaundice as traditional. At the same time, it has been investigated in terms of *in vivo* hepatoprotective activity (Rahmouni et al. 2019). For pregnancy use, the toxic effect of *T. polium* had investigated via a chick extra-embryonic membrane model. Results showed that *T. polium* has anti-angiogenic activity due to causing vascular defects in embryos. Therefore, using this plant during pregnancy or lactation is not recommended for vascular toxicity reasons. According to the findings of Moeini and Tavakkoli, this plant's consumption should be limited to dosages less than 3 mg/kg in pregnant women during embryonic development (Moeini and Tavakkoli 2020). Additionally, three hepatotoxicity cases have been reported in women who are in the last months of pregnancy and postpartum periods who showed jaundice and severely elevated liver enzymes due to *T. polium* consumption (Dag et al. 2014).

12.6 SUMMARY POINTS

- This chapter focuses on the effects of *T. polium* on various diseases and cancer.
- *T. polium* is used widely as a traditional medicine to treat various diseases such as gastrointestinal diseases, and diabetes.
- Cancer is one of the diseases that *T. polium* was reported to be used traditionally for the treatment.
- The main phytochemical content of aerial parts of *T. polium* includes terpenoids, steroids, flavonoids, iridoids, clerodanes, phenylethanoid glycosides, and essential oil.
- Essential oil of the plant reported to has antimicrobial activity.
- *T. polium* can cause liver toxicity with long-term use, especially in women.

REFERENCES

Abadian, K., Z. Keshavarz, F. Mojab, H. A. Majd, and N. M. Abbasi. 2016. "Comparison the effect of mefenamic acid and *Teucrium polium* on the severity and systemic symptoms of dysmenorrhea." *Complementary Therapies in Clinical Practice* 22:12–15. doi:10.1016/j.ctcp.2015.09.003

Abdollahi, M., H. Karimpour, and H. R. Monsef-Esfehani. 2003. "Antinociceptive effects of *Teucrium polium* L. total extract and essential oil in mouse writhing test." *Pharmacological Research* 48 (1):31–35. doi:10.1016/S1043-6618(03)00059-8

Abu-Darwish, M. S., and T. Efferth. 2018. "Medicinal plants from near East for cancer therapy." *Frontiers in Pharmacology* 9. ARTN 56. doi:10.3389/fphar.2018.00056

Abu-rish, E. Y., V. Kasabri, M. M. Hudaib, S. H. Mashalla, L. H. AlAlawi, K. Tawaha, M. K. Mohammad, Y. S. Mohamed, and Y. Bustanji. 2016. "Evaluation of antiproliferative activity of some traditional anticancer herbal remedies from Jordan." *Tropical Journal of Pharmaceutical Research* 15 (3):469–474. doi:10.4314/tjpr.v15i3.6

Alachkar, A., A. Jaddouh, M. S. Elsheikh, A. R. Bilia, and F. F. Vincieri. 2011. "Traditional medicine in syria: Folk medicine in aleppo governorate." *Natural Product Communications* 6 (1):79–84.

Al-Asmari, A. K., A. Al-Elaiwi, M. T. Athar, M. Tariq, A. Al Eid, and S. M. Al-Asmary. 2014. "A review of hepatoprotective plants used in Saudi traditional medicine." *Evidence-Based Complementary and Alternative Medicine*. Artn 890842. doi:10.1155/2014/890842

Ali-Shtayeh, M. S., Z. Yaniv, and J. Mahajna. 2000. "Ethnobotanical survey in the Palestinian area: A classification of the healing potential of medicinal plants." *Journal of Ethnopharmacology* 73 (1–2):221–232. doi:10.1016/S0378-8741(00)00316-0

Alreshidi, M., E. Noumi, L. Bouslama, O. Ceylan, V. N. Veettil, M. Adnan, C. Danciu, S. Elkahoui, R. Badraoui, K. A. Al-Motair, M. Patel, V. De Feo, and M. Snoussi. 2020. "Phytochemical screening, antibacterial, antifungal, antiviral, cytotoxic, and anti-quorum-sensing properties of *Teucrium polium* L. aerial parts methanolic extract." *Plants-Basel* 9 (11). ARTN 1418. doi:10.3390/plants9111418

Altanlar, N., G. S. Citoglu, and B. S. Yilmaz. 2006. "Antilisterial activity of some plants used in folk medicine." *Pharmaceutical Biology* 44 (2):91–94. doi:10.1080/13880200600591907

Alzweiri, M., A. Al Sarhan, K. Mansi, M. Hudaib, and T. Aburjai. 2011. "Ethnopharmacological survey of medicinal herbs in Jordan, the Northern Badia region." *Journal of Ethnopharmacology* 137 (1):27–35. doi:10.1016/j.jep.2011.02.007

Benali, T., K. Habbadi, A. Bouyahya, A. Khabbach, I. Marmouzi, T. Aanniz, H. Chtibi, H. N. Mrabti, E. Achbani, and K. Hammani. 2021. "Phytochemical analysis and study of antioxidant, anticandidal, and antibacterial activities of *Teucrium polium* subsp. *polium* and *Micromeria graeca* (Lamiaceae) essential oils from Northern Morocco." *Evidence-Based Complementary and Alternative Medicine*. Artn 6641720 doi:10.1155/2021/6641720

Ben-Arye, E., E. Schiff, E. Hassan, K. Mutafoglu, S. Lev-Ari, M. Steiner, O. Lavie, A. Polliack, M. Silbermann, and E. Lev. 2012. "Integrative oncology in the Middle East: From traditional herbal knowledge to contemporary cancer care." *Annals of Oncology* 23 (1):211–221. doi:10.1093/annonc/mdr054

Bendjabeur, S., O. Benchabane, C. Bensouici, M. Hazzit, A. Baaliouamer, and A. Bitam. 2018. "Antioxidant and anticholinesterase activity of essential oils and ethanol extracts of *Thymus algeriensis* and *Teucrium polium* from Algeria." *Journal of Food Measurement and Characterization* 12 (4):2278–2288. doi:10.1007/s11694-018-9845-x

Candela, R. G., S. Rosselli, M. Bruno, and G. Fontana. 2021. "A review of the phytochemistry, traditional uses and biological activities of the essential oils of genus *Teucrium*." *Planta Medica* 87 (06):432–479. doi:10.1055/a-1293-5768

Chitturi, S., and G. C. Farrell. 2008. "Hepatotoxic slimming aids and other herbal hepatotoxins." *Journal of Gastroenterology and Hepatology* 23 (3):366–373. doi:10.1111/j.1440-1746.2008.05310.x

Dafni, A., Z. Yaniv, and D. Palevitch. 1984. "Ethnobotanical survey of medicinal plants in northern Israel." *Journal of Ethnopharmacology* 10 (3):295–310. doi:10.1016/0378-8741(84)90017-5

Dag, M., Z. Ozturk, M. Aydinli, I. Koruk, and A. Kadayifci. 2014. "Postpartum hepatotoxicity due to herbal medicine *Teucrium polium*." *Annals of Saudi Medicine* 34 (6):541–543. doi:10.5144/0256-4947.2014.541

Ekim, T. 1982. "*Teucrium* L." In *Flora of Turkey and the East Aegean Islands*, edited by P.H. Davis, 53–75. Edinburgh: Edinburgh University Press.

El Beyrouthy, M., W. Dhifi, and N. Arnold-Apostolides. 2013. "Ethnopharmacological survey of the indigenous Lamiaceae from Lebanon." *International Symposium on Medicinal and Aromatic Plants: Sipam 2012* 997:257–275.

Essid, R., F. Z. Rahali, K. Msaada, I. Sghair, M. Hammami, A. Bouratbine, K. Aoun, and F. Limam. 2015. "Antileishmanial and cytotoxic potential of essential oils from medicinal plants in Northern Tunisia." *Industrial Crops and Products* 77:795–802. doi:10.1016/j.indcrop.2015.09.049

Gharaboghaz, M. N. Z., M. R. Farahpour, and S. Saghaie. 2020. "Topical co-administration of *Teucrium polium* hydroethanolic extract and aloe vera gel triggered wound healing by accelerating cell proliferation in diabetic mouse model." *Biomedicine & Pharmacotherapy* 127. doi:10.1016/j.biopha.2020.110189

Ghasemi, T., H. Sohanaki, M. Keshavarz, E. Ghasemi, and M. Parviz. 2019. "Low dose *Teucrium polium* hydro-alcoholic extract treatment effects on spatial memory and hippocampal neuronal count of rat A beta 25–35 model of Alzheimer's disease." *Archives of Neuroscience* 6 (3). doi:10.5812/ans.90893

Hasanein, P., and S. Shahidi. 2012. "Preventive effect of *Teucrium polium* on learning and memory deficits in diabetic rats." *Medical Science Monitor* 18 (1):Br41–Br46. doi:10.12659/Msm.882201

Hashem-Dabaghian, F., A. Shojaii, J. Asgarpanah, and M. Entezari. 2020. "Anti-mutagenicity and apoptotic effects of *Teucrium polium* L. essential oil in HT29 cell line." *Jundishapur Journal of Natural Pharmaceutical Products* 15 (3). doi:10.5812/jjnpp.79559

Huseini, H. F., A. H. Abdolghaffari, M. Ahwazi, E. Jasemi, M. Yaghoobi, and M. Ziaee. 2020. "Topical application of *Teucrium polium* can improve wound healing in diabetic rats." *International Journal of Lower Extremity Wounds* 19 (2):132–138. doi:10.1177/1534734619868629

Kandouz, M., A. Alachkar, L. Zhang, H. Dekhil, F. Chehna, A. Yasmeen, and A. E. Al Moustafa. 2010. "*Teucrium polium* plant extract inhibits cell invasion and motility of human prostate cancer cells via the restoration of the E-cadherin/catenin complex." *Journal of Ethnopharmacology* 129 (3):410–415. doi:10.1016/j.jep.2009.10.035

Khodadadi, S., N. A. Zabihi, S. Niazmand, A. Abbasnezhad, M. Mahmoudabady, and S. A. Rezaee. 2018. "*Teucrium polium* improves endothelial dysfunction by regulating eNOS and VCAM-1 genes expression and vasoreactivity in diabetic rat aorta." *Biomedicine & Pharmacotherapy* 103:1526–1530. doi:10.1016/j.biopha.2018.04.158

Khodaei, F., K. Ahmadi, H. Kiyani, M. Hashemitabar, and M. Rezaei. 2018. "Mitochondrial effects of *Teucrium polium* and *Prosopis farcta* extracts in colorectal cancer cells." *Asian Pacific Journal of Cancer Prevention* 19 (1):103–109. doi:10.22034/APJCP.2018.19.1.103

Khoshnood-Mansoorkhani, M. J., M. R. Moein, and N. Oveisi. 2010. "Anticonvulsant activity of *Teucrium polium* against seizure induced by PTZ and MES in mice." *Iranian Journal of Pharmaceutical Research* 9 (4):395–401.

Mehrabani, D., A. Rezaee, N. Azarpira, M. R. Fattahi, M. Amini, N. Tanideh, M. R. Panjehshahin, and M. Saberi-Firouzi. 2009. "The healing effects of *Teucrium polium* in the repair of indomethacin-induced gastric ulcer in rats." *Saudi Medical Journal* 30 (4):494–499.

Milutinovic, M. G., V. M. Maksimovic, D. M. Cvetkovic, D. D. Nikodijevic, M. S. Stankovic, M. Pesic, and S. D. Markovic. 2019. "Potential of *Teucrium chamaedrys* L. to modulate apoptosis and bio-transformation in colorectal carcinoma cells." *Journal of Ethnopharmacology* 240. doi:10.1016/j.jep.2019.111951

Moeini, E., and H. Tavakkoli. 2020. "*Teucrium polium* alters the vascular branching pattern and VEGF-a expression in the chick extra-embryonic membrane model." *Jundishapur Journal of Natural Pharmaceutical Products* 15 (4). doi:10.5812/jjnpp.68649

Mousavi, S. E., A. Shahriari, A. Ahangarpour, H. Vatanpour, and A. Jolodar. 2012. "Effects of *Teucrium polium* ethyl acetate extract on serum, liver and muscle triglyceride content of sucrose-induced insulin resistance in rat." *Iranian Journal of Pharmaceutical Research* 11 (1):347–355.

Movahedi, A., R. Basir, A. Rahmat, M. Charaffedine, and F. Othman. 2014. "Remarkable anticancer activity of *Teucrium polium* on hepatocellular carcinogenic rats." *Evidence-Based Complementary and Alternative Medicine*. doi:10.1155/2014/726724

Naghibi, F., M. Mosaddegh, S. M. Motamed, and A. Ghorbani. 2005. "Labiatae family in folk medicine in Iran: From ethnobotany to pharmacology." *Iranian Journal of Pharmaceutical Research* 2:63–79.

Nematollahi-Mahani, S. N., M. Rezazadeh-Kermani, M. Mehrabani, and N. Nakhaee. 2007. "Cytotoxic effects of *Teucrium polium* on some established cell lines." *Pharmaceutical Biology* 45 (4):295–298. doi:10.1080/13880200701214904

Niazmand, S., M. Esparham, T. Hassannia, and M. Derakhshan. 2011. "Cardiovascular effects of *Teucrium polium* L. extract in rabbit." *Pharmacognosy Magazine* 7 (27):260–264. doi:10.4103/0973-1296.84244

Niazmand, S., E. Fereidouni, M. Mahmoudabady, and M. Hosseini. 2017. "*Teucrium polium*-induced vasore-laxation mediated by endothelium-dependent and endothelium-independent mechanisms in isolated rat thoracic aorta." *Pharmacognosy Research* 9 (4):372–377. doi:10.4103/pr.pr_140_16

Nor, N. H. M., F. Othman, E. R. M. Tohit, S. M. Noor, R. Razali, H. A. Hassali, and H. Hassan. 2019. "In vitro antiatherothrombotic effects of extracts from *Berberis vulgaris* L., *Teucrium polium* L., and *Orthosiphon stamineus* Benth." *Evidence-Based Complementary and Alternative Medicine*. doi:10.1155/2019/3245836

Noumi, E., M. Snoussi, E. Anouar, M. Alreshidi, V. N. Veettil, S. Elkahoui, M. Adnan, M. Patel, A. Kadri, K. Aouadi, V. De Feo, and R. Badraoui. 2020. "HR-LCMS-based metabolite profiling, antioxidant, and anticancer properties of *Teucrium polium* L. methanolic extract: Computational and *In Vitro* study." *Antioxidants* 9 (11). doi:10.3390/antiox9111089

Orhan, I., and M. Aslan. 2009. "Appraisal of scopolamine-induced antiamnesic effect in mice and *in vitro* anti-acetylcholinesterase and antioxidant activities of some traditionally used Lamiaceae plants." *Journal of Ethnopharmacology* 122 (2):327–332. doi:10.1016/j.jep.2008.12.026

Panicker, N. G., S. O. M. S. Balhamar, S. Akhlaq, M. M. Qureshi, T. S. Rizvi, A. Al-Harrasi, J. Hussain, and F. Mustafa. 2019. "Identification and characterization of the caspase-mediated apoptotic activity of *Teucrium mascatense* and an isolated compound in human cancer cells." *Molecules* 24 (5). doi:10.3390/molecules24050977

Rahmouni, F., R. Badraoui, N. Amri, A. Elleuch, A. El-Feki, T. Rebai, and M. Saoudi. 2019. "Hepatotoxicity and nephrotoxicity in rats induced by carbon tetrachloride and the protective effects of *Teucrium polium* and vitamin C." *Toxicology Mechanisms and Methods* 29 (5):313–321. doi:10.1080/15376516.2018.1519864

Rahmouni, F., M. Saoudi, and T. Rebai. 2021. "Therapeutics studies and biological properties of *Teucrium polium* (Lamiaceae)." *Biofactors* 47 (6):952–963. doi:10.1002/biof.1782

Rajabalian, S. 2008. "Methanolic extract of *Teucrium polium* L. potentiates the cytotoxic and apoptotic effects of anticancer drugs of vincristine, vinblastine and doxorubicin against a panel of cancerous cell lines." *Experimental Oncology* 30 (2):133–138.

Sadeghi, Z., J. L. Yang, A. Venditti, and M. M. Farimani. 2021. "A review of the phytochemistry, ethnopharmacology and biological activities of *Teucrium* genus (Germander)." *Natural Product Research*. doi:10.10 80/14786419.2021.2022669

Sevindik, E., Z. T. Abaci, C. Yamaner, and M. Ayvaz. 2016. "Determination of the chemical composition and antimicrobial activity of the essential oils of *Teucrium polium* and *Achillea millefolium* grown under North Anatolian ecological conditions." *Biotechnology & Biotechnological Equipment* 30 (2):375–380. doi:10.1080/13102818.2015.1131626

Sezer, R. G., and A. Bozaykut. 2012. "Pediatric hepatotoxicity associated with Polygermander (*Teucrium polium*)." *Clinical Toxicology* 50 (2):153–153. doi:10.3109/15563650.2011.645487

Sheikhbahaei, F., S. N. Nematollahi-Mahani, M. Khazaei, M. R. Khazaei, and S. Khazayel. 2021. "*Teucrium polium* extract enhances the anti-angiogenic effect of tranilast in a three-dimensional fibrin matrix model." *Asian Pacific Journal of Cancer Prevention* 22 (8):2471–2478. doi:10.31557/APJCP.2021.22.8.2471

Simonyan, K. V., and V. A. Chavushyan. 2016. "Protective effects of hydroponic *Teucrium polium* on hippocampal neurodegeneration in ovariectomized rats." *Bmc Complementary and Alternative Medicine* 16. doi:10.1186/s12906-016-1407-3

Simonyan, K. V., H. M. Galstyan, and V. A. Chavushyan. 2019. "Post-tetanic potentiation and depression in hippocampal neurons in a rat model of Alzheimer's disease: effects of *Teucrium Polium* extract." *Neurophysiology* 51 (5):332–343. doi:10.1007/s11062-020-09827-8

Tabatabaie, P. S., and R. Yazdanparast. 2017. "*Teucrium polium* extract reverses symptoms of streptozotocin-induced diabetes in rats via rebalancing the Pdx1 and FoxO1 expressions." *Biomedicine & Pharmacotherapy* 93:1033–1039. doi:10.1016/j.biopha.2017.06.082

Tafrihi, M., S. Toosi, T. Minaei, A. R. Gohari, V. Niknam, and S. M. A. Najafi. 2014. "Anticancer properties of *Teucrium persicum* in PC-3 prostate cancer cells." *Asian Pacific Journal of Cancer Prevention* 15 (2):785–791. doi:10.7314/Apjcp.2014.15.2.785

Tusi, S. K., A. Jafari, S. M. A. Marashi, S. F. Niknam, M. Farid, and M. Ansari. 2020. "The effect of antimicrobial activity of *Teucrium polium* on oral *Streptococcus mutans*: A randomized cross-over clinical trial study." *Bmc Oral Health* 20 (1). ARTN 130. doi:10.1186/s12903-020-01116-4

Tuzlacı, E. 2016. *Türkiye Bitkileri Geleneksel İlaç Rehberi*. Istanbul: Istanbul Tıp Kitabevleri.

Zendehdel, M., M. Taati, M. Jadidoleslami, and A. Bashiri. 2011. "Evaluation of pharmacological mechanisms of antinociceptive effect of *Teucrium polium* on visceral pain in mice." *Iranian Journal of Veterinary Research* 12 (4):292–297.

13 Giant Angelica
Angelica gigas *Nakai – Herbal Giant's Anticancer Potential*

Junxuan Lü, Cheng Jiang, Monika Joshi
and Joseph J. Drabick

ABBREVIATIONS

AGN	*Angelica gigas* Nakai
AR	androgen receptor
AUC	area under the curve
CES	carboxylesterase
CRPC	castration resistant prostate cancer
Cyp	cytochrome P450
D	decursin
DA	decursinol angelate
DOH	decursinol
GC/MS	gas chromatography/mass spectrometry
HPLC	high-performance liquid chromatography
IL-1β	interleukin-1 beta
iNOS	inducible nitric oxide synthase
LC-MS	liquid chromatography–mass spectrometry
LPS	lipopolysaccharide
NK	natural killer cell
NMR	nuclear magnetic resonance
PK	pharmacokinetics
PSA	prostate specific antigen
TME	tumor microenvironment
TNF-α	tumor necrosis factor alpha
UHPLC	ultra-high-performance liquid chromatography

13.1 INTRODUCTION

Three major species of *Angelica* are used in herbal medicine in China, Korea and Japan: *Angelica sinensis* (Chinese Dang-gui), *A. gigas* Nakai (Korean or Cham Dang-gui), and *A. acutiloba* (Japanese). The *gigas* in the Korean Dang-gui binomial is for *gigantus*, an appropriate reference to its tall above-ground vegetative parts, which top 6 feet. Molecule-based classification in addition to morphology is very crucial to detecting and preventing adulteration of the dried roots of different *Angelica* species in the herbal markets. Genetic differences among *A. sinensis, A. gigas*, and *A. acutiloba* have been documented, including 5S-rRNA spacers (Zhao et al., 2003). Phylogenetically, AGN is more closely related to *A. acutiloba* than to *A. sinensis* (Zhao et al., 2003). Chemically, the contents of ferulic acid and Z-ligustilide in the root of *A. sinensis* were much higher than those of *A. acutiloba* and AGN (Zhao et al., 2003). Gas chromatographic/mass spectrometry (GC/MS)

DOI: 10.1201/9781003260028-15

was used to profile the volatile components in *Angelica* species (Kim et al., 2006a, 2006b) and as a pattern recognition method for the quality control of AGN (Piao et al., 2007). Profiling chemical components of AGN from different geographical origins using ^{1}H NMR and UPLC-MS analyses identified pyranocoumarins decursin (D) and its isomer decursinol angelate (DA) (see structures in Figure 13.1), and furanocoumarins nodakenin, marmesin, and 7-hydroxy-6-(2R-hydroxy-3-methyl-but-3-ethyl)coumarin as major phytochemicals that contributed to the discrimination factor (Kim et al., 2011). D and DA are the most unique signature chemicals to distinguish AGN from other oriental *Angelica* species.

The anticancer bioactivities of AGN root extracts and signature pyranocoumarin compounds D, DA, and their botanical synthesis precursor and mammalian hepatic metabolite decursinol (DOH) (see structures in Figure 13.1) were reviewed a decade ago (Zhang et al., 2012) and updated in 2015 (Lu et al., 2015) and 2022 (Lu et al., 2022). In addition to anticancer activities, the reader is directed to a most recent comprehensive review of many other potential health benefits including memory enhancement, pain relief, and preventing or treating cerebral ischemia/stroke, anxiety, sleep disorder, epilepsy, inflammatory bowel disease, sepsis, metabolic disorders (syndrome), osteoporosis, osteoarthritis, and male infertility (Lu et al., 2022). In the last decade, significant progress has been made in understanding the pharmacokinetics (PK) and metabolism of these signature compounds in animal models. Two human single-dose PK studies have been published with very discordant PK outcomes (Zhang et al., 2015a; Kim et al., 2018b). The second study had apparently tested a questionable AGN of extremely low total D + DA content and atypical D/DA ratio, as critiqued in the recent review (Lu et al., 2022). This chapter will focus on the anticancer activities in animal models, discuss challenges, and identify strategies for human translational studies aiming to unlock the anticancer potential from this "sleeping" giant.

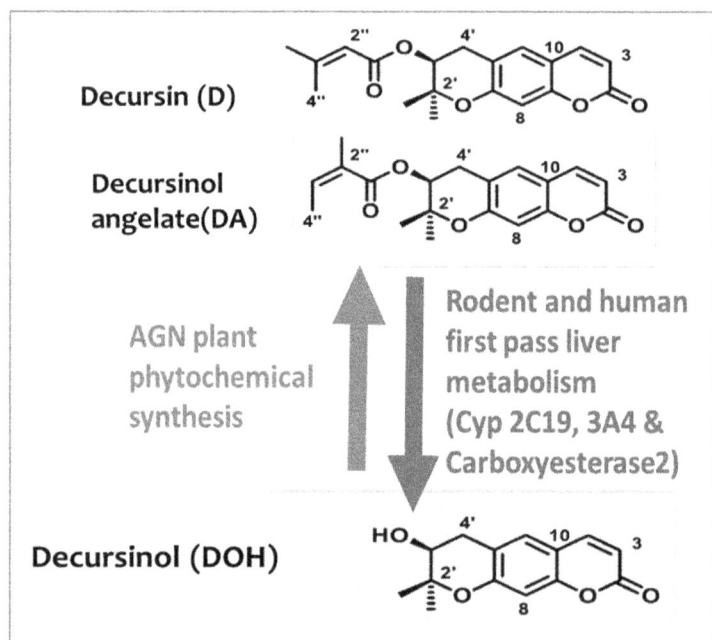

FIGURE 13.1 Chemical structure of signature pyranocoumarins in *Angelica gigas* Nakai root and their interrelationship in botanical synthesis (up arrow) and hepatic metabolism in rodents and humans (down arrow). Cyp = cytochrome P450.

13.2 AGN NUTRACEUTICAL PREPARATIONS AND PHYTOCHEMICALS

In traditional herbal medicine, dried AGN roots are used to treat anemia, cold, pain, and other diseases and known to Korean herbalists as "female ginseng" (Zhang et al., 2012). However, these traditional medicinal properties were mostly based on using boiling water to extract the active ingredients. Pyranocoumarin compounds could not be extracted by water. Chemical compositions of roots of the *Angelica* genus have been extensively studied and reviewed (Zhang et al., 2012). The different types of AGN root preparations and extracts and their respective signature phytochemicals are summarized below.

Alcohol extracts: Pyranocoumarins are the major chemicals identified in the ethanolic or methanolic extracts of dried AGN root. Decursin (D) (Figure 13.1) was first isolated from the root of *A. decursiva* Fr. et Sav. and later from AGN in the 1960s. Decursinol angelate (DA) (Figure 13.1) is a structural isomer of D on the side chain and about 50%–70% as abundant as D in the root of AGN. The pyranocoumarin core decursinol (DOH) (Figure 13.1) can be detected with a much lower abundance, if at all. D/DA may constitute 3.0%–8.2% of dried AGN root or as high as 60% of the ethanol extract, depending on the extraction protocols and source of AGN roots. The botanical biosynthetic pathways for DOH core and the more complex pyranocoumarins have been reviewed (Zhang et al., 2012). The sources of variability in the chemical composition of the resultant extracts have been discussed (Lu et al., 2022).

Water extracts: Typically, root powder was soaked and agitated in a sufficient volume of warmed or boiling water and filtered to eliminate particulates. The ethanol-precipitable (insoluble) components of the aqueous extracts of AGN root were used either directly (e.g., Immuno-Stimulatory component of A. *gigas*, or ISAg) (Kim et al., 2018a; Lee et al., 2019) or further subfractionated into more refined polysaccharides (e.g., angelan) (Han et al., 1998; Han et al., 2006; Kim et al., 2008) for studies of immune regulatory activities and cancer control in syngeneic mouse models. These preparations contain predominantly polysaccharides and 9%–17% proteins. One AGN water extract (condensed volume without further organic solvent partitioning) was tested for cerebral ischemia stroke protection in rats (Oh et al., 2015). All these water extracts should not contain pyranocoumarins or hydrophobic secondary metabolites.

Whole root powders: Finely ground powders of AGN root have been tested in ovariectomized rats against ovarian hormone–deficient osteoporosis (Choi et al., 2012). Nanoparticle formulations of AGN root powder was also tested for memory benefit (Piao et al., 2015). These herbal preparations should contain both the primary fibrous structural components (cellulose) and secondary phytochemical metabolites, including D/DA.

13.3 PHARMACOKINETICS OF D, DA, AND DOH

Rodent PK model studies have shown a rapid and extensive conversion of D and DA to DOH, as reviewed previously (Lu et al., 2015) (Lu et al., 2022). Figure 13.2 summarizes the latest metabolism knowledge based on rodent models and *in vitro* human microsomal preparation testing. The extensive conversion has been confirmed in a human PK study (Zhang et al., 2015a), as highlighted next.

Human PK studies: A single oral dose human PK study of D and DA delivered through an AGN-based dietary supplement Cogni.Q (obtained from Quality of Life Labs, Purchase, NY) in ten men and ten women was carried out in Amarillo, Texas, USA (Zhang et al., 2015a). Each subject consumed 119 mg D and 77 mg DA from four capsules. Figure 13.3 panels illustrate the concentration-time curves of D, DA, and DOH in plasma. The mean C_{max} were 5.3, 48.1, and 2,480 nmol/L, and the mean AUC_{0-48h} for D, DA, and DOH were 37, 335, and 27,579 h·nmol/L, respectively. The human data supported an extensive conversion of D and DA to DOH ($AUC_{DOH}/AUC_{total} = 98.7\%$) at the dietary supplement dose tested.

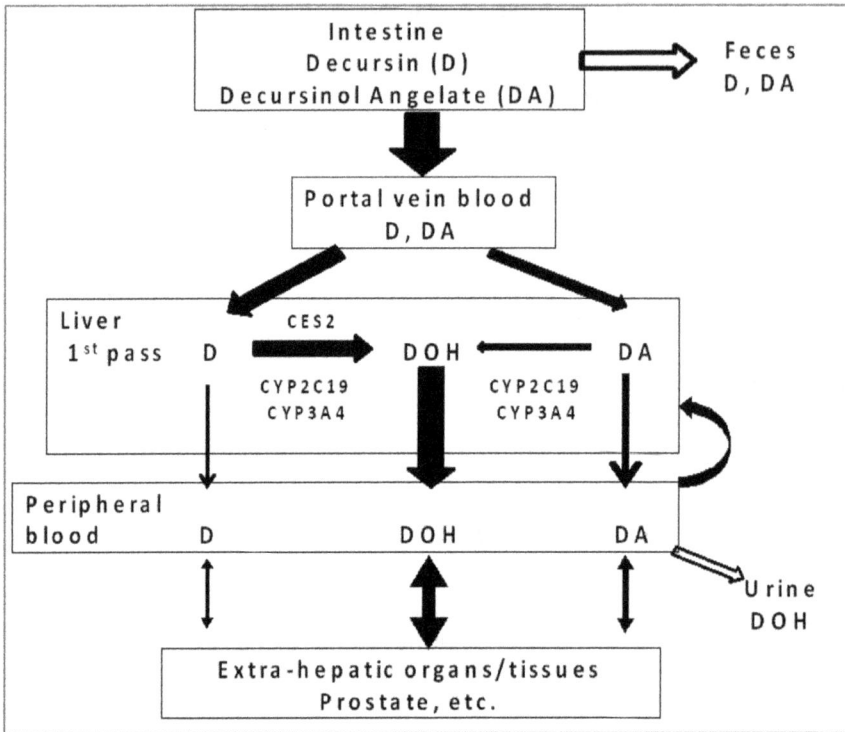

FIGURE 13.2 Current knowledge of metabolism of gavage/supplement–delivered pyranocoumarins in rodents and humans. Peripheral peak blood levels of decursin (D) and decursinol angelate (DA) after *Angelica gigas* Nakai alcoholic extract oral intake would be expected to be two to three orders of magnitude lower (nM to single-digit μM) than that of decursinol (DOH) (double- to triple-digit μM). The portal vein entry of D/DA also applies to *i.p.* injection delivery. CES2 = carboxylesterase-2; CYP = cytochrome P450.

Source: Adapted from a recent review (Lu et al., 2022).

CYP2C19 and 3A4 were identified as the major human isoforms for D and DA metabolism to DOH (Zhang et al., 2015b). In addition, a strong selectivity was observed for carboxylesterase-2 (CES-2) to catalyze D to DOH conversion, but DA was resistant to this enzyme (Zhang et al., 2015b). The differential substrate specificity to CES-2 may account for the reversed D/DA ratio in plasma compared to that in Cogni.Q.

A Korean group carried out a PK study in ten healthy men by oral dosing of 4.6 g of "AGN" root powder containing 0.055 mg of D and 0.184 mg of DA (Kim et al., 2018b). They reported values of the elimination $t_{1/2}$ for D, DA, and DOH of 3.03, 4.04, and 2.62 hours, respectively and t_{max} of 0.44, 0.31, and 0.64 hours, respectively. These PK metrics were obviously different from those of the male American subjects ($n = 10$) receiving Cogni.Q (119 mg D and 77 mg DA) (Zhang et al., 2015a). Two major differences are noted for the test articles. The first was the ratio of D/DA in Cogni.Q was roughly 1/0.65 (Zhang et al., 2015a), which has been reported consistently for ethanolic or methanolic extracts of AGN by many groups. The "AGN" powder used to dose the Korean men yielded a reversed D/DA ratio of 1/3.3 (Kim et al., 2018b). The second difference was that the total D+DA dosage for the Cogni.Q study was 196 mg, whereas that for the Korean trial was only 0.24 mg. Therefore, the authenticity of the "AGN" powder for the Korean study is highly questionable.

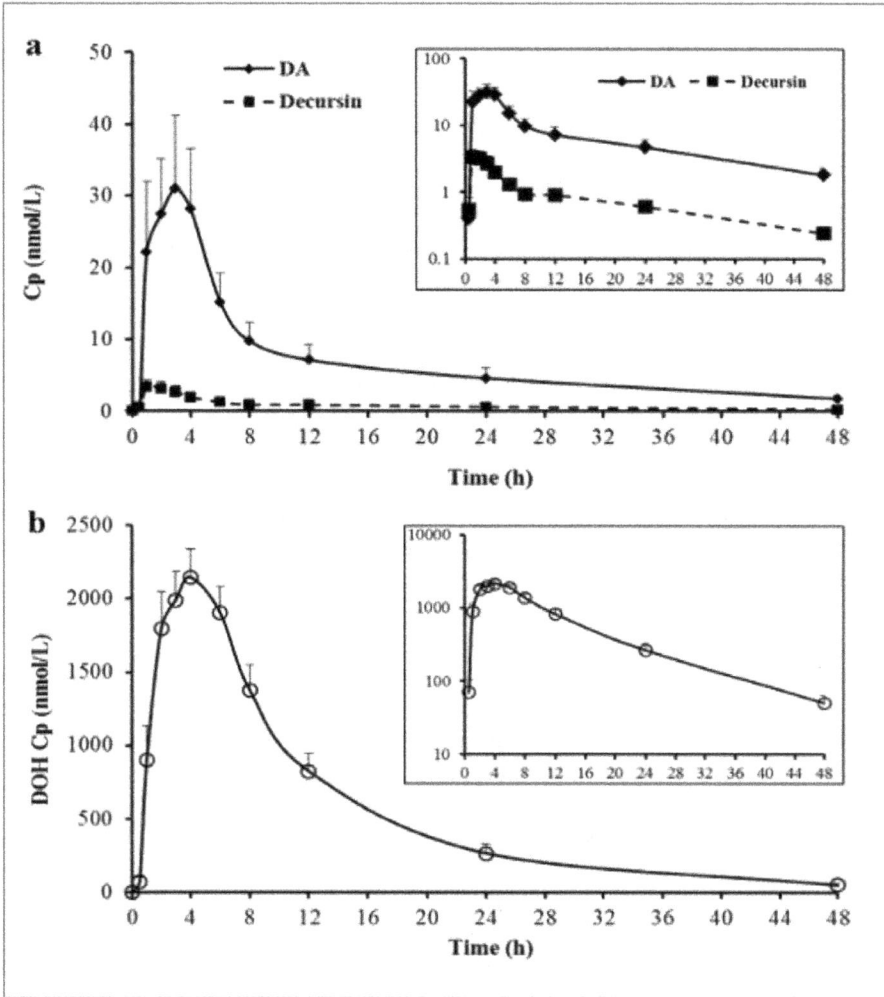

FIGURE 13.3 First-in-human PK data. Human plasma (A) Decursin (D), decursinol angelate (DA) and (B) Decursinol (DOH) concentration (nM) vs. time. Insets are data presented on semi-log scale. Mean + sem, *n* = 20. Each person took four *Angelica gigas* Nakai–CognI.Q capsules (800 mg INM-176 AGN) at time 0.

Source: Adapted from Zhang et al. (2015a).

Knowledge gaps for PK and metabolism: So far, only single-dose PK studies have been reported in human subjects (Zhang et al., 2015a; Kim et al., 2018b) with a serious authenticity concern as noted above of "AGN" for the Korean study (Kim et al., 2018b). The pattern of PK dose-response to increasing dosages of AGN supplements has not been reported. In addition, PK study after repeated AGN exposure in humans or in animal models will need to be carried out to determine whether metabolic adaptation occurs over chronic intake, especially whether the extent of D/DA conversion to DOH would be modified. Furthermore, since hepatic CYPs are principally involved in controlling D/DA conversion to DOH, how CYP geno/phenotypes are related to the above PK metrics could guide personalizing dosages to achieve desired health benefits. Moreover, whether and how DOH may be further metabolized should be investigated.

13.4　*IN VIVO* ANTICANCER ACTIVITIES OF AGN ALCOHOLIC EXTRACTS

Table 13.1 provides a summary of reported studies in animal cancer models. Intervention information includes dosage, frequency, and route of administration and duration of treatment.

Xenograft models in immunocompromised mice: Although limited in number and heavily focused on cancers of human prostate origin, these reported studies have documented *in vivo* inhibitory efficacy of AGN ethanol extracts without an adverse impact on the body weight of the host mice. The target cancer cells included androgen-independent DU145 and PC3 xenografts (Lee et al., 2009) and LNCaP-derived androgen receptor (AR) positive models (Wu et al., 2017). In the LNCaP-AR-luc model, metastasis to lung and liver detectable by ex vivo bioluminescence of the harvested organs was decreased by AGN in a dose-dependent manner.

Transgenic mouse prostate carcinogenesis model: In immune competent transgenic mice, the TRAMP (Transgenic Adenocarcinoma Mouse Prostate) model, AGN gavage decreased growth of lesions in two lineages of diseases (Zhang et al., 2015c). Male C57BL/6 TRAMP mice and wild type littermates were given a daily gavage (5 mg/mouse [~200 mg/kg] AGN or 1% Tween 80 vehicle, beginning at 8 weeks of age (WOA). All mice were terminated at 24 WOA. The AGN-treated TRAMP mice experienced less dorsolateral prostate (DLP) lesion growth by 30% ($p = 0.009$) and developed fewer and smaller neuroendocrine-carcinomas (NE-Ca) (0.12 g/mouse) than vehicle-treated counterparts (0.81 g/mouse, $p = 0.037$). Proteomic and transcriptomic analyses of NE-Ca suggest not only multiple cancer cell targeting actions of AGN but also impacts on the tumor microenvironments (TME) such as angiogenesis, inflammation, and immune surveillance.

The efficacy was replicated for AGN ethanolic extract (a different batch from above; D/DA content as high as 60%) in a follow-up experiment in the TRAMP model (Tang et al., 2015) and compared side by side with D/DA at equimolar dosage. Three cohorts of male C57BL/6 TRAMP mice (35–36 mice per group) were fed AIN93M purified diet and gavaged with a new vehicle (ethanol: PEG400: Tween 80: 5% glucose = 3:6:1:20), AGN (5 mg per mouse) or D/DA (3 mg per mouse, equimolar to that in AGN) 5 days per week from 8 weeks of age (WOA). Mice were euthanized at either 16 WOA ($n = 12$ mice per group) or 28 WOA unless large tumors necessitated earlier sacrifice. Measurement of plasma and NE-Ca D, DA, and their common metabolite DOH indicated similar retention from AGN versus D/DA dosing. The growth of TRAMP DLP in AGN- and D/DA-treated mice was inhibited by 66% and 61% at 16 weeks and by 67% and 72% at 28 weeks, respectively. Survival of mice bearing NE-Ca to 28 weeks was improved by AGN, but not by D/DA. Nevertheless, AGN- and D/DA-treated mice had lower NE-Ca burden than vehicle group. Immunohistochemical and mRNA analyses of DLP showed that AGN and D/DA exerted similar inhibition of TRAMP epithelial lesion progression and key cell-cycle genes. Profiling of NE-Ca mRNA showed a greater scope of modulating angiogenesis, epithelial–mesenchymal transition, invasion-metastasis, and inflammation genes by AGN than D/DA. The data support D/DA as probable active/prodrug compounds against TRAMP epithelial lesions, and they cooperate with non-pyranocoumarin compounds to exert AGN efficacy against NE-Ca.

13.5　*IN VIVO* ANTICANCER ACTIVITIES OF D, DA, OR DOH

Cell culture models have been primarily used as screening tools and cellular targets for studying potential anticancer activities and "mechanisms" of these compounds. The laboratory of the primary authors (JL and CJ) discovered a potent anti–AR-prostate specific antigen (PSA) axis signaling activity of D and DA at exposure concentrations that were at least one order of magnitude lower than apoptotic level using the LNCaP cells as the *in vitro* screening model (Jiang et al., 2006; Guo et al., 2007). They also examined the structure activity relationship (SAR) of D, DA, and DOH. DOH exhibited a biphasic effect on AR signaling in the presence of androgen and a partial agonist role in the absence of androgen (Guo et al., 2007). At the single-digit micromolar subapoptotic concentrations, D and DA promoted neuroendocrine differentiation of LNCaP cells to distinctive

TABLE 13.1

Studies of *Angelica gigas* Nakai Root Ethanol Extracts and Signature Pyranocoumarins in Mouse Cancer Models

Mouse Strain	N per Group	Cancer Model	Drug Dose (mg/kg)	Dose Interval	Route	Duration	Anticancer Efficacy	References
Mouse, athymic nude	10–15	Xenograft, human DU145 PCa, prophylactic	AGN 100	Once daily	PO IP	8 weeks	Tumor wt −64%; −72%	Lee et al., 2009
Mouse, athymic nude	10–15	Xenograft, human PC3 PCa, prophylactic	AGN 100	Once daily	IP	8 weeks	Tumor wt −51%	Lee et al., 2009
Mouse, SCID NSG	10	Xenograft	AGN 200, 400 DOH 160	Once daily	PO	10 weeks	Tumor wt −50%; −70% by two doses of AGN	Wu et al., 2017
Mouse, SCID NSG	6–7	Human LNCaP-AR PCa, prophylactic	DOH 120	Once daily	PO	4 weeks	Tumor wt −50%	Lu lab TBP
Mouse, SCID NSG	17	Xenograft LNCaP PCa, treatment	DOH 120	Once daily	PO	4.5 weeks	Tumor wt −50%	Lu lab TBP
Mouse, transgenic	15	TRAMP NE carcinoma, prophylactic	AGN 200	Once daily	PO	16 weeks	NE Tumor wt −80%	Zhang et al., 2015c
Mouse, transgenic	12–20	TRAMP NE carcinoma and metastasis, prophylactic	AGN 200	Once daily	PO	8 and 20 weeks	NE Tumor wt −70% Improved survival to 28 weeks	Tang et al., 2015
Mouse, transgenic	12–20	TRAMP NE carcinoma and metastasis, prophylactic	D/DA 120	Once daily	PO	8 and 20 weeks	NE Tumor wt −50% No survival benefit	Tang et al., 2015
Mouse, syngeneic	10	Allograft, lung Ca, LLC, prophylactic	D 4	Every other day	IP	2 weeks	Tumor wt −65%	Jung et al., 2009
Mouse, syngeneic	6	Allograft, lung Ca, LLC, prophylactic	D or DOH 50	Once daily	IP	2 weeks	Tumor wt −40%	Lee et al., 2009
Mouse, syngeneic	5	Allograft, lung Ca, LLC, intervention	D 10	Every other day	IP	9 days	Tumor wt −40%	Ge et al., 2020
Mouse, syngeneic	10	Allograft, colon Ca, CT-26 metastasis, prophylactic	D or DOH 10	Once daily	PO	2 weeks	Lung metastasis −50%	Son et al., 2011
Mouse, syngeneic	10	Allograft Sarcoma-180, treatment	D or DA 50, 100	Once daily	IP	9 days, Observe survival	Increased host survival +50%, +77%	Lee et al., 2003
Mouse, athymic nude	5	Xenograft, B16F10 melanoma intervention	DA 100, 200	Every other day	PO	4 weeks	Tumor wt −40, −64%	Chang et al., 2021

Abbreviations: D = decursin; DA = decursinol angelate; DOH = decursinol; IP = intraperitoneal; PO = oral route (gavage, gastric intubation with feeding needle); TBP = to be published from Lu lab.

Source: From Lu et al. (2022).

neurite-bearing morphology. This SAR applied to estrogen-dependent breast cancer MCF-7 cells as well as estrogen receptor negative MDA-MB-231 breast cancer cells (Jiang et al., 2007). Cell culture models of other organ sites included lung, colon, bladder, sarcoma, and blood cancers and were extensively reviewed in our article a decade ago (Zhang et al., 2012). In the last decade, additional cancer cell lines have been studied and reported. Unfortunately, these papers rarely justified the relevance of pyranocoumarin exposure levels, "ignoring" PK and metabolism knowledge as summarized in Figure 13.2.

The following focuses on organ sites with available *in vivo* efficacy information: prostate cancer, lung cancer, colon cancer, sarcoma, and melanoma. Overall, the data support efficacy against a wide spectrum of cancers in the animal models for D/DA, most probably through DOH or its combined action with the parent compounds that survived hepatic degradation.

Prostate cancer: D/DA mixture was compared at equimolar dosage with AGN dose of 5 mg per mouse in the TRAMP model (Tang et al., 2015). Measurement of plasma and NE-Ca D, DA, and their common metabolite DOH indicated similar retention from AGN versus D/DA dosing. The growth of TRAMP dorsolateral prostate (DLP) was equally and substantially inhibited by AGN or D/DA at 18 and 28 weeks. However, the survival of mice bearing NE-Ca to 28 weeks was improved by AGN, but not by D/DA. Focused detection of NE-Ca mRNA showed a wider scope of modulating angiogenesis, epithelial–mesenchymal transition, invasion-metastasis, and inflammation genes by AGN than D/DA. The data therefore support superiority of AGN to D/DA against TRAMP NE-Ca, and that D/DA were probable "active" prodrug compounds through DOH against the epithelial lesions.

Purified DOH had been tested for suppressing xenograft growth of human prostate cancer cells expressing AR in SCID-NSG mice (Wu et al., 2017). In mice carrying subcutaneously inoculated human LNCaP/AR-luc cells overexpressing the wild type AR, 4.5 mg DOH per mouse dosing was compared with an equimolar dose of 6 mg D/DA per mouse. DOH decreased xenograft tumor growth by 75% and the associated lung metastasis, yet D/DA exerted little suppressing effect. The plasma DOH concentration at 3 hours after the last dose showed a higher circulating level in the DOH-treated NSG mice than in the D/DA-treated mice. The DOH bioavailability advantage over D/DA was supported by a single-dose PK experiment that showed that DOH dosing led to 3.7-fold area under curve (AUC) of plasma DOH over that achieved by equimolar D/DA dosing.

Sarcoma: In a mouse allograft study, D or DA, at doses of 50 and 100 mg/kg by IP injection daily for 9 days, significantly suppressed Sarcoma-180 tumor growth in syngeneic ICR mice (Lee et al., 2003). Compared with the median survival time for the control group of 22 days, those for 50 and 100 D mg/kg treated groups were 29 and 40 days, and those for 50 and 100 mg DA/kg treated groups were 32 and 34 days, respectively.

Lung cancer: In the mouse LLC lung cancer allograft model, D or DA exerted notable growth inhibitory activity. An anti-neoangiogenesis activity of D and DA was observed and attributed to their inhibition of VEGFR2 signaling (Jung et al., 2009). The microvessel density in tumors treated with D (IP, 4 mg per kg, every other day) for 14 days was significantly decreased compared with a vehicle control group.

Ge et al. recently reported immune involvement in the hypoxic tumor microenvironment (TME) by D in the LLC allograft model (Ge et al., 2020). Treatment with D (IP, 10 mg/kg, every other day) reduced tumor size and the hypoxic area. They observed reduced HIF-1α and PD-L1 expression in the treated tumors. IHC detected increased infiltrating T cells (CD3+), helper T cells (CD4+), and cytotoxic (CD8+) T cells and fewer regulatory T cells (Foxp3) and myeloid-derived suppressor (arginase-1 positive) cells.

Murine colon cancer metastasis to lung: In a mouse CT-26 colon cancer model, oral administration of D and DOH (10 mg/kg) given 30 minutes before the tail vein injection of the cancer cells and followed by daily oral dosing of D or DOH for 14 days reduced the number of tumor nodules in the lungs and blunted the increase in lung weight caused by CT-26 metastases (Son et al., 2011).

Melanoma: DA was tested by gavage administration for efficacy against mouse melanoma cell line (B16.F10) SC xenograft in athymic nude mice (Chang et al., 2021) in a "therapy" model. Treatment was started after tumors had reached 50 cubic mm 3 times per week for 4 weeks. The tumor weight was decreased in a dose-dependent manner for 100 and 200 mg/kg dosages. Biomarker analysis of the tumors showed dose-dependent increase of apoptosis related to mitochondria intrinsic signaling (cytochrome C, Bax/Bcl2 proteins).

Knowledge gaps and challenges: As the PK and metabolism studies of D and DA have supported their pro-drug role and rapid conversion to DOH (Figure 13.2), DOH is the probable principal *in vivo* chemical mediator for their anticancer activities. Depending on the dosage and metabolic adaptation upon chronic intake, if any, the overall anticancer efficacy outcome would be expected to be the integrated actions of the three pyranocoumarin species. With a paradoxical lack of direct cytocidal and cytostatic activity of DOH against cancer cells in cell culture (Yim et al., 2005; Jiang et al., 2006; Guo et al., 2007; Jiang et al., 2007), future cell culture modeling should emphasize the *in vivo* achievable concentrations of each entity and TME cells as well in order to be relevant.

13.6 IMMUNE REGULATORY AND ANTICANCER ACTIVITIES OF AGN WATER EXTRACTS

Compared to alcoholic extracts, much less has been published with AGN water extracts or their subfractions. *Angelan* is a refined subfraction of a water extract of AGN root that was precipitated out with ethanol and contains mostly polysaccharides (90%) (Han et al., 1998). Angelan is approximately 10 kDa and composed of arabinose, galactose, and galacturonic acid but not glucose (Han et al., 1998). Angelan treatment lengthened the survival time of B16F10 melanoma-bearing syngeneic mice when administered *i.p.* at a dose of 30 mg/kg (Han et al., 2006). Angelan most likely targets macrophages and natural killer (NK) cells which are involved in the innate immunity against cancer cells or virally-infected cells (Han et al., 1998; Han et al., 2006). In a cell culture model, angelan induced transcription of inducible nitric oxide synthase (iNOS), interleukin-1 beta (IL-1β) and tumor necrosis factor alpha (TNF-α) in murine macrophage RAW 264.7 cells, mediated by specific activation of NF-κB/Rel (Jeon et al., 1999; Jeon et al., 2001). Another study claimed the macrophage activation by angelan differed from that induced by bacterial lipopolysaccharide (LPS) (Jeon et al., 2000). Angelan activated NF-κB/Rel through the CD14 and complement receptor type 3 (CR3) membrane receptor and p38 mitogen activated protein kinase (P38MAPK) in murine macrophages (Jeon and Kim, 2001). Subsequently, the same group investigated the effects of angelan on dendritic cell (DC) maturation and found a crucial role of toll-like receptor 4 (TLR4) signaling pathways (Kim et al., 2007).

ISAg was prepared with a similar procedure to angelan, minus the ethanol precipitation step, and therefore was less refined than angelan (Kim et al., 2018a). ISAg contains glucose which accounts for 70% of total carbohydrate. ISAg also contained more protein than did angelan (17% vs. 8%). In the murine macrophage RAW264.7 cell culture model, ISAg treatment induced nitric oxide (NO) production and cytokine gene expression involved in innate immune responses much like angelan and LPS.

Gavage treatment in the dose range of 1, 2, and 4 mg ISAg per mouse, every other day for 4 weeks activated macrophages and DCs to secrete cytokine IL-12 (Kim et al., 2018a). Consistent with IL-12 playing a crucial role in NK and NKT cell activation, the authors reported increased activation of NK and NKT cells producing IFN-γ and TNF-α by ISAg supplement in the mice. The immune stimulatory effects were probably mediated through the TLR4 and IL-12 signaling pathway because their respective-knockout mice diminished response to ISAg. In syngeneic mice bearing *s.c.* B16 melanoma cell allografts, the gavage treatment with 4 mg ISAg 3 times per week for 2 weeks decreased tumor weight by more than 60%. The efficacy was accompanied by increased infiltrating NK and NKT cells in the tumors.

The same group examined whether ISAg affected *in vivo* differentiation of T cells (Lee et al., 2019). They found that the oral administration of 4 mg ISAg 3 times per week for 4 weeks induced the polarization of CD4+ T cells toward the Th1 phenotype *in vivo*. Additionally, in mice treated with ISAg, CD8+ cytotoxic T cells produced more IFNγ than in control mice treated with PBS. Moreover, treatment with ISAg activated CD4+ and CD8+ T cells and NK and NKT cells, resulting in the secretion of Th1-type cytokines in a TLR4-dependent manner. ISAg treatment increased the number of Foxp3+ Treg cells, but not Th2 cells than PBS treatment, indicating that ISAg possesses an immunomodulatory capacity that could also control adaptive immune responses in addition to the innate NK and NKT cells. However, how much of the immune stimulating substance like angelan or ISAg is present in the alcohol extract of AGN sold as dietary supplements is not known.

13.7 HUMAN CLINICAL TRANSLATION CHALLENGES

Human clinical trial status: No human trial has been reported to assess the utility of AGN alcoholic extracts or pyranocoumarins or water extract preparations for cancer prevention or treatment. We discuss the challenges and opportunities for human cancer trials next.

AGN herbal products: The major challenges for cancer indication and in other diseases for clinical trials are the source of raw materials, the standardization of AGN extraction procedures, and the formulation and dosing regimens for future studies. These issues are not unique to AGN trials as all herbal/botanical investigations face the same problems of quality control (QC) and quality assurance (QA) for product consistency. Therefore, many research and development opportunities open up for horticulture and harvest, postharvest processing, and storage to ensure relatively uniform raw source materials, standardization of protocols of extraction, and manufacturing for AGN extracts and QC/QA practices. It will be very desirable for consensus to be built around these issues with a global herbal industry-wide effort.

Optimizing trial design: Properly powered, randomized, blinded, and placebo-controlled trials are the best approach to support cancer treatment or interception indications. However, choosing the optimal dosages for testing will be crucial. Insufficient dosage to deliver the "active" principles of any given extract type will lead to false-negative outcomes that may prematurely shortchange a beneficial indication if properly tested at the correct dosages. We recommend Phase I dose-escalation trials to determine Phase II recommended doses for each type of extract in the intended target subject/patient populations prior to efficacy testing in Phase II trials. Such staged progression of trials ensures that the efficacy testing conditions in Phase II trials are maximized for positive signals.

A case for early-stage trials in niche cohort of prostate cancer patients to estimate "effect size": Early-stage operable prostate cancer of high and intermediate risk of progression is frequently treated with radical prostatectomy (RP) and radiation therapy (RT) with curative intent (Figure 13.4A). Since the prostate along with the localized cancer lesion has been removed from these patients, their blood PSA level serves as a "clean" reliable metric of recurrent prostate cancer burden (Pound et al., 1999; Maffezzini et al., 2007). From clinical experience, these patients will rarely (if not never) undergo spontaneous PSA decline or stabilization. When indicated by rapid PSA rise and unfavorable risk factors, the standard of care for managing these patients is androgen deprivation therapy (ADT) (Figure 13.4A). ADT is non-curative with a median relapse time for castration resistant prostate cancer (CRPC) of about 18 months. It is not only expensive, but ADT also causes many serious and unpleasant side effects including sexual dysfunction, impotence, osteoporosis and bone fractures, mode swings, hot flashes, fatigue, loss of lean body mass, gynecomastia, and anemia. In spite of multiple next-generation androgen synthesis and AR-targeting blocker drugs (e.g., abiraterone acetate, enzalutamide), DNA-repair drugs (PARP inhibitors) and microtubule-targeting taxane drugs indicated for managing the more advanced stage CRPC diseases (Figure 13.4A), there is currently no FDA-approved modality before ADT to intercept or delay disease progression in the clinic practice.

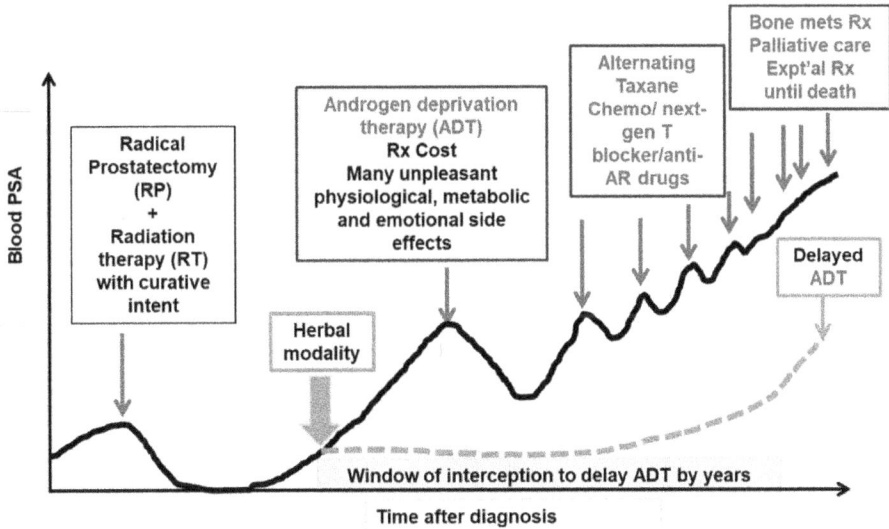

FIGURE 13.4A Stylized blood prostate specific antigen changes during the course of prostate cancer treatments and an anticipated interception effect of an herbal supplement on delaying biochemical recurrent disease progression to postpone or avoid androgen deprivation therapy.

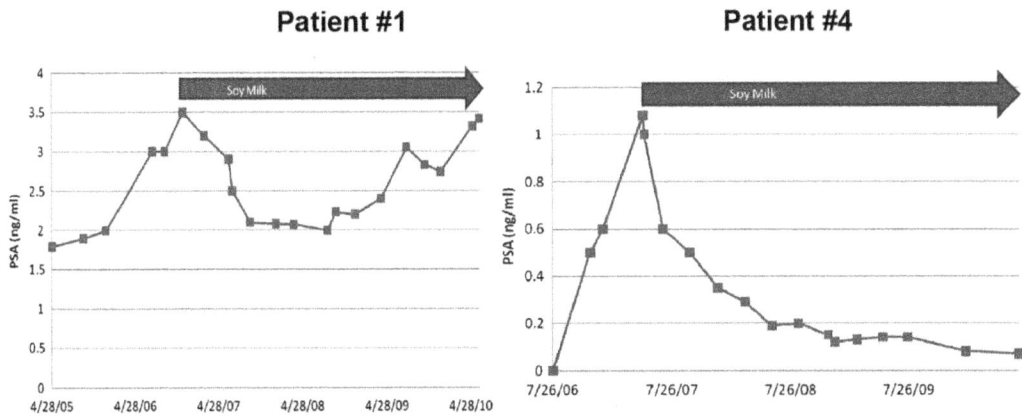

FIGURE 13.4B Serum prostate specific antigen changes in two responding patients before and after taking soy milk in Joshi-Drabick study.

Source: Adapted from Joshi et al. (2011).

Earlier studies with dietary components and botanicals in prostate cancer patients inspire a creative use of the niche patient cohort to estimate interception "effect size." At Hershey Medical Center, Drs. Joshi and Drabick and co-workers showed that daily consumption of 24 oz. of soy milk caused a PSA decline or stabilization in three of seven patients with ADT-naive disease and one of three patients with castration resistant (CR) disease (see response profiles of two patients in Figure 13.4B) (Joshi et al., 2011). A similar extent of PSA control with soy beverage was reported in two other papers with a total of 49 evaluable patients (8/29 Kwan 2010 study [Kwan et al., 2010]; 6/20 Pendleton 2008 study [Pendleton et al., 2008]). Soy isoflavones have been shown to antagonize AR axis signaling (Bektic et al., 2004) and are structurally different from pyranocoumarins in AGN.

Given these "successes," we hypothesize that the "clean PSA" post-RP and post-RT patient cohort would be ideal for the first step of clinical translation of AGN supplement. The following PK dose

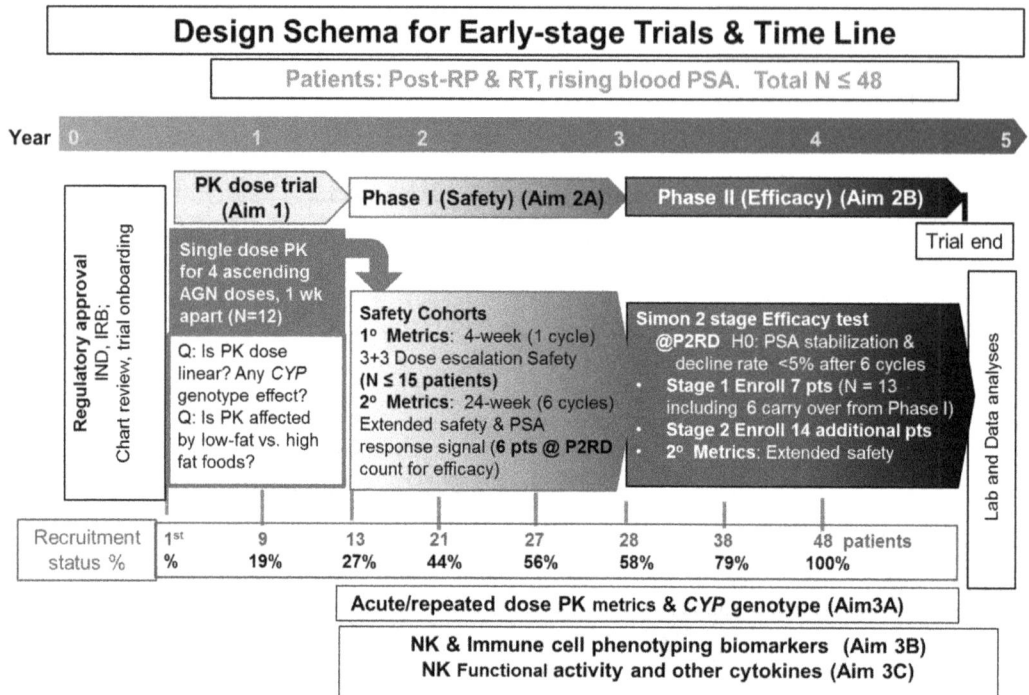

FIGURE 13.5   Proposed early-stage clinical trials in prostate cancer patients to define the PK dose response pattern and estimate the "effect size" of *Angelica gigas* Nakai supplement to intercept biochemically recurrent prostate cancer. NK = natural killer cell; PK = pharmacokinetics.

and Phase I/II trials have been planned with NCI grant funding (R01CA260901, NCT05375539) (Figure 13.5).

These proposed trials were designed in stages, that is, with single ascending dose SAD PK trial for acute dose safety and PK metrics, followed by Phase I dose escalation in target patient cohorts to study dose safety information for subchronic intake to establish maximally tolerated dose (MTD) as well as the Phase II recommended dosage (P2RD). The open label design is appropriate to gauge the likely "effect size" to enable decision for future double-blinded, randomized, placebo-controlled trials with sufficient statistical power. Cogni.Q made with proprietary extract of AGN root has been chosen as the test article. It has been marketed in the United States for more than 2 decades with remarkable safety. It possesses a chemical profile that matched AGN extract studied in the animal cancer models (Zhang et al., 2015a), and its single-dose human PK has been studied in the United States with favorable half-life for DOH (Zhang et al., 2015a) and Figure 13.3.

The trials will provide the first of their kind knowledge of safety and preliminary efficacy of an AGN herbal supplement against prostate cancer at therapeutic dosages. The information from these trials will guide future phase II/III trials in prostate cancer patients at different malignancy stages. They will also be applicable to the prevention and therapy of cancers of other organ sites and non-malignant diseases including pain, neurodegeneration, stroke, and other conditions (Lu et al., 2022).

13.8   DISTINCTIONS FROM OTHER FOODS, HERBS, SPICES, AND BOTANICALS USED IN CANCER

The pyranocoumarins belong to a new class of "active" phytochemicals *distinct* from those in other herbal or nutraceutical "remedies" or their combinations, including soy (e.g., isoflavones), tea (e.g., polyphenols), fish oil (omega-3 polyunsaturated fatty acids), raspberries (e.g., anthocyanins), cannabis (e.g., cannabinoids) or mushrooms, and so forth. Their chemical structure uniqueness offers research opportunity to complement and synergize with other herbal or nutraceutical remedies.

13.9   TOXICITY AND CAUTIONARY NOTES

Based on reported adverse events in the Korean Phase II study of 3 months' duration of supplement at the dose 800 mg per day (Kim et al., 2003), anorexia, nausea, and indigestion might be low-frequency events linked to CognI.Q (INM176) use. No documented AGN toxicity has been reported. The safety profile, especially in patients, of higher than dietary supplement dosages should be carefully investigated in Phase I dose escalation studies, as outlined in this chapter.

A couple of publications explored potential AGN pyranocoumarin-drug interactions in animal PK models (Chae et al., 2012a, 2012b) using theophylline as a model drug, which is a phosphodiesterase inhibitor bronchial dilator and a substrate for CYP 1A2. After pretreatment with D or DA (vehicle vs. 5 and 25 mg/kg by oral administration) for 3 days, the rats were given the respective D or DA dosage and theophylline (10 mg/kg, oral route) concomitantly on the fourth day. The blood theophylline and its major metabolites (1-methylxanthine (1-MX), 3-methylxanthine (3-MX), 1-methyluric acid (1-MU), and 1,3-dimethyluric acid (1,3-DMU)) levels were monitored with LC-MS/MS. The results indicated increased the area under concentration-time curve (AUC) or C_{max} in D or DA pretreatment at the higher dose, not the lower dose. The higher dose of D or DA pretreatment affected the AUC_{24h} of three metabolites and other PK metrics. The authors cautioned that patients receiving CYP1A2-metabolized drugs, such as caffeine and theophylline, should be advised of the potential herb-drug interaction to reduce the risk of therapeutic failure or increased toxicity of conventional drug therapy. In hindsight, as D and DA are metabolized by CYP 2C19 and 3A4 to decursinol in first-pass metabolism (Figure 13.3), the slower breakdown of theophylline by D and DA could reflect a competition of CYP isoforms and/or co-substrate NADPH.

13.10   SUMMARY POINTS

- This chapter focuses on *A. gigas* Nakai (AGN) root and its signature phytochemical pyranocoumarins decursin and decursinol angelate in terms of their metabolism/metabolite, and pharmacokinetics and their anticancer efficacy in animal models.
- AGN is cultivated in the Korean peninsula as a medicinal herb and grows as a wild plant in the northeastern Chinese provinces contiguous with North Korea.
- AGN differs from *A. sinensis* (Chinese) and *A. acutiloba* (Japanese) with its unique possession of pyranocoumarins.
- Alcoholic extracts of AGN and pyranocoumarins have multiple health benefits in animal models, including anticancer activities.
- Clinical translation requires careful choice of AGN source, dosage, and forms amid numerous challenges.
- Early-stage clinical trials (PK dose trial and Phase I/II) are under way to address these issues to advance evidence-based herbal oncology and beyond.

13.11   ACKNOWLEDGMENTS

Work cited from Lu/Jiang laboratory has been supported by National Center for Complementary and Integrative Health (NCCIH) grants R21 AT005383 and R01 AT007395 and Penn State College of Medicine startup fund and Penn State Cancer Institute Developmental fund. Composition of this review chapter has been supported in part by National Cancer Institute (NCI) multi-PI grant R01CA260901 (Lu, Joshi).

REFERENCES

Bektic, J., A.P. Berger, K. Pfeil, G. Dobler, G. Bartsch and H. Klocker. Androgen receptor regulation by physi-ological concentrations of the isoflavonoid genistein in androgen-dependent LNCaP cells is mediated by estrogen receptor beta. *Eur Urol* 45: 245–251, discussion 251, 2004.

Chae, J.W., J.H. An, W. Kang, J. Ma and K.I. Kwon. Effect of decursinol angelate on the pharmacokinetics of theophylline and its metabolites in rats. *Food Chem Toxicol* 50: 3666–3672, 2012a.

Chae, J.W., I.H. Baek and K.I. Kwon. Effect of decursin on the pharmacokinetics of theophylline and its metabolites in rats. *Journal of Ethnopharmacology* 144: 248–254, 2012b.

Chang, S.N., I. Khan, C.G. Kim, S.M. Park, D.K. Choi, H. Lee, B.S. Hwang, S.C. Kang and J.G. Park. Decursinol angelate arrest melanoma cell proliferation by initiating cell death and tumor shrinkage via induction of apoptosis. *Int. J. Mol. Sci.* 22, 2021.

Choi, K.O., I. Lee, S.Y. Paik, D.E. Kim, J.D. Lim, W.S. Kang and S. Ko. Ultrafine *Angelica gigas* powder nor-malizes ovarian hormone levels and has antiosteoporosis properties in ovariectomized rats: Particle size effect. *J. Med. Food* 15: 863–872, 2012.

Ge, Y., S.H. Yoon, H. Jang, J.H. Jeong and Y.M. Lee. Decursin promotes HIF-1alpha proteasomal degradation and immune responses in hypoxic tumor microenvironment. *Phytomed* 78: 153318, 2020.

Guo, J., C. Jiang, Z. Wang, H.J. Lee, H. Hu, B. Malewicz, J.H. Lee, N.I. Baek, J.H. Jeong, D.K. Kim, K.S. Kang, S.H. Kim and J. Lu. A novel class of pyranocoumarin anti-androgen receptor signaling com-pounds. *Mol. Cancer Ther.* 6: 907–917, 2007.

Han, S.B., Y.H. Kim, C.W. Lee, S.M. Park, H.Y. Lee, K.S. Ahn, I.H. Kim and H.M. Kim. Characteristic immu-nostimulation by angelan isolated from *Angelica gigas* Nakai. *Immunopharmacol* 40: 39–48, 1998.

Han, S.B., C.W. Lee, M.R. Kang, Y.D. Yoon, J.S. Kang, K.H. Lee, W.K. Yoon, S.K. Park and H.M. Kim. Pectic polysaccharide isolated from *Angelica gigas* Nakai inhibits melanoma cell metastasis and growth by directly preventing cell adhesion and activating host immune functions. *Cancer Lett* 243: 264–273, 2006.

Jeon, Y.J., S.B. Han, K.S. Ahn and H.M. Kim. Activation of NF-kappaB/Rel in angelan-stimulated macro-phages. *Immunopharmacol* 43: 1–9, 1999.

Jeon, Y.J., S.B. Han, K.S. Ahn and H.M. Kim. Differential activation of murine macrophages by angelan and LPS. *Immunopharmacology* 49: 275–284, 2000.

Jeon, Y.J., S.B. Han, S.H. Lee, H.C. Kim, K.S. Ahn and H.M. Kim. Activation of mitogen-activated protein kinase pathways by angelan in murine macrophages. *Int. Immunopharmacol.* 1: 237–245, 2001.

Jeon, Y.J. and H.M. Kim. Experimental evidences and signal transduction pathways involved in the activation of NF-kappa B/Rel by angelan in murine macrophages. *Int. Immunopharmacol.* 1: 1331–1339, 2001.

Jiang, C., J. Guo, Z. Wang, B. Xiao, H.J. Lee, E.O. Lee, S.H. Kim and J. Lu. Decursin and decursinol angelate inhibit estrogen-stimulated and estrogen-independent growth and survival of breast cancer cells. *Breast Cancer Res.* 9: R77, 2007.

Jiang, C., H.J. Lee, G.X. Li, J.M. Guo, B. Malewicz, Y. Zhao, E.O. Lee, J.H. Lee, M.S. Kim, S.H. Kim and J.X. Lu. Potent antiandrogen and androgen receptor activities of an *Angelica gigas*–containing herbal formulation: Identification of decursin as a novel and active compound with implications for prevention and treatment of prostate cancer. *Cancer Res* 66: 453–463, 2006.

Joshi, M., N.M. Agostino, R. Gingrich and J.J. Drabick. Effects of commercially available soy products on PSA in androgen-deprivation-naive and castration-resistant prostate cancer. *South Med J* 104: 736–740, 2011.

Jung, M.H., S.H. Lee, E.M. Ahn and Y.M. Lee. Decursin and decursinol angelate inhibit VEGF-induced angio-genesis via suppression of the VEGFR-2-signaling pathway. *Carcinog* 30: 655–661, 2009.

Kim, E.J., J. Kwon, S.H. Park, C. Park, Y.B. Seo, H.K. Shin, H.K. Kim, K.S. Lee, S.Y. Choi, D.H. Ryu and G.S. Hwang. Metabolite profiling of *Angelica gigas* from different geographical origins using (1)H NMR and UPLC-MS analyses. *J Agric Food Chem* 59: 8806–8815, 2011.

Kim, H.M., J.S. Kang, S.K. Park, K. Lee, J.Y. Kim, Y.J. Kim, J.T. Hong, Y. Kim and S.B. Han. Antidiabetic activity of angelan isolated from *Angelica gigas* Nakai. *Arch. Pharm. Res.* 31: 1489–1496, 2008.

Kim, J.H., S.K. Koh, H.J. Koh, Y.A. Kwon, S.H. Kim, J.G. Kim, T.E. Kim, J.W. Park, M.Y. Seo and Y.R. Song. A three month placebo-controlled clinical trial of INM 176 in the old aged subjects with memory impair-ment. *J. Korean Neuropsychiatric Assn* 42: 254–262, 2003.

Kim, J.Y., Y.D. Yoon, J.M. Ahn, J.S. Kang, S.K. Park, K. Lee, K. Bin Song, H.M. Kim and S.B. Han. Angelan isolated from *Angelica gigas* Nakai induces dendritic cell maturation through toll-like receptor 4. *Int. Immunopharmacol.* 7: 78–87, 2007.

Kim, M.R., A.M.A. Abd El-Aty, J.H. Choi, K.B. Lee and J.H. Shim. Identification of volatile components in *Angelica* species using supercritical-CO2 fluid extraction and solid phase microextraction coupled to gas chromatography-mass spectrometry. *Biomed. Chromatog. BMC* 20: 1267–1273, 2006a.

Kim, M.R., A.M.A. Abd El-Aty, I.S. Kim and J.H. Shim. Determination of volatile flavor components in dang-gui cultivars by solvent free injection and hydrodistillation followed by gas chromatographic-mass spectrometric analysis. *J. ChromAtogr. A* 1116: 259–264, 2006b.

Kim, S.H., S.W. Lee, H.J. Park, S.H. Lee, W.K. Im, Y.D. Kim, K.H. Kim, S.J. Park, S. Hong and S.H. Jeon. Anti-cancer activity of *Angelica gigas* by increasing immune response and stimulating natural killer and natural killer T cells. *BMC Complement. Altern. Med.* 18: 218, 2018a.

Kim, S.J., S.M. Ko, E.J. Choi, S.H. Ham, Y.D. Kwon, Y.B. Lee and H.Y. Cho. Simultaneous determination of decursin, decursinol angelate, nodakenin, and decursinol of *Angelica gigas* Nakai in human plasma by UHPLC-MS/MS: Application to pharmacokinetic study. *Molecules* 23, 2018b.

Kwan, W., G. Duncan, C. Van Patten, M. Liu and J. Lim. A phase II trial of a soy beverage for subjects without clinical disease with rising prostate-specific antigen after radical radiation for prostate cancer. *Nutr Cancer* 62: 198–207, 2010.

Lee, H.J., E.O. Lee, J.H. Lee, K.S. Lee, K.H. Kim, S.H. Kim and J. Lu. In vivo anti-cancer activity of Korean *Angelica gigas* and its major pyranocoumarin decursin. *Am. J. Chin. Med.* 37: 127–142, 2009.

Lee, S., Y.S. Lee, S.H. Jung, K.H. Shin, B.K. Kim and S.S. Kang. Anti-tumor activities of decursinol angelate and decursin from *Angelica gigas*. *Arch. Pharm. Res.* 26: 727–730, 2003.

Lee, S.W., H.J. Park, S.H. Kim, S. Shin, K.H. Kim, S.J. Park, S. Hong and S.H. Jeon. TLR4-dependent effects of ISAg treatment on conventional T cell polarization in vivo. *Anim. Cells Syst. (Seoul)* 23: 184–191, 2019.

Lu, J., C. Jiang, T.D. Schell, M. Joshi, J.D. Raman and C. Xing. Angelica gigas: Signature Compounds, In Vivo Anticancer, Analgesic, Neuroprotective and Other Activities, and the Clinical Translation Challenges. *Am J Chin Med* Vol. 50, No. 6, 1475–1527, 2022.

Lu, J., J. Zhang, L. Li, C. Jiang and C. Xing. Cancer chemoprevention with Korean *Angelica*: Active compounds, pharmacokinetics, and human translational considerations. *Curr. Pharmacol. Rep.* 1: 373–381, 2015.

Maffezzini, M., A. Bossi and L. Collette. Implications of prostate-specific antigen doubling time as indicator of failure after surgery or radiation therapy for prostate cancer. *Eur Urol* 51: 605–613, discussion 613, 2007.

Oh, T.W., K.H. Park, H.W. Jung and Y.K. Park. Neuroprotective effect of the hairy root extract of *Angelica gigas* Nakai on transient focal cerebral ischemia in rats through the regulation of angiogenesis. *BMC Complement. Altern. Med.* 15: 101, 2015.

Pendleton, J.M., W.W. Tan, S. Anai, M. Chang, W. Hou, K.T. Shiverick and C.J. Rosser. Phase II trial of iso-flavone in prostate-specific antigen recurrent prostate cancer after previous local therapy. *BMC Cancer* 8: 132, 2008.

Piao, J., J.Y. Lee, J.B. Weon, C.J. Ma, H.J. Ko, D.D. Kim, W.S. Kang and H.J. Cho. *Angelica gigas* Nakai and Soluplus-based solid formulations prepared by hot-melting extrusion: Oral absorption enhancing and memory ameliorating effects. *PLoS One* 10: e0124447, 2015.

Piao, X.L., J.H. Park, H. Cui, D.H. Kim and H.H. Yoo. Development of gas chromatographic mass spectrometry-pattern recognition method for the quality control of Korean *Angelica*. *J. Pharm. Biomed. Anal.* 44: 1163–1167, 2007.

Pound, C.R., A.W. Partin, M.A. Eisenberger, D.W. Chan, J.D. Pearson and P.C. Walsh. Natural history of progression after PSA elevation following radical prostatectomy. *JAMA* 281: 1591–1597, 1999.

Son, S.H., K.K. Park, S.K. Park, Y.C. Kim, Y.S. Kim, S.K. Lee and W.Y. Chung. Decursin and decursinol from *Angelica gigas* inhibit the lung metastasis of murine colon carcinoma. *Phytother. Res.* 25: 959–964, 2011.

Tang, S.N., J. Zhang, W. Wu, P. Jiang, M. Puppala, Y. Zhang, C. Xing, S.H. Kim, C. Jiang and J. Lu. Chemopreventive effects of Korean *Angelica* versus its major pyranocoumarins on two lineages of transgenic adenocarcinoma of mouse prostate carcinogenesis. *Cancer Prev. Res. (Phila)* 8: 835–844, 2015.

Wu, W., S.N. Tang, Y. Zhang, M. Puppala, T.K. Cooper, C. Xing, C. Jiang and J. Lu. Prostate cancer xenograft inhibitory activity and pharmacokinetics of decursinol, a metabolite of *Angelica gigas* pyranocoumarins, in mouse models. *Am. J. Chin. Med.* 45: 1773–1792, 2017.

Yim, D., R.P. Singh, C. Agarwal, S. Lee, H. Chi and R. Agarwal. A novel anticancer agent, decursin, induces G1 arrest and apoptosis in human prostate carcinoma cells. *Cancer Res.* 65: 1035–1044, 2005.

Zhang, J., L. Li, T.W. Hale, W. Chee, C. Xing, C. Jiang and J. Lu. Single oral dose pharmacokinetics of decursin and decursinol angelate in healthy adult men and women. *PLoS One* 10: e0114992, 2015a.

Zhang, J., L. Li, C. Jiang, C. Xing, S.H. Kim and J. Lu. Anti-cancer and other bioactivities of Korean *Angelica gigas* Nakai (AGN) and its major pyranocoumarin compounds. *Anticancer Agents Med. Chem.* 12: 1239–1254, 2012.

Zhang, J., L. Li, S. Tang, T.W. Hale, C. Xing, C. Jiang and J. Lu. Cytochrome P450 isoforms in the metabolism of decursin and decursinol angelate from Korean *Angelica. Am. J. Chin. Med.* 43: 1211–1230, 2015b.

Zhang, J., L. Wang, Y. Zhang, L. Li, S. Tang, C. Xing, S.H. Kim, C. Jiang and J. Lu. Chemopreventive effect of Korean *Angelica* root extract on TRAMP carcinogenesis and integrative "omic" profiling of affected neuroendocrine carcinomas. *Mol. Carcinog.* 54: 1567–1583, 2015c.

Zhao, K.J., T.T. Dong, P.F. Tu, Z.H. Song, C.K. Lo and K.W. Tsim. Molecular genetic and chemical assessment of radix *Angelica* (Danggui) in China. *J. Agric. Food. Chem.* 51: 2576–2583, 2003.

14 Ginger (*Zingiber officinale*) and Biomedical Applications to Cancer
Cellular and Molecular Targets of Extracts

Somayyeh Ghareghomi, Salar Hafez Ghoran,
Fatemeh Taktaz and Ali Hosseini

ABBREVIATIONS

AMPK	AMP-activated protein kinase
Caspase	cysteine-aspartate protease
CAT	catalase
CDKs	cyclin-dependent kinases
CKIs	CDK inhibitors
DR5	death receptor 5
eIF-2α	eukaryotic initiation factor 2-alpha
EMT	epithelial–mesenchymal transition
ERK	extracellular signal–regulated kinase
GPx	glutathione peroxidase
GSK	glycogen synthase kinase
IL-8	interleukin-8
JNK	c-Jun NH 2-terminal kinase
MAPK	mitogen-activated protein kinase
MMP	matrix metalloproteinase
MRP1	multidrug resistance protein 1
NF-κB	nuclear factor kappa B
PGE-2	prostaglandin E-2
ROS	reactive oxygen species
SOD	superoxide dismutase
STAT3	signal transducer and activator of transcription 3
TIMP-1	tissue inhibitor of matrix metalloproteinase 1
VEGF	vascular endothelial growth factor

14.1 INTRODUCTION

With regard to changing lifestyles and using everyday synthetic drugs, turning to inherent health is a big challenge. Controlling disease development and progression, on the other hand, resolving lifestyle-related disarray calls for researchers to shift their attention more to natural products causing health-boosting activity. Therefore, the approaches of using medicinal plants come to help humanity to solve the undesired drawbacks to control disorders through

DOI: 10.1201/9781003260028-16

181

alleviation of pharmacological activities. In particular, ginger is a perennial flowering medicinal plant that belongs to the Zingiberaceae family, mainly native to East and Southern Asia, consisting of 49 genera along with 1300 species, 80–90 of which are in the genus *Zingiber*. Generically known as *Zingiber officinale* Roscoe, the plant has been conventionally consumed in Arabic, Ayurvedic, Chinese, Tibetan, Unani-Tibb, and various folkloric systems of ethnomedicine. An age-old herb with an aromatic odor and pungent taste that is utilized by human beings is a plant of particular interest not only in the culinary industry as a food additive, condiment, and spice, but also in pharmaceutical attitudes (Remadevi et al. 2016). In general, herbalists and traditional healers are believed that various ginger preparations including tea, infusion, decoction, tincture, and spice are used for nausea, vomiting, abdominal pain, arthritis, cystic fibrosis, hyperglycemia, hypercholesterolemia, atonic dyspepsia, anorexia, carminative, stimulant, common cold, cough, sore throat, and applied for indigestion, stomachache, and fevers (Moghaddasi and Kashani 2012). Documented healing effects together with potent nutraceutical impacts encourage ethnobotanists and ethnopharmacologists to till ginger worldwide and use it traditionally in cancer management. Therefore, its rhizomes are commercially cultivated in the Middle East, Japan, China, India, Brazil, Mexico, Australia, Africa, and the United States for medicinal purposes (Mahomoodally et al. 2021). This chapter will provide a piece of current knowledge of traditional uses of ginger and its derived phytochemicals that are useful in either cancer prevention or cancer treatment.

14.2 TRADITIONAL USES AND ETHNOPHARMACOLOGY

Associated with population-based studies in Southeast Asian countries, scientists realized that the occurrence of gastrointestinal, prostate, breast, colon, and other cancers was less than the risk of cancer in Western countries. This is reflected in the rich dietary and traditional use of plants which promote human health (Ma et al. 2021). The use of ginger in China dates back at least 2500 years when local people consumed ginger roots for digestive and bleeding problems, treatment of nausea, and rheumatism. The plant materials were also utilized for the treatment of respiratory complications and snakebite. In Malaysia and Indonesia, a kind of ginger soup is given to new mothers for 30 days after their successful natural childbirth in order to warm the body and sweat out the impurities. The use of ginger rhizomes in cancer treatment is not a newcomer approach; however, ethnomedicine uses it as a daily practice from ancient times. In the Ayurvedic medicinal system, the Indian people orally take its juice and decoction to decrease blood cholesterol, hinder excessive clotting (heart problem), and ameliorate arthritis (Moghaddasi and Kashani 2012). In Palestine, not only both infusion and decoction (preparing by soaking 100 g dried ginger root in boiled water) are prescribed traditionally toward breast, liver, and stomach cancers, but also the decoction of ginger rhizome mixed with turmeric and honey is used for a general treatment of cancer. A decoction of ginger roots plus *Nigella sativa* seeds and camel milk used daily before breakfast is a recipe having been reported. In Ghana, a fresh paste of powdered ginger roots and rhizomes is taken for stomach and brain cancer. In addition, some African people believe that daily consumption of ginger will help ward off mosquitoes. In order to cancer prevention, Singaporean people apply cooked ginger roots, while in Morocco, the ground rhizomes are orally administered with honey (Mahomoodally et al. 2021).

14.3 PHYTOCHEMICAL CONSTITUENTS

Diverse bioactive natural products, called specialized (or secondary) metabolites, are biosynthesized by the plant kingdom, in addition to bacteria, fungi, and marine organisms. Interestingly, many of these potential metabolites are utilized in clinical therapeutics. As a worthwhile medicinal herb, ginger roots are included a variety of primary and secondary metabolites consisting of proteins, carbohydrates, minerals, vitamins (B_1, B_2, B_3, B_6, B_9, C, E, and K), fats and fatty acids, phytosterols, and volatile and phenolic compounds like flavonoids that are responsible for a myriad of biological and pharmacological activities (Shahrajabian et al. 2019). In the following, the species-specific and high value-added bioactive compounds that act as anticancer agents are described.

14.3.1 GINGEROLS

Gingerols are classified as volatile phenolic compounds causing the strong taste of fresh and dried ginger and contribute to human health and nutrition (see Figure 14.1, no. 1). However, in the ginger plant, the complete biosynthesis pathway of gingerol has not been distinguished and it still needs to be researched. Among gingerols, [6]-gingerol, a potential candidate for the development of lead compounds for cancer therapy, is responsible for the pungent taste of the rhizomes. To a lesser extent, other gingerols such as [4]-, [8]-, [10]-, and [12]-gingerol can also be found in ginger root, which shows biological activities (Semwal et al. 2015).

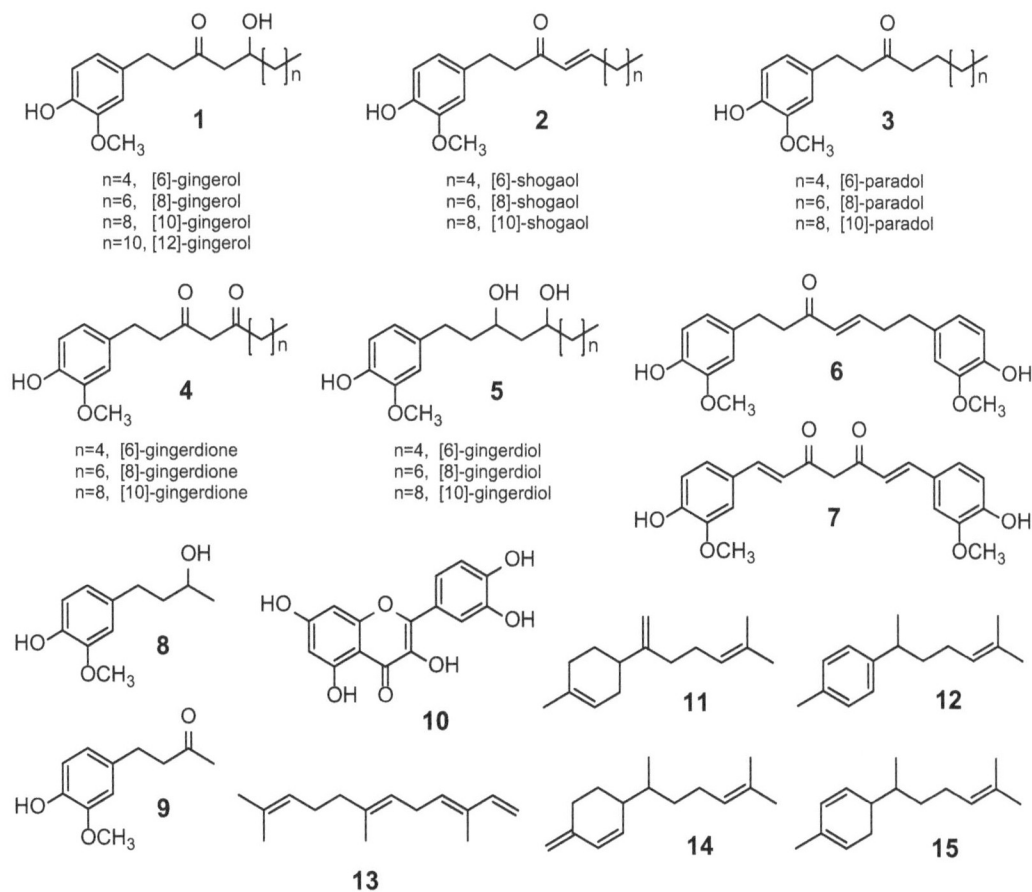

FIGURE 14.1 Ginger secondary metabolites. Chemical structure of some important ginger secondary metabolites including (1) gingerols, (2) shogaols, (3) paradols, (4) gingerdiones, (5) gingerdiols, (6) gingerenone-A, (7) curcumin, (8) zingerol, (9) zingerone, (10) quercetin, (11) β-bisabolene, (12) α-curcumene, (13) α-farnesene, (14) β-sesquiphellandrene, and (15) zingiberene.

14.3.2 Shogaols

Exposed to high temperatures, low pH (2.5–7.2), and long-time storage, gingerol analogues easily lose a water molecule because of the β-hydroxy keto group. This feature corresponds to shogaol metabolites that give ginger its spicy-sweet fragrance (see Figure 14.1, no. 2). Semwal et al. have expertly reviewed that the ginger phenolic compounds (e.g., [6]-gingerol and [6]-shogaol) have promising cytotoxicity toward a range of human cancer cells (Semwal et al. 2015).

14.3.3 Paradols

Hydrogenation of shogaols resulted in biosynthesis of paradols, which are similar to the corresponding gingerols (see Figure 14.1, no. 3). Biologically, the most considered paradols are [6]-, [8]-, and [10]-paradol (Ma et al. 2021). Associated with suppressive behavior in proliferation and metastases of pancreatic cancer, [6]-paradol and its synthetic derivatives have also displayed antioxidative promoting and chemoprotective potential in cancer (Chung et al. 2001).

14.3.4 Other Phytochemicals

Ginger rhizomes also contain other phenolic metabolites including gingerdiones, gingerdiols, gingerenone-A, curcumin, zingerol, zingerone, and quercetin (see Figure 14.1, nos. 4–10). It is believed that ginger phenolics effectively contribute to promoting human health ranging from anticancer, anti-inflammatory, antimicrobial, antidiabetic ability to the improvement of neural disorders (Ali et al. 2008). On the other hand, several sesquiterpene metabolites, including β-bisabolene, α-curcumene, α-farnesene, β-sesquiphellandrene, and zingiberene, have been recorded as the main active compositions found in ginger essential oil, which attribute diverse biological activities (see Figure 14.1, nos. 11–15) (Yeh et al. 2014).

14.4 GINGER IN CANCER TREATMENT

14.4.1 Ginger Nanoparticles in Cancer

With the aid of the nanotechnology approach using micelles, liposomes, inorganic nanoparticles, and nano-emulsion, some intrinsic behavior of ginger derivatives, namely low bioavailability together with poor solubility, is having potential promise to apply for better ADME (adsorption, desorption, metabolism, and elimination) performance in clinical applications. In this respect, nanomedicine has a unique advantage for making drug delivery to serve cancer therapy. Zhang et al. synthesized nanocarrier lipids and reassembled the lipids into ginger-derived nanovectors (GDNVs) for loading the doxorubicin in colon cancer therapy. Compared with free drug, the conjugated GDNVs with folic acid increased the chemotherapeutic inhibition of Colon-26 tumor growth (Zhang et al. 2016). In order to prevent inflammatory bowel disorder together with colitis-associated cancer, the same authors designed a new approach using edible ginger-derived nanoparticles. The synthesized nanoparticles containing a large number of lipids along with high concentrations of [6]-gingerol and [6]-shogaol potentially increased the repair of the intestine, decreased chronic colitis, and also avoided acute colitis together with colitis-associated cancer (Zhang et al. 2016). Further research about fucoidan/poly-lysine-functionalized layer-by-layer ginger-derived lipid vectors (LbL-GDLVs) targeting P-selectin reported that these molecules can deliver loaded doxorubicin into vascularized colon cancer. In addition to a selective bound of LbL-GDLVs to P-selectin and excellent biocompatibility, experimental results showed that the fucoidan degradation caused the rapid attachment of cancer cells. In *in vivo* studies on HCT-116 and Luc-HT-29 xenografts, Dox-loaded LbL-GDLVs exhibited much better therapeutic efficiency and significant inhibition of colon tumor growth when compared with free doxorubicin (Zhang et al. 2019). Evaluated the cytotoxicity of PEGylated nano-niosomal gingerol against T47D breast cancer cells using MTT assay, Behroozeh et al., realized that better performance of prepared nanoparticles is due to the efficient stability and slower drug release. These properties made a potent IC_{50} value of 0.44 ng/mL toward T47D cells *in vitro* when compared with standard drug (IC_{50} value of 3.804 ng/mL) (Behroozeh et al. 2018).

14.4.2 CELLULAR AND MOLECULAR TARGETS

Cancer, a multifactorial disease, is the second-most prevalent reason for death in both developed and developing countries despite an excessive development of various types of its treatment. There is a wide range of therapeutic options to deal with cancer including surgical procedures, radiation, chemotherapy, and gene therapy because the presently accessible drugs are often accompanied by acute toxicity and diverse side effects. However, replacing these methods with more efficient approaches is the main goal of various studies. Plant preparations along with their natural metabolites have shown remarkable performance as anticancer and chemo-preventive components. The agents with more functional advantages have wider molecular targets in cells. Possessing a vast variety of biological activity, ginger nutraceutical compounds can present novel and captivating inhibitory/therapeutic alternatives for several cancers (Zadorozhna and Mangieri 2021). Therefore, ginger as a well-recognized anticancer agent has various ranges of target molecular mechanisms in the cells, including cell cycle arrest, promotion of cancer cell death, disruption of cellular redox homeostasis, drug sensitivity, and suppression of angiogenesis and metastasis of cancer cells (Figure 14.2).

Modulation of various factors referred to the cell cycle by ginger and its derivatives is a targeted strategy in cancer therapy. Due to the special importance of the cell cycle for cell proliferation and tissue entirety, it is highlighted to specific points by various proteins and kinases that include

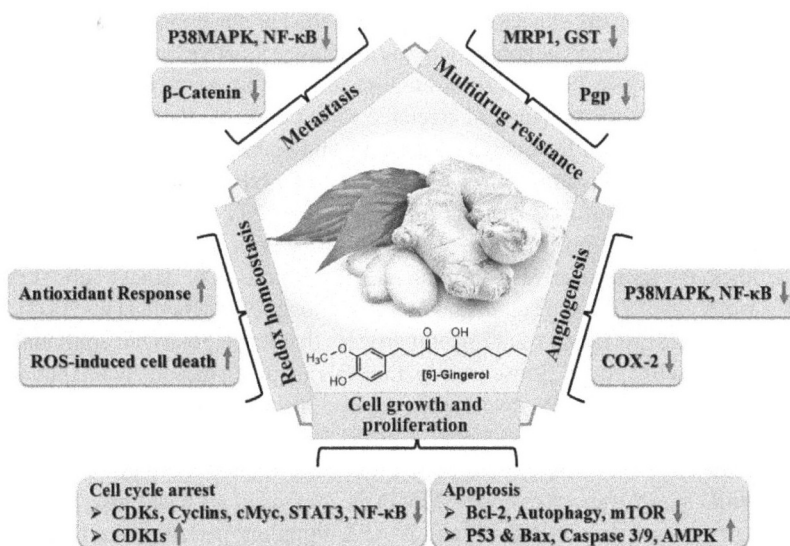

FIGURE 14.2 Molecular targets of ginger. Various cell signaling pathways and biomolecules are affected by ginger and its potent components including the arrest of the cell cycle, induction of cancer cell death, disruption of cellular redox homeostasis, drug sensitivity, and inhibition of angiogenesis and metastasis of cancer cells.

cyclins, cyclin-dependent kinases (CDKs), and CDK inhibitors (CKIs). Upregulation of the cell cycle often stimulates tumorigenesis and cancer development (Vermeulen et al. 2003). As well, the modulation of signal transducer and activator of transcription 3 (STAT3), nuclear factor kappa B (NF-κB), and AKT/mTOR signaling pathways are related to the regulation of the cell cycle (Wani et al. 2018). Apoptosis, commonly known as programmed cell death, is a vital procedure for the efficient removal of dysfunctional cells, carried out by cysteine-aspartate proteases (caspases) and the Bcl-2 family proteins. Two leading apoptotic pathways, the death receptor (extrinsic) and mitochondrial (intrinsic) pathways, are triggered by caspase-8 and caspase-9, respectively. Moreover, ER-stress-related apoptosis is the third pathway that induces apoptosis in cells. Surprisingly, in various cancer cells mutation in the p53 gene is an important cause of apoptosis changes. Ginger and its derivatives induce apoptosis through various pathways in cancer cells. Increased level of death receptor 5 (DR5) in a p53-related manner and pro-apoptotic protein (Bax and truncate Bid) via a reduced level of anti-apoptotic proteins (XIAP, Bcl-2, c-FLIP, and survivin) induce apoptosis process in cells treated with ginger (Lee et al. 2014). On contrary, induction of apoptosis is related to various cell-signaling pathways including the mitogen-activated protein kinase (MAPKs) family, c-Jun N-terminal kinase (JNK), p38 MAPK (p38), and extracellular signal–regulated kinase (ERK). Oxidative stress along with reactive oxygen species (ROS) repletion in cells promote autophagy followed by caspase-independent apoptosis. Therefore, ROS accumulation presents an impressive role in programmed cell death (Luna-Dulcey et al. 2018). The high levels of ROS generation have been identified in all types of cancers supporting some features of tumor formation and development. Despite the increased production of antioxidant proteins in cancer cells to maintain cellular redox balance, a high level of ROS can eventually stimulate cancer progression. One of the most efficient approaches for cancer therapy is to excite the ROS signaling to ROS-induced apoptosis. Increased production of non-enzymatic and enzymatic antioxidant systems by various plant preparations and natural compounds like ginger can enhance the detoxification, therewith inhibiting carcinogenesis (Kathiresan and Govindhan 2016). Therefore, ROS with the dual function can (1) induce an antioxidant response to prevent cancer and (2) utilize the effects of high ROS in inducing cancer cell death (Figure 14.2).

Due to a complex metabolism, cancer cells are in dire need of developing new blood vessels from preexisting endothelium, a phenomenon called angiogenesis. Positive and negative regulators are needed to control this process. In the case of angiogenesis for tumor development and metastatic cascade, many strategies are focused on tumor-related vasculature. On the other hand, NF-κB, COX-2, and p38 MAPK are important factors involved in the angiogenesis and their suppression through various pathways can affect the angiogenesis of cancer cells. NF-κB signaling pathway including IL-8 shows a crucial effect in tumorigenesis through its capacity to regulation the expression of several genes involved in cell proliferation, survival, and angiogenesis. Associated with various documented studies, ginger derivatives can reduce the proliferation of cancer cells through downregulation of various pathways and proteins involving angiogenesis (Rhode et al. 2007). Epithelial–mesenchymal transition (EMT) is a fundamental process that lets a polarized epithelial cell endure various biochemical modifications. Subsequently, the cells acquire a mesenchymal phenotype which contains boosted migratory capacity, invasiveness, raised resistance to apoptosis, and significantly incremented production of ECM components. Cancer metastasis is created by numerous genes and follows various stages. Degradation of the extracellular matrix by matrix metalloproteinases (MMPs) is the initial step. Overexpression of MMPs is associated with cell growth and metastasis. Various signaling pathways such as NF-κB and MAPK signaling pathways are involved in MMPs regulation (Kim et al. 2017). Meanwhile, the Wnt/β-catenin signaling is a main inducer of the EMT event and is imperative in preserving cancer stem cell features. Therefore, targeting Wnt/β-catenin signaling by numerous agents can be an efficient strategy to combat the metastatic power of several types of cancer cells. MicroRNAs (miRs) as non-coding RNAs can posttranscriptionally regulate various gene expressions to control normal cellular acts. Some studies have revealed that the miR-200 family has a critical role in the suppression of Wnt/β-catenin signaling, thereby inhibiting EMT and cancer cell metastasis (Ghahhari and Babashah 2015). Sometimes, cancer cells can use various strategies to increase survival and escape apoptosis. P-glycoprotein (Pgp) overexpression or drug detoxifying proteins, such as glutathione-*S*-transferase (GST) and multidrug resistance-associated protein 1 (MRP1), are responsible for multidrug resistance (MDR) mechanisms in cancer cells. Downregulation of these proteins is related to the sensitivity of cancer cells to chemotherapeutic drugs (Liu et al. 2017). Various researches have been concentrated on ginger function and its potent ingredients in relation to various types of cancers, which are described below.

14.4.2.1 Breast Cancer

As mentioned, ginger ingredients have various molecular targets that inhibit the growth of cancer cells. Bernard et al. have shown that ginger has an inhibitory effect on the growth of human and mouse mammary carcinoma cells. In this study, the inhibitory effects of ginger derivatives were compared and then the effect of [10]-gingerol as the most effective component was determined against T47D, MCF-7, and SK-BR-3 breast cancer cell lines. In addition to the promotion of cell cycle arrest in the S-phase, apoptosis was the related mechanism reported by the authors (Bernard et al. 2017). The ginger ethanolic extract has an effect on various MMP gene expression; thereby, the MMP-9 was found to be the main target gene. Downregulation of MMPs, especially MMP-9 gene expression, can suppress the growth of breast cancer cells and prevent metastasis (Meysami et al. 2021). Compared to HF normal cells, da Silva et al. concluded that [8]- and [10]-gingerols have an inhibitory effect on MDA-MB-231 cell proliferation (da Silva et al. 2012).

14.4.2.2 Colon Cancer

According to various studies, ginger root and its derivatives act as potential agents in the suppression of growth and proliferation of colon cancer cells. Ginger administration in the early and poststages of carcinogenesis considerably decreased circulating lipid peroxidation and significantly promoted the enzymatic (CAT, GST, GPx, GR, and SOD) and non-enzymatic (vitamins A, C, E, and GSH) antioxidants. The Ras-ERK (extracellular signal–regulated kinase) and PI3K/AKT signaling together play a critical role in colorectal carcinogenesis. Thus, they are targets to reveal complicated mechanisms, which are involved in inducing colon cancer cell death. In a synergistic model, combined ginger and Gelam honey treatment cause a cell death indicating the upregulation of caspase 9 and IκB genes complemented by downregulation of KRAS, ERK, AKT, Bcl-xL, and NF-κB (p65) genes (Tahir et al. 2015). At the G_0/G_1 and G_2/M phases, ginger extract induces cell cycle arrest attributing in the S-phase and apoptosis in HCT-116 and HT-29 colon cancer cell lines (Abdullah et al. 2010). Zingerone, an active phenylpropanoid isolated from ginger, considerably increases the production of ROS and lipid peroxidation but decreases cell viability and mitochondrial membrane potential. Moreover, zingerone treatment efficiently increases Bax, caspase-9, and caspase-3 expressions and reduces the expression of Bcl-2 in HCT-116 colon cancer cells (Su et al. 2019).

14.4.2.3 Leukemia Cancer

Obtained results from various studies revealed that supplementation of plant extracts might be a safer method to discover a lasting therapy for leukemia. Induction of cell death, DNA fragmentation and inhibition of Bcl-2 expression has been determined as the main mechanism of action of [6]-gingerol. Suppression of Bcl-2 expression in HL-60 cells might be a reason for the mechanism of [6]-gingerol-induced apoptosis. Meanwhile, [6]-gingerol prompts cell death by interceding ROS species such as hydrogen peroxide (H_2O_2) and superoxide anion ($O_2^{\cdot-}$) (Wang et al. 2003). A novel antileukemic peptide, P2 (sequence: RALGWSCL), isolated from ginger roots has shown acute cytotoxicity. This peptide causes apoptosis via modulation of Bax/Bcl-2 expression and p53 in leukemia cell lines (Chatupheeraphat et al. 2021). Recently, researchers have shown that [6]-shogaol is safe for normal cells but is toxic for primary leukemia cells through inducing apoptosis. This ginger-derived component also induces apoptosis by affecting eukaryotic translation initiation factor 2 alpha (eIF2α) as the main regulator. [6]-Shogaol binds to eIF2α at the N-terminal domain of Ser51 and induces apoptosis through a manner relating dephosphorylation and inactivation of eIF2α (Liu et al. 2013).

14.4.2.4 Liver Cancer

Evidence obtained from some studies suggests the effective action of ginger and its phytochemicals against liver cancer cells. A study has shown that ginger extract suppressed cell proliferation of the HepG-2 cell line through ROS-induced apoptosis (Vijaya Padma et al. 2007). According to another study, [6]-shogaol could efficiently target ROS-mediated apoptosis through caspase activation in the hepatoma cell line (Chen et al. 2007). Weng et al. suggested that pure ginger-derived constituents, [6]-shogaol and [6]-gingerol, have an antimetastatic impact in liver cancer cells by downregulation of MMP-9, urokinase-type plasminogen, and upregulation of TIMP-1 (Weng et al. 2010).

14.4.2.5 Lung Cancer

Various molecular targets have been reported in lung cancer therapy using ginger and its bioactive components. Ginger extract interacts with microtubules and consequently disturbs their structures leading to inducing apoptosis. p53 upregulation and alteration of normal Bax/Bcl-2 ratio are two mechanisms of promoting apoptosis in A549 cancer cells as well. Some morphological changes have been observed after A549 cell treatment using ginger extract (Choudhury et al. 2010). Cellular aging, which is triggered by telomere shortening, is deliberated as one of the main tumor-suppressor mechanisms in eukaryotes. Both [6]-paradol and [6]-shogaol compounds inhibit the human telomerase reverse transcriptase (hTERT) expression as well as telomerase activity in A549 cancer cells (Kaewtunjai et al. 2018). In addition to suppressing hTERT, the ginger extract could repress the expression of c-Myc in A549 lung cancer cells as well. Therefore, the reduction of c-Myc as an hTERT transcription factor reduces the hTERT expression in cells (Ghareghomi et al. 2021). [6]-Shogaol prevented cell proliferation through death promoting and autophagy, but not mainly the apoptosis process. Meanwhile, this component suppressed survival signaling via the AKT/mTOR pathway by delaying the activation of AKT and downstream targets, including the mammalian target of rapamycin (mTOR), forkhead transcription factors (FKHR), and glycogen synthase kinase-3β (GSK-3β) (Hung et al. 2009).

14.4.2.6 Ovarian Cancer

Researches on the antitumor effects of ginger and its related phytoconstituents are ongoing, and researchers are trying to either identify or target the various mechanisms of these nutraceuticals in ovarian cancer cell lines. [6]-Gingerol has been exerted an anti-inflammatory activity through modulation of NF-κB pathway. This pathway can be essentially triggered in ovarian cancer cells and involved in the increase of production of angiogenic factors. Ginger treatment causes suppression of NF-κB signaling as well as reduced secretion of VEGF and IL-8 (Rhode et al. 2007). Also, obtained results from a study have shown that ginger extract exerts anti-ovarian cancer activities via the p53 pathway leading to apoptosis in SKOV-3 cells (Pashaei-Asl et al. 2017). As discussed, ginger extract induces cell death in ovarian cancer cells through apoptosis as well as the promotion of autophagy. Furthermore, its administration resulted in reduced generation of IL-8, PGE-2, and VEGF in ovarian cancer cells (Rhode et al. 2006).

14.4.2.7 Pancreas Cancer

Pancreatic cancer cells, like those of other cancers, can be treated with natural compounds derived from ginger. The ethanolic extract of ginger inhibited cell-cycle development and subsequently prompted human pancreatic cancer cell death. Ginger extract not only can induce autosis, an autophagy-dependent cell death, but also activates AMPK and mTOR as a positive and negative regulator of autophagy, respectively. However, the plant extract increases ROS generation and shows effective anticancer activity through ROS-mediated autosis. [6]-Gingerol suppressed the cell growth through cell cycle arrest at the G1 phase and decreased cyclin A and CDK expression in human pancreatic cancer cells (Park et al. 2006). Numerous mechanisms participate in cell arrest and promotion of apoptosis; thereby, p53 has a pivotal role in the induction of apoptosis in pancreatic cancer cell lines caused by the treatment of ginger extract (Sarami et al. 2020). Zerumbone, a component derived from a kind of subtropical ginger, could inhibit the production of angiogenic factors and NF-κB activity. Further investigations recognized zerumbone as an anti-angiogenic phytochemical in pancreatic cancer (Shamoto et al. 2014).

14.4.2.8 Prostate Cancer

Inhibition of prostate cancer cells is another therapeutic target of ginger natural products. Ginger extract shows a considerable inhibitory effect on cell growth and induces cell death in a variety of prostate cancer cells. It also modulates cell-cycle development and apoptosis regulatory factors, subsequently inducing a caspase-driven, mitochondrially associated apoptosis in human prostate cancer cells (Karna et al. 2012). In addition, Brahmbhatt et al. concluded that a dual combination of ginger secondary metabolites synergistically suppresses PC-3 cell proliferation (Brahmbhatt et al. 2013). A variety of ginger compounds including gingerols [6] and [10] and shogaols [6] and [10] suppresses the PC3R cell growth through the downregulation of glutathione-*S*-transferase (GST) protein and multidrug resistance-associated protein 1 (MRP1) expression (Liu et al. 2017). In prostate cancer cells, [6]-shogaol decreased the activity of interleukin-6–induced STAT3 and suppressed both constitutive and TNF-α–induced NF-κB activity. Furthermore, it also reduced the STAT3 levels and NF-κB-related target genes at the protein level counting cyclin D1, survivin, and c-Myc and controlled mRNA amounts of chemokine, cytokine, cell cycle, and apoptosis-directing genes (Saha et al. 2014).

14.4.2.9 Other Cancer

In addition to the common cancers treated with ginger preparation and its secondary metabolites, few studies have been performed on other cancers; confirming the anticancer properties of ginger. In this context, aqueous extract of ginger reduces oxidative stress along with the level of pro-inflammatory markers in gastric cancer cells. To more extent, [6]-gingerol promotes TRAIL-induced apoptosis through an increase of TRAIL-related caspase-3/7 activation. Also, the compound exhibits a downregulation of cIAP1 expression, which inhibits caspase-3/7 activity by blocking TRAIL-related NF-κB activation (Ishiguro et al. 2007). [6]-Gingerol decreases phosphorylation of AKT Ser473, cyclin-dependent kinases (CDK4), and cyclin D1 and, meantime, increment glycogen synthase kinase (GSK-3β) protein levels. It also prompts cell-cycle arrest and cell-growth suppression via an AKT-GSK3β-cyclin D1 pathway in renal cell carcinoma treatment (Xu et al. 2020). [6]-Shogaol could inhibit HeLa and SiHa cell proliferation and metastasis causing cell cycle arrest in the G2/M phase. Furthermore, [6]-shogaol prompted apoptosis through the mitochondrial pathway by modulation of the p-PI3K, p-Akt, and p-mTOR expression levels (Pei et al. 2021). According to the obtained outcomes recorded by Nazhvani et al., 1′-acetoxychavicol acetate, an isolated phytoconstituent of Malaysian ginger, had an inhibitory impact on the growth of oral squamous cell carcinoma (OSCC) through prompting apoptosis, suppression of NF-κB activation, and reducing the COX-2 and cyclin D1 expression (Nazhvani et al. 2020).

14.5 CLINICAL TRIALS AND CHEMOTHERAPY

Nausea and vomiting are the most prevalent and irritating side properties of chemotherapy. These may lead to various unfavorable effects in patients treated with chemotherapeutic drugs. The adding of ginger (1.5 g/day) to typical anti-emetic therapy (granisetron plus dexamethasone) in patients with progressive breast cancer efficiently decreases the occurrence of nausea for 24 hours postchemotherapy (Panahi et al. 2012). Combined ginger administration with typical anti-emetic agents helps chemotherapy-related vomiting and chemotherapy-induced nausea and vomiting (CINV)-related effects. Also, it has beneficial effects on the possibility of severe vomiting, as well as considerable enhancements on weakness between persons having chemotherapy (Crichton et al. 2019). Ginger and its related phytochemicals potentially affect various pathways involved in the physiological characteristics of CINV. These pathways contain the alterations of significant neuropeptides, vasopressin release, and redox and anti-inflammatory signaling; however, the clinical proof for its usage in treating CINV is presently unclear (Marx et al. 2017). Incidentally, ginger consumption at a dose of 0.5–1.0 g/day meaningfully benefits patients with cancer by decreasing acute chemotherapy-related nausea (Ryan et al. 2012). A randomized, double-blind, and placebo-controlled clinical trial showed that ginger has no obvious impact on CINV improvement in patients with lung cancer receiving cisplatin-based regimes (Li et al. 2018). In recent years, some clinical investigations have been dedicated to fatty acid anabolism contributing not only to various malignancies but also to acute lymphoblastic leukemia (ALL). Ghaeidamini and coworkers designed a study involving 65 clinical samples (40 newly diagnosed ALL children plus 22 healthy control cases). Having cultured the primary cells obtained from the patients, the cancer cells were treated with ginger extract. Results showed that ginger phytochemicals including gingerols, shogaols, paradols, along with zingerone could effectively prevent the activity of fatty acid synthase. These results led to proposing the ability of ginger in the induction of dexamethasone susceptibility and consequent decrease of fatty acid synthase activity (Ghaeidamini et al. 2020).

14.6   TOXICITY AND CAUTIONARY NOTES

According to the US Food and Drug Administration (FDA), ginger is commonly known to be a nontoxic and safe food additive. However, few scientific reports have described some adverse effects related to ginger compositions. A study has reported that [6]-shogaol was established to be less mutagenic when compared with [6]-gingerol (Nakamura and Yamamoto 1983). However, there have not been any new reports proposing the mutagenic manner of ginger. Based on safety evaluation studies, ginger is fully safe even at a very high amount (Kumar et al. 2013). Also, another study in humans shows no record of teratogenicity from usages for early pregnancy nausea that included ginger (Jewell and Young 2003). Concerning the valuable points obtained from various studies, ginger does not have significant cytotoxicity on normal cells. Therefore, ginger and its related phytochemicals are safe with minimal side effects.

14.7   SUMMARY POINTS

- This chapter focuses on anticancer effects of *Z. officinale* (ginger) along with its related phytoconstituents.
- Southeast Asians are less prone to cancer than European people because they use ginger in their daily diet.
- Traditional healers believe that ginger preparations such as tea, infusion, decoction, tincture, and spice are used for nausea, vomiting, abdominal pain, stomachache, arthritis, cystic fibrosis, hyperglycemia, atonic dyspepsia, anorexia, carminative, stimulant, common cold, cough, sore throat, and fevers.
- Besides gingerdiones and gingerdiols, gingerols, shogaols, and paradols are the main bioactive components in ginger rhizomes.
- Nanoparticles as smart nanocarriers enhance the performance of ginger in the ADME (adsorption, desorption, metabolism, and elimination) processes.

- Ginger extract together with its secondary metabolites represses a panel of cancer cells through the following mechanisms: cell cycle arrest, apoptosis, interfering in the redox homeostasis of the cell, drug sensitivity, and deterrence of angiogenesis and metastasis.
- NF-κB, PI3K/AKT/mTOR, and Wnt/β-catenin are significant signaling pathways that are involved in ginger anticancer activity.
- The scientific studies approve the FDA claim regarding ginger safety and its uses in the diet.

REFERENCES

Abdullah, S., S. A. Z. Abidin, N. A. Murad, S. Makpol, W. Z. W. Ngah, and Y. A. M. Yusof. 2010. Ginger extract (*Zingiber officinale*) triggers apoptosis and G0/G1 cells arrest in HCT 116 and HT 29 colon cancer cell lines. *African Journal of Biochemistry Research*:134–142.

Ali, B. H., G. Blunden, M. O. Tanira, and A. Nemmar. 2008. Some phytochemical, pharmacological and toxicological properties of ginger (*Zingiber officinale* Roscoe): A review of recent research. *Food and Chemical Toxicology* 46:409–420.

Behroozeh, A., M. M. Tabrizi, S. M. Kazemi, E. Choupani, N. Kabiri, D. Ilbeigi, A. Heidari Nasab, A. Akbarzadeh Khiyavi, and A. S. Kurdi. 2018. Evaluation the anti-cancer effect of pegylated nano-niosomal gingerol, on breast cancer cell lines (T47D), *in-vitro*. *Asian Pacific Journal of Cancer Prevention* 19:645–648.

Bernard, M. M., J. R. McConnery, and D. W. Hoskin. 2017. [10]-Gingerol, a major phenolic constituent of ginger root, induces cell cycle arrest and apoptosis in triple-negative breast cancer cells. *Experimental and Molecular Pathology* 102:370–376.

Brahmbhatt, M., S. R. Gundala, G. Asif, S. A. Shamsi, and R. Aneja. 2013. Ginger phytochemicals exhibit synergy to inhibit prostate cancer cell proliferation. *Nutrition and Cancer* 65:263–272.

Chatupheeraphat, C., S. Roytrakul, N. Phaonakrop, K. Deesrisak, S. Krobthong, U. Anurathapan, and D. Tanyong. 2021. A novel peptide derived from ginger induces apoptosis through the modulation of p53, BAX, and BCL2 expression in leukemic cell lines. *Planta Medica* 87:560–569.

Chen, C.-Y., T.-Z. Liu, Y.-W. Liu, W.-C. Tseng, R. H. Liu, F.-J. Lu, Y.-S. Lin, S.-H. Kuo, and C.-H. Chen. 2007. 6-shogaol (alkanone from ginger) induces apoptotic cell death of human hepatoma p53 mutant Mahlavu subline via an oxidative stress-mediated caspase-dependent mechanism. *Journal of Agricultural and Food Chemistry* 55:948–954.

Choudhury, D., A. Das, A. Bhattacharya, and G. Chakrabarti. 2010. Aqueous extract of ginger shows antiproliferative activity through disruption of microtubule network of cancer cells. *Food and Chemical Toxicology* 48:2872–2880.

Chung, W.-Y., Y.-J. Jung, Y.-J. Surh, S.-S. Lee, and K.-K. Park. 2001. Antioxidative and antitumor promoting effects of [6]-paradol and its homologs. *Mutation Research/Genetic Toxicology and Environmental Mutagenesis* 496:199–206.

Crichton, M., S. Marshall, W. Marx, A. L. McCarthy, and E. Isenring. 2019. Efficacy of ginger (*Zingiber officinale*) in ameliorating chemotherapy-induced nausea and vomiting and chemotherapy-related outcomes: A systematic review update and meta-analysis. *Journal of the Academy of Nutrition and Dietetics* 119:2055–2068.

da Silva, J. A., A. B. Becceneri, H. S. Mutti, A. C. B. M. Martin, J. B. Fernandes, P. C. Vieira, and M. R. Cominetti. 2012. Purification and differential biological effects of ginger-derived substances on normal and tumor cell lines. *Journal of Chromatography B* 903:157–162.

Ghaeidamini, M. H., S. Rahgozar, S. B. Rahimi, A. Safavi, and E. S. Ghodousi. 2020. Fatty acid synthase, a novel poor prognostic factor for acute lymphoblastic leukemia which can be targeted by ginger extract. *Scientific Reports* 10:20952.

Ghahhari, N. M., and S. Babashah. 2015. Interplay between microRNAs and WNT/β-catenin signalling pathway regulates epithelial: Mesenchymal transition in cancer. *European Journal of Cancer* 51:1638–1649.

Ghareghomi, S., S. Ahmadian, N. Zarghami, and H. Kahroba. 2021. Fundamental insights into the interaction between telomerase/TERT and intracellular signaling pathways. *Biochimie* 181:12–24.

Hung, J.-Y., Y.-L. Hsu, C.-T. Li, Y.-Ch. Ko, W.-C. Ni, M.-S. Huang, and P.-L. Kuo. 2009. 6-Shogaol, an active constituent of dietary ginger, induces autophagy by inhibiting the AKT/mTOR pathway in human non–small cell lung cancer A549 cells. *Journal of Agricultural and Food Chemistry* 57:9809–9816.

Ishiguro, K., T. Ando, O. Maeda, N. Ohmiya, Y. Niwa, K. Kadomatsu, and H. Goto. 2007. Ginger ingredients reduce viability of gastric cancer cells via distinct mechanisms. *Biochemical and Biophysical Research Communications* 362:218–223.

Jewell, D., and G. Young. 2003. Interventions for nausea and vomiting in early pregnancy. *Cochrane Database of Systematic Reviews* (4):CD000145. doi:10.1002/14651858.CD000145

Kaewtunjai, N., R. Wongpoomchai, A. Imsumran, W. Pompimon, A. Athipornchai, A. Suksamrarn, T. R. Lee, and W. Tuntiwechapikul. 2018. Ginger extract promotes telomere shortening and cellular senescence in A549 lung cancer cells. *ACS Omega* 3:18572–18581.

Karna, P., S. Chagani, S. R. Gundala, P. C. G. Rida, G. Asif, V. Sharma, M. V. Gupta, and R. Aneja. 2012. Benefits of whole ginger extract in prostate cancer. *British Journal of Nutrition* 107:473–484.

Kathiresan, S., and A. Govindhan. 2016. [6]-Shogaol, a novel chemopreventor in 7, 12-dimethylbenz [a] anthracene-induced hamster buccal pouch carcinogenesis. *Phytotherapy Research* 30:646–653.

Kim, Y.-J., Y. Jeon, T. Kim, W.-C. Lim, J. Ham, Y. N. Park, T.-J. Kim, and H. Ko. 2017. Combined treatment with zingerone and its novel derivative synergistically inhibits TGF-β1 induced epithelial-mesenchymal transition, migration and invasion of human hepatocellular carcinoma cells. *Bioorganic & Medicinal Chemistry Letters* 27:1081–1088.

Kumar, S., K. Saxena, U. N. Singh, and R. Saxena. 2013. Anti-inflammatory action of ginger: A critical review in anemia of inflammation and its future aspects. *International Journal of Herbal Medicine* 1:16–20.

Lee, D.-H., D.-W. Kim, C.-H. Jung, Y. J. Lee, and D. Park. 2014. Gingerol sensitizes TRAIL-induced apoptotic cell death of glioblastoma cells. *Toxicology and Applied Pharmacology* 279:253–265.

Li, X., Y. Qin, W. Liu, X.-y. Zhou, Y.-n. Li, and L.-y. Wang. 2018. Efficacy of ginger in ameliorating acute and delayed chemotherapy-induced nausea and vomiting among patients with lung cancer receiving cisplatin-based regimens: A randomized controlled trial. *Integrative Cancer Therapies* 17:747–754.

Liu, C.-M., C.-L. Kao, Y.-T. Tseng, Y.-C. Lo, and C.-Y. Chen. 2017. Ginger phytochemicals inhibit cell growth and modulate drug resistance factors in docetaxel resistant prostate cancer cell. *Molecules* 22:1477. doi:10.3390/molecules22091477

Liu, Q., Y.-B. Peng, Z. Zhou, L.-W. Qi, M. Zhang, N. Gao, E.-H. Liu, and P. Li. 2013. 6-Shogaol induces apoptosis in human leukemia cells through a process involving caspase-mediated cleavage of eIF2α. *Molecular Cancer* 12:1–12.

Luna-Dulcey, L., R. Tomasin, M. A. Naves, J. A. da Silva, and M. R. Cominetti. 2018. Autophagy-dependent apoptosis is triggered by a semi-synthetic [6]-gingerol analogue in triple negative breast cancer cells. *Oncotarget* 9:30787–30804.

Ma, R.-H., Z.-J. Ni, Y.-Y. Zhu, K. Thakur, F. Zhang, Y.-Y. Zhang, F. Hu, J.-G. Zhang, and Z.-J. Wei. 2021. A recent update on the multifaceted health benefits associated with ginger and its bioactive components. *Food & Function* 12:519–542.

Mahomoodally, M. F., M. Z. Aumeeruddy, K. R. R. Rengasamy, S. Roshan, S. Hammad, J. Pandohee, X. Hu, and G. Zengin. 2021. Ginger and its active compounds in cancer therapy: From folk uses to nano-therapeutic applications. *Seminars in Cancer Biology* 69:140–149.

Marx, W., K. Ried, A. L. McCarthy, L. Vitetta, A. Sali, D. McKavanagh, and L. Isenring. 2017. Ginger-Mechanism of action in chemotherapy-induced nausea and vomiting: A review. *Critical Reviews in Food Science and Nutrition* 57:141–146.

Meysami, M., M. Rahaie, A. Ebrahimi, and F. Samiee. 2021. Four matrix metalloproteinase genes involved in murine breast cancer affected by ginger extract. *Gene Reports* 25:101332.

Moghaddasi, M. S., and H. H. Kashani. 2012. Ginger (*Zingiber officinale*): A review. *Journal of Medicinal Plants Research* 6:4255–4258.

Nakamura, H., and T. Yamamoto. 1983. The active part of the [6]-gingerol molecule in mutagenesis. *Mutation Research Letters* 122:87–94.

Nazhvani, A. D., N. Sarafraz, F. Askari, F. Heidari, and M. Razmkhah. 2020. Anti-cancer effects of traditional medicinal herbs on oral squamous cell carcinoma. *Asian Pacific Journal of Cancer Prevention* 21:479–484.

Panahi, Y., A. Saadat, A. Sahebkar, F. Hashemian, M. Taghikhani, and E. Abolhasani. 2012. Effect of ginger on acute and delayed chemotherapy-induced nausea and vomiting: A pilot, randomized, open-label clinical trial. *Integrative Cancer Therapies* 11:204–211.

Park, Y. J., J. Wen, S. Bang, S. W. Park, and S. Y. Song. 2006. [6]-Gingerol induces cell cycle arrest and cell death of mutant p53-expressing pancreatic cancer cells. *Yonsei Medical Journal* 47:688–697.

Pashaei-Asl, R., F. Pashaei-Asl, P. M. Gharabaghi, K. Khodadadi, M. Ebrahimi, E. Ebrahimie, and M. Pashaiasl. 2017. The inhibitory effect of ginger extract on ovarian cancer cell line; application of systems biology. *Advanced Pharmaceutical Bulletin* 7:241–249.

Pei, X.-D., Z.-L. He, H.-L. Yao, J.-S. Xiao, L. Li, J.-Z. Gu, P.-Z. Shi, J.-H. Wang, and L.-H. Jiang. 2021. 6-Shogaol from ginger shows anti-tumor effect in cervical carcinoma via PI3K/Akt/mTOR pathway. *European Journal of Nutrition* 60:2781–2793.

Remadevi, R., E. Surendran, and P. N. Ravindran. 2016. Properties and medicinal uses of ginger. In *Ginger*, pp. 509–528. CRC Press.

Rhode, J., S. Fogoros, S. Zick, H. Wahl, K. A. Griffith, J. Huang, and J. R. Liu. 2007. Ginger inhibits cell growth and modulates angiogenic factors in ovarian cancer cells. *BMC Complementary and Alternative Medicine* 7:1–9. doi:10.1186/1472-6882-7-44

Rhode, J. M., J. Huang, S. Fogoros, L. Tan, S. Zick, and J. R. Liu. 2006. Ginger induces apoptosis and autophagocytosis in ovarian cancer cells. *American Association for Cancer Research* 47:1058.

Ryan, J. L., C. E. Heckler, J. A. Roscoe, S. R. Dakhil, J. Kirshner, P. J. Flynn, J. T. Hickok, and G. R. Morrow. 2012. Ginger (*Zingiber officinale*) reduces acute chemotherapy-induced nausea: A URCC CCOP study of 576 patients. *Supportive Care in Cancer* 20:1479–1489.

Saha, A., J. Blando, E. Silver, L. Beltran, J. Sessler, and J. DiGiovanni. 2014. 6-Shogaol from dried ginger inhibits growth of prostate cancer cells both *in vitro* and *in vivo* through inhibition of STAT3 and NF-κB signaling. *Cancer Prevention Research* 7:627–638.

Sarami, S., M. Dadmanesh, Z. M. Hassan, and K. Ghorban. 2020. Study on the effect of ethanol ginger extract on cell viability and p53 level in breast and pancreatic cancer. *Archives of Pharmacy Practice* 1:115.

Semwal, R. B., D. K. Semwal, S. Combrinck, and A. M. Viljoen. 2015. Gingerols and shogaols: Important nutraceutical principles from ginger. *Phytochemistry* 117:554–568.

Shahrajabian, M. H., S. U. N. Wenli, and Q. Cheng. 2019. Pharmacological uses and health benefits of ginger (*Zingiber officinale*) in traditional Asian and ancient Chinese medicine, and modern practice. *Notulae Scientia Biologicae* 11:309–319.

Shamoto, T., Y. Matsuo, T. Shibata, K. Tsuboi, T. Nagasaki, H. Takahashi, H. Funahashi, Y. Okada, and H. Takeyama. 2014. Zerumbone inhibits angiogenesis by blocking NF-κB activity in pancreatic cancer. *Pancreas* 43:396–404.

Su, P., V. P. Veeraraghavan, S. K. Mohan, and W. Lu. 2019. A ginger derivative, zingerone: A phenolic compound-induces ROS-mediated apoptosis in colon cancer cells (HCT-116). *Journal of Biochemical and Molecular Toxicology* 33:e22403.

Tahir, A. A., N. F. A. Sani, N. A. M. S. Makpol, W. Z. W. Ngah, and Y. A. M. Yusof. 2015. Combined ginger extract & Gelam honey modulate Ras/ERK and PI3K/AKT pathway genes in colon cancer HT29 cells. *Nutrition Journal* 14:1–10.

Vermeulen, K., Z. N. Berneman, and D. R. Van Bockstaele. 2003. Cell cycle and apoptosis. *Cell Proliferation* 36:165–175.

Vijaya Padma, V., S. A. D. Christie, and K. M. Ramkuma. 2007. Induction of apoptosis by Ginger in HEp-2 cell line is mediated by reactive oxygen species. *Basic & Clinical Pharmacology & Toxicology* 100:302–307.

Wang, C. C., L. G. Chen, L. T. Lee, and L.-L. Yang. 2003. Effects of 6-gingerol, an antioxidant from ginger, on inducing apoptosis in human leukemic HL-60 cells. *In Vivo* 17:641–645.

Wani, N. A., B. Zhang, K.-y. Teng, J. M. Barajas, T. Motiwala, P. Hu, L. Yu, R. Brüschweiler, K. Ghoshal, and S. T. Jacob. 2018. Reprograming of glucose metabolism by zerumbone suppresses hepatocarcinogenesis. *Molecular Cancer Research* 16:256–268.

Weng, C.-J., C.-F. Wu, H.-W. Huang, C.-T. Ho, and G.-C. Yen. 2010. Anti-invasion effects of 6-shogaol and 6-gingerol, two active components in ginger, on human hepatocarcinoma cells. *Molecular Nutrition & Food Research* 54 (11):1618–1627.

Xu, S., H. Zhang, T. Liu, W. Yang, W. Lv, D. He, P. Guo, and L. Li. 2020. 6-Gingerol induces cell-cycle G1-phase arrest through AKT-GSK 3β-cyclin D1 pathway in renal-cell carcinoma. *Cancer Chemotherapy and Pharmacology* 85:379–390.

Yeh, H.-y., C.-h. Chuang, H.-c. Chen, C.-j. Wan, T.-l. Chen, and L.-y. Lin. 2014. Bioactive components analysis of two various gingers (*Zingiber officinale* Roscoe) and antioxidant effect of ginger extracts. *LWT-Food Science and Technology* 55:329–334.

Zadorozhna, M., and D. Mangieri. 2021. Mechanisms of chemopreventive and therapeutic proprieties of ginger extracts in cancer. *International Journal of Molecular Sciences* 22:6599. doi:10.3390/ijms22126599

Zhang, M., E. Viennois, M. Prasad, Y. Zhang, L. Wang, Z. Zhang, M. K. Han, B. Xiao, C. Xu, and S. Srinivasan. 2016. Edible ginger-derived nanoparticles: A novel therapeutic approach for the prevention and treatment of inflammatory bowel disease and colitis-associated cancer. *Biomaterials* 101:321–340.

Zhang, M., B. Xiao, H. Wang, M. K. Han, Z. Zhang, E. Viennois, C. Xu, and D. Merlin. 2016. Edible ginger-derived nano-lipids loaded with doxorubicin as a novel drug-delivery approach for colon cancer therapy. *Molecular Therapy* 24:1783–1796.

Zhang, M., C. Yang, X. Yan, J. Sung, P. Garg, and D. Merlin. 2019. Highly biocompatible functionalized layer-by-layer ginger lipid nano vectors targeting p-Selectin for delivery of doxorubicin to treat Colon Cancer. *Advanced Therapeutics* 2:1900129.

15 Love Apple (*Paris polyphylla* Smith) and Oral Cancer Investigations
Antiproliferative and Apoptosis-Inducing Effects of Phytochemical Agents on Oral Cancer Cells

Arcadius Puwein and Shiny C. Thomas

15.1 INTRODUCTION

Medicinal plants play a major role in the primary health care of many developing countries. They are widely exploited for their curative potential. Jeyachandran et al. (2010) and Saslis-Lagoudakis et al. (2014) estimated that about 80% of the world's population relies on traditional medicine for their primary health care. In fact, numerous modern medicines were developed from many years of beliefs and practices of plant-based traditional medicine (Aburjai et al. 2007). Medicinal plants contain rich sources of secondary metabolites like flavonoids, alkaloids, glycosides, amines, steroids, fatty acids, and related constituents. These secondary metabolites have been extensively used in the drug and pharmaceutical industry. Such secondary metabolites are distributed in various parts of the plant such as the root, stem, leaves, fruits, and flowers. Traditionally, there are numerous species of plants and herbs that are known worldwide to have medicinal value but are not validated. There are about 6000 medicinal plants in India, of which only 3000 have been proven to have medicinal value, and still many remain unexplored (Jagatheeswari et al. 2013).

Some medicinal plants exhibit anticancer bioactivities. The search for anticancer agents from medicinal plants started in the early 1950s (Cragg and Newman 2005). In our modern era, investigations on natural products have gained momentum for biological significance. It was reported that over 3000 species of medicinal plants possess anticancer properties (Graham et al. 2000). The surveys of the National Cancer Institute (USA) showed that 75% of all anticancer drugs are in one way or another based on natural resources (Newman et al. 2016). Northeast India is particularly rich in medicinal plants which exhibit anticancer activities. *Paris polyphylla* Smith is one of the numerous herbs that are available in the region that possess anticancer agents.

15.2 BACKGROUND

P. polyphylla was documented for the first time in the Chinese Pharmacopeia in 1985 (Liang et al. 2000). It is an erect and herbaceous plant that thrives well in an environment where human interference is almost negligible. The herb has a spider-like flower that throws out long, thread-like, yellowish-green petals throughout most of the warm summer months and into the autumn. The genus name is derived from *pars*, referring to the symmetry of the plant. The species *polyphylla* means "many leaves"; *poly* means "many" and *phyla* means "leaves" (Shah et al. 2012). *P. polyphylla*, which is known in English as "love apple," belongs to the family of Melanthiaceae (earlier

Trilliaceae or Liliaceae), as reported by Long et al. (2003). The classification of this herb is complicated and remains unresolved to date.

P. polyphylla has been traditionally used to relieve various ailments. The people of Meghalaya in the northeastern part of India have been using the paste of rhizomes to treat cuts, snake bites, and relieve and cure bone fractures. It is popularly known as *sohbsein* in the local (Khasi) language, although the local name *sohbsein* represents also other species like *Arisaema tortuosum* (Puwein and Thomas 2020). The herb is well-known in traditional Chinese medicine (TCM). It was reported to have been used for traumatic injuries, abscess, parotitis, hemostatic analgesia, anti-inflammation, relieving sore throat, snake bites, and bruises (Yun et al. 2007; Chinese Pharmacopoeia 2010).

P. polyphylla is a shade-loving plant and grows under a canopy closure of more than 80%, at an altitude of 1300–2500 m above sea level (Deb et al. 2015). The herb grows mainly in a forest where bamboo groves, grassy or rocky slopes, stream-sides, mixed conifer forests, and scrub thickets thrive abundantly. It is a slow-germinating herb that takes about 7 months to sprout from the seed. *P. polyphylla* was found to grow well inside the deep forest where anthropogenic activities (e.g., timbering, shifting cultivation) and other interventions are insignificant or absent. It grows in humus-rich and well-drained soil. Waterlogging is found to be toxic for the germination and flowering of the herb. The plant can rehabilitate in artificial habitats while maintaining similar temperatures and at similar altitudes. It was observed that plants that lack inflorescence are usually shorter in height. The research on its adaptability has displayed that when the whole plant was taken outside its natural habitat, it showed signs of growth in the initial year but failed to flower in an artificial habitat. Even if the plant flowered, it rapidly withered without seed formation. It was also observed that this species thrives well in the presence of some commonly associated plants within a 5 m perimeter. These commonly associated plants include trees, herbs, and climbers. Further research is required to understand agronomy, the conditions for their growth, and their mode of interaction with one another (Deb et al. 2015).

15.3 PHYTOCHEMICAL COMPOUNDS OF *P. POLYPHYLLA*

Most bioactive compounds of *P. polyphylla* were isolated from the rhizomes, but recently few chemical constituents were also extracted from the stems and leaves. Many bioactive compounds isolated from the herb are vital for various cancer treatments. Medicinal plants contain various phytochemical compounds such as alkaloids, flavonoids, saponins, carbohydrates, glycosides, cardiac glycosides, terpenoids, sterols, quinones, phenols, and tannins (Cragg and Newman 2001). It was reported that nearly 98 compounds were isolated and identified from the rhizome of the herb, which includes more than 30 steroidal saponins (Rajsekhar et al. 2016).

15.4 PHYTOCHEMICAL COMPOUNDS ISOLATED FROM RHIZOMES AND LEAVES

The rhizomes of *P. polyphylla* are rich in active components such as steroidal saponins, dioscin, polyphyllin D, and balanitin 7 (Fu et al. 2007). Paris saponins account for more than 80% of the total compounds of *P. polyphylla*. Some important saponin compounds isolated from this plant are Paris saponin I, Paris saponin II, Paris saponin III, polyphyllin VI, and polyphyllin VII (Wu et al. 2004). It has been observed that rhizomes collected from different geographical locations showed some variations in the types of compounds isolated and identified. This might be due to the influence of biotic and abiotic factors. Rhizomes collected from Nepal were seen to contain active compounds such as Saponin-1, Polyphyllin C, Polyphyllin D, Przewalskinone B, Stigmasterol, and Stigmasterol-3-*O*-β-D-glucoside (Devkota 2005). The rhizomes collected from China showed the presence of bioactive compounds such as diosgenin, pennogenin, steroid saponins, dioscin, polyphyllin D, balanitin 7, saponin I, saponin II, and saponin III, polyphyllin VI, and polyphyllin VII (Yun et al. 2007; Fu et al. 2007; Wu *et al.* 2004). Recently, the isolation of compounds from the stems and leaves was reported. This is significant, as leaves and stems can regenerate every year. Photochemical analysis of the ethanol extracts of stems and leaves of *P. polyphylla* var. *yunnanensis* has yielded six new spirostanol saponins, named chonglouosides SL-1 to SL-6 (1–6), along with one sapogenin and 24 steroidal saponins (Qin et al. 2012).

15.5 EFFECT OF BIOTIC AND ABIOTIC FACTORS IN ACCUMULATION OF SECONDARY METABOLITES

Recently, the rhizomes of *P. polyphylla* collected from Meghalaya in the northeastern part of India indicated the presence of fatty acid esters and other steroidal saponins, as indicated in Table 15.1. The identification of novel compounds from *P. polyphylla* Smith collected from Meghalaya could be due to various factors. It was reported that the accumulation of secondary metabolites in medicinal plants is influenced by both abiotic and biotic factors (Ma and Zhang 2010; Wink 2008). Many plants depend on various external factors such as light, temperature, soil water, soil fertility, and salinity for growth, development, their ability to synthesize secondary metabolites, and eventually leading to the change of overall production of active constituents as investigated by Verma and Shukla (2015) and Ferrandino and Lovisolo (2014). Further, it was observed that medicinal plants require an appropriate intensity of light for photosynthesis, and this affects the quality and accumulation of total alkaloid yields, total flavonoids, and phenolic acids. For example, *Centilla asiatica* produced high contents of secondary metabolites when grown under 70% shade conditions (Li et al. 2018). It was reported that when *Camptotheca acuminate* was grown in 27% sunlight, it can elevate the concentration of camptothecin (Liu et al. 1997). *P. polyphylla* was observed as a shade-loving plant and grows under the canopy closure of more than 80%, at an altitude of 1300–2500 m above sea level (Liang et al. 2000). It grows mainly in a forest with bamboo groves, grassy or rocky slopes, stream-sides, mixed conifer forests, and shrub thickets.

Moreover, the interactions of *P. polyphylla* with the associated plants also have a vital role in the production of secondary metabolites of this plant. Biotic interactions with plant biochemistry and plant physiology affect the synthesis of active compounds (Briskin 2000). This species thrives well in the presence of some commonly associated species (*Dioscorea* sp. *Bidens pilosa*, *Curculigo capitulate*, *Eupatorium adenophorum*, *Hottuynia cordata*, *Lycopodium* sp., and *Smilax* sp.) within a 5 m perimeter (Deb et al. 2015).

The phytochemical investigation of *P. polyphylla* Smith collected from Meghalaya contains bioactive compounds such as fatty acid esters, phytosterols, and steroidal saponins that showed anticancer activities. The novel compounds isolated and identified from *P. polyphylla* Smith collected from Meghalaya have their unique phytoconstituents as compared to those investigated in China. This study also suggests that the same species collected from different locations could show variation in the content of bioactive constituents due to the influence of biotic and abiotic factors.

TABLE 15.1
Compounds Identified with Reported Bioactivity from Fraction of *Paris polyphylla* by GC-MS

Name of Compound	Molecular Structure	Biological Activity
Heptadecanoic acid, ethyl ester	$C_{18}H_{36}O_2$	Antimicrobial
10-Bromodecanoic acid, ethyl ester	$C_{12}H_{23}BrO_2$	Antimicrobial and antioxidant
10-Undecenoic acid, ethyl ester	$C_{13}H_{24}O_2$	Antioxidant, anticancer
Octadecanoic acid, 17-methyl-, methyl ester	$C_{27}H_{42}O_2$	Anti-inflammatory, anti-arthritis
Diosgenin	$C_{27}H_{42}O_3$	Anticancer
Des-n-solasodine	$C_{27}H_{42}O_2$	Anticancer

The presence of the novel compounds as indicated by the GC-MS analysis (Table 15.1) will boost future research toward exploring new bioactive compounds that are yet to be identified. These phytochemical compounds isolated and identified from *P. polyphylla* could be assayed to treat various types of cancer which have become a global burden of disease.

15.6 CANCER: A COMPLEX AND GLOBAL BURDEN OF DISEASE

Cancer is a complex genetic disease. It arises from a single cell that has undergone mutation. Cancer cells contain many alterations which accumulate as tumors develop. Alteration of genes is due to the mutations that occurred in two broad classes of genes: proto-oncogenes and tumor suppressor genes. The proto-oncogenes encode proteins that control cell proliferation, differentiation, cell cycle control, and apoptosis. The tumor suppressor genes restrain cell proliferation by arresting progression through the cell cycle and block differentiation. The complex process of proliferation is controlled and regulated through the cell cycle. The cell cycle involves a series of events that result in DNA duplication and cell division. In normal cells, the process is carefully regulated. On the other hand, in tumor cells, the process results in the progression of cells with damaged DNA through the cell cycle due to mutations in the genes associated with the cell cycle (Macdonald et al. 2004). Based on the GLOBOCAN 2018 estimation of cancer incidence and mortality produced by the International Agency for Research on Cancer (IARC), there were 18.1 million new cancer cases and 9.6 million cancer deaths in 2018. Lung cancer is the most commonly diagnosed cancer in both sexes (11.6% of the total cases) and mortality of 18.4% of the total cancer deaths. Lung cancer has the highest mortality death rate among males, and breast cancer is the most commonly diagnosed cancer and the leading cause of death in females. However, these incidences and mortality rates of cancer vary across and within countries (Bray et al. 2018). This complex disease has become a global burden. The increasing burden due to cancer disease poses a threat to human health. Different countries are threatened by different types of cancer, depending mainly on their lifestyle and food habits.

15.7 ORAL CANCER: A BURDEN IN NORTHEAST INDIA

Oral cancer represents one of the most common types and yet scarcely known malignancies worldwide (Bray et al. 2018). It is the predominant cancer in the Indian subcontinent, ranking among the top three types of cancer in the country. Oral cancer has been reported to be the most commonly diagnosed cancer in India among males. Sankaranarayanan et al. (2005) have reported that oral cancer accounts for about 30% of all types of cancer in India. Oral cancer is the most commonly diagnosed cancer (16.1% of the total cases) among males in India (Bray et al. 2018). This is mainly due to smoking and chewing tobacco-related products, alcohol consumption, human papilloma virus (HPV), and exposure to ultraviolet radiation as investigated by Petti (2008).

The northeastern region has the highest incidence of cancer in India (Dutta et al. 2019). The incidence and death rate due to oral cancer is very high in Northeast India because of smoked and smokeless tobacco use (Sapkota et al. 2007). Mathur et al. (2020) have reported in the national cancer registry program that the East Khasi Hills district of Meghalaya had the highest relative proportion of cancers associated with the use of tobacco, with 70.4% and 46.5% for males and females, respectively. Despite the remarkable advancements made in the major clinical treatments for oral cancer such as surgery, chemotherapy, and radiotherapy, these non-selective treatments cause serious side effects and show minimal improvement (Cosgrove and Salani 2018). Further, oral cancer in Northeast India is interrelated with factors like nutrition, health care, and poor living conditions. Aggravating to these factors, according to Rao et al. (2013), oral cancer is mostly diagnosed at later stages which results in low treatment outcomes and high costs. This prompts numerous researchers to look for alternative treatments which are effective, devoid of side effects, and have low-cost treatment. Apoptosis occurs normally during development and aging to maintain cell populations or as a defense mechanism against some agents and is a well-established effective treatment against cancers.

15.8 INHIBITION OF ORAL CANCER VIA APOPTOSIS

Apoptosis, or programmed cell death, is a series of genetically controlled events that result in the removal of unwanted cells without disruption of tissues. It differs from cell necrosis, where cells swell and burst, spilling their contents over their neighbors and eliciting an inflammatory response (Kerr et al. 1972). Cancer treatment therapies target apoptotic pathways by increasing apoptosis in cells and thus preventing cancer, as reported by Kalimuthu and Se-Kwon (2013) and Zhao et al. (2014). Antioxidants and phytochemicals present in medicinal plants have been found to arrest the growth of cancer cells by promoting apoptosis, thus preventing the proliferation of cancer (Alok et al. 2014). The mechanism of such antioxidants and phytochemicals in the process of apoptosis is highly complex and sophisticated.

Inhibition of apoptotic cell death is a highly regulated process via a complex signaling cascade. Apoptosis is featured by cell shrinkage, plasma membrane blebbing, cell detachment, externalization of phosphatidylserine, nuclear condensation, and ultimately DNA fragmentation (Taylor et al. 2008; Henry et al. 2013). A large number of assays are available to detect the above-mentioned features and count apoptotic cells. Most apoptosis assays detect cytomorphological alterations, DNA fragmentation, detection of caspases, cleaved substrates, regulators and inhibitors, membrane alterations, detection of apoptosis in whole mounts, and mitochondrial assays. However, many features of apoptosis and necrosis can overlap, so it is necessary to employ two or more distinct assays to confirm if cell death is occurring through apoptosis (Elmore 2007).

Inhibition of apoptotic cells death consists of two main apoptotic pathways: the extrinsic or death receptor pathway and the intrinsic or mitochondrial pathway. However, it is evidenced that the two pathways are linked and that molecules in one pathway can influence the other, as demonstrated by Igney and Krammer (2002). There is an additional pathway called the perforin/granzyme pathway that can induce apoptosis via either granzyme B or granzyme A. The three pathways converge on the execution pathway. The pathway is initiated by the cleavage of caspase-3 and undergoes a series of events leading to the uptake by the phagocytic cells (Martinvalet et al. 2005).

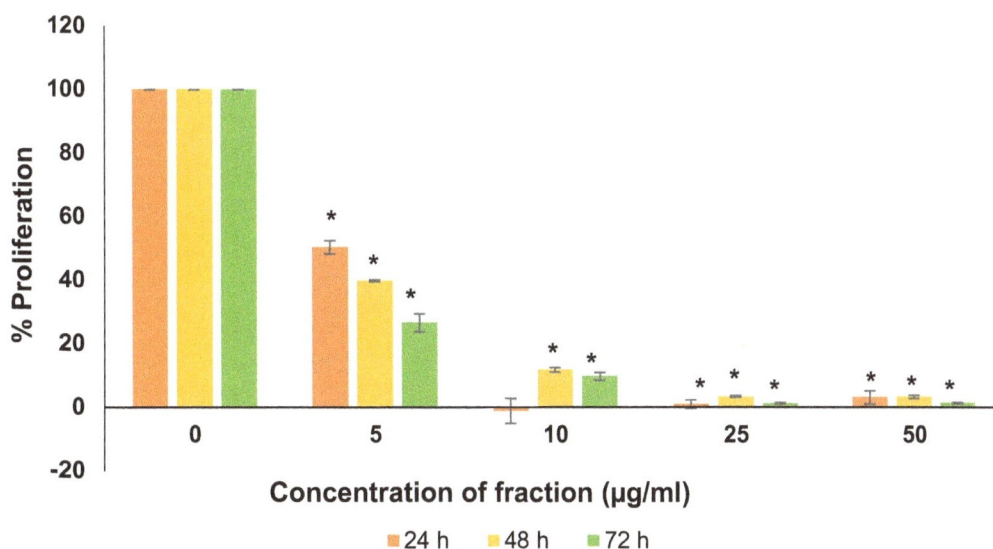

FIGURE 15.1 MTT assay showing the proliferation of SAS cells after exposure to increasing concentrations for 24, 48, and 72 hours. * = $p \leq 0.05$ vs. control.

15.9   *P. POLYPHYLLA* COMPOUNDS INHIBIT PROLIFERATION OF ORAL CANCER CELL

The main mechanism of inhibition of *P. polyphylla* against various types of cancer is apoptosis. The rhizome of *P. polyphylla* contains several active compounds which showed anticancer activity on several cell lines (Ji et al. 2001). Compounds such as diosgenin, pennogenin, steroid saponins, dioscin, polyphyllin D, balanitin 7, saponin I, saponin II, and saponin III, polyphyllin VI, and polyphyllin VII decreased proliferation of cancerous cells (Yun et al. 2007; Fu et al. 2007; Wu et al. 2004). Steroidal saponins are the main antitumor active components that inhibit the proliferation of oral cancer. The induction of apoptosis is triggered through different mechanisms in different types of cancers. The increased percentage of apoptosis of cancer cells is confirmed by different markers. These different markers are confirmed by increased expression of pro-apoptotic and apoptotic proteins, activation of caspase, DNA damage, increased expression of connexion 26, cell cycle arrest, the polarization of mitochondrial membrane potential, and DNA fragmentation (Yang et al. 2016; Ke et al. 2016; Li et al. 2012; Gao et al. 2011).

15.10   EFFECT OF *P. POLYPHYLLA* EXTRACTS ON PROLIFERATION AND APOPTOSIS OF SAS ORAL CELLS

When MTT assay was performed to examine the effect of ethanol and methanol crude extracts of the herb, the extracts decreased the cells' viability rate in a concentration-dependent manner. When plant extracts were exposed to SAS cells at various concentrations (10, 50, 250, 500, and 1000 µg/mL), the extracts inhibited the growth of the cells from 90.17% ± 2.30% to 3.12% ± 0.08%. Ethanol crude extract significantly decreased the proliferation of SAS cells with an IC_{50} value of 25.84 µg/mL. To confirm if the inhibition of proliferation that was observed in MTT assay was caused by apoptosis, an Annexin V-FITC/PI double-staining assay was performed. When SAS cells were treated with crude extracts at 250 and 500 µg/mL, the apoptotic cells increased up to 34% ± 3.1% (Puwein et al. 2021).

Further, we noticed the effect of the fraction on SAS cell proliferation when treated at different (5, 10, 25, 50 µg/mL) for 24, 48, and 72 hours, as presented in Table 15.2 and Figure 15.1. The isolated fraction of *P. polyphylla* inhibited the percentage of the proliferation of SAS oral cells significantly ($p \leq 0.05$) in a dose-dependent manner (50.42% ± 3.54% at 5 µg/mL, 1.17% ± 6.88% at 10 µg/mL, 0.99% ± 2.32% at 25 µg/mL, and 3.12% ± 3.80% at 50 µg/mL) and time-dependent manner (50.42% ± 3.54% for 24 hours, 39.73% ± 0.51% for 48 hours, and 26.56% ± 4.92% at 72 hours), as indicated in Table 15.2 and Figure 15.1. To examine whether the isolated fraction can induce apoptosis in SAS oral cells, we analyzed SAS cells by flow cytometry after staining with Annexin V-FITC and PI. Annexin V-FITC-positive and PI-negative cells were considered to be early apoptotic, whereas Annexin V-FITC-positive and PI-positive cells were considered to be late apoptotic

---

TABLE 15.2

MTT Assay Showing the Percentage of Proliferation of SAS Cells after Exposure to Increasing Concentrations of *Paris polyphylla* Fraction at 24, 48, and 72 Hours

% Proliferation	24 Hours	48 Hours	72 Hours
0	100	100	100
5	50.42 ± 3.54	39.73 ± 0.51	26.56 ± 4.92
10	1.17 ± 6.88	11.86 ± 1.24	9.80 ± 2.088
25	0.99 ± 2.32	3.45 ± 0.57	1.26 ± 0.33
50	3.12 ± 3.80	3.25 ± 0.89	1.33 ± 0.32

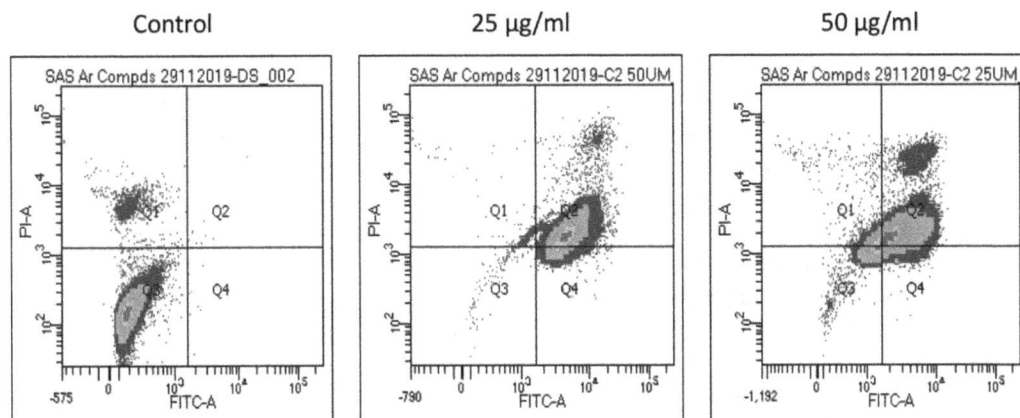

FIGURE 15.2 Annexin V-FITC/PI apoptosis assay carried out on SAS cells treated with different concentrations (25 and 50 µg/mL) of *Paris polyphylla* fraction.

Source: All data are represented as mean ± SD from experiments performed in triplicate.

cells. SAS cells were treated with 25 µg/mL and 50 µg/mL of fraction for 72 hours, after which apoptosis was determined by flow cytometry analysis. The SAS oral cells undergoing apoptosis after being exposed to the isolated fractions at 25 µg/mL and 50 µg/mL were compared with the control (DMSO). As shown in Figures 15.1 and Table 15.2, treatment of SAS cells with 25 µg/mL and 50 µg/mL of isolated fraction for 72 hours resulted in cell death. The percentage of apoptotic cells (Q2 + Q4) increased from 0.17% ± 0.06% (control) to 69.60% ± 2.07% and 91.77% ± 4.55% at 25 µg/mL and 50 µg/mL, respectively, for 72 h.

The assay with a flow cytometer using propidium iodide (PI) and fluorescein isothiocyanate (FITC)-conjugated Annexin V (Annexin V-FITC) has a great advantage in detecting early apoptotic and late apoptotic cells. Early apoptotic cells are Annexin V-positive and PI-negative (Annexin V-FITC$^+$/PI$^-$), whereas late apoptotic cells are Annexin V/PI double-positive (Annexin V-FITC$^+$/PI$^+$), as elucidated by Henry et al. (2013). Further, Bossy-Wetzel and Green (2000) have reported that detection of the externalization of phosphatidylserine residues on the outer plasma membrane of apoptotic cells via Annexin V is very sensitive. It can detect a single apoptotic cell. Fractions from *P. polyphylla* induced apoptosis on SAS oral cells, and it is confirmed by the annexin V-FITC/PI double staining.

15.11 TOXICITY AND CAUTIONARY NOTES

P. polyphylla is known to have caused vascular malady, antifertility, spermicidal enhancement, and sedation (Cheng et al. 2008). The extract of this herb was reported to have effective spermicidal activity against rat and human sperms (Devkota et al. 2005). Oral toxicity of the fruits of the plant is well-known locally in Meghalaya. There were sporadic reports where individuals consumed the herb by accident, which caused vomiting and an uneasy feeling with the formation of foam in the mouth. This is the reason that the herb is widely used as a painkiller and poison. The herb is unsafe when taken orally. The fruit contains poisonous chemicals and can cause nausea, vomiting, diarrhea, and headache. Saponins are the main chemical constituents of *P. polyphylla* (Shah et al. 2012). The toxicity of the herb might be due to the presence of a high content of saponins. Some plants produce saponins to serve as potential chemical barriers against pathogens. The saponins in *P. polyphylla* are present in the rhizomes, leaves, and fruits (Zaynab et al. 2021).

15.12   OTHER FOODS, HERBS, SPICES, AND BOTANICALS USED IN CANCER

Northeast India is one of the richest repositories of medicinal and aromatic plants in the world. Some of the herbs are endemic and known to certain tribes of the region only for their effective uses. Herbs such as *Centella asiatica, Curcuma aromatic, Potentilla fulgens, Prunella vulgaris, Fagopyrum esculentum, Rubus setchuenensis, Hedychium coronarium,* and *Molineria capitulata* are being used by the Khasi tribes for medicinal purposes and as food. In recent years, various herbs have been utilized not only as herbal medicines but for their health benefits and as food products. Many herbs were utilized as supplements, since herbs showed no or minimal side effects. *P. polyphylla* is a well-known medicinal herb but is not known to be an edible plant. In fact, accidental consumption of the herb in a few localities in northeast India was reported to cause an anaphylactic reaction.

However, *P. polyphylla* is demonstrated to have great potential for cancer treatment. Numerous studies have been reported on the chemical compounds of this herb to have triggered anticancer properties. The chemical compounds of the herb showed anticancer properties against various cell lines (Ji et al. 2001). The anticancer activity of this herb is indicated by the increased apoptotic cells. The bioactive compounds of *P. polyphylla* were assayed mainly for morphological changes (histopathology, cytopathology), cytotoxicity, and apoptosis. Cancer cell lines were confirmed to undergo apoptosis by the presence of markers such as decreased expression of anti-apoptotic proteins, upregulation of tumor suppressers genes, caspase activation cascade, depolarization of mitochondrial membrane potential (MMP), DNA fragmentation, DNA damage, increased expression of pro-apoptotic proteins, increased expression of connexin 26, and cell cycle arrest (Puwein et al. 2018).

15.13   SUMMARY

- Traditional herbs have become the preferred and effective treatments for cancer, as plant-derived drugs are comparatively less toxic.
- *P. polyphylla* has been traditionally used to relieve various ailments. The people of Meghalaya in the northeastern part of India have been using the paste of rhizomes to treat cuts, snake bites, and to cure bone fractures. It is popularly known as *sohbsein* in the local language (Khasi), although the local name *sohbsein* also includes other species like *Arisaema tortuosum.*
- *P. polyphylla* contains phytochemical compounds such as steroidal saponins and fatty acid esters that induce antiproliferative activity against oral cancer cells as observed in MTT assay.
- Further, when cancer cells were treated with extracts and fraction from *P. polyphylla,* the percentage of apoptotic cells (Q2 + Q4) increased from 0.17% ± 0.06% (control) up to 91.77% ± 4.55% (50 µg/mL), respectively, for 72 hours.
- Therefore, *P. polyphylla* collected from Meghalaya possesses several bioactive constituents that could be utilized for the therapeutic treatment of oral cancer.

REFERENCES

Aburjai, T. et al. 2007. Ethnopharmacological survey of medicinal herbs in Jordan, the Ajloun Heights region. *Journal of Ethnopharmacology* 110: 294–304.
Alok, S. et al. 2014. Herbal antioxidant in clinical practice: A review. *Asian Pacific Journal of Tropical Biomedicine* 4: 78–84.
Bossy-Wetzel, E. and D.R. Green. 2000. Detection of apoptosis by Annexin V labeling. *Methods Enzymology* 322: 15–18.
Bray, F. et al. 2018. Global cancer statistics 2018: Globocan estimates of incidence and mortality worldwide for 36 cancers in 185 countries. *CA: A Cancer Journal of Clinicians* 68: 394–424.

Briskin, D.P. 2000. Medicinal plants and phytomedicines: Linking plant biochemistry and physiology to human health. *Plant Physiology* 124: 507–514.

Cheng, Z.X. et al. 2008. *Journal of Ethnopharmacology* 120(2): 129–137.

Cosgrove, C.M. and R. Salani. 2018. Ovarian effects of radiation and cytotoxic chemotherapy damage. *Best Practice & Research Clinical Obstetrics & Gynaecology* 55: 37–48.

Cragg, G.M. and D.J. Newman. 2001. Natural product drug discovery in the next millennium. *Pharmaceutical Biology* 39: 8–17.

Cragg, G.M. and D.J. Newman. 2005. Plants as a source of anti-cancer agents. *Journal of Ethnopharmacology* 100(1–2): 72–79.

Deb, C.R. et al. 2015. Studies on vegetative and reproductive ecology of *Paris polyphylla* Smith: A vulnerable medicinal plant. *American Journal of Plant Sciences* 6: 2561–2568.

Devkota, K.P. 2005. Bioprospecting studies on *Sarcococca hookeriana* Bail, *Sonchus wightianus* DC, *Paris polyphylla* Smith and related Medicinal Herbs of Nepal: Ph D Thesis, HEJ Research Institute of Chemistry, International Centre for Chemical Science, University of Karachi: Karachi-75270, Pakistan.

Dutta, U. 2019. Epidemiology of gallbladder cancer in India. *Chin Clin Oncol* 8: 33.

Elmore, S. 2007. Apoptosis: A review of programmed cell death. *Toxicologic Pathology* 35: 495–516.

Ferrandino, A. and C. Lovisolo. 2014. Abiotic stress effects on grapevine (*Vitis vinifera* L.): Focus on abscisic acid-mediated consequences on secondary metabolism and berry quality. *Environmental and Experimental Botany* 103: 138–147.

Fu, Y.L. et al. 2007. Inducing effect of total steroid saponins from *Paris polyphylla* on platelet aggregation *in vitro* and its potential mechanism. *Bulletin of the Academy of Military Medical Sciences* 31: 416–419.

Gao, L.L. et al. 2011. *Paris chinensis* dioscin induces G2/M cell cycle arrest and apoptosis in human gastric cancer SGC-7901 cells. *World Journal of Gastroenterology: WJG* 17: 4389–4395.

Graham, J.G. et al. 2000. Plants used against cancer-an extension of the work of Jonathan Hartwell. *Journal of Ethnopharmacology* 73: 347–377.

Henry, C.M. et al. 2013. Measuring apoptosis by microscopy and flow cytometry. *Methods* 61: 90–97.

Igney, F.H. and P.H. Krammer. 2002. Death and anti-death: Tumor resistance to apoptosis. *Nature Reviews Cancer* 2: 277–288.

Jagatheeswari, D. et al. 2013. *Acalypha indica* L – an important medicinal plant: A review of its traditional uses and pharmacological properties. *International Journal of Research in Botany* 3: 19–22.

Jeyachandran, R. et al. 2010. *In vitro* antibacterial activity of three Indian medicinal plants. *International Journal of Biological Technology* 1: 103–106.

Ji, S. et al. 2001. Determination of antitumor cytotoxic active substance gracillin in *Rhizoma paridis* and Yunnan white. *Chinese Traditional Patent Medicine* 23: 212–215.

Kalimuthu, S. and K. Se-Kwon 2013. Cell survival and apoptosis signaling as therapeutic target for cancer: Marine bioactive compounds. *International Journal of Molecular Sciences* 14: 2334–2354.

Ke, J.Y. et al. 2016. A monomer purified from *Paris polyphylla* (PP-22) triggers S and G2/M phase arrest and apoptosis in human tongue squamous cell carcinoma SCC-15 by activating the p38/cdc25/cdc2 and caspase 8/caspase 3 pathways. *Tumor Biology* 37: 14863–14872.

Kerr, J.F.R. et al. 1972. *British Journal of Cancer* 26: 239.

Li, F.R. et al. 2012. *Paris polyphylla* Smith extract induces apoptosis and activates cancer suppressor gene connexin26 expression. *Asian Pacific Journal Cancer Prevention* 13: 205–209.

Li, Y.Q. et al. 2018. Alkaloid content and essential oil composition of *Mahonia breviracema* cultivated under different light environments. *Journal of Applied Botany and Food Quality* 91: 171–179.

Liang, S.Y. et al. 2000. *Flora of China, Volume 24 Flagellariceae through Marantaceae*. Wu Z.Y. and P.H. Raven (eds.). Beijing, China: Science Press and St Louis, USA: Botanical Garden Press, 88–95.

Liu, Z. et al. 1997. Camptothecin production in Camptotheca acuminata seedlings in response to shading and flooding. *Canadian Journal of Botany* 75: 368–373.

Long, C.L. et al. 2003. Strategies for agrobiodiversity conservation and promotion: A case from Yunnan, China. *Biodivers. Conserv.* 12: 1145–1156.

Ma, Z.Q. and S.S. Zhang. 2010. Light intensity affects growth, photosynthetic capability, and total flavonoid accumulation of *Anoectochilus* plants. *HortScience* 45: 863–867.

Macdonald, F. et al. 2004. *Molecular Biology of Cancer* (2nd Ed.). London and New York: Bios Scientific Publishers.

Martinvalet, D. et al. 2005. Granzyme A induces caspase independent-mitochondrial damage, a required first step for apoptosis. *Immunity* 22: 355–370.

Mathur, P. et al. 2020. Cancer statistics, 2020: Report from national cancer registry programme, India. *JCD Global Oncology* 6: 1063–1075.

Newman, D.J. and G.M. Cragg. 2016. Natural products as sources of new drugs from 1981 to 2014. *Journal of Natural Products* 79: 629–661.

Petti, S. 2008. Lifestyle risk factors for oral cancer. *Oral Oncology* 45: 340–350.

The Pharmacopoeia Committee of China. *Chinese Pharmacopoeia.* 2010 ed. Beijing: The People's Medical Publishing House, 243–244.

Puwein, A. and S.C. Thomas. 2020. An overview of *Paris polyphylla*, a highly vulnerable medicinal herb of Eastern Himalayan Region for sustainable exploitation. *The Natural Products Journal* 10: 3–14.

Puwein, A., Thomas, S.C., Singha, L.I. 2018. A review on *Paris Polyphylla* smith: As an effective and alternative treatment of Cancer. *International Journal of Pharmaceutical Science Invention* 6–12.

Puwein, A. et al. 2021. Anti-proliferative and apoptosis induction activity of rhizome extracts of *Paris polyphylla* Smith on oral cancer cell. *Current Cancer Therapy Reviews* 17: 82–86.

Qin, X.J. et al. 2012. Steroidal saponins from stems and leaves of *Paris polyphylla* var. *yunnanensis. Steroids* 77: 1242–1248.

Rajsekhar, P.B. et al. 2016. Extraction of *Paris polyphylla* rhizome using different solvents and its phytochemical studies. *International Journal of Pharmacognosy and Phytochemical Researc* 8: 18–21.

Rao, S.V. et al. 2013. Epidemiology of oral cancer in Asia in the past decade – an update (2000–2012). *Asian Pacific Journal of Cancer Prevention* 14: 5567–5577.

Sankaranarayanan, R. et al. 2005. Effect of screening on oral cancer mortality in Kerala, India: A cluster-randomised controlled trial. *The Lancet* 365: 1927–1933.

Sapkota, A. et al. 2007. Smokeless tobacco and increased risk of hypopharyngeal and laryngeal cancers: A multicentric case-control study from India. *International Journal of Cancer* 121: 1793–1798.

Saslis-Lagoudakis, C.H. et al. 2014. The evolution of traditional knowledge: Environment shapes medicinal plant use in Nepal. *Proceedings of the Royal Society B: Biological Sciences*, 281 (1780): 20132768.

Shah, A.S., Mazumder, P.B., Choudhury, M.D. 2012. Medicinal properties of *Paris polyphylla* smith: A review. *J. Herb. Med. Toxicol.* 6 (1): 27–33.

Taylor, R.C. et al. 2008. Apoptosis: Controlled demolition at the cellular level. *Nature Reviews Molecular Cell Biology* 9: 231–241.

Verma, N. and S. Shukla. 2015. Impact of various factors responsible for fluctuation in plant secondary metabolites. *Journal of Applied Research on Medicinal and Aromatic Plants* 2: 105–113.

Wink, M. 2008. Evolution of secondary plant metabolism. *eLS*: 1–11.

Wu, S.S. et al. 2004. Advances in studies on chemical constituents and pharmacological activities of *Rhizoma paridis. Chinese Traditional and Herbal Drugs* 35: 344–347.

Yang, C. et al. 2016. Polyphyllin D induces apoptosis and differentiation in K562 human leukemia cells. *International Immunopharmacology* 36: 17–22.

Yun, H. et al. 2007. Separation and identification of steroidal compounds with cytotoxic activity against human gastric cancer cell lines in vitro from the rhizomes of *Paris polyphylla* var. *chinensis. Chemistry of Natural Compounds* 43: 672–677.

Zaynab, M et al. 2021. Saponin toxicity as key player in plant dense against pathogens. *Toxicon* 193: 21–27.

Zhang, W. et al. 2014. Paris saponin VII suppressed the growth of human cervical cancer HeLa cells. *European Journal of Medical Research* 19: 1–7.

16 Papaya (*Carica papaya* L.) as an Effective Adjuvant to Cancer Therapy
Phytochemical Profile, Cellular and Molecular Targets

Salar Hafez Ghoran, Fatemeh Taktaz and Seyed Abdulmajid Ayatollahi

ABBREVIATIONS

AgNP	silver nanoparticle
AMPK	AMP-activated protein kinase
AuNP	gold nanoparticle
BG	benzyl glucosinolate
BITC	benzyl isothiocyanate
CAT	catalase
CA15–3	antigen 15
CIT	chemotherapy-induced thrombocytopenia
COX-2	cyclooxygenase 2
CRD	carbohydrate recognition domain
FPP	fermented papaya preparation
GPx	glutathione peroxidase
GSH	glutathione
HG	homogalacturonan
IC_{50}	half maximal inhibitory concentration
IL-6	interleukin-6
iNOS	inducible nitric oxide synthase
JNK	c-Jun N-terminal kinase
LDH	lactate dehydrogenase
MβCD	methyl-β-cyclodextrin
MDA	malondialdehyde
MMP	mitochondrial membrane potential
MTT	3-(4,5-dimethylthiazol-2-yl)-2,5-diphenyl tetrazolium bromide
NF-κB	nuclear factor kappa B
PI3K	phosphoinositide 3-kinase
RG	rhamnogalacturonan
ROS	reactive oxygen species
SCC25	squamous cell carcinoma
SeNPs	selenium nanoparticles
SOD	superoxide dismutase
TNF-α	tumor necrosis factor alpha

DOI: 10.1201/9781003260028-18

16.1   INTRODUCTION

Cancer remains the leading cause of death worldwide despite advancements in diagnosis and treatment. As a result of tumor heterogeneity, many targeted therapies and personalized medicines are ineffective (Heung et al. 2021). Meanwhile, uncontrolled proliferation, genetic instability, and alterations accumulate within normal cells turning them into malignant cells. The genetic instabilities include mutations in DNA repair genes (p2, p21, p27, p51, p53, and tool box for DNA), tumor suppressor genes (p53, NF1, NF2, RB, and biological breaks), oncogenes (MYC.RAF.Bcl-2, RAS), and genes involved in cell growth metabolism. Besides external factors such as radiation, smoking, tobacco, pollutants in drinking water, food, and air, chemicals, certain metals, and infection agents, there are internal factors like genetic mutations, immune system dysfunction, and hormonal imbalance that contribute to cancer development (Iqbal et al. 2017). A variety of cancer remedies are currently available based on the type, stage, and location of cancer, including chemotherapy, widely used for metastatic stages of cancer, surgery, radiotherapy, immunotherapy, vaccination, and combination therapy (Weaver 2014). Plant-derived drugs, for example, vincristine, vinblastine, etoposide, and taxol, are used to treat cancer. Dose-associated side effects and the toxicity to non-tumor tissues negatively affect their usage. Because of this, alternative therapies against cancer cells with minimal or no effect on healthy tissues are highly desirable against cancer cells. Scientific studies have shown that plant extracts, herbal preparations, and their secondary metabolites appear to be the best option for treating cancer without causing noticeable side effects (Singh et al. 2016). Plant secondary metabolites are recognized to exhibit antitumor effects via cell cycle arrest, inhibition of enzymes and protein pathways that stimulate cancer cell proliferation and enhance DNA repair. The pleiotropic actions of phytochemicals on cancer targets make them salient candidates in pharmaceutical development as anticancer drugs. Therefore, anticancer phytoconstituents are being investigated that might be able to either slow or block cancer cell growth without any serious side effects (Iqbal et al. 2017). Papaya (*Carica papaya* L.) is a member of the Caricaceae family, a native plant to Mexico, northern South America, and other tropical and subtropical regions. Since ancient times, various parts of the papaya plant have been used for their therapeutic and nutritional properties worldwide. All papaya parts, such as fruit, leaf, seed, root, bark, and latex, play a vital role in the treatment of human diseases. Due to the presence of alkaloids, glycosides, tannins, saponins, and flavonoids reported in the leaf of *papaya*, several medicinal properties, such as antioxidant, anti-inflammatory, antibacterial, antidiabetic, anticancer, antifertility, and hepatoprotective have been reported (Singh et al. 2020). This calls for researchers to develop a strategy, which is eco-friendly, biocompatible, and cost-effective, to combat the rising incidence of cancer, the high cost of conventional therapy, and the high toxicity of present anticancer drugs. In light of this, phytomolecules could revolutionize cancer prevention and treatment in the next decade, providing a promising alternative to conventional drugs. This chapter will provide a piece of current knowledge of traditional uses of papaya and its derived secondary metabolites that are appropriate in either cancer prevention or cancer treatment.

16.2   TRADITIONAL USES AND ETHNOPHARMACOLOGY

It is well documented that the whole parts of papaya such as fruit, flowers, latex, leaves, roots, bark, and seeds have diverse medicinal applications in folk medicine. For example, in Jamaica, the ripe fruit of papaya is applied for reducing the smell of chronic skin ulcers, healing, and topical ulcer dressings. In Pakistan, India, and Sri Lanka, the juice of green fruit is prescribed by traditional healers for various human and veterinary diseases, and in Nigeria, the plant is used for malaria, hypertension, diabetes mellitus, jaundice, and intestinal helminthiasis. Most significantly, the infusion/decoction of papaya leaves and roots/bark is used for sore teeth, colic, fever, beriberi, abortion, asthma in India, syphilis in Africa, and digestive, tonic, abortifacient, and cancer in Australia. The latex of papaya is applied as an external remedy to treat burns, scalds, and as a styptic agent. Latex is also used by people in Laos, Cambodia, and Vietnam for the treatment of eczema and psoriasis. Local people also use the seeds for the purpose of vermifuge, for bleeding piles, as a thirst quencher, and as a painkiller. In some parts of Asia, especially in Ayurvedic medicine, either an infusion or decoction of the papaya flowers is administered for jaundice, cough, respiratory disorders, hoarseness, bronchitis, low digestion strength, and tracheitis (Nguyen et al. 2013).

16.3 PHYTOCHEMICAL CONSTITUENTS

Up to now, several studies have been reported dealing with the chemical constituents of papaya. The plant's leaves contain several active specialized (or secondary) metabolites, such as fatty acids, flavonoids, glycosides, simple phenolics, saponins, and tannins and to a lesser amount alkaloids and anthraquinones, which are in charge of anticancer and chemopreventive properties. On the other hand, the aerial parts not only contain minerals, such as Ca, Fe, K, Mg, Mn, and Zn, but also are a source of fiber. The plant also includes enzymes like papain, chymopapain, caricain, and protease omega (Fauziya and Krishnamurthy 2013). Interestingly, papaya seeds contain phenolic compounds, which are known for their potent antioxidant and anticancer activity, benzyl isothiocyanate, glucosinolates, carotenoids, β-cryptoxanthin, oleic acids, and stearic acids (Santana et al. 2019; Kumar and Devi 2017). In the following sections, the major bioactive compounds in papaya that play as anticancer agents are described.

16.3.1 CAROTENOIDS

Carotenoids, belonging to the tetraterpenoid compounds (C_{40}), are natural pigments in plants, fungi, marine algae, and cyanobacteria. The most well-known pigment carotenoids reported from the fruit of papaya are lycopene, α- and β-carotene, α- and β-cryptoxanthin, neoxanthin, zeaxanthin, and violaxanthin, which have high reactivity against oxygen and free radicals and also cytotoxicity against various cancer cell lines, such as colon, prostate, liver, breast, gastric, breast, skin, and leukemia (Sharma et al. 2020). The structure of some of these metabolites is shown in Figure 16.1.

16.3.2 FLAVONOIDS

As diverse and eminent biological activities, flavonoids, with a C_6-C_3-C_6 skeleton, are a group of secondary metabolites that not only play an essential role against cancer but also increase the whole body's immunity. Despite quenching the harmful free radicals and active oxygen, the flavonoid content of papaya might be a salient candidate against different types of cancer cell lines and even for cancer prevention (Sharma et al. 2020). Apigenin, rutin, kaempferol, kaempferol-*O*-rutinoside, quercetin, isorhamnetin, and myricetin are examples of flavonoids reported in papaya. The structures of flavonoids are shown in Figure 16.1.

16.3.3 GLUCOSINOLATES

Glucosinolates, also known as thioglycosides, differ in the aglycon part's structure, somewhat having no biological activity. However, after physiological hydrolysis, glucosinolates provide a broad spectrum of biological activity. For instance, besides thiocyanate ions and nitriles, many isothiocyanate compounds produced in papaya are toxic to the intestinal, liver, lung, pancreatic, urinary bladder, breast, colon, gastric, and prostate cancer cell lines (Sharma et al. 2020). The seeds and pulp of papaya possess the thiol/nitrogen-containing metabolites like benzyl glucosinolate and benzyl isothiocyanate presented in Figure 16.1.

16.3.4 OTHER PHENOLIC COMPOUNDS

The main phenolic compounds in papaya's leaf, peel, flesh, and ripe fruit comprise the three classes of phenylpropanoids, coumarins, and simple phenolics, showing diverse cytotoxic activity against various types of cancer cell lines. Cinnamic acid, *p*-coumaric acid, caffeic acid, ferulic acid, chlorogenic acid, protocatechuic acid, and 5,7-dimethoxy coumarin are examples of some major phenolics in papaya (Sharma et al. 2020). Figure 16.1 covers some of these compounds.

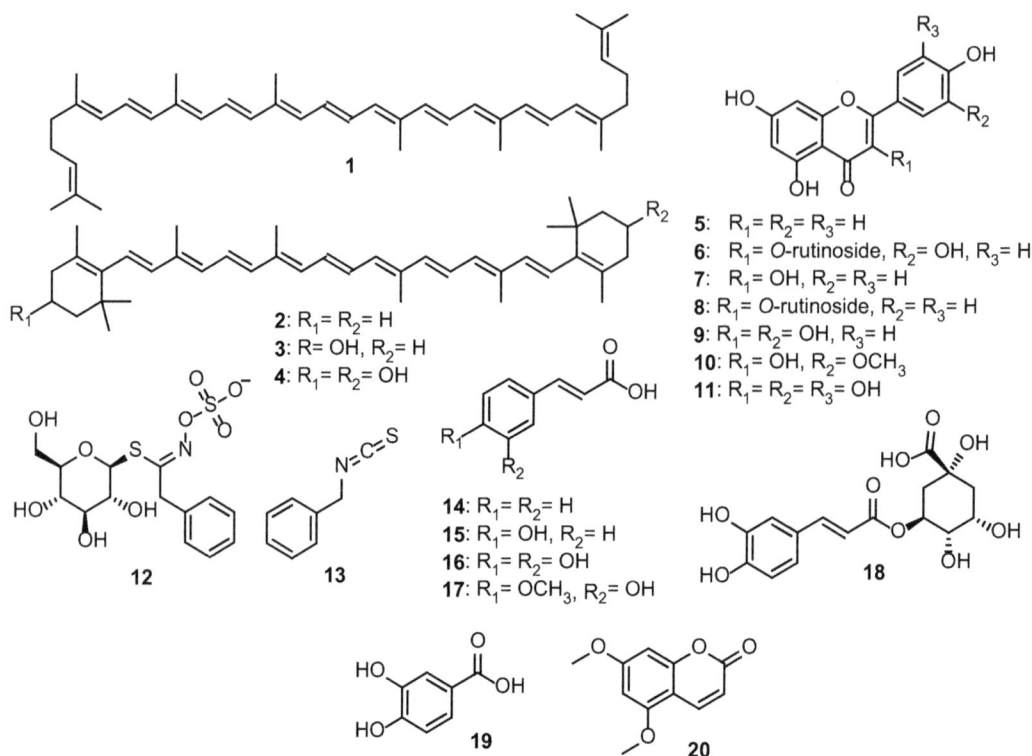

FIGURE 16.1 Papaya secondary metabolites. The chemical structures of some important papaya secondary metabolites include (1) lycopene, (2) β-carotene, (3) β-cryptoxanthin, (4) zeaxanthin, (5) apigenin, (6) rutin, (7) kaempferol, (8) kaempferol-*O*-rutinoside, (9) quercetin, (10) isorhamnetin, (11) myricetin, (12) benzyl glucosinolate, (13) benzyl isothiocyanate, (14) cinnamic acid, (15) *p*-coumaric acid, (16) caffeic acid, (17) ferulic acid, (18) chlorogenic acid, (19) protocatechuic acid, and (20) 5,7-dimethoxy coumarin.

16.4 PAPAYA IN CANCER TREATMENT

16.4.1 CELLULAR AND MOLECULAR TARGETS

Most types of cancers are caused by genetic abnormalities promoting cell proliferation. Apoptosis occurs naturally in malignant tumors and significantly delays their progression. It can be either induced or suppressed by the proto-oncogene and tumor suppressor gene p53. On the other hand, Bcl-2 one of the genes that regulate cell homeostasis during cancer development. Some members of this family include Bcl-2a, Bcl-xL (causing the inhibition of apoptosis), Bax, and Bclxs (causing the stimulation of apoptosis). Anilkumar and Bhanu (2022) reported that papaya dark seeds could be a promising tonic in the liver and malignant growth treatment through the possibility to prompt apoptotic changes via downregulation of Bcl-2 and upregulation of p53 and caspase-3 genes. A flavonoid compound, quercetin, derived from the leaf extract of papaya, displayed apoptosis induction in MCF-7 breast cancer cell lines by decreasing Bcl-2 expression (Astuti and Murdiati 2017). In an animal model, lycopene extracted from red papaya also had positive effects on HT-29 colorectal cancer cell lines with its inhibitory activity on cell viability and progression by different cellular pathways like nuclear factor kappa B (NF-κB) and c-Jun N-terminal kinase (JNK) (Carini et al. 2017). Furthermore, lycopene could suppress NF-κB and JNK activation in human SW480 colorectal cancer cell lines and decrease inflammation. The pure lycopene also inhibited cyclooxygenase-2 (COX-2), inducible nitric oxide synthase (iNOS), interleukin-6 (IL-6), and tumor necrosis factor alpha (TNF-α) (Cha et al. 2017).

Having extracted the papaya's pectin, caused the most effective cell death and increased expression of pAkt and pErk in HCT116 cells. This phenomenon might be related to cell migration and survival. The pectin content could also stimulate the cleaved caspase 3 in HCT116 cell lines and eventually induction of apoptosis. Additional activation of p21 has stimulated apoptosis by both p53-dependent and p53-independent mechanisms (Xue and Hemmings 2013; Prado et al. 2017). Methyl-β-cyclodextrin (MβCD) is effective in reducing plasma membrane cholesterol levels. A recent study examined the modulation effects of MβCD on the antiproliferation induced by benzyl isothiocyanate (BITC), which was derived from papaya seeds. BITC effectively increased the phosphoinositide 3-kinase (PI3K)/Akt pathway in human colorectal cancer cells, and MβCD inhibited the Akt phosphorylation. As a result, MβCD treatment not only induces phosphorylation of mitogen-activated protein kinases but also stimulates BITC anticancer activity by cholesterol depletion (Yang et al. 2018). BITC also activates the phosphorylation of ERK in the MEK/ERK signaling pathway that is involved in cell survival and proliferation. It is noteworthy to mention that BITC potentiated the JNK, AMP-activated protein kinase (AMPK), and p38 MAPK signaling pathways (Nakamura and Miyoshi 2010). In a variety of cancer types, PI3K/AKT may contribute to resistance to apoptosis induced by chemotherapy and radiation (Boreddy et al. 2011). Cancer initiates and progresses by reactive oxygen species (ROS) generated by metabolic reactions in the mitochondria. If ROS levels are low enough to be tolerated by body cells, cancer progression could occur by either altering genomic DNA or causing DNA damage that alters normal physiological signaling pathways. Generally, cancer cells are more resistant to oxidative stress than normal cells to allow uncontrolled proliferation and to survive during metastasis (Saha et al. 2017). An *in vivo* study reported that 500 mg/kg of fermented papaya preparation (FPP) significantly increases enzymatic antioxidant status, including glutathione peroxidase (GPx), superoxide dismutase (SOD), and catalase (CAT). In addition to preventing DNA structural damage caused by genotoxins, FPP also prevented DNA damage caused by free radicals (Somanah et al. 2016). In another study, papaya peel extract sufficiently increased glutathione (GSH) levels, whereas it decreased the levels of reactive oxygen species (ROS) and malondialdehyde (MDA) (Waly et al. 2014). Aruoma and colleagues showed that fermented papaya preparation inhibited the phosphorylation of Akt and p38 by H_2O_2 and downregulated the MAPK pathway (Aruoma et al. 2006). There is a comparative study of antitumor effects of bromelain, a proteolytic enzyme in pineapple juice and stem, and papain in human cholangiocarcinoma (CC) cell lines that showed bromelain effectively inhibits the NF-κB/AMPK pathway, an important pathway in carcinogenesis of several tumor diseases. In addition, the cytotoxic effect of bromelain and papain seemed to be caused by apoptotic cell death (MüLLER et al. 2016). Researchers found that ascorbic acid, quercetin, riboflavin, and lycopene, derived from the papaya leaves, could attenuate angiogenesis in pathological conditions and are also useful in the development of anticancer drugs (Tayal et al. 2019). A review of previous studies has shown that increased galectin-3 expression enhances tumor growth, invasiveness, and metastatic potential during cancer progression (Farhad et al. 2018). There are several biological processes involving galectin-3 expression, including cell-cell interaction, proliferation, differentiation, apoptosis, and mRNA maturation. Pectin-containing fractions may reduce carcinogenesis by interacting with galectin-3, a pro-metastatic protein, through its carbohydrate recognition domain (CRD) (Prado et al. 2020). Hence, the consumption of papaya at the intermediate stages of ripening is advisable due to the presence of pectin-containing homogalacturonans (HGs) and rhamnogalacturonans (RGs) and could be structurally compatible with inhibiting the galectin-3 expression and inhibition of colon cancer (Zhang et al. 2017). The general overview of the cellular and molecular targets of papaya is shown in Figure 16.2. Several kinds of research have been concentrated on papaya and its bioactive phytoconstituents' function against cancers described below.

16.4.1.1 Prostate Cancer

The most common malignancy among men is prostate cancer (PCa). The leaf extract of papaya has been used traditionally in Australia for its anticancer properties (Pandey et al. 2018). In this respect, papaya seeds might have anticancer effects against cancer of the prostate gland, a vital organ of the

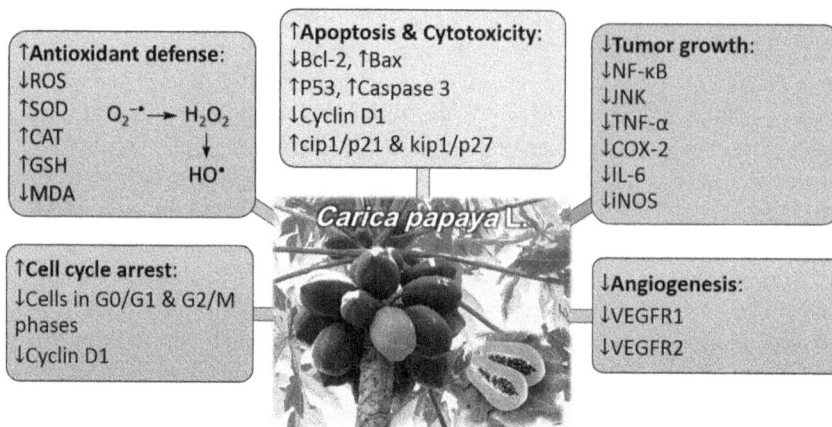

FIGURE 16.2 Molecular targets of papaya in cancer. Various cell signaling pathways and biomolecules are affected by papaya and its bioactive compositions by reducing the tumor growth and angiogenesis, enhancing antioxidant defense, apoptosis, and cytotoxicity, as well as cell cycle arrest in cancer cell lines.

male reproductive system. According to a study, the methanol extract of black seeds obtained from yellow ripe papaya directly inhibits prostate cancer cell growth and proliferation of PC-3 cells. It is noted that black seed extracts inhibit prostate cancer cells, whereas white seed extracts stimulate preexisting prostate cancer cells and should be avoided for consumption (Alotaibi et al. 2017). Also, the juice of papaya leaves (JPL) and its extracts were investigated for antiproliferative activity against benign hyperplasia cells, tumorigenic cells, and normal prostate cells. The proliferation of all cell lines tested was inhibited by JPL in a dose- and time-dependent manner (Pandey et al. 2017).

16.4.1.2 Breast Cancer

There is a significant mortality rate among females who are suffering from breast cancer around the globe, making it one of the most deadly forms of cancer. Many research reported druggable targets for breast cancer such as ERa, FGRF1, VEGFR2, HER2, and COX-2 (Maran et al. 2022). Papaya leaf aqueous extract could inhibit the proliferation of MCF-7 breast cancer cell lines and induce apoptosis. Compared with doxorubicin and quercetin, the plant extract has a low percentage of cell apoptosis (Astuti and Murdiati 2017). Besides the antioxidant ability of leaves, skin, pulp, and seeds extracts from green papaya, the water extract of leaves and seeds had modest cytotoxic effects on ER-negative breast cancer cells (Hadadi et al. 2018). The antigen 15 (CA15–3) and lactate dehydrogenase (LDH) have a crucial role in providing biochemical insight into the progression and proliferation of cancer cells. Aqueous extract of papaya leaves in a dose of 200 mg/kg body weight decreased CA15–3 and LDH levels and prevented the progression of cancer growth (Gurudatta et al. 2015). Jayakumar and Kanthimathi (2011) used ethanolic extracts of papaya pericarp at doses between 50 and 640 g/mL, and the result showed a significant decrease in cell viability in MCF-7 cell lines. There is also evidence that flavonoids derived from papaya leaves possess anticancer properties in human breast cancer cells by inhibiting cell cycle progression at the G2/M phase, which plays a crucial role in downregulating signaling pathways. Furthermore, it induces cell death through apoptosis and autophagy (Abotaleb et al. 2018). García-Solís et al. concluded the significant inhibitory effect of aqueous extract of papaya flesh, consumed in Mexico, on the proliferation of breast cancer MCF-7 cell lines (García-Solís et al. 2009).

16.4.1.3 Liver Cancer

One of the cancer types with a poor prognosis is hepatocellular carcinoma (HCC), the third leading cause of cancer death and the fifth most common cancer type (Huang et al. 2020). The methanolic extract of papaya black seeds showed potent inhibitory activity against cell viability and migration of HepG2 cell lines (liver cancer) (Anilkumar and Bhanu 2022). Both papaya juice and pure lycopene caused cell death in the liver cancer cell lines (HepG2) with half maximal inhibitory concentration (IC_{50}) of 20 and 22.8 mg mL^{-1}, respectively (Nguyen et al. 2013). The further study evaluated the antitumor effect of an alkaloidal extract derived from papaya seeds using rodent models of HCC. The extract significantly reduced tumor multiplicity (Kyei-Barffour et al. 2021). In liver cancer, FPP appears to modulate immune defenses by preserving liver integrity against oxidative damage and preventing irreversible DNA structural changes caused by *N*-methyl-*N*-nitrosourea-induced hepatocellular carcinoma (Somanah et al. 2016).

16.4.1.4 Colon Cancer

Papaya pulp, containing a water-soluble fraction of pectin, has been shown already to have positive effects on colon cancer cell lines. Despite this, it is still unknown what mechanisms can cause these beneficial effects and what characteristics of pectin cause them (Prado et al. 2020). A recent study has reported that galectin-3 overexpression is related to a progression in colorectal cancer as a biomarker for cancer development. The consumption of papaya fibers like pectin, as a type of dietary fiber containing the β-galactosidase part, can decrease the risk of colon cancer and inhibit galectin-3 mediated effects (do Prado et al. 2019). There is a different effect between neutral and acidic fractions of pectins isolated from ripe and overripe papaya on galectin-3 inhibition and colon cancer cell growth (de Freitas Pedrosa et al. 2020). The CT-26 colorectal malignant growth cell lines viability and migration were decreased effectively by papaya dark seed extracts (Chang et al. 2020). The positive anticarcinogenic effect of papaya peel extract may be attributed to the antioxidant phytochemical contents. It is also worth mentioning that the plant extract ameliorates damage by azoxymethane, a potent carcinogenic agent commonly used to induce colon cancer, by reducing oxidative stress (Waly et al. 2014).

16.4.1.5 Lung Cancer

Li et al. have demonstrated the content of benzyl glucosinolate (BG) in the pulp and seed of papaya showing anti–lung cancer activity. The pulp contains more BG before the maturation of papaya and it nearly disappeared after papaya matured, while the seeds contain BG at every stage. According to an experimental test, a higher concentration of benzyl isothiocyanate (BITC) showed a better inhibition rate of cell proliferation on H69 cells. BG can also be produced in the pulp of papaya and it will be stored in the seed after the fruit has matured. The hydrolysis product of BG has certain anticancer activities for humans (Li et al. 2012).

16.4.1.6 Pancreatic Cancer

According to Vuong et al. study, saponins extracted from papaya leaves exhibit antioxidant capacity and anti–pancreatic cancer activity when extracted under optimized conditions. Phenolic compounds together with saponins displayed antioxidant, free radical scavenging, ion-reducing capacities, and anti–pancreatic cancer activity. In addition, the ethanolic extract has more efficiency, and the study revealed that bioactive compounds in papaya leaves warrant further studies on the anticancer activity (Vuong et al. 2015).

16.4.1.7 Skin Cancer

The papaya plant has been used by people for centuries to treat wounds and skin infections, and this widespread application has been scientifically validated. A cytotoxicity study on four fractions of papaya leaves correlated positively with cell viability on human oral squamous cell carcinoma (SCC25) cells. It is relieved that papaya leaf acidic extracts contain many bioactive compounds that have selective interactions with SCC25 cell lines (Nguyen et al. 2015). The *in vitro* cytotoxicity of decoction of papaya leaves and juice of leaves was analyzed by metabolomics profiling. As shown by tests on non-cancerous human keratinocyte HaCaT cells, the leaf juice exhibited a selective cytotoxic effects on SCC25 cancer cells, whereas no cytotoxicity was observed toward HaCaT cells (Nguyen et al. 2016).

16.4.2 PAPAYA NANOPARTICLES WITH ANTICANCER ACTIVITIES

Nanotechnology is a fast-growing field in medicine due to its potential for improving diagnostic, imaging, and drug delivery. Biomedical research is undergoing a rapid shift to the green synthesis of gold nanoparticles (AuNPs). It has been reported that papaya fruit (CPf) extract can synthesize the AuNPs, which have antioxidant and anticancer properties. The antiproliferative activity of CPf and CPf-AuNPs was tested against a variety of cancer cell lines using 3-(4,5-dimethylthiazol-2-yl)-2,5-diphenyl tetrazolium bromide (MTT) reduction assay. Interestingly, the CPf-AuNPs showed cytotoxic effects against different cancer cells, especially HT-29 and MDA-MB-231 cell lines (Anadozie et al. 2022). Singh et al. investigated the anticancer properties of silver nanoparticles (AgNPs), synthesized by papaya leaf extract (PLE), against a variety of human cancer cells. The authors reported the inhibition of cell proliferation by cell cycle arrest at the G2/M phase at 24 hours also the arrests at G0/G1 and G2/M at 48 hours. Additionally, suppressing cyclin D1 (checkpoint marker) with upregulation in cip1/p21 and kip1/p27 (tumor suppressor proteins) caused by AgNPs-PLE (Singh et al. 2021). The biologically active molecules, di-methyl flubendazole isolated from the extract of papaya leaves, were used to synthesize silver nanoparticles (AgNPs). Regarding the antiproliferative effects of AgNPs on cancer cell lines, it is reported that the antiproliferative activity of AgNPs against HepG2 cell lines was significantly stronger than that of MCF-7 and A549 cell lines. However, AgNPs exhibited a less cytotoxic effect on normal cells. AgNPs-treated cells showed necrosis, and apoptotic morphology was evidenced by cell shrinkage, membrane blebbing, and cell decay. In HepG2 cells, AgNPs blocked the G0/G1 phase and downregulated the Bcl-2 expression (Devanesan et al. 2021). In another research using papain for nanoparticle synthesis, the gold nanoparticles encored with flutamide increased the cytotoxicity against prostate cancer cell lines (Xu and Man 2021). Researchers demonstrated that selenium nanoparticles synthesized by the latex of papaya have significant cytotoxicity against MDA-MB-231 human breast cancer cells (Rajasekar and Kuppusamy 2021). Vundela et al. examined the synthesized selenium nanoparticles (SeNPs) by papaya extract against the growth of cancer cells compared to normal cells through evaluation of mitochondrial membrane potential (MMP), caspase-3, and lactate dehydrogenase (LDH). The *in vitro* anticancer activity of SeNPs showed cytotoxic activity toward RAW 264.7, Caco-2, MCF-7, and IMR-32 cell lines. Also, based on their experiment, SeNPs were less toxic and did not cause death in zebrafish (*Danio rerio*) embryos at a lower concentration, suggesting that low doses of SeNPs could be beneficial (Vundela et al. 2021).

16.5 CHEMOPREVENTIVE PROPERTIES

A randomized open clinical trial demonstrated that an enzyme preparation containing chymotrypsin and papain derived from papaya latex was effective on patients suffering from advanced uterine cervix cancer. Results showed that the patients experienced fewer acute side effects from radiation therapy. As a result of using this preparation orally, the side effects of acute radiation therapy, such as skin reactions, gastrointestinal discomfort, and mucosal reactions at specific sites could be significantly decreased. Moreover, unpleasant side effects that are common during chemotherapy like acute headaches, vomiting, nausea, and bouts of unconsciousness were found to be reduced through treatment of fermented papaya preparation (FPP) in children with acute myeloleukemia (Aruoma et al. 2014). Aqueous extracts of papaya were chromatographically fractionated into petroleum ether, benzene, chloroform, ethyl acetate, and methanol. The molecular mechanisms of the flavonoid-rich benzene fraction demonstrated significant cytoprotective activity, which was correlated with proliferative indexes, cell cycle regulators, anti-inflammatory effects, reversal of stress-induced senescence, and genoprotection (Pathak et al. 2014). Several mechanisms are responsible for the chemoprevention effects, such as deactivating oncogene products, simulated tumor-suppressor genes, and decreasing oxidative stress damage. In an animal model study, it was found that the benzene fraction of the aqueous extract of papaya demonstrated chemoprotective effects against induced carcinogenic exposure to benzo(a)pyrene and 7,12-dimethyl benz(a)anthracene (Pathak et al. 2014). Chemotherapy-induced thrombocytopenia (CIT) occurs when platelet counts are abnormally reduced following chemotherapeutic treatment. Papaya leaf extract (CPLE) may be a good herbal preparation for patients with low or mid-platelet counts. It was reported that CPLE could be used to boost platelet in patients with CIT (Koehler et al. 2022).

16.6 TOXICITY EFFECT

According to the World Health Organization's Global Report on Traditional and Complementary Medicine, herbal medicine safety must be thoroughly assessed in most countries, under similar processes to conventional medicine, including postmarketing surveillance (WHO 2019). The potency of papaya as a medicinal product has been proven by emerging evidence; however, the use of this product in different medical conditions still requires more safety data. It is well-known that many plants, despite having therapeutic benefits, can be toxic to cells (Bussmann et al. 2011). The extract of papaya leaves tested in an acute toxicity study showed that it had no significant toxic effects at a concentration up to 2 g/kg of body weight (Afzan et al. 2012). In addition, different methods of papaya extraction, such as using ethanol and aqueous solvents, may have different safety profiles (Yamthe et al. 2012). It is noteworthy to mention that there is a potential herb-drug interaction with oral hypoglycemic agents, p-glycoprotein substrates, and antibiotics with cation-chelating properties. The consumption of papaya leaves by adults is generally safe for short-term use, whereas pregnant women and people with liver impairment should avoid it (Lim et al. 2021).

16.7 SUMMARY POINTS

- This chapter provides the anticancer properties of *C. papaya* L. (papaya) along with its phytochemical constituents.
- With the growing body of science, a well-balanced diet including a wide range of vegetables, fruits, and whole grains not only enhances the immune system but also helps one avoid the development of cancer.
- Different parts of papaya, such as ripe fruit, green fruit, latex, seeds, leaves, flowers, roots, and bark, are traditionally used across the world to treat a wide range of human disorders from the simplest (cough) to the most complicated (cancer).
- Because of the presence of glucosinolates, phenolics (phenylpropanoids, flavonoids, and coumarins), and carotenoids, the papaya plant is a salient candidate for evaluation of anticancer activity.
- The papaya's anticancer effects are associated with PI3/AKT, JNK, NF-κB, and AMPK pathways.
- In various cancers, papaya significantly increases antioxidant enzyme levels, such as glutathione peroxidase (GPx), superoxide dismutase (SOD), and catalase (CAT), preventing DNA damage caused by free radicals. As a useful nanocarrier, nanoparticles enhance papaya's anticancer properties.
- It has been shown that papaya can provide chemoprotection against radiation therapy side effects including skin reaction, gastrointestinal discomfort, mucosal reactions, acute headaches, vomiting, nausea, and unconsciousness.
- Despite emerging evidence of papaya's potential as a medicine, more safety evidence is still needed to use this product for different medical conditions.
- Several clinical studies are required before applying papaya's phytochemicals to patients.

REFERENCES

Abotaleb, M., S. M. Samuel, E. Varghese, S. Varghese, P. Kubatka, A. Liskova, and D. Büsselberg. 2018. Flavonoids in cancer and apoptosis. *Cancers* 11:28.

Afzan, A., N. R. Abdullah, S. Z. Halim, B. A. Rashid, R. H. R. Semail, N. Abdullah, I. Jantan, H. Muhammad, and Z. Ismail. 2012. Repeated dose 28-days oral toxicity study of *Carica papaya* L. leaf extract in Sprague Dawley rats. *Molecules* 17:4326–4342.

Alotaibi, K. S., H. Li, R. Rafi, and R. A. Siddiqui. 2017. Papaya black seeds have beneficial anticancer effects on PC-3 prostate cancer cells. *Journal of Cancer Metastasis and Treatment* 3:161–168.

Anadozie, S. O., O. B. Adewale, A. O. Fadaka, O. B. Afolabi, and S. Roux. 2022. Synthesis of gold nanoparticles using extract of *Carica papaya* fruit: Evaluation of its antioxidant properties and effect on colorectal and breast cancer cells. *Biocatalysis and Agricultural Biotechnology* 42:102348.

Anilkumar, A., and A. Bhanu. 2022. *In vitro* anticancer activity of methanolic extract of papaya blackseeds (MPB) in Hep G2 cell lines and its effect in the regulation of bcl-2, caspase-3 and p53 gene expression. *Advances in Cancer Biology-Metastasis* 4:100025.

Aruoma, O. I., R. Colognato, I. Fontana, J. Gartlon, L. Migliore, K. Koike, S. Coecke, E. Lamy, V. Mersch-Sundermann, and I. Laurenza. 2006. Molecular effects of fermented papaya preparation on oxidative damage, MAP Kinase activation and modulation of the benzo[a]pyrene mediated genotoxicity. *Biofactors* 26:147–159.

Aruoma, O. I., J. Somanah, E. Bourdon, P. Rondeau, and T. Bahorun. 2014. Diabetes as a risk factor to cancer: Functional role of fermented papaya preparation as phytonutraceutical adjunct in the treatment of diabetes and cancer. *Mutation Research/Fundamental and Molecular Mechanisms of Mutagenesis* 768:60–68.

Astuti, M., and A. Murdiati. 2017. Anti-proliferation and apoptosis induction of aqueous leaf extract of *Carica papaya* L. on human breast cancer cells MCF-7. *Pakistan Journal of Biological Sciences* 20:36–41.

Boreddy, S. R., K. C. Pramanik, and S. K. Srivastava. 2011. Pancreatic tumor suppression by benzyl isothiocyanate is associated with inhibition of PI3K/AKT/FOXO pathway. *Clinical Cancer Research* 17:1784–1795.

Bussmann, R. W., G. Malca, A. Glenn, D. Sharon, B. Nilsen, B. Parris, D. Dubose, D. Ruiz, J. Saleda, and M. Martinez. 2011. Toxicity of medicinal plants used in traditional medicine in Northern Peru. *Journal of Ethnopharmacology* 137:121–140.

Carini, F., S. David, G. Tomasello, M. Mazzola, P. Damiani, F. Rappa, L. Battaglia, F. Cappello, A. Jurjus, and A. G. Geagea. 2017. Colorectal cancer: An update on the effects of lycopene on tumor progression and cell proliferation. *Journal of Biological Regulators and Homeostatic Agents* 31:769–774.

Cha, J. H., W. K. Kim, A. W. Ha, M. H. Kim, and M. J. Chang. 2017. Anti-inflammatory effect of lycopene in SW480 human colorectal cancer cells. *Nutrition Research and Practice* 11:90–96.

Chang, Y.-X., Y.-T. Liu, C.-C. Chen, Y.-S. Lin, Y.-C. Hung, C.-Y. Lin, T.-Y. Chi, H.-Y. Chen, P.-M. Huang, and Y.-H. Chen. 2020. Inhibition activities of papaya black seed extracts on colorectal cancer cell viability and migration. *Adaptive Medicine* 12:59–63.

de Freitas Pedrosa, L., R. G. Lopes, and J. P. Fabi. 2020. The acid and neutral fractions of pectins isolated from ripe and overripe papayas differentially affect galectin-3 inhibition and colon cancer cell growth. *International Journal of Biological Macromolecules* 164:2681–2690.

Devanesan, S., M. Jayamala, M. S. AlSalhi, S. Umamaheshwari, and A. J. A. Ranjitsingh. 2021. Antimicrobial and anticancer properties of *Carica papaya* leaves derived di-methyl flubendazole mediated silver nanoparticles. *Journal of Infection and Public Health* 14:577–587.

do Prado, S. B. R., G. R. C. Santos, P. A. S. Mourão, and J. P. Fabi. 2019. Chelate-soluble pectin fraction from papaya pulp interacts with galectin-3 and inhibits colon cancer cell proliferation. *International Journal of Biological Macromolecules* 126:170–178.

Farhad, M., A. S. Rolig, and W. L. Redmond. 2018. The role of Galectin-3 in modulating tumor growth and immunosuppression within the tumor microenvironment. *Oncoimmunology* 7:e1434467.

Fauziya, S., and R. Krishnamurthy. 2013. Papaya (*Carica papaya*): Source material for anticancer. *CIBTech Journal of Pharmaceutical Sciences* 2:25–34.

García-Solís, P., E. M. Yahia, V. Morales-Tlalpan, and M. Díaz-Muñoz. 2009. Screening of antiproliferative effect of aqueous extracts of plant foods consumed in Mexico on the breast cancer cell line MCF-7. *International Journal of Food Sciences and Nutrition* 60:32–46.

Gurudatta, M., Y. A. Deshmukh, and A. A. Naikwadi. 2015. Anticancer effects of *Carica papaya* in experimental induced mammary tumors in rats. *International Jounal of Medical Research & Health Scinces* 4:667–671.

Hadadi, S. A., H. Li, R. Rafie, P. Kaseloo, S. M. Witiak, and R. A. Siddiqui. 2018. Anti-oxidation properties of leaves, skin, pulp, and seeds extracts from green papaya and their anti-cancer activities in breast cancer cells. *Journal of Cancer Metastasis and Treatment* 4:25.

Heung, T. Y., J. Y. S. Huong, W. Y. Chen, Y. W. Loh, K. Y. Khaw, B.-H. Goh, and Y. S. Ong. 2021. Anticancer potential of *Carica papaya* through modulation of cancer hallmarks. *Food Reviews International*: 1–19.

Huang, C.-C., J.-M. Hwang, J.-H. Tsai, J. H. Chen, H. Lin, G.-J. Lin, H.-L. Yang, J.-Y. Liu, C.-Y. Yang, and J.-C. Ye. 2020. Aqueous *Ocimum gratissimum* extract induces cell apoptosis in human hepatocellular carcinoma cells. *International Journal of Medical Sciences* 17:338.

Iqbal, J., B. A. Abbasi, T. Mahmood, S. Kanwal, B. Ali, S. A. Shah, and A. T. Khalil. 2017. Plant-derived anticancer agents: A green anticancer approach. *Asian Pacific Journal of Tropical Biomedicine* 7:1129–1150.

Jayakumar, R., and M. S. Kanthimathi. 2011. Inhibitory effects of fruit extracts on nitric oxide-induced proliferation in MCF-7 cells. *Food Chemistry* 126:956–960.

Koehler, A., R. Rao, Y. Rothman, Y. M. Gozal, T. Struve, L. Alschuler, and S. Sengupta. 2022. A case study using papaya leaf extract to reverse chemotherapy-induced thrombocytopenia in a GBM patient. *Integrative Cancer Therapies* 21:15347354211068417.

Kumar, N. S., and P. S. S. Devi. 2017. The surprising health benefits of papaya seeds: A. *Journal of Pharmacognosy and Phytochemistry* 6:424–429.

Kyei-Barffour, I., R. K. B. Kwarkoh, D. O. Acheampong, A. S. Brah, S. A. Akwetey, and B. Aboagye. 2021. Alkaloidal extract from *Carica papaya* seeds ameliorates CCl_4-induced hepatocellular carcinoma in rats. *Heliyon* 7:e07849.

Li, Z.-Y., Y. Wang, W.-T. Shen, and P. Zhou. 2012. Content determination of benzyl glucosinolate and anti: Cancer activity of its hydrolysis product in *Carica papaya* L. *Asian Pacific Journal of Tropical Medicine* 5:231–233.

Lim, X. Y., J. S. W. Chan, N. Japri, J. C. Lee, and T. Y. C. Tan. 2021. *Carica papaya* L. Leaf: A systematic scoping review on biological safety and herb-drug interactions. *Evidence-Based Complementary and Alternative Medicine* 2021:Article ID 5511221. doi: https://doi.org/10.1155/2021/5511221

Maran, M., S. Gangadharan, and I. A. Emerson. 2022. Molecular dynamics study of quercetin families and its derivative compounds from *Carica papaya* leaf as breast cancer inhibitors. *Chemical Physics Letters* 793:139470.

Müller, A., S. Barat, X. Chen, K. C. Bui, P. Bozko, N. P. Malek, and R. R. Plentz. 2016. Comparative study of antitumor effects of bromelain and papain in human cholangiocarcinoma cell lines. *International Journal of Oncology* 48:2025–2034.

Nakamura, Y., and N. Miyoshi. 2010. Electrophiles in foods: The current status of isothiocyanates and their chemical biology. *Bioscience, Biotechnology, and Biochemistry* 74:242–255.

Nguyen, T. T., M.-O. Parat, M. P. Hodson, J. Pan, P. N. Shaw, and A. K. Hewavitharana. 2015. Chemical characterization and *in vitro* cytotoxicity on squamous cell carcinoma cells of *Carica papaya* leaf extracts. *Toxins* 8:7.

Nguyen, T. T., M.-O. Parat, P. N. Shaw, A. K. Hewavitharana, and M. P. Hodson. 2016. Traditional aboriginal preparation alters the chemical profile of *Carica papaya* leaves and impacts on cytotoxicity towards human squamous cell carcinoma. *PLoS One* 11:e0147956.

Nguyen, T. T., P. N. Shaw, M.-O. Parat, and A. K. Hewavitharana. 2013. Anticancer activity of *Carica papaya*: A review. *Molecular Nutrition & Food Research* 57:153–164.

Pandey, S., C. Walpole, P. J. Cabot, P. N. Shaw, J. Batra, and A. K Hewavitharana. 2017. Selective antiproliferative activities of *Carica papaya* leaf juice extracts against prostate cancer. *Biomedicine & Pharmacotherapy* 89:515–523.

Pandey, S., C. Walpole, P. N. Shaw, P. J. Cabot, A. K. Hewavitharana, and J. Batra. 2018. Bio-guided fractionation of papaya leaf juice for delineating the components responsible for the selective anti-proliferative effects on prostate cancer cells. *Frontiers in Pharmacology* 9:1319.

Pathak, N., S. Khan, A. Bhargava, G. V. Raghuram, D. Jain, H. Panwar, R. M. Samarth, S. K. Jain, K. K. Maudar, and D. K. Mishra. 2014. Cancer chemopreventive effects of the flavonoid-rich fraction isolated from papaya seeds. *Nutrition and Cancer* 66:857–871.

Prado, S. B. R., M. Beukema, E. Jermendi, H. A. Schols, P. de Vos, and J. P. Fabi. 2020. Pectin interaction with immune receptors is modulated by ripening process in papayas. *Scientific Reports* 10:1–11.

Prado, S. B. R., G. F. Ferreira, Y. Harazono, T. M. Shiga, A. Raz, N. C. Carpita, and J. P. Fabi. 2017. Ripening-induced chemical modifications of papaya pectin inhibit cancer cell proliferation. *Scientific Reports* 7:1–17.

Rajasekar, S., and S. Kuppusamy. 2021. Eco-friendly formulation of selenium nanoparticles and its functional characterization against breast cancer and normal cells. *Journal of Cluster Science* 32:907–915.

Saha, S. K., S. B. Lee, J. Won, H. Y. Choi, K. Kim, G.-M. Yang, A. A. Dayem, and S.-g. Cho. 2017. Correlation between oxidative stress, nutrition, and cancer initiation. *International Journal of Molecular Sciences* 18:1544.

Santana, L. F., A. C. Inada, B. L. S. do E. Santo, W. F. O. Filiú, A. Pott, F. M. Alves, R. de C. A. Guimarães, K. de C. Freitas, and P. A. Hiane. 2019. Nutraceutical potential of *Carica papaya* in metabolic syndrome. *Nutrients* 11:1608.

Sharma, A., A. Bachheti, P. Sharma, R. K. Bachheti, and A. Husen. 2020. Phytochemistry, pharmacological activities, nanoparticle fabrication, commercial products and waste utilization of *Carica papaya* L.: A comprehensive review. *Current Research in Biotechnology* 2:145–160.

Singh, S. P., S. Kumar, S. V. Mathan, M. S. Tomar, R. K. Singh, P. K. Verma, A. Kumar, S. Kumar, R. P. Singh, and A. Acharya. 2020. Therapeutic application of *Carica papaya* leaf extract in the management of human diseases. *DARU Journal of Pharmaceutical Sciences* 28:735–744.

Singh, S. P., A. Mishra, R. K. Shyanti, R. P. Singh, and A. Acharya. 2021. Silver nanoparticles synthesized using *Carica papaya* leaf extract (AgNPs-PLE) causes cell cycle arrest and apoptosis in human prostate (DU145) cancer cells. *Biological Trace Element Research* 199:1316–1331.

Singh, S. P., B. Sharma, S. S. Kanwar, and A. Kumar. 2016. Lead phytochemicals for anticancer drug development. *Frontiers in Plant Science* 7:1667.

Somanah, J., S. Ramsaha, S. Verma, A. Kumar, P. Sharma, R. K. Singh, O. I. Aruoma, E. Bourdon, and T. Bahorun. 2016. Fermented papaya preparation modulates the progression of *N*-methyl-*N*-nitrosourea induced hepatocellular carcinoma in Balb/c mice. *Life Sciences* 151:330–338.

Tayal, N., P. Srivastava, and N. Srivastava. 2019. Anti angiogenic activity of *Carica papaya* leaf extract. *Journal of Pure and Applied Microbiology* 13:567–571.

Vundela, S. R., N. K. Kalagatur, A. Nagaraj, K. Kadirvelu, S. Chandranayaka, K. Kondapalli, A. Hashem, E. F. Abd-Allah, and S. Poda. 2021. Multi-biofunctional properties of phytofabricated selenium nanoparticles from *Carica papaya* fruit extract: Antioxidant, antimicrobial, antimycotoxin, anticancer, and biocompatibility. *Frontiers in Microbiology* 12:769891.

Vuong, Q. V., S. Hirun, T. L. K. Chuen, C. D. Goldsmith, S. Murchie, M. C. Bowyer, P. A. Phillips, and C. J. Scarlett. 2015. Antioxidant and anticancer capacity of saponin-enriched *Carica papaya* leaf extracts. *International Journal of Food Science & Technology* 50:169–177.

Waly, M. I., A. S. Al-Rawahi, M. Al-Riyami, M. A. Al-Kindi, H. K. Al-Issaei, S. A. Farooq, A. Al-Alawi, and M. S. Rahman. 2014. Amelioration of azoxymethane induced-carcinogenesis by reducing oxidative stress in rat colon by natural extracts. *BMC Complementary and Alternative Medicine* 14:1–10.

Weaver, B. A. 2014. How Taxol/paclitaxel kills cancer cells. *Molecular Biology of the Cell* 25:2677–2681.

World Health Organization. 2019. *WHO global report on traditional and complementary medicine 2019*. World Health Organization.

Xu, X., and L. Man. 2021. Papain mediated synthesized gold nanoparticles encore the potency of bioconjugated flutamide. *Current Pharmaceutical Biotechnology* 22:557–568.

Xue, G., and B. A. Hemmings. 2013. PKB/Akt: Dependent regulation of cell motility. *Journal of the National Cancer Institute* 105:393–404.

Yamthe, L. R., K. David, and Y. M. Ngadena. 2012. Acute and chronic toxicity studies of the aqueous and ethanol leaf extracts of *Carica papaya* Linn in Wistar rats. *Journal of Natural Product and Plant Resources* 2:617–627.

Yang, Q., M. Miyagawa, X. Liu, B. Zhu, S. Munemasa, T. Nakamura, Y. Murata, and Y. Nakamura. 2018. Methyl-β-cyclodextrin potentiates the BITC-induced anti-cancer effect through modulation of the Akt phosphorylation in human colorectal cancer cells. *Bioscience, Biotechnology, and Biochemistry* 82:2158–2167.

Zhang, T., M. C. Miller, Y. Zheng, Z. Zhang, H. Xue, D. Zhao, J. Su, K. H. Mayo, Y. Zhou, and G. Tai. 2017. Macromolecular assemblies of complex polysaccharides with galectin-3 and their synergistic effects on function. *Biochemical Journal* 474:3849–3868.

17 Plum Mango (*Bouea macrophylla*) Compositional Profile and Usage in Cancer

Jiraporn Kantapan and Nathupakorn Dechsupa

ABBREVIATIONS

Akt	protein kinase B
CDK	cyclin-dependent kinase
COX-2	cyclooxygenase 2
CSC	cancer stem cell
EG	ethyl gallate
EMT	epithelial–mesenchymal transition
GA	gallic acid
GC-MS	gas chromatography–mass spectrometry
HNSCC	head and neck squamous cell carcinoma
HPLC	high-performance liquid chromatography
IP	intraperitoneal
IR	irradiation
LC-MS	liquid chromatography–mass spectrometry
MAPK	mitogen-activated protein kinase
MMP	matrix metalloproteinase
MPSE	Maprang seed extract/plum mango seed extract
NF-κB	nuclear factor kappa B
NMR	nuclear magnetic resonance spectroscopy
PGG	pentagalloyl glucose
PI3K	phosphatidylinositol 3-kinase
ROS	reactive oxygen species
STAT3	signal transducer and activator of transcription 3
UPLC-Q-TOF-MS	ultra-performance liquid chromatography–quadrupole–time-of-flight–mass spectrometry
UV-Vis	ultraviolet-visible spectrophotometry
VEGF	vascular endothelial growth factor

17.1 INTRODUCTION

17.1.1 *Bouea macrophylla*: Taxonomy and General Properties

Plum mango or Marian plum (*Bouea* genus), a tropical fruit tree, is native to Southeast Asia, including the Philippines, Indonesia, Malaysia, Thailand, Cambodia, Myanmar, Laos, Vietnam, and South China. The genus *Bouea* is a member of the family Anacardiaceae, as is *Mangifera indica* (mango). The tree bears a mango-like fruit, known as plum mango, but its taste is notably

DOI: 10.1201/9781003260028-19

different. As of 2016, there were three specific plant species belonging to the genus *Bouea*: (1) *B. macrophylla* Griffith, (2) *B. oppositifolia* (Roxb.) Adelb., and (3) *B. microphylla* Griffith (Lim 2012a, 2012b; Harsono et al. 2017; Norfaizal et al. 2016). *Bouea* has various names in different regions (Table 17.1), such as *Maprang* or *Mayong* (Thailand), *Gandaria* (Indonesia and the Philippines), and *Kundang* (Malaysia) (Lim 2012a, 2012b; Dechsupa et al. 2019; Fu'adah et al. 2022; Rajan and Bhat 2016). In Thailand, plum mango flowering occurs during the cool, dry season (November–December) and the fruits mature in February and March (Subhadrabandhu 2001). The immature fruit is pale green when small; the green color darkens as the fruit develops. The ripe fruit is yellow-orange and a roundish to ovate shape (Figure 17.1). The fruit size averages 3.5–3.8 cm wide and 4.9–7.2 cm long. The fruit is juicy, with a sour-sweet taste, with the sweetness ranging from 15.6 to 23.7 Brix, according to the variety. It has a faint turpentine smell. The fruit contains one seed like the mango, albeit smaller. The seed kernel is white and pinkish-purple and has a bitter and astringent taste (Figure 17.1) (Office of Agricultural and Development Region 2 2022). These seeds represent about 60–150 g/kg (6–15% w/w) of the fruit (Dechsupa et al. 2019).

17.1.2 *B. macrophylla*: Cultivation and Uses

Plum mango is cultivated widely as a fruit tree, especially in Thailand, Malaysia, and Indonesia. In Thailand, Maprang is divided into three groups according to the taste of fruits, including Maprang wan (sweet), Maprang prieyo (sour), and Mayong, that is well-known as Mayong Chid (sweet with some sourness) (Dechsupa et al. 2019; Subhadrabandhu 2001). In Thailand, two species, *B.*

TABLE 17.1
The Taxonomical Classification and Vernacular Names of *Bouea*

Taxonomical Classification of Plum Mango

Kingdom	Plantae		
Division	Magnoliophyta		
Class	Magnolipsida		
Order	Sapindales		
Family	Anacardiaceae		
Genus	*Bouea*		
Species	*B. macrophylla* Griff.	*B. oppositifolia* (Roxb.) Adelb.	*B. microphylla* Griff.
Synonyms	*B. gandaria* Blume ex Miq., *Tropidopetalum javanicum* Turcz.	*B. oppositifolia* (Roxb.) Meisn., *B. burmanica* Griff., *B. angustifolia* Bl.	*B. oppositifolia* var. *microphylla* (Griff.), *B. burmanica* var. microphylla (Griff.) Engl.
Country/Language:	Vernacular Names:		
English	Plum mango, Marian plum, Gandaria	Marian plum, Marian tree, Plum-mango	
Thailand	*Maprang*	*Mayong Chid*	*Mapring*
Indonesia	*Gandaria,* *Pao Gandoriah, Kundangan,* *Remie, Ramen*	*Kunangan,* *Gandaria,* *Raman, Ramania, Uris*	
Malaysia	*Kundang, Kondongan,* *Pako Kundangan, Rembunia,* *Remenya, Rumenia, Rumia, Setar*	*Kundang,* *Kundang Siam, Kundang* *Rumenia, Rumenia, Rumia*	*Remia*

Source: Lim (2012a, 2012b); Rajan and Bhat (2016); Norfaizal et al. (2016); Dechsupa et al. (2019); Fu'adah et al. (2022).

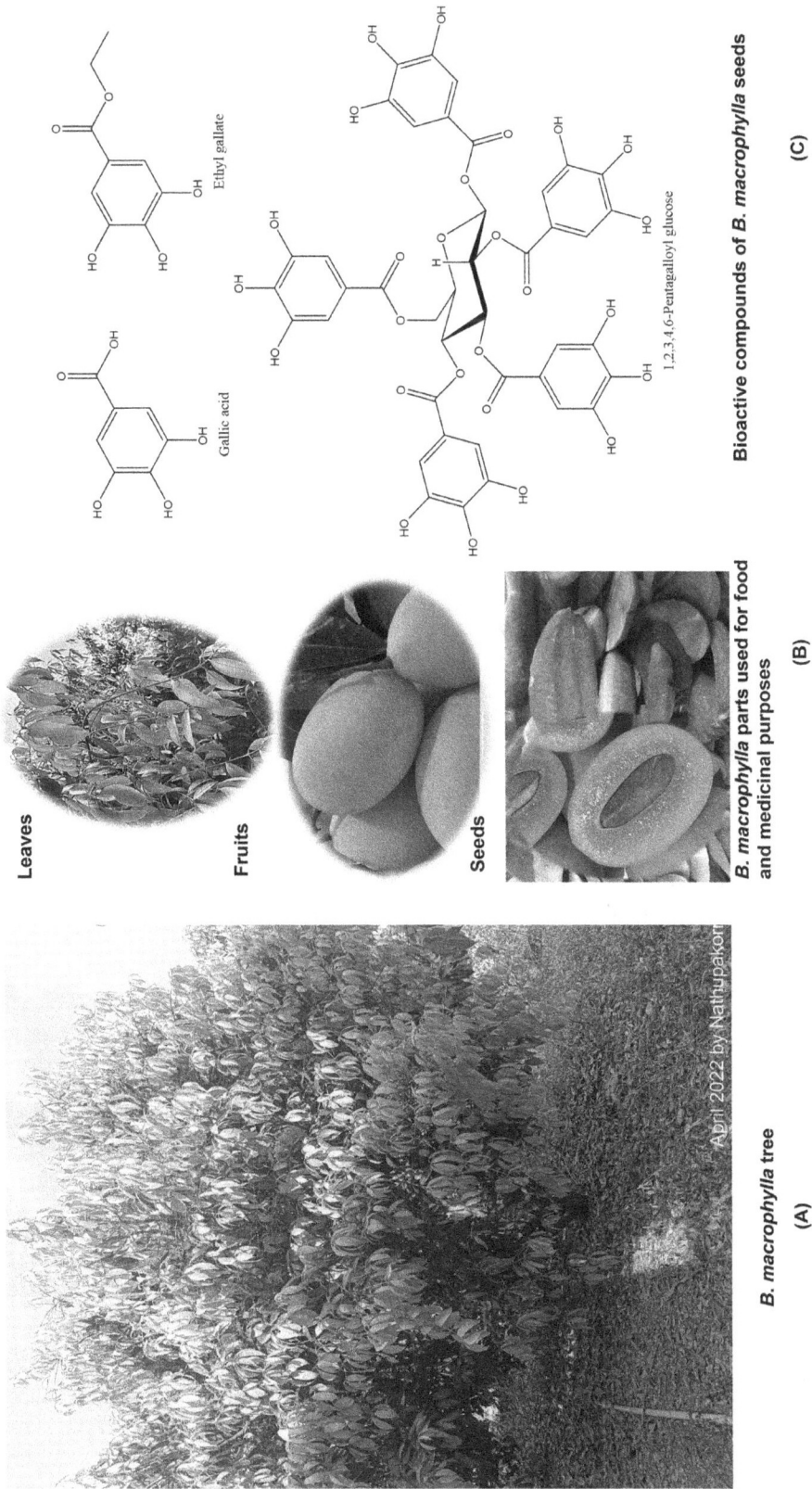

FIGURE 17.1 *Bouea macrophylla* Griffith: (A) tree after postharvest season (April); (B) parts used for food and medicinal purposes; and (C) chemical structures of bioactive compounds of seeds.

macrophylla (Maprang wan) and *B. oppositifolia* (Mayong Chid), were developed and collected for commercial cultivation with (Office of Agricultural and Development Region 2 2022). In 2022, the Department of Agricultural Extension, Thailand, recorded the cultivation area and production yield for 2021 for species *B. oppositifolia* as 4,261 hectares and 9,763 metric tons. In contrast, species *B. macrophylla* was 2,965 hectares and 8,225 metric tons. Currently, plum mango has been rapidly gaining popularity in Thailand. The planting area and production of the two species (*B. oppositifolia* and *B. macrophylla*) summation increased from 5,949 hectares and 4,890 metric tons in 2017 to 7,226 hectares and 17,988 metric tons in 2021 (Department of Agricultural Extension 2022). Traditionally, almost all the parts of the plum mango plant (leaves, unripe and ripe fruits, and seeds (Figure 17.1) are edible. Regularly, ripe fruits are used in jam, refreshing drinks, syrups, stews, and bakeries. Normally, the plum mango fruit is either consumed fresh or pickled. Regionally, this unripe fruit can be made into a compote or used in *sambal* (Indonesia), *rujak* (Indonesia), *rojak* (Malaysia), and *nam-pla wan* (Thailand). The young leaves of this plant are also edible, and they can be added to salads or served alongside vegetables, usually with chilies and shrimp paste (Lim 2012a, 2012b; Subhadrabandhu 2001; Rajan and Bhat 2019). The leaves have been used as poultice for headaches and their juice as a gargle for thrush in traditional medicine (Lim 2012a). While the seed of this plant with its bitter and astringent taste is rarely consumed and often left as waste from consumption and processing. However, Dechsupa et al. (2019) demonstrate that plum mango seed is a novel source of polyphenols with antioxidants, and antibacterial and anticancer properties (Dechsupa et al. 2019).

17.2 PHYTOCHEMICAL COMPOSITION OF PLUM MANGO

Evidence suggests that consuming a diet high in fruits and vegetables has long been associated with lowered risk of chronic diseases, such as cardiovascular disease and cancer (Aune et al. 2017). The disease-preventing abilities of fruits and vegetables are mainly due to the presence of several phytochemicals (Zhang et al. 2015; Jideani et al. 2021). Scientific data collected from the literature have documented that the plum mango plant contains several potentially bioactive components from several parts of the plant, including the stem, leaves, fruits, and seeds (Table 17.2).

17.2.1 STEM

The sequential maceration of the *B. macrophylla* stem in hexane, ethyl acetate, and methanol indicated that stigmasterol, fustin, garbanzole, methyl gallate, luteolin, and naringenin were the major phytoconstituents (Rudiana et al. 2019; Rudiana et al. 2021).

TABLE 17.2

Potential Bioactive Compounds Identified from Different Parts of *Bouea macrophylla* Griffith

Plant Part	Phytochemicals	Extraction/Isolation Methods	Characterization Methods	Reference
Stem	Stigmasterol	Sequential maceration	NMR,	Rudiana et al.
	Fustin	in hexane, ethyl	UPLC-Q-TOF-MS	2021
	Garbanzole	acetate, and		
	Methyl gallate	methanol/column		
		chromatography		
	Luteolin	Ethyl acetate	LC-MS/MS	Rudiana et al.
	Naringenin	extraction/column		2019
		chromatography		

TABLE 17.2
(Continued)

Plant Part	Phytochemicals	Extraction/Isolation Methods	Characterization Methods	Reference
Leaves	Caryophyllene	Maceration in 70% ethanol	GC-MS	Nguyen et al. 2020
	Humulene			
	Caryophyllene oxide			
	2-Methyl-*cis*-7,8-epoxynonadecane			
	Hexadecanoic acid, ethyl ester			
	Phytol			
	Oxiraneundecanoic acid, 3-pentyl-, methyl ester, *trans-*			
	Hexadecanoic acid, ethyl ester			
	Diisooctyl phthalate			
	Squalene			
	trans-Geranylgeraniol			
	Vitamin E			
	Retinol, acetate			
	γ-Himachalene			
	Quercetin	Sequential maceration in hexane, hiethyl ether, and ethyl acetate	UV-Vis	Hardinsyah et al. 2019
Fruits		Continuous hydrodistillation using a Likens-Nickerson distillation unit	GC-MS	Rajan and Bhat 2017
–Ripe	Terpene hydrocarbons (29.28%): α-terpineol, E, E-alpha-farnesene, 1,10-di-epi-cubenol, cadin-4-en-10-ol			
	Ketones (27.27%): acetyl valeryl, acetophenone			
	Esters (20.73%): pentanoic acid, 2-propenyl ester, hexanedioic acid, bis(2-ethylhexyl) ester			
	Acids (9.68%): dodecanoic acid, *N*-hexadecanoic acid			
	Alcohols (9.35%)			
–Unripe	Terpene hydrocarbons (32.89%): delta-cadinene, tumerone, α-cadinol, cubenol			
	Acids (29.72%)			
	Esters (17.32%): hexanedioic acid, bis(2-ethylhexyl) ester, decanedioic acid, bis(2-ethylhexyl) ester			
	Ketones (16.85%): 5,6-decanedione, acetophenone			
	Alcohols (2.83%): trimethylacetic anhydride, margaric acid, palmitic acid			
Seeds	Gallic acid	Ethanol maceration/ colum chromatography	HPLC, LC-MS	Dechsupa et al. 2019; Kantapan et al. 2020
	Ethyl gallate			
	Pentagalloyl glucose			
	Ellagic acid			
	High molecular weight gallotannins			

17.2.2 LEAVES

The phytochemical screening conducted on methanolic extract of plum mango leaves was rich in alkaloids, flavonoids, anthraquinones, saponins, total phenols, tannins, sterols, triterpenes, and vitamin C (Sukalingam 2018), while the ethanolic extract of *B. macrophylla* leaves also found secondary metabolites such as phenols, flavonoids, steroids, and terpenoids (Fitri et al. 2018). Nguyen et al. (2020) investigated the bioactive components of ethanolic extract of *B. macrophylla* leaves by GC-MS analysis. It was found that the ethanolic extracts contained various bioactive compounds, including polyphenols, flavonoids, caryophyllene, phytol, and *trans*-geranylgeraniol (Nguyen et al. 2020).

17.2.3 FRUITS

The ethanolic extract of unripe and ripe fruits, identified by GC-MS methods, reported the isolation of volatile compounds, such as terpene hydrocarbons, ketones and esters, acetophenone, and acetylvaleryl, as the main bioactive compounds (Nguyen et al. 2020).

17.2.4 SEEDS

The ethanolic extract of plum mango seed is a rich source of hydrolyzable gallotannin. This gallotannin exerts attractive pharmacological activities, including anticancer, anti-angiogenic, antioxidant, anti-inflammatory, and anti-ulcerative properties (Torres-León et al. 2017). Example gallotannins found in plum mango seed extract include pentagalloyl glucose (PGG; 50%), ethyl gallate (EG; 36%), and gallic acid (GA; 0.5%). The other 13.5% is composed of high molecular weight gallotannins (such as hexa-, hepta-, and octa-galloyl moieties) (Kantapan et al. 2020). *B. macrophylla* seed extract has demonstrated various pharmacological activities, including antioxidant, antimicrobial, antihyperglycemic, and anticancer activities (Dechsupa et al. 2019; Fu'adah et al. 2022). However, studies have been dominated by anticancer activities.

17.3 ANTICANCER ACTIVITIES OF *B. MACROPHYLLA* EXTRACT AND ITS PHYTOCHEMICALS

Relevant scientific literature collected from the scientific database documented that *B. macrophylla* extracts exhibited anticancer effects against several types of cancers. *In vitro* cell proliferation inhibitory effects of various *B. macrophylla* plant parts have been reported against breast cancer, lung cancer, leukemia, head and neck squamous cell carcinoma (HNSCC), colorectal carcinoma, and Vero cells. These have been addressed in further detail in the following sections.

17.3.1 LEAF EXTRACT

A study showed that the ethanolic extract of plum mango leaves exhibited excellent antiproliferative activity against cervical cancer (HeLa) and colorectal carcinoma (HCT116) cell lines with IC_{50} values at 24 ± 0.8 and 28 ± 0.9 µg/mL, respectively. In this study, the main bioactive constituents, such as caryophyllene, squalene, and phytol, were believed to be the main mediated links to the antiproliferative activity of the extract (Nguyen et al. 2020). Another study reported that the ethanolic extract of *B. macrophylla* leaf decreased the cell viability of Vero cells with the IC_{50} value at 35.81 µg/mL. Moreover, it was observed that the extract induced cell morphology changes, including membrane blebbing and chromatin condensation, which suggested that the extract induced Vero cells to undergo apoptosis (Fitri et al. 2018).

17.3.2 STEM EXTRACT

The stem extract of *B. macrophylla* contains four main compounds: stigmasterol, fustin, garbanzole, and methyl gallate. All compounds were assayed for their anticancer property against MCF-7,

A549, HCC-1954, and MDA-MB231 cell lines. All the isolated compounds exhibited moderate anticancer activities against almost cell lines tested. Among them, fustin and methyl gallate were more active on HCC-1954 cells, with IC_{50} values of 134.35 ± 44.62 and 153.69 ± 12.54 µg/mL, respectively, than other isolated compounds (Rudiana et al. 2021).

17.3.3 FRUIT EXTRACT

To the authors' knowledge, to date no studies of the anticancer activities of the fruit extract of *B. macrophylla* have been reported in any scientific database.

17.3.4 SEED EXTRACT

An emerging body of evidence has suggested that *B. macrophylla* seed extract (MPSE) possesses excellent anticancer activities against various cancer cells, including leukemia, lung cancer, breast cancer, and head and neck squamous cell carcinoma (HNSCC). The cytotoxicity test results of the ethanolic seed extracts against four cancer cell lines, including doxorubicin-sensitive and doxorubicin-resistant leukemic (K562, K562/ADR) and lung cancer (GLC4 and GLC4/ADR) cells, showed that the seed extracts dose-dependently inhibited the proliferation of cancer cells, with IC_{50} values varying between 4 and 35 µg/mL. It should be noted that MPSE had a more toxic effect on the drug-resistant cell lines than the parental cell lines, suggesting that MPSE targeted drug-resistant cancers (Dechsupa et al. 2019). Furthermore, Kantapan et al. reported the ability of MPSE, to inhibit cell proliferation of breast cancer cells (MCF-7 and MDA-MB231). Fortunately, MPSE showed lower toxicity on normal breast mammary epithelial cells (MCF-10A). The IC_{50} value of MPSE was significantly lower for the cancer cells than the normal cells, which had IC_{50} values of 6.94, 18.92, and 30.08 µg/mL for MCF-7, MDA-MB231, and MCF-10A, respectively. The results from this study suggested that MPSE was a cancer-selective agent (Kantapan et al. 2020).

Radiation therapy is one of the core treatments for cancer treatment. However, the effectiveness is limited by the tumor radioresistance. It was found that MPSE, significantly improved radiation-induced DNA damage and reduced cell survival. Combined treatment with MPSE and irradiation revealed an enhanced radiosensitivity of breast cancer cell lines with sensitization enhancement ratios of 2.33 and 1.35 for MCF-7 and MDA-MB231 cells, respectively. It is believed that cancer stem cells (CSCs) are the main contributor to the development of therapeutic resistance, recurrence, and metastasis (Kantapan et al. 2021b). Thus, developing novel strategies that target the elimination of CSCs is essential for cancer treatment. Recently, a study revealed that radiation directly contribute to the generation of novel CSCs via radiation-induced epithelial–mesenchymal transition (EMT) during the fractionate of radiotherapy (Kim et al. 2016). It revealed that pretreatment with MPSE before irradiation attenuated the radiation-induced EMT process and decreased stemness-like properties in the radiation-surviving MCF-7 cells. Moreover, another study by the same research group reported the ability of MPSE and PGG, the pure bioactive compound isolated from MPSE, to suppress the stemness properties. As a consequence of MPSE and PGG attenuating CSCs, the radiosensitivity of irradiated HNSCC cell lines was promoted (Kantapan et al. 2021b).

Kantapan et al. demonstrated that the MPSE contained higher levels of PGG, EG, and GA, which could have contributed to its high anticancer activity. As described below, various studies have demonstrated the anticancer activity of the individual phytochemical compounds contained in MPSE.

17.3.4.1 Pentagalloylglucose

Pentagalloylglucose (1,2,3,4,6-penta-O-galloyl-β-d-glucose [PGG]), a main bioactive compound in *B. macrophylla* seed extract (Kantapan et al. 2020), is a water-soluble phenolic compound consisting of the glucose core and saturated with five galloyl groups. PGG is a natural abundance and is mainly found in medicinal herbs and plants (Torres-León et al. 2017) such as *Rhus chinensis* Mill.

(Huh et al. 2005), *Paeonia suffruticosa* (Liu et al. 2018; Oh et al. 2001), *Paeonia lactiflora* (Kim et al. 2016), *Schinus terebinthifolius* (Rosas et al. 2015), *Pelargonium inquinans* Ait. (Piao et al. 2008), *Terminalia chebula* (Saleem et al. 2002), and *Mangifera indica* (Nithitanakool et al. 2009). The anticancer activity of PGG has been extensively studied against several types of cancer, including prostate cancer, lung cancer, breast cancer, sarcoma, leukemia, melanoma, liver cancer, and HNSCC.

As reported by Hu et al., PGG exhibited a dose-dependent inhibition of the cell viability of prostate cancer cells (LNCaP and DU145). PGG caused the induction of intracellular reactive oxygen species (ROS) production, leading to cell cycle arrest at the G1 and S-phases, consequently inducing caspase-mediated apoptosis. In addition, a daily intraperitoneal (IP) injection of PGG (20 mg/kg) led to a significant reduction in tumor growth in the DU145 xenograft model. This reduction was mainly associated with the decreasing of phosphorylation of signal transducers and activators of transcription 3 (STAT3) (Hu et al. 2008a). Moreover, PGG was also reported to induce autophagic cell death in aggressive prostate cancer cells (PC-3). This study suggested that PGG may induce cell death by caspase-independent programmed cell death. These results supported its merit as a potential drug candidate for caspase-resistant recurrent prostate cancer therapy (Hu et al. 2009b). The anti-invasive effects of PGG were also reported; an IP injection, at a dose of 25 mg/kg of PGG for 28 days, reduced the tumor weight of PC-3 tumor in a xenograft mouse and suppressed cancer cell invasion into bone via the inhibition of matrix metalloproteinase-9 (MMP-9) expression, stemming from the suppression of the EGFR/JNK pathway. Their results suggested that PGG suppressed invasion and tumorigenesis of aggressive prostate cancer PC-3 xenografts model and PGG could be a therapeutic candidate for the treatment of advanced prostate cancer (Kuo et al. 2009).

The *in vitro* and *in vivo* studies of anticancer effects of PGG have also been reported in breast cancer. Chen et al. revealed the growth inhibitory effect of PGG on MCF-7 cells through a perturb in the cell cycle at the G1 phase (Chen et al. 2003). In another study, Lee et al. reported the remarkable *in vivo* efficacy of an orally administered PGG at 10 or 20 mg/kg to inhibit the growth and metastasis of a very aggressive triple-negative breast cancer MDA-MB231 xenograft in nude mice. PGG treatment also decreased the incidence of lung metastasis, decreased the phosphorylation of STAT3 and its downstream target proteins (VEGF, Bcl-2, and cyclin D1), and induced caspase activation. The suppression of pSTAT3 resulted in the occurrence of cellular processes, including anti-angiogenesis, anti-invasion, and apoptosis induction in the PGG-treated nude mice model. These findings suggested a potential role for PGG as a natural therapeutic agent for breast cancer treatment (Lee et al. 2011). Vascular endothelial growth factor (VEGF) and matrix metalloproteinases (MMPs) are the key molecules contributing to the regulation of angiogenesis, invasion, and metastasis. Huh et al. reported that a once-daily IP injection of PGG (20 mg/kg) significantly inhibited tumor growth and decreased the microvessel density of a highly angiogenesis-dependent lung cancer (Lewis lung cancer) allograft. In this study, PGG effectively inhibited proliferation and tube formation of human umbilical vein endothelial cells treated with fibroblast growth factor. PGG revealed a decrease in microvessel density via suppressed expression of cyclooxygenase-2 (COX-2) and VEGF (Huh et al. 2005). These results strongly supported the anti-angiogenesis effect of PGG.

Kantapan et al. isolated PGG from *B. macrophylla* seed extraction and then tested cellular effects *in vitro* biological assays. PGG was able to inhibit the growth of HNSCC cell lines (CAL27 and FaDu) in a dose-dependent manner and exhibited effective antimigration activity on those cells. A combination of PGG and cisplatin synergism inhibited the growth of cancer cells and enhanced the apoptotic cell death induced by cisplatin (Kantapan et al., unpublished data). These results demonstrated that cisplatin synergized with PGG to promote potent apoptosis in HNSCC cells. Furthermore, the dose of the chemotherapeutic drug could be reduced without reducing antitumor activity by using it in combination with PGG to reduce the severe side effect of chemotherapeutic drugs.

17.3.4.2 Ethyl Gallate

Ethyl gallate (EG), one of the most abundantly bioactive compounds found in *B. macrophylla* seed extract, is a phenolic compound and has been used extensively as a food additive. EG has demonstrated various pharmacological activities, including anticancer, antioxidant, anti-inflammatory, and free radical scavenging. Its anticancer activity has been extensively studied in several cancer types. Cui et al. reported that EG extract from the roots of *Euphorbia fischeriana* Steud. could inhibit cell proliferation of breast cancer cells (MCF-7 and MDA-MB231) in both a dose- and time-dependent manner (Cui et al. 2015). Notably, highly invasive and metastatic breast cancer cells (MDA-MB231) were more sensitive to the EG treatment. Additionally, EG treatment significantly inhibited the cell motility of MDA-MB231 via decreasing the expression of MMP-2 and MMP-9, a critical enzyme for tumor invasion. Moreover, EG treatment decreased PI3K/Akt and nuclear factor kappa B (NF-κB) activation in MDA-MB231 cells. These findings suggested that EG-induced suppressed proliferation and invasion in human breast cancer cells, involving the modulation of the PI3K/Akt pathway, which could inhibit their downstream targets (e.g., NF-κB p-65, Bcl-2/Bax, MMP-2, and MMP-9) in breast cancer cells (Cui et al. 2015). Another study reported the ability of EG to suppress esophageal cancer cell growth via induced G2/M phase cell cycle arrest upon reducing the expression of cyclin A2 and cyclin B1. Further, EG directly bound to and inhibited ERK1/2 activities and their downstream signaling, which could contribute to stimulated apoptosis and suppress esophageal tumor growth. These results suggested that EG was a novel ERK1/2 inhibitor and potentially developed for treating esophageal cancer (Liu et al. 2019).

17.4 MECHANISM INSIGHTS INTO THE ANTICANCER ACTIONS OF *B. MACROPHYLLA* EXTRACT AND ITS PHYTOCHEMICALS

Evidence from *in vitro* and *in vivo* studies suggested that *B. macrophylla* extract and its phytochemicals could exert an anticancer effect. A gallotannin-enrich extract may act individually or synergistically to prevent cancer cell growth. Possible mechanisms underlying the anticancer activity of *B. macrophylla* extract, supported by the evidence from an *in vitro* experiment, include the induction of reactive oxygen species' generation – leading to cell cycle arrest and apoptosis induction, decreased migration and invasion – and the inhibition of STAT3/Akt pathways, contributing to the observed reduced in-cell survival, cell migration, and metastasis.

17.4.1 Generation of Reactive Oxygen Species

Reactive oxygen species (ROS) play a dual role in cancer biology and require tight regulation of ROS levels for cellular life. A moderately elevated ROS level can promote tumorigenesis, facilitating cancer cell proliferation, survival, and adaptation to hypoxia. On the other hand, elevated ROS levels above the threshold can promote antitumorigenic activity and induced cancer cell death. Recently, anticancer strategies that focus on oxidative stress-induced cell death have drawn the attention and interest of scientists. As reported by Kantapan et al., MPSE inhibited cell growth and induced apoptotic cell death in MCF-7 cells via induction of oxidative stress (Kantapan et al. 2020). As shown through observation, a dose-dependent elevated level of intracellular ROS production in MCF-7 cells treated with MPSE, followed by depolarization of mitochondrial membrane potential, led to an increase in the Bax/Bcl-2 gene expression ratio, suggesting MPSE-induced apoptosis as a mitochondria-dependent pathway (Figure 17.2).

17.4.2 Induction of Cell Cycle Arrest and Apoptosis

It is well-known that cell cycle arrest in response to DNA damage or cellular stress is integral to maintaining genomic integrity. On the other hand, in cancer cells, cell cycle arrest represents a

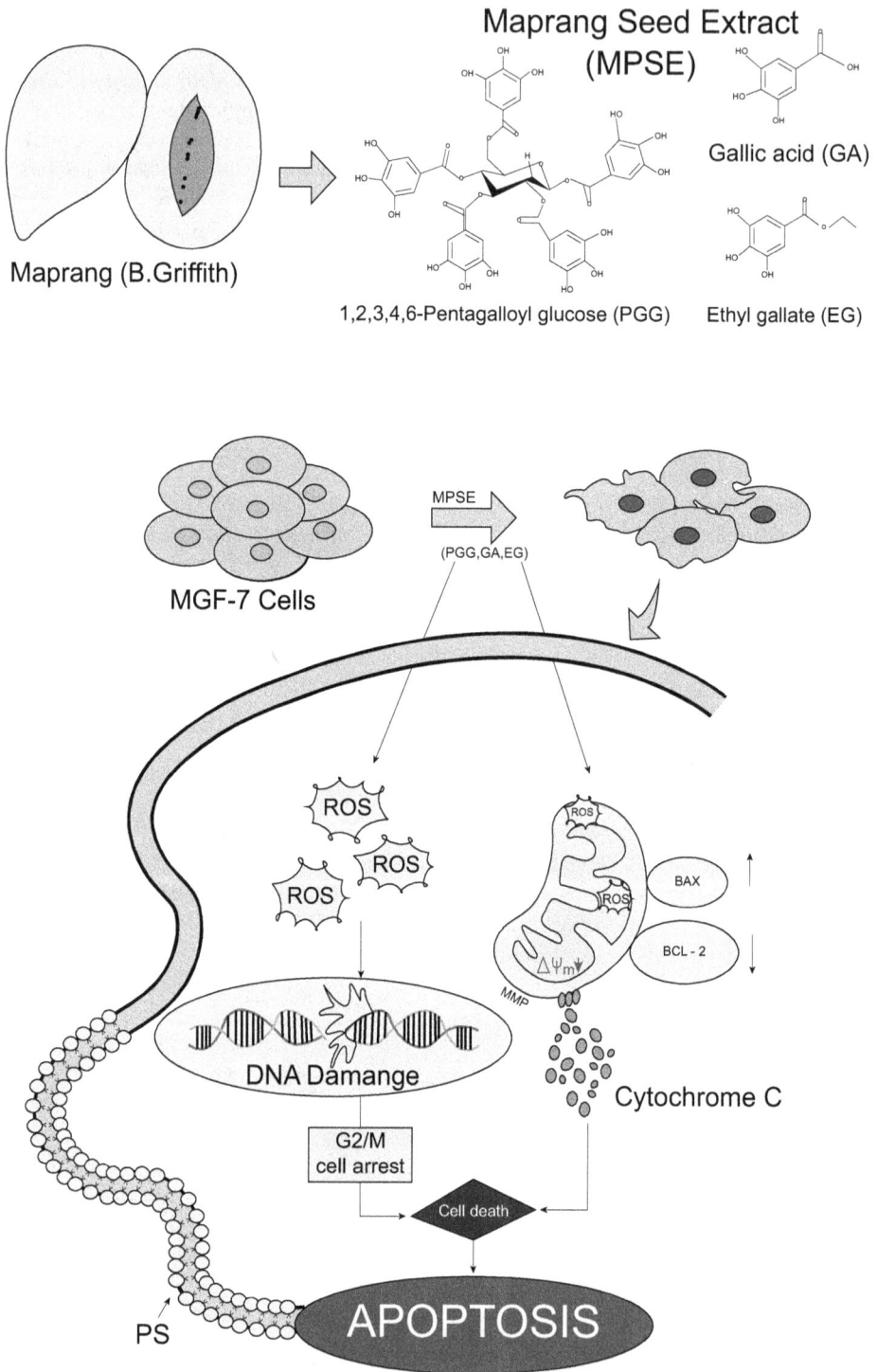

FIGURE 17.2 Anticancer mechanism of *Bouea macrophylla* Griffith. *B. macrophylla* Griffith seed extract (MPSE) inhibits cancer cell growth and induces apoptotic cell death in MCF-7 cells via oxidative stress (ROS) induction and the consequent mitochondrial-dependent apoptosis. BAX = Bcl-2-associated X; Bcl-2 = B-cell lymphoma protein 2; MMP = mitochondrial membrane permeability; $\Delta\psi_m$ = mitochondrial membrane potential; PS = phosphatidylserine; ROS = reactive oxygen species.

survival mechanism that allows cancer cells to repair their own damaged DNA (Otto and Sicinski 2017). Thus, cell cycle checkpoints play a crucial role in controlling the mechanisms that restrain cell cycle transition; abrogation of cell cycle checkpoints can activate the apoptotic cascade, leading to cell death.

MPSE was reported to induce a G2/M phase arrest in MCF-7 cells following MPSE treatment for 24 h. It has long been known that the cell cycle phase also determines a cell's relative radiosensitivity, with cells being most radiosensitive in the G2-M phase (Kantapan et al. 2020). Therefore, the targeted drugs, when combined with radiation therapy that can synchronize tumor cells to accumulate in radiosensitive cell cycle phases, work better by altering the radiosensitivity. As mentioned above, MPSE induced MCF-7 cells to accumulate in the G2/M phase cell cycle arrest; pretreatment of breast cancer cells with MPSE followed by irradiation resulted in increased radiosensitivity and enhanced radiation-induced cell death. Thus, MPSE-induced cell cycle arrest at the G2/M phase may be one mechanism underlying the radiosensitizing effects of MPSE.

17.4.3 ATTENUATE THE ACTIVATION OF CRITICAL SURVIVAL PATHWAYS

The activation of critical survival pathways – such as the PI3K/Akt and MAPK signaling pathways – following exposure to radiation of cancer cells led to the development of radioresistance (Ouellette et al. 2022). Therefore, targeting these survival pathways in combination with radiotherapy is a means to enhance therapeutic efficacy by attenuating cellular defense in response to treatment. The radiosensitizing effects of MPSE on breast cancer cells have been linked to attenuation in the IR-induced activation of the survival pathway. Kantapan et al. analyzed the protein expression levels of various PI3K/Akt and MAPK pathway components in breast cancer cells treated with MPSE combined with radiation. It was observed that pretreatment with MPSE before irradiation markedly decreased the phosphorylation of Akt, ERK1/2, and JNK in MCF7 and MDA-MB231 cells compared to IR treatment alone, and further sensitized cancer cells to radiation (Kantapan et al. 2021a).

17.4.4 INHIBITION OF THE EPITHELIAL–MESENCHYMAL TRANSITION

Epithelial–mesenchymal transition is a reversible process in which the cellular phenotype in epithelial cells transforms into a mesenchymal state. EMT is known to drive differentiation of non–stem cancer cells into cancer stem cells that remain after cancer treatment and contribute to intratumor heterogeneity. The cells exhibiting EMT features exist in the cancer stem cell population, which is involved in therapeutic resistance, recurrence, and metastasis. In addition, ample evidence has shown that a cancer treatment–induced EMT program is an essential process in therapeutic resistance (Smith and Bhowmick 2016). A study showed that MCF-7 cell pretreatment with MPSE before irradiation attenuated the stemness phenotypic characteristics of the radiation-survived population of MCF-7 cells. This led to a decrease in the number of tumor mammospheres, the downregulation of stemness- or EMT-associated markers (ZEB-1, vimentin) and migratory ability, and a reduced ability of cells to form colonies in an anchorage-independent fashion (Kantapan et al. 2021a).

Interestingly, the population of radiation-surviving MCF-7 cells showed an EMT phenotype and overexpressed multidrug resistance proteins. It was reported that MPSE could suppress the expression of multidrug resistance proteins in the surviving population of MCF-7 cells (Paksee et al. 2019).

17.4.5 SUPPRESSING CANCER STEM CELLS

Similarly, the same research group reported suppressing cancer stemness properties using MPSE and a purified PGG isolated from MPSE in HNSCC. This study found that MPSE and PGG were able to suppress tumor sphere formation and decrease protein expression of CSC markers, including Oct4, SOX-2, and CD44, all of which were associated with a decrease in phosphorylated STAT3 protein expression (Kantapan et al. 2021b). This was not surprising, because it has long been known that the activation of STAT3 contributes to the critical regulation and maintenance of CSC characteristics (Geiger et al. 2016). Moreover, it was reported that highly activated STAT3 was positively correlated with high-grade HNSCC tissue containing CSC traits and the radioresistance ability of HNSCC (Bu et al. 2015). In the same study, HNSCC cell treatment with MPSE or PGG was shown to downregulate the expression of phosphorylated STAT3. Subsequently, it downregulated CSC-related proteins, Oct4, SOX2, and CD44, and further conferred the radiosensitivity of the HNSCC cell line. Collectively, these results suggested the effectiveness of MPSE and PGG in suppressing activities on critical oncogenic pathway STAT3 signaling (Kantapan et al. 2021b).

17.4.6 Inhibition of the STAT3 Signaling Pathway

A mounting body of evidence has demonstrated that aberrant activation of the STAT3 signaling pathway is significantly associated with aggressive cancer phenotypes, including angiogenesis, migration, and metastasis. It has been demonstrated that STAT3 directly regulated the expression of VEGF, a key angiogenic protein, and matrix metalloproteinases such as MMP-2 and MMP-9. The expression of VEGF and MMPs proteins promotes angiogenesis and invasive processes, all of which contribute to cancer metastasis. A study by Kantapan et al. found that PGG, a bioactive compound isolated from plum mango seed extract, suppressed the phosphorylation of STAT3 and consequently reduced VEGF expression in HNSCC cells (Kantapan et al., unpublished data). Moreover, PGG also inhibited cell migration and invasion in HNSCC cells. Similarly, as reported by another study, PGG also exerted an anti-invasive effect by suppressing the epidermal growth factor receptor (EGFR)/c-Jun N-terminal kinases (JNK) pathway and controlling MMP-9 expression, resulting in the suppression of bone metastasis in nude mice treated with an intratibial injection of PC-3 prostate cancer cells (Kuo et al. 2009).

17.4.7 Other Foods, Herbs, Spices, and Botanicals Used in Cancer

Many medicinal herbs and plants show promising anticancer activity. The beneficial effects of natural products are attributable to their rich phytochemical contents, which are believed to be attributed to their potent, widely pharmacological activities. In particular, *B. macrophylla* seed extract is a rich source of hydrolyzable gallotannins, which contributes to its potent anticancer properties. In addition to plum mango seed gallotannin, other plants also contain gallotannin and have been extensively studied for their anticancer activities (Table 17.3).

17.4.8 Toxicity and Cautionary Notes

Nearly all parts of the plum mango plant (seeds, unripe and ripe fruits, leaves) have been used for various culinary purposes. They have been known to be safe for centuries. To date, however, no published study on the safety and efficacy of *B. macrophylla* extract in humans has been reported. Nevertheless, MSN Nature Solution Co., Ltd. (Thailand) conducted acute and subchronic oral toxicity studies on *B. macrophylla* seed extract (MPSE under trademark NATURE U, data with permission) in Wistar rats. The acute oral toxicity of MPSE reported the LD50 as >5000 mg/kg body weight. Subchronic toxicity was tested in Wistar rats given MPSE orally for 90 days. MPSE was not found to be toxic in rats. There were no side effects of MPSE (either mortalities or abnormalities in body weight and hematology) in the MPSE-treated group. No significant hepatic or renal toxicity was seen in rats given the maximum dose level of MPSE at 2000 mg/kg body weight.

TABLE 17.3

Summary of *In Vitro* Anticancer Potential Evaluations of Herbs and Plants Containing Gallotannin Constituents

Plants/Herbs	Phytochemical Constituent	Cancers/Cell Lines	*In Vitro* Results	Reference
Mango (*M. indica*)	Gallotannin (pentagalloyl glucose)	Breast cancer/MCF-7	↓ Cell viability ↑ G1-phase arrest	Chen et al. 2003
Mango (*M. indica*) kernel extract	Gallotannin (gallic acid)	Breast cancer/MCF-7 and MDA-MB231	↑ ROS and MDA ↓ GSH level ↑ p53 level ↑ Mitochondrial-dependent apoptosis pathway	Abdullah et al. 2015a; Abdullah et al. 2015b
Galla chinensis extract	Gallotannin (pentagalloyl glucose)	Breast cancer/ MDA-MB231	↓ Cell viability ↓ Lactic acid production	Deiab et al. 2015
Paeonia suffruticosa extracts	Gallotannin (pentagalloyl glucose)	Pancreatic/AsPC1	↓ Cell viability ↑ Mitophagy ↑ Apoptotic cell death	Liu et al. 2018
T. chebula Retz. fruit extract	Gallotannin (pentagalloyl glucose, gallic acid)	Human breast cancer (MCF-7)/mouse breast cancer(S115)/ osteosarcoma (HOS-1)/ prostate cancer (PC-3)	↓ Cell viability ↑ Apoptotic cell death	Saleem et al. 2002
Rhus chinensis Mill.	Gallotannin (pentagalloyl glucose)	Lewis lung carcinoma (LLC)	↓ Cell viability ↑ Apoptotic cell death ↓ Angiogenesis ↓ VEGF and COX-2 expression	Huh et al. 2005
Paeonia suffruticosa root extract	Gallotannin (pentagalloyl glucose)	Hepatocellular carcinoma/SK-HEP-1	↓ Cell viability ↑ G1-phase arrest ↑ Apoptotic cell death ↓ Activation of nuclear factor-kappa B	Oh et al. 2001

Nevertheless, additional data are needed for *in vivo* study of MPSE–drug interactions and human safety in a clinical trial.

17.5   SUMMARY POINTS

- This chapter focused on plum mango (*B. macrophylla* Griffith) and its anticancer activities.
- Plum mango is widely cultivated in Thailand.
- Almost all parts of the plum mango are edible, including fruits, leaves, and seeds.
- Plum mango seeds are a waste product from consumption and agricultural processing.
- Pentagalloyl glucose, ethyl gallate, and gallic acid are potent anticancer constituents of plum mango seeds.
- Plum mango seed extracts inhibit cancer cell growth, proliferation, migration, and invasion. They also trigger apoptosis and cell cycle arrest against various cancers.
- Plum mango seed extracts and PGG show additive and synergistic effects in relation to anticancer drugs and radiation therapies in cancer treatment.

- Plum mango seed extract is safe as a continuous, long-term dietary supplement according to animal studies.
- Plum mango seed extract may be a promising adjunct drug for use with conventional cancer therapies.
- Further *in vivo* studies and clinical trials are needed for MPSE–drug interactions to ensure human safety.

REFERENCES

Abdullah, A.S.H., Mohammed, A.S., Rasedee, A., Mirghani, M.E.S., and Al-Qubaisi, M.S. 2015a. Induction of apoptosis and oxidative stress in estrogen receptor-negative breast cancer, MDA-MB231 cells, by ethanolic mango seed extract. BMC Complement Altern Med, 15: 45. doi:10.1186/s12906-015-0575-x

Abdullah, A.S.H., Mohammed, A.S., Rasedee, A., and Mirghani, M.E. 2015b. Oxidative stress-mediated apoptosis induced by ethanolic mango seed extract in cultured estrogen receptor positive breast cancer MCF-7 cells. International Journal of Molecular Sciences, 16(2), 3528–3536. doi:10.3390/ijms16023528

Aune, D., Giovannucci, E., Boffetta, P., Fadnes, L.T., Keum, N., Norat, T., Greenwood, D.C., Riboli, E., Vatten, L.J., and Tonstad, S. 2017. Fruit and vegetable intake and the risk of cardiovascular disease, total cancer and all-cause mortality – a systematic review and dose-response meta-analysis of prospective studies. International Journal of Epidemiology, 46(3): 1029–1056. doi:10.1093/ije/dyw319

Bu, L.L., Zhao, Z.L., Liu, J.F., Ma, S.R., Huang, C.F., Liu, B., Zhang, W.F., and Sun, Z.J. 2015. STAT3 blockade enhances the efficacy of conventional chemotherapeutic agents by eradicating head neck stemloid cancer cell. Oncotarget, 6(39): 41944–41958. doi:10.18632/oncotarget.5986

Chen, W.J., Chang, C.Y., and Lin, J.K. 2003. Induction of G1 phase arrest in MCF human breast cancer cells by pentagalloylglucose through the down-regulation of CDK4 and CDK2 activities and up-regulation of the CDK inhibitors p27(Kip) and p21(Cip). Biochemical Pharmacology, 65(11): 1777–1785.

Cui, H., Yuan, J., Du, X., Wang, M., Yue, L., and Liu, J. 2015. Ethyl gallate suppresses proliferation and invasion in human breast cancer cells via Akt-NF-κB signaling. Oncology Reports, 33(3): 1284–1290.

Dechsupa, N., Kantapan, J., Tungjaj, M., and Intorasoot, S. 2019. Maprang "Bouea macrophylla Griffith" seed: The proximate composition, HPLC fingerprints, the antioxidation, anticancer, and antimicrobial properties of ethanolic seed extracts. Heliyon, 5: e02052. doi:10.1016/j.heliyon.2019.e02052

Deiab, S., Mazzio, E., Eyunni, S., McTier, O., Mateeva, N., Elshami, F., and Soliman, K.F. 2015. 1,2,3,4,6-penta-O-galloylglucose within Galla chinensis inhibits human LDH-A and attenuates cell proliferation in MDA-MB-231 breast cancer cells. Evidence-Based Complementary and Alternative Medicine, 2015: 276946. doi:10.1155/2015/276946

Department of Agricultural Extension. 2022. Agricultural production data base. https://production.doae.go.th/ (In Thai, Accessed April 20, 2022).

Fitri, L., Taufiqurrahman, I., and DH, I. 2018. Phytochemical and cytotoxicity testing of ramania leaves (Bouea macrophylla Griffith) ethanol extract toward Vero cells using MTT assay method (Preliminary study of adjuvant therapy materials to the preparation of the drug). Dentino Jurnal Kedokteran Gigi, 3: 51–56.

Fu'adah, I.T., Sumiwi, S.A., and Wilar, G. 2022. The evolution of pharmacological activities Bouea macrophylla Griffith in vivo and in vitro study: A review. Pharmaceuticals (Basel) 15(2): 238. doi:10.3390/ph15020238

Geiger, J.L., Grandis, J.R., and Bauman, J.E. 2016. The STAT3 pathway as a therapeutic target in head and neck cancer: Barriers and innovations. Oral Oncology, 56: 84–92.

Hardinsyah, H., Windardi, I.K., Aries, M., and Damayanthi, E. 2019. Total phenolic content, quercetin, and antioxidant activity of gandaria (Bouea Macrophylla Griff.) leaf extract at two stages of maturity. Jurnal Gizi dan Pangan, 14(2): 61–68. doi:10.25182/jgp.2019.14.2.61-68

Harsono, T., Pasaribu, N., Sobir, S., Fitmawati, F., and Prasetya, E. 2017. Phylogenetic analysis of Indonesian gandaria (Bouea) using molecular markers of cpDNA trnL-F intergenic spacer. Biodiversitas, 18: 51–57.

Hu, H., Chai, Y., Wang, L., Zhang, J., Lee, H.J., Kim, S.H., and Lü, J. 2009b. Pentagalloylglucose induces autophagy and caspase-independent programmed deaths in human PC-3 and mouse TRAMP-C2 prostate cancer cells. Molecular Cancer Therapeutics, 8(10): 2833–2843. doi:10.1158/1535-7163.MCT-09-0288

Hu, H., Lee, H.J., Jiang, C., Zhang, J., Wang, L., Zhao, Y., Xiang, Q., Lee, E.O., Kim, S.H., and Lü, J. 2008a. Penta-1,2,3,4,6-O-galloyl-beta-D-glucose induces p53 and inhibits STAT3 in prostate cancer cells in vitro and suppresses prostate xenograft tumor growth in vivo. Molecular Cancer Therapeutics, 7(9): 2681–2691.

Huh, J.E., Lee, E.O., Kim, M.S., Kang, K.S., Kim, C.H., Cha, B.C., Surh, Y.J., and Kim, S.H. 2005. Penta-O-galloyl-beta-D-glucose suppresses tumor growth via inhibition of angiogenesis and stimulation of apoptosis: Roles of cyclooxygenase-2 and mitogen-activated protein kinase pathways. Carcinogenesis, 26(8): 1436–1445.

Jideani, A.I.O., Silungwe, H., Takalani, T., Omolola, A.O., Udeh, H.O., and Anyasi, T.A. 2021. Antioxidant-rich natural fruit and vegetable products and human health. International Journal of Food Properties, 24(1): 41–67. doi:10.1080/10942912.2020.1866597

Kantapan, J., Dechsupa, N., Tippanya, D., Nobnop, W., and Chitapanarux, I. 2021b. Gallotannin from *Bouea macrophylla* seed extract suppresses cancer stem-like cells and radiosensitizes head and neck cancer. International Journal of Molecular Sciences, 22(17): 9253. doi:10.3390/ijms22179253

Kantapan, J., Paksee, S., Chawapun, P., Sangthong, P., and Dechsupa, N. 2020. Pentagalloyl glucose- and ethyl gallate–rich extract from maprang seeds induce apoptosis in MCF-7 breast cancer cells through mito-chondria-mediated pathway. Evidence-Based Complementary and Alternative Medicine, 2020: 5686029. doi:10.1155/2020/5686029

Kantapan, J., Paksee, S., Duangya, A., Sangthong, P., Roytrakul, S., Krobthong, S., Suttana, W., and Dechsupa, N. 2021a. A radiosensitizer, gallotannin-rich extract from *Bouea macrophylla* seeds, inhibits radiation-induced epithelial-mesenchymal transition in breast cancer cells. BMC Complementary Medicine and Therapies, 21(1): 189. doi:10.1186/s12906-021-03363-6

Kim, R.K., Kaushik, N., Suh, Y., Yoo, K.C., Cui, Y.H., Kim, M.J., Lee, H.J., Kim, I.G., and Lee, S.J. 2016. Radiation driven epithelial-mesenchymal transition is mediated by Notch signaling in breast cancer. Oncotarget, 7(33): 53430–53442. doi:10.18632/oncotarget.10802

Kuo, P.T., Lin, T.P., Liu, L.C., Huang, C.H., Lin, J.K., Kao, J.Y., and Way, T.D. 2009. Penta-O-galloyl-beta-D-glucose suppresses prostate cancer bone metastasis by transcriptionally repressing EGF-induced MMP-9 expression. Journal of Agricultural and Food Chemistry, 57(8): 3331–3339. doi:10.1021/jf803725h

Lee, H.J., Seo, N.J., Jeong, S.J., Park, Y., Jung, D.B., Koh, W., Lee, H.J., Lee, E.O., Ahn, K.S., Ahn, K.S., Lü, J., and Kim, S.H. 2011. Oral administration of penta-O-galloyl-β-D-glucose suppresses triple-negative breast cancer xenograft growth and metastasis in strong association with JAK1-STAT3 inhibition. Carcinogenesis, 32(6): 804–811. doi:10.1093/carcin/bgr015

Lim, T.K. 2012a. *Bouea macrophylla*. In: Edible medicinal and non-medicinal plants. Springer, Dordrecht. doi:10.1007/978-90-481-8661-7_7

Lim, T.K. 2012b. *Bouea oppositifolia*. In: Edible medicinal and non-medicinal plants. Springer, Dordrecht. doi:10.1007/978-90-481-8661-7_8

Liu, F., Zu, X., Xie, X., Liu, K., Chen, H., Wang, T., Liu, F., Bode, A.M., Zheng, Y., Dong, Z., and Kim, D.J. 2019. Ethyl gallate as a novel ERK1/2 inhibitor suppresses patient-derived esophageal tumor growth. Molecular Carcinogenesis, 58(4): 533–543. doi:10.1002/mc.22948

Liu, Y.H., Weng, Y.P., Tsai, H.Y., Chen, C.J., Lee, D.Y., Hsieh, C.L., Wu, Y.C., and Lin, J.Y. 2018. Aqueous extracts of *Paeonia suffruticosa* modulates mitochondrial proteostasis by reactive oxygen species-induced endoplasmic reticulum stress in pancreatic cancer cells. Phytomedicine: International Journal of Phytotherapy and Phytopharmacology, 46: 184–192. doi:10.1016/j.phymed.2018.03.037

Nguyen, N.H., Nguyen, T.T., Ma, P.C., Ta, Q.T.H., Duong, T.-H., and Vo, V.G. 2020. Potential antimicrobial and anticancer activities of an ethanol extract from *Bouea macrophylla*. Molecules, 25: 1996. doi:10.3390/molecules25081996

Nithitanakool, S., Pithayanukul, P., and Bavovada, R. 2009. Antioxidant and hepatoprotective activities of Thai mango seed kernel extract. Planta Medica, 75(10): 1118–1123. doi:10.1055/s-0029-1185507

Norfaizal, G.M., Latiff, A., Masrom, H., and Fahmi, Y.M. 2016. *Bouea microphylla* Griff. (Anacardiaceae) reinstated. The Malayan Nature Journal, 67(4): 480–485.

Office of Agricultural and Development Region 2, Thailand. 2022. KM2564 เทคโนโลยีการผลิตพืชอัตลักษณ์ในเขตพื้นที่ภาคเหนือตอนล่าง, Chapter 5, p. 59–72. www.doa.go.th/oard2/?page_id=63. (In Thai, Accessed April 10, 2022).

Oh, G.S., Pae, H.O., Oh, H., Hong, S.G., Kim, I.K., Chai, K.Y., Yun, Y.G., Kwon, T.O., and Chung, H.T. 2001. In vitro anti-proliferative effect of 1,2,3,4,6-penta-O-galloyl-beta-D-glucose on human hepatocellular carcinoma cell line, SK-HEP-1 cells. Cancer Letters 174(1): 17–24. doi:10.1016/s0304-3835(01)00680-2

Otto, T., and Sicinski, P. 2017. Cell cycle proteins as promising targets in cancer therapy. Nature Reviews Cancer, 17(2): 93–115. doi:10.1038/nrc.2016.138

Ouellette, M.M., Zhou, S., and Yan, Y. 2022. Cell signaling pathways that promote radioresistance of cancer cells. Diagnostics (Basel), 12(3): 656. doi:10.3390/diagnostics12030656

Paksee, S., Kantapan, J., Chawapun, P., Sangthong, P., and Dechsupa, N. 2019. Maprang seed extracts suppressed chemoresistant properties of breast cancer cells survived from ionizing radiation treatment via the regulation of ABCB1 genes. Journal of Associated Medical Sciences, 52(3): 185–192. https://he01.tci-thaijo.org/index.php/bulletinAMS/article/view/183869 (Accessed April 24, 2022).

Piao, X., Piao, X.L., Kim, H.Y., and Cho, E.J. 2008. Antioxidative activity of geranium (*Pelargonium inquinans* Ait) and its active component, 1,2,3,4,6-penta-O-galloyl-beta-D-glucose. Phytotherapy Research, 22(4): 534–538. doi:10.1002/ptr.2398

Rajan, N.S., and Bhat, R. 2016. Antioxidant compounds and antioxidant activities in unripe and ripe kundang fruits (*Bouea macrophylla* Griffith). Fruits, 71: 41–47. doi:10.1051/fruits/2015046

Rajan, N.S., and Bhat, R. 2017. Volatile constituents of unripe and ripe kundang fruits (*Bouea macrophylla* Griffith). International Journal of Food Properties, 20(8): 1751–1760. doi:10.1080/10942912.2016.1218892

Rajan, N.S., and Bhat, R. 2019. Bioactive compounds of plum mango (*Bouea microphylla* Griffith). In: Murthy, H., Bapat, V. (eds.), Bioactive compounds in underutilized fruits and nuts. Reference Series in Phytochemistry. Springer, Cham. doi:10.1007/978-3-030-06120-3_36-1

Rosas, E., Correa, L., Pádua, T., Costa, T., Mazzei, L., Heringer, A., Carlos Alberto Bizarro, C., Kaplan, M., Figueiredo, M., and Henriques, M. 2015. Anti-inflammatory effect of *Schinus terebinthifolius* Raddi hydroalcoholic extract on neutrophil migration in zymosan-induced arthritis. Journal of Ethnopharmacology, 175: 490–498. doi:10.1016/j.jep.2015.10.014

Rudiana, T., Suryani, N., Indriatmoko, D.D., Yusransyah, Y., Amelia, A., Noviany, N., and Hadi, S. 2019. Characterization of antioxidative fraction of plant stem *Bouea macrophylla* Griff. Journal of Physics: Conference Series, 1341: 072008. https://iopscience.iop.org/article/10.1088/1742-6596/1341/7/072008/pdf.

Rudiana, T., Suryani, N., Indriatmoko, D.D., Yusransyah, Y., Hardiyanto, M.A., Yohanes, R., Nurbayti, S., Nurdiansyah, E., Fajri, H., Noviany, N., and Hadi, S. 2021. The anticancer activity of phytoconstituents of the stem of *Bouea macrophylla*. Biomedical and Pharmacology Journal, 14(4).

Saleem, A., Husheem, M., Härkönen, P., and Pihlaja, K. 2002. Inhibition of cancer cell growth by crude extract and the phenolics of *Terminalia chebula* retz. fruit. Journal of Ethnopharmacology, 81(3): 327–336. doi:10.1016/s0378-8741(02)00099-5

Smith, B.N., and Bhowmick, N.A. (2016). Role of EMT in metastasis and therapy resistance. Journal of Clinical Medicine, 5(2): 17. doi:10.3390/jcm5020017

Subhadrabandhu, S. 2001. Part 1: Species with potential for commercial development. Under-Utilized Tropical Fruits of Thailand. www.fao.org/docrep/004/ab777e/ab777e04.htm#bm4.3. (Accessed April 10, 2022).

Sukalingam, K. 2018. Preliminary phytochemical analysis and in vitro antioxidant properties of Malaysian 'Kundang' (*Bouea macrophylla* Griffith). Trends in Phytochemical Research, 2(4): 261–266.

Torres-León, C., Ventura-Sobrevilla, J., Serna-Cock, L., Ascacio-Valdés, J.A., Contreras-Esquivel, J., and Aguilar, C.N. 2017. Pentagalloylglucose (PGG): A valuable phenolic compound with functional properties. Journal of Functional Foods, 37: 176–189. doi:10.1016/j.jff.2017.07.045

Zhang, Y.J., Gan, R.Y., Li, S., Zhou, Y., Li, A.N., Xu, D.P., and Li, H.B. 2015. Antioxidant phytochemicals for the prevention and treatment of chronic diseases. Molecules (Basel, Switzerland), 20(12): 21138–21156. doi:10.3390/molecules201219753

18 Sabah Snake Grass (*Clinacanthus nutans*) and Its Anticancer Activity
Phytochemical Composition and Signaling Pathways

Yoke Keong Yong, Nozlena Abdul Samad and Vuanghao Lim

ABBREVIATIONS

AVO	acidic vesicular organelle
Bad	Bcl-2-associated death promoter
Bax	Bcl-2-associated X
Bcl-2	B-cell lymphoma 2
Bcl-XL	B-cell lymphoma-extra large
CAM	chorioallantoic membrane
Caspase-10	cysteine-aspartic proteases-10
Caspase-3	cysteine-aspartic proteases-3
Caspase-8	cysteine-aspartic proteases-8
Caspase-9	cysteine-aspartic proteases-9
CN	*Clinacanthus nutans*
DR 5	death receptor 5
FADD	Fas-associated death domain
LC3-II	LC3-phosphatidylethanolamine conjugate
p53	tumor protein 53
ROS	reactive oxygen species
VEGF	vascular endothelial growth factor

18.1 INTRODUCTION

Clinacanthus nutans (CN) (Figure 18.1) is a member of the Acanthaceae family and a well-known traditional herb in Southeast Asia with various names such as "Sabah snake grass" or *belalai gajah* in Malaysia, *phya yo* or *phya plongthong* in Thailand, *dandang gendis* in Indonesia, *you dun cao* or *ee zui hua* in China, and *xuong khi* or *manh cong* in Vietnam. CN is scientifically known as *C. nutans* var. robinsonii Benoist, *C. burmanni* Nees, and *Justicia nutans* (Burm.f.). Although it can be cultivated from stem cuttings, CN can also be found widely distributed in tropical forests (Khoo et al., 2018; Tan et al., 2020). CN is commonly cultivated as an herb for its medicinal properties. It has a long petiole (0.3–2.0 cm), lanceolate leaves that are bifariously pubescent, a central or acuminate base, and terete stems with pubescent branches. The plant can reach a height of 1–3 m and has glabrescent green leaves. CN's leaves are narrow, lanceolate, or linear in shape. They range in length from 2 to 12 cm and in width from 0.5 to 1.5

DOI: 10.1201/9781003260028-20

233

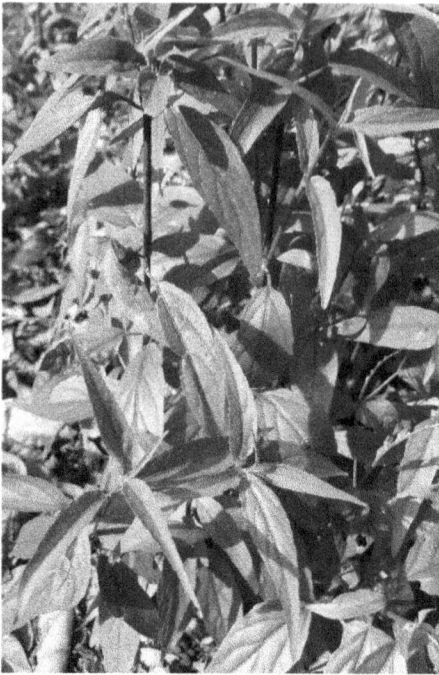

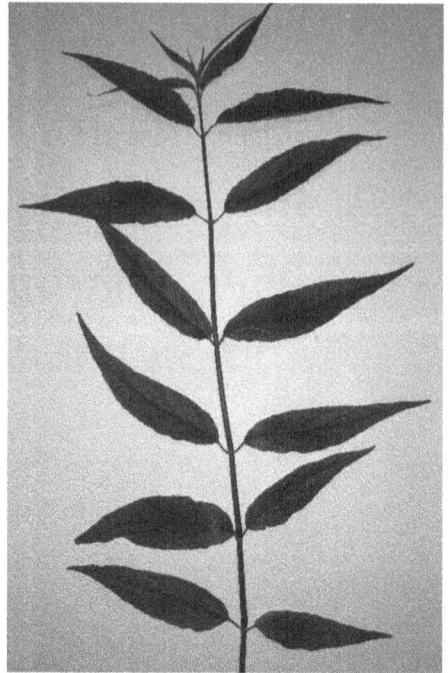

(A)   (B)

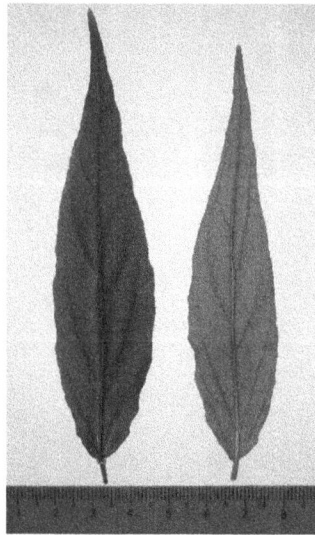

(C)

FIGURE 18.1 *Clinacanthus nutans* (Burm. F.) Lindau: (A) plant, (B) leaves with stem, and (C) leaves. The *C. nutans* plant has glabrescent green leaves and grows to a height of 1–3 m. The leaves are narrow, lanceolate, or linear.

Order	Lamiales
Family	Acanthaceae
Genus	*Clinacanthus*
Species	*nutans*
Scientific name	*Clinacanthus nutans* (Burm.f.) Lindau
Common name	Sabah snake grass, *phya yo, belalai gajah, dandang gendis, ee zui hua, xuong khi*

cm (Zulkipli et al., 2017; Tan et al., 2020). Flowers are developed by thick cymes on the tops of their branches and appear a greenish yellow. The flower's calyx is approximately 1 cm long and the stamen is linked to the corolla's neck. The ovaries are divided into two cells, each of which contains two ovules (Kamarudin et al., 2017). CN is classified taxonomically as shown in Figure 18.1.

18.2 BACKGROUND

CN has been used for a long time in many parts of Asia due to its diverse pharmacological properties. It is a prominent medicinal plant that Southeast Asians cultivate and use for several medical applications (Chiu et al., 2021). The vernacular name, Sabah snake grass, is derived from the form of its leaf, which resembles the leaf of Kalmegh (*Andrographis paniculata*), which is also known as snake grass among the Malaysian Chinese. Furthermore, the plant was discovered in Sabah, a Malaysian state located in the East Malaysia region on the northern portion of Borneo. Young leaves of CN are commonly consumed as vegetables because of their ability to maintain general health. They are commonly mixed with various juices to give flavor to cold drinks. In Malaysia, fresh leaves are often boiled with water and used to make herbal tea (Kamarudin et al., 2017).

In most maritime Southeast Asian countries, including Thailand, CN is used to treat snake bites, herpes infections, various skin infections, burns, and diabetes. Since 1967, Thai researchers have published numerous studies of the plant. Since 1987, it is known to have been used in hospitals and other medical facilities. The plant's main component is the leaf, which is commonly ingested orally, but it is also applied topically to inflamed areas and used widely by traditional healers in Thailand as a snake antivenom (Khoo et al., 2018). The mode of action is anti–cell lysis rather than as an antineuromuscular transmission blocker (Alam et al., 2016). In Indonesia, a sprig of fresh leaves is boiled until the water level is reduced. To treat diabetes, the leaves are boiled and served in glasses of water twice a day. Additionally, to cure fever and dysuria, 15 g of fresh leaves are boiled for 15 minutes and taken daily. Chinese healers use the plant for various purposes such as pain relief, digestion improvement, and fractured bone repositioning (Alam et al., 2016).

The plant's leaves are also traditionally consumed as part of an herbal combination or tea, and it is one of the ingredients in Ya-tan-mareng, an anticancer medicine from the province of Singburi (Kamarudin et al., 2017). Some cancer patients in Malaysia, Thailand, Singapore, and Indonesia have claimed that their treatments were successful due to the high consumption of the plant. Furthermore, CN's leaves can be used to treat various skin diseases, including allergic reactions and sunburn. They are also used to treat various insect and animal bites. The plant can be used to treat a wide range of injuries and conditions, such as fractures, bruises, and rheumatism. Its highquality medicinal use is evidenced in its recognition by Thailand's National Drug Committee as an essential medicine (Kamarudin et al., 2017).

According to various studies, CN has a variety of biological activities that can be utilized for a wide range of applications (Devasvaran et al., 2020). Some of these include antimicrobial, antiinflammatory, and antihyperlipidemic properties. Its versatility has garnered the attention of scientists, especially those who work in anticancer therapy. Although it has been known to cure certain types of liver cancer, this claim is only made after standard treatment methods such as chemotherapy and radiotherapy have been used (Khoo et al., 2018). Studies have shown that patients who were given CN extract for cancer treatment were able to recover from various cancers. In addition, its properties are nontoxic to some extent. Several studies have investigated the extract's effects on human cancer cells, resulting in suggestions that it could potentially be used as a cancer treatment. Therefore, to keep track of CN's anticancer activities, this chapter will review their current status and highlight future potential.

18.3 PHYTOCONSTITUENTS

The CN plant contains a wide range of bioactive compounds (Table 18.1) that can be used for various purposes. However, many of these compounds have not been tested for anticancer properties. Understanding CN's anticancer effects necessitates additional research to provide a more complete and accurate understanding of these compounds' properties. The anticancer effects of CN extracts and/or compounds have been demonstrated through various mechanisms, including cell cycle arrest, apoptosis induction, and antimigration, which are discussed in the section "Mechanisms of Antitumor Effects."

TABLE 18.1

Isolated Phytoconstituents and Their Cytotoxicity Activities from *Clinacanthus nutans*

Phytoconstituent	Chemical Group	Observations	References
Aurantiamide	Alkaloids	IC_{50}: A549 = 64.82 μM MCF-7 = 53.11 μM HeLa = 58.16 μM	(Diao et al., 2019; Tan et al., 2020)
Aurantiamide acetate	Alkaloids	IC_{50}: A549 = >100 μM MCF-7 = 71.17 μM HeLa = 85.09 μM	
Lupeol	Triterpenoid	IC_{50}: MCF-7 = 16.813 ± 1.316 μg/mL	(Cheng et al., 2021)
Nigramide B	Alkaloids	IC_{50}: A549 = >100 μM MCF-7 = >100 μM HeLa = 58.88 μM	(Diao et al., 2019; Tan et al., 2020)

TABLE 18.1
(Continued)

Phytoconstituent	Chemical Group	Observations	References
Pheophorbide A	Pheophorbide	CC_{50}: A549 = 25 µg/mL	(Sakdarat et al., 2018; Zulkipli et al., 2017)
Purpurin 18 phytyl ester		CC_{50}: A549 = 50 µg/mL	
13^2-Hydroxy-(13^2-S)-chlorophyll B	Phaeophytins	CC_{50}: A549 = 50 µg/mL	(Sakdarat et al., 2018; Tan et al., 2020)
13^2-Hydroxy-(13^2-S)-pheophytin B	Phaeophytins	CC_{50}: A549 = 50 µg/mL	

(Continued)

TABLE 18.1
(Continued)

Phytoconstituent	Chemical Group	Observations	References
	Furofuran lignans	IC_{50}: A549 = 59.17 μM MCF-7 = 60.00 μM HeLa = 68.55 μM	(Diao et al., 2019; Zulkipli et al., 2017)

2-methoxy-9β-hydroxydiasesamin

Abbreviations: CC_{50}: 50% cytotoxic concentration; IC_{50} = 50% inhibitory concentration.

18.4 TYPES OF ANTICANCER STUDIES

Various studies have been successfully conducted on CN's anticancer activities. According to these studies, the plant could be a natural nutraceutical that could be used for cancer prevention and treatment (Table 18.2). Despite the abundance of *in vitro* experimental data supporting CN's cancer-causing properties, the evaluation of its *in vivo* anticancer effects remains limited. Different methods of extraction also have an impact on CN's various characteristics. Therefore, *in vitro* anticancer studies on this plant should follow a standard design to ensure that the right drugs are used. This process should be carried out in conjunction with the current clinical drugs used to treat cancer. The potential use of CN could be accelerated through *in vivo* and clinical studies to improve cancer patients' treatments.

18.5 MECHANISMS OF ANTITUMOR EFFECTS

18.5.1 INDUCTION OF CANCER CELL DEATH

18.5.1.1 Cytotoxicity and Antiproliferative Effect

Direct cytotoxicity of compounds eliminates intracellular foreign bodies and cancer cells by interfering with DNA synthesis or synthesizing chemicals capable of damaging DNA (Bracci et al., 2014), whereas antiproliferative compounds have the potential to suppress the growth of abnormal cells, such as cancer cells. Both effects are common in current cancer treatment and extensive studies on CN have been conducted. A study of CN extract on several cancer cell lines revealed that the aqueous extract efficiently decreased the growth of HeLa (36%) and K-562 (41%) cells. Surprisingly, CN-chloroform extract inhibited the most cell lines, including K-562 (IC_{50} = 48 μg/mL)

TABLE 18.2

Anticancer Activities of *Clinacanthus nutans* (2018 to 2022)

Experimental Model (*In vitro / Ex Vivo/In vivo*)	Samples (Crude/ Fraction/Active Compound)	Observations	Part Utilized	References
In vitro MTT assay MOLT-4, SUP-T1	Crude methanol extract, further fractionated by hexane, ethyl acetate, and butanol Subfractionation of hexane fraction into hexane and acetone	i. IC_{50} SUP-T1 = 37.5 µg/mL for subfraction acetone from hexane (MHA) after 48h. ii. MHA from hexane increased expression in SUP-T1 cells at a 50 µg/mL concentration. iii. MHA significantly reduced the cell viability of MOLT-4 cells. iv. In SUP-T1 cells, the MHA promoted apoptosis, ROS, and calcium ions; however, it decreased the mitochondrial membrane potential.	Leaf	(Lu et al., 2018)
In vitro MTT assay HeLa L929 NIH 3T3	Hexane (soaked) and chloroform (Soxhlet) crude extracts Bioassay-guided fractionation: Column chromatography: Gradient mobile phase Total 16 fractions	The IC_{50} of fraction 11 exhibited the most significant 27 ± 2.6 µg/mL after 72 hours of incubation.	Leaf	(Roslan et al., 2018)
In vitro SRB assay MDA-MB-231	Ethanol, aqueous extract	i. Synergistic effect of ethanolic extract (0.125–0.5 mg/mL) and paclitaxel were observed at 0.028 µg/mL for 72h. ii. For 72h, aqueous extract (0.5–1 mg/mL) worked synergistically with paclitaxel (0.028 µg/mL).	Leaf	(Mohd Rosli et al., 2018)
In vitro Cell counting kit-8 assay D24 NHDF	Aqueous extracts: Cold (22°C) Hot (100°C)	i. Cell death was triggered by cold (57.6%) and hot (48.6%) aqueous extracts at 200 µg/mL. ii. Apoptosis was triggered by cold aqueous extracts.	Leaf	(Fong et al., 2019)
In vitro SRB assay HeLa	80% methanolic crude extract Fractionated into hexane, dichloromethane, and aqueous	i. All the extracts have antiproliferative effects on HeLa cells. ii. Dichloromethane fraction showed the highest antiproliferative activity (IC_{50}: 70 µg/mL) at 48 h.	Leaf	(Haron et al., 2019)
In vitro MTT assay HCT116, HT-29, CaSki, NCL-H23, HepG2, MCF-7, CCD-18Co	70% ethanolic crude extract (soaked) Fractionated into hexane, ethyl acetate, and aqueous	i. The ethyl acetate fraction (CNEAF) exhibited the greatest cytotoxicity (IC_{50} = 48.81 ± 1.44 µg/mL) against HCT-116 cells.	Leaf	(Wang et al., 2019)

(Continued)

TABLE 18.2
(Continued)

Experimental Model (*In vitro / Ex Vivo/In vivo*)	Samples (Crude/ Fraction/Active Compound)	Observations	Part Utilized	References
		ii. The CNEAF triggered apoptosis with rising ROS and Bax expression but reduced the mitochondrial membrane's potential, Bcl-2, and Bcl-X2 expression. iii. CNEAF induced autophagy with upregulation in LC-3 and downregulated in p62 level).		
In vitro MTT assay Hep-G2	Methanolic crude extract (maceration, room temperature) Fractionated with hexane: ethyl acetate = 7:3 Triterpenes-containing fraction	Fraction 2 showed the lowest IC_{50} = 1.73 µg/mL at 24h (triterpenes).	Leaf	(Zakaria et al., 2019)
In vitro Colorimetric assay (neutral red dye) ORL-48	Aqueous (decoction, boiled)	The extract exhibited an IC_{50} = 49.8 µg/mL.	Leaf	(Zulkapli & Razak, 2019)
In vitro MTT assay MDA-MB-231 MCF-7	Hexane and methanolic crude extracts Fractionation of methanolic crude extract using column chromatography Isolation of entadamide C and clinamide D	Fractions A12 and A17 exhibited the highest activity for both cancer cells: A12: MDA-MB231; IC_{50} = 8.394 ± 0.086 µg/mL; MCF-7; IC_{50} = 8.007 ± 0.043 µg/mL. A17: MDA-MB231; IC_{50} = 5.683 ± 0.064 µg/mL; MCF-7; IC_{50} = 5.048 ± 0.083 µg/mL.	Bark	(Mutazah et al., 2020)
In vitro and *in vivo* 4 T1 Female BALB/c mice	Methanolic crude extract (room temperature)	At 1000 mg/kg extract, a significant reduction in mitotic cells, tumor weight, and tumor volume.	Leaf	(Nik Abd Rahman et al., 2019)
In vitro, ex vivo and *in vivo* MTT assay (*in vitro*) HSC-4 Rat aortic ring assay (ex vivo) Chick embryo chorioallantoic membrane assay (*in vivo*)	50, 70, and 100% ethanolic and aqueous crude extracts (sonication, room temperature)	i. The aqueous extract was shown to have the highest activity in an *in vitro* assay. ii. In the absence and presence of VEGF, aqueous extract substantially reduced endothelial cell proliferation and migration. iii. The sprouting of arteries in aortic rings and chick embryo chorioallantoic membrane assay was reduced considerably by the aqueous extract.	Leaf	(Ng et al., 2018)

Note: The table summarizes the anticancer activity of *C. nutans* as determined by various experimental designs and extract types.

and Raji (IC_{50} = 47 µg/mL). However, CN-methanol extract exhibited very weak cytotoxicity and antiproliferative activities against most of the cancer cell lines tested in the study (Yong et al., 2013). CN-petroleum ether extract demonstrated enormously important cytotoxicity and antiproliferative activity against the cancer cell lines HeLa (IC_{50} = 18 µg/mL) and K-562 (IC_{50} = 20 µg/mL) (Arullappan et al., 2014). Aside from the cancer cell lines mentioned above, the cytotoxicity and antiproliferative effect of CN were tested on the cells of the following cancers: breast (MCF-7 and MDA-MB-231), colorectal (HCT-116), gastric (SGC-7901), liver (HepG2), lung (A549), lymphoma and leukemia (SUP-T1 and MOLT-4), head and neck (CNE-1 and HSC-4), and skin (D24) (Lin et al., 2021). CN's cytotoxicity and antiproliferative activities are strongly associated with the various active phytocompounds listed in Table 18.1.

18.5.1.2 Apoptosis Effect

A breakdown in the dynamic equilibrium between cell growth and cell death is one of the primary causes of cancer. When cells fail to die owing to a lack of apoptotic signals, they proliferate uncontrollably, culminating in cancer. The intrinsic and extrinsic systems are the two primary mechanisms that generate apoptotic signals. Extrinsic ligands connect to death receptors, activating caspase-8. This pathway is activated by CN by upregulating DR 5 expression and activating caspase-8 and caspase-10 (Wang et al., 2019).

In contrast, the role of reactive oxygen species (ROS) in cellular metabolism is crucial. ROS generation is known to enhance apoptosis in many chemotherapy treatments. Caspase-3 and caspase-9 activation by CN generates ROS and promotes apoptosis (Wang et al., 2019). The ethanolic extract of CN was found to have potent tumoricidal effects in tumor-bearing mice after Western blot analysis, as evidenced by high expression of caspase-3, an apoptotic executioner protein, in tumors from CN-treated tumor-bearing Hep-A mice (Figure 18.2) (Huang et al., 2015).

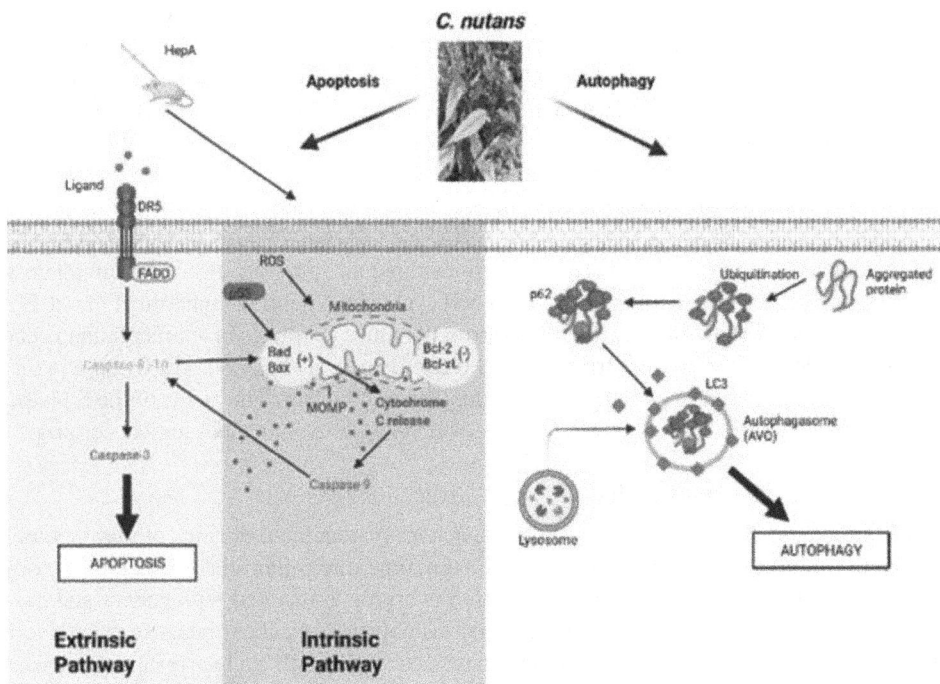

FIGURE 18.2   The cell death pathways of *Clinacanthus nutans*. Protein involvement in the intrinsic and extrinsic of apoptotic and autophagic pathways.

Source: Created in Biorender.com.

The intrinsic route decreases Bcl-2 and Bcl-XL production, which can be pro- or anti-apoptotic. Bcl-2 deficiency may cause the outer mitochondrial membrane to permeabilize, enabling mitochondrial cytochrome c to be released into the cytoplasm. Cytochrome c forms an apoptosome complex with protease activating factor 1 and deoxyadenosine triphosphate as part of the apoptotic process. CN was discovered to be capable of suppressing breast, colon, skin, and liver carcinogenesis. In many cases, CN extract promotes apoptotic cell death by inhibiting Bcl2 and Bcl-XL and activating Bad, Bax, caspase-3, caspase-9, and FADD via multiple survival signaling pathways (Yong et al., 2013).

According to extensive research, CN can disrupt the equilibrium in the mitochondrial membrane potential, resulting in increased suppression of the Bcl-XL protein. Growth of the MDA-MB-231 triple-negative breast cancer cell line was inhibited by a crude aqueous extract of CN leaves. The extract also stimulated apoptosis in the treated cells by facilitating both intrinsic and extrinsic apoptotic mechanisms. These findings were reflected by increased mRNA expression of Bad, Bax, and FADD and decreased Bcl-2 and Bcl-XL levels. As a result, CN was identified as a potential candidate for breast cancer therapy and intervention (Yong et al., 2020). It also caused apoptosis in hepatoma cells by increasing Bax expression while decreasing Bcl2 expression. A real-time polymerase chain reaction (RT-PCR) study revealed that the presence of ethyl acetate and methanol root extracts increases the production of the pro-apoptotic gene Baxn in MCF-7 cells (Teoh et al., 2017). The increased Bax synthesis by CN was expected to activate p53, causing cytochrome c to be released from mitochondria into the cytosol (Zainuddin et al., 2019). Several prior investigations on CN indicated that apoptosis was directly generated in human cervical cancer by increasing Bax, decreasing Bcl-2, and cytochrome c release via activation of the mitochondrial-dependent pathway (Figure 18.2) (Teoh et al., 2017; Lin et al., 2021).

18.5.1.3 Cell Cycle Arrest

The cell cycle is a series of interrelated steps that allows a cell to divide and grow while remaining intact. When activated, cyclin-dependent kinases (CDKs) can help a cell move from one phase to the next. In brief, there are five phases: G1 and G2 phase (cell growth), S phase (replication of DNA), M phase (mitosis), and G0 phase (cease to proliferate and enter quiescence) (Whittaker et al., 2017). Cells that overexpress cyclins or lack CDKs continue to grow uncontrollably in pathological conditions, which can lead to the development and progression of cancer. Additionally, the cell cycle arrest process helps to protect the cell's DNA and allows a cell to repair it (Whittaker et al., 2017). Apoptotic cascades are activated when cell cycle checkpoints are disrupted before DNA repair is complete. The CN standard fraction demonstrated an apoptotic effect on human cervical cancer cells, and SiHa through an arrested G1/S cell cycle checkpoint (Zainuddin et al., 2019). On the contrary, CN-dichloromethane extract was shown to induce apoptosis in another human cervical cancer cell line, HeLa, via cell cycle arrest at the S phase (Haron et al., 2019). The S phase in the cell cycle is vital for DNA synthesis or chromosome duplication to occur. The arrest of the S phase cell cycle suggested a decrease in DNA synthesis rate, which might explain CN's anticancer property.

18.5.1.4 Reactive Oxygen Species

ROS, including radical and non-radical oxygen species, are generated during cellular metabolism and contribute significantly to cell proliferation, signaling, and inflammation-related factor production (Dayem et al., 2017). Apart from this, ROS is highly associated with cancer and has two faces: ROS can be carcinogenic, causing genomic instability and cancer because excessive ROS damages lipids, proteins, and DNA, but it may also cause cancer cell cycle arrest, senescence, and cell death via the ASK1/JNK and ASK1/p38 signaling pathways (Reczek & Chandel, 2017). It is worth noting that most current chemotherapeutics cause cancer cell damage by inducing oxidative stress and ROS-mediated cell injury. According to research, CN hexane extract interfered with the oxidative homeostasis of several cancer cell lines, including non–small cell lung cancer

(A549), nasopharyngeal cancer (CNE1), and liver cancer cells (HepG2), by elevating the ROS level in the cancer cell lines, resulting in cell death (Ng et al., 2017). In addition, the CN ethyl acetate fraction can induce cancer cell death in ROS-dependent apoptosis and autophagy in HCT 116 (Wang et al., 2019).

18.5.1.5 Autophagy

Autophagy is a type II programmed cell death process in which cellular material is sequestered within autophagosomes before being degraded by lysosomes. Acidic vesicular organelle (AVO) formation, which can be detected and measured using acridine orange vital staining, is a hallmark of autophagy. Light chain 3 (LC3) and p62/SQSTM1 (p62) proteins are connected to autophagosomal membranes that absorb cytoplasmic substances for degradation. CN ethyl acetate fraction (CNEAF) increased AVOs in HCT116 cells, indicating that it stimulated autophagy. Furthermore, one of the essential autophagy determinants, the LC3-II protein, was found to significantly accumulate concurrently with p62 protein degradation in CNEAF-treated HCT116 cells. Conversely, ROS serves as an important signaling mediator in governing a wide range of signal transduction pathways, making cells more vulnerable to DNA damage, drug sensitivity, and cell death (Figure 18.2). CNEAF-induced ROS generation was responsible for the initiation of autophagic cell death. As a result, it is concluded that CNEAF promotes autophagy, as evidenced by the accumulation of AVO and LC3-II, as well as the degradation of ROS-dependent and p62 proteins (Lin et al., 2021).

18.5.2 INHIBITION OF ANGIOGENESIS, INVASION, AND METASTASIS

Angiogenesis inhibition is a critical component of cancer treatment and prevention. One potential approach is to inhibit angiogenesis by targeting vascular endothelial growth factor (VEGF). Angiogenesis and vasculogenesis are controlled by the VEGF signaling molecule. Anti-angiogenic therapy based on VEGF suppression has been reported to be effective in oncology and ophthalmology. The initiation of angiogenesis requires an increase in the expression of angiogenic cytokines such as VEGF. For example, in tumor-induced angiogenesis (TIA), VEGF increases endothelial cell permeability, proliferation, and angiogenesis. VEGF promotes the production of enzymes involved in the degradation of the basement membrane and extracellular matrix. Existing blood vessels are stimulated to grow new ones during these procedures (Samad et al., 2017).

CN has an anti-angiogenesis effect by regulating one of the most important pro-angiogenesis factors, VEGF ex vivo, *in vivo*, and *in vitro*, and these factors could promote angiogenesis under certain circumstances (Figure 18.3). The rat aortic ring test is commonly used to assess the angiogenesis activity of potential therapeutic compounds because it allows for rapid induction of angiogenesis. Assaying the aortic ring in rats is quantitative, and the microvessel that forms from the aorta can be easily measured. In the rat aortic ring assay, CN water extract significantly inhibits VEGF-induced microvessel outgrowth. Suramin, an established anti-angiogenic drug, produces a similar effect (Ng et al., 2018).

A conducive microenvironment, including the availability of extracellular tissue matrix, is required for the formation and anchorage of new blood vessels. CN's anti-angiogenic activity is reflected in its ability to impede matrix formation for endothelial cell growth. The chorioallantoic membrane assay confirmed this effect, indicating that CN had a significant inhibitory effect on neovascularization (Ng et al., 2018).

In a dose-dependent manner, CN caused severe disturbances in the vasculature pattern impacting primary vessels, as well as a decrease in the amount of newly formed secondary and tertiary capillaries. CN's anti-neovascularization action was more pronounced at higher concentrations (Ng et al., 2018). This could be explained by the fact that tumors are not always angiogenic from the start. Only after a specific mass of tumor has formed will it begin promoting angiogenesis to assist development and spread (Samad et al., 2017).

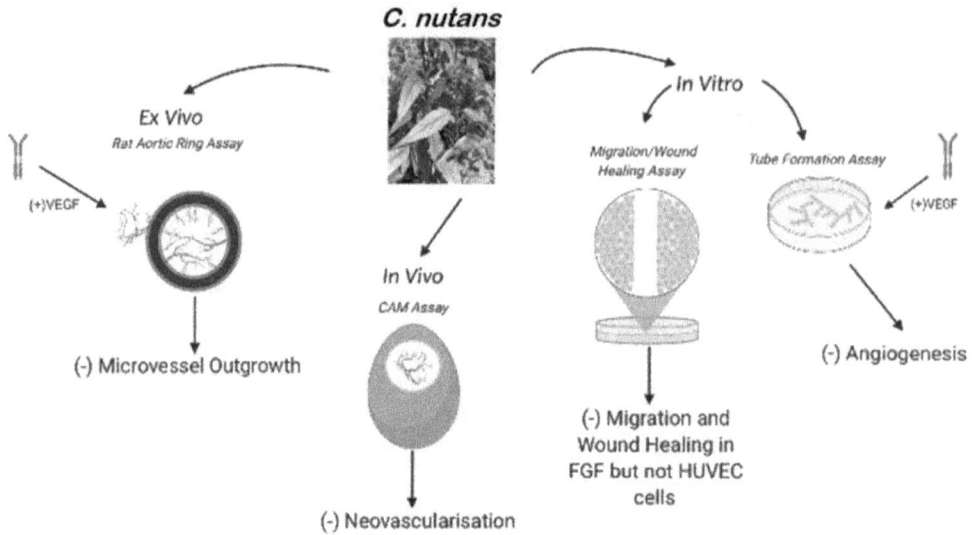

FIGURE 18.3 The role of *Clinacanthus nutans* in regulating angiogenesis. The angiogenesis regulation by *C. nutans* in *in vitro*, *in vivo*, and ex vivo studies.

Source: Created in Biorender.com.

The ability of tumor cells to metastasize is also linked to VEGF expression, which can be inhibited to suppress tumor development and invasion. CN has been shown to inhibit VEGF-stimulated angiogenesis by targeting structure tubes, endothelial cell proliferation, and microvessel formation (Ng et al., 2018).

In addition to the widely studied activities, a few other potential pharmacological activities of CN have been reported. For instance, when compared to hexane extract, chloroform extract generated the greatest improvement in the migration rate of human gingival fibroblast (HGF) and wound recovery during six hours of observation (Khoo et al., 2018). A similar *in vitro* wound healing assay claimed that supplementing CN with chloroform and hexane extracts did not affect the migration rate of HGF (Kamarudin et al., 2017). Conversely, the incapacity of CN water extract to change human umbilical vein endothelial cell (HUVEC) chemotaxis in response to VEGF was verified (Figure 18.3) (Ng et al., 2018).

18.5.3 IMMUNOREGULATION IN CANCER GROWTH

The immune system, particularly innate and adaptive immune cells, plays a crucial role in the origin and development of cancer. Innate and adaptive immune cells collaborate to create an inflammatory milieu that can either promote or inhibit cancer growth. Cancer is an inflammatory disease that involves innate and adaptive immune responses. There is evidence that a tumor's microenvironment is full of inflammatory cells that regulate tumor formation. For instance, innate immune cells such as neutrophils, macrophages (M2), and myeloid-derived suppressor cells stimulate cancer growth, whereas dendritic cells (both stimulation and inhibition) and macrophages (M1) inhibit cancer growth (Disis, 2010). However, Th2 CD4+ T cell, CD4+ T regulatory cells from adaptive immune cells are known to stimulate cancer growth, whereas cytotoxic CD8+ T cells, Th1 CD4+ T cells, and Th17 CD4+ T cells showed cancer inhibition activity (Disis, 2010).

A hepatoma (Hep-A) tumor-bearing mouse treated with CN enhanced CD8+ T cell infiltration promoted Th1 cell differentiation. Data showed that tumor tissues had an abundance of CD8+ T cells after receiving CN for 10 consecutive days (Huang et al., 2015). Infiltration of CD8⁺ T cells to the tumor site could lead to cytotoxicity by releasing perforin and granzymes from the CD8⁺ T cells. Furthermore, CN demonstrated the ability to promote Th1 cell differentiation, which involved the secretion of IL-2 and IFN-γ (Huang et al., 2015). Indeed, serum levels of IL-2 and IFN-γ were significantly increased in Hep-A tumor-bearing mice treated with CN. IL-2, accelerating lymphocyte mitosis, improving killer cell osmotic lysis, and helping to generate antibodies, all result in tumor inhibition. Incremental levels of IFN-γ in cancer were found to aid in the enhancement of immune functions by activating macrophages (Huang et al., 2015).

A similar pattern of data was reported with levels of IL-2 and IFN-γ expression significantly increasing in tumor-bearing mice treated with CN in the murine mammary carcinoma cell line (4T1). In addition, the percentage of CD3⁺ T, CD8⁺ T, and NK1.1 cells increased significantly in the CN-treated group (Nik Abd Rahman et al., 2019). Several studies have documented that increasing the levels of these immune cells inhibits tumor metastasis and progression, potentially improving cancer survival rates. For instance, CD8⁺ T and NK1.1 cells mediated the cytotoxic effect on cancer cells through the direct or indirect killing of damaged cells by producing IFN-γ and perforin/granzyme (Figure 18.4) (St. Paul & Ohashi, 2020; Steiger et al., 2015).

A more recent study showed that CN exhibited immunomodulatory potential in the tumor microenvironment *in vitro* (Nordin et al., 2021). Chronic inflammation is linked to multiple cellular changes in breast cancer, including cancer-related lymphocytes, macrophages, and tumor cells, and contributes to the malignant progression of several types of cancer (Danforth, 2021). As a result, inhibiting inflammation in the tumor microenvironment may help in slowing cancer progression, particularly in breast cancer. CN has successfully reduced pro-inflammatory cytokines, such as IL-6, IL-1, and TNF-α, in the MDA-MB-231 microenvironment, potentially slowing cancer progression (Figure 18.4) (Nordin et al., 2021).

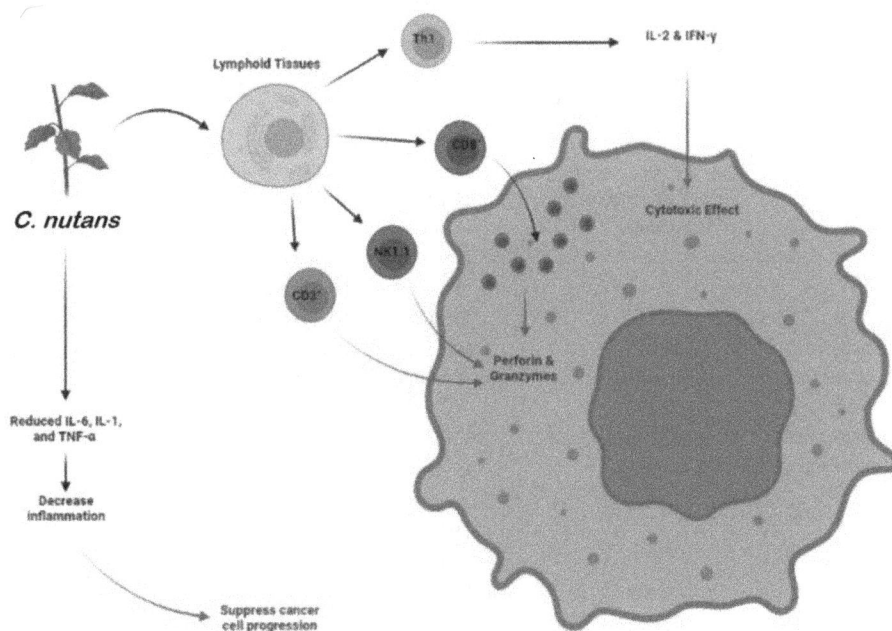

FIGURE 18.4 Immunoregulatory activity of *Clinacanthus nutans* towards cancer cells. *C. nutans* suppresses cancer progression by reducing inflammation in the microenvironment or by releasing enzymes and cytokines that are toxic to cancer cells.

Source: Created in Biorender.com.

18.6 OTHER FOODS, HERBS, SPICES, AND BOTANICALS USED IN CANCER

Natural products such as spices, food, and herbs have surpassed pharmaceuticals as the primary source of cancer chemoprevention. They have been completely safe for human consumption for thousands of years. They contain potential phytochemical compounds that have shown promising anticancer activity in preclinical studies. Their development was then completed to evaluate their potential as agents for new cancer therapies. Various phenolic compounds, such as sulforaphane, curcumin, and phenols, are tabulated in Table 18.3. Numerous clinical trials are currently being conducted on these compounds.

TABLE 18.3
Phytoconstituents from Various Natural Products for Anticancer Activity

Plants	Phytoconstituents	Types of Cancer (Experiment)	References
Turmeric *Curcuma longa*	Curcuma longa A2	ROS-dependent endothelial cell (HUVECs)	(Choudhari et al., 2020; Ma et al., 2021)
	Curcumin	Liver cancer (Transgenic mice)	
		Ovarian cancer (Hens)	
		Lung cancer (H1299, A549)	
		Advanced and metastatic breast cancer (Clinical trial)	
Garlic, allium	Allicin	Thyroid cancer (SW1736 and Hth-7 cells)	(Ma et al., 2021)
	Diallyl tetrasulfide Diallyl disulfide Diallyl trisulfide	Colon cancer (CoLo 205)	
Green tea	(−)-Epicatechin	Prostate cancer (Clinical trial)	(Ma et al., 2021; Rashidi et al., 2017)
	(−)-Epigallocatechin	Breast cancer (MCF10A)	
	(−)-Epicatechin-3-gallate	Liver cancer (HepG2)	
		Osteosarcoma cancer (U2OS)	
	(−)-Epigalocatachin-3-gallate	Hepatocellular carcinoma (HuH7)	
		Breast cancer (Tumorigenic breast epithelial cells)	
		Prostate cancer (Clinical trial)	
Broccoli, onions, tomatoes, apples, leek, corn, pumpkin, papaya, grapefruit, watermelon, spinach, wolfberry, peach	Lutein Zeaxanthin Lycopene Apo-10-lycopenoic Sulforaphane	Lung, colon cancers, and benign prostatic hyperplasia (Clinical trial)	(Ma et al., 2021)
		Liver tumors (Mice)	
		Breast cancer (Rats)	
		Triple-negative breast cancer (Orthotopic mouse xenograft model)	
	Quercetin	Oral squamous cell carcinoma (Hamster)	
		Melanoma (SK-MEL-28)	

Source: Adapted from Ma et al. (2021). Article printed under a CC-BY 4.0 license.

18.7 TOXICITY AND CAUTIONARY NOTES

The combined treatment of CN methanolic extract with cisplatin had a strong antagonistic effect on MCF-7 cells. The combination of leaf and stem extract with gemcitabine on several cancer cell lines can potentiate the killing of cancer cells by upregulating Bax and cIAP-2 (Lin et al., 2021). A 90-day *in vivo* subchronic study on rats revealed that the ethanol extract did not cause toxicity but did alter the levels of certain markers. In addition, a 14-day subacute toxicity investigation on CN extract revealed no toxic effects on rats (P'ng et al., 2012). Despite having higher levels of the cholinergic enzyme in their liver, kidney, and heart, mice fed 1000 mg/kg of CN crude extract for the same duration showed no aberrant behavior. The effects of long-term CN exposure and dose on rats revealed that the longer the treatment period, the lower the ALP levels became, but the group with 2000 mg/kg showed no significant changes. Although the plant's polar fraction is nontoxic, the non-polar extract is harmful (Aliyu et al., 2020). The LC_{50} of the CN *n*-hexane fraction was found to be 75.49 g/mL, with noticeable morphological defects on zebrafish (Murugesu et al., 2019). Small-scale clinical trials with a topical preparation of CN extract revealed that it significantly improved the symptoms of genital herpes and herpes zoster infections (Alam et al., 2016). Although CN has been shown to reduce the period of ulcers and pain in patients with recurrent aphthous stomatitis, its potential synergistic effect has been overshadowed by questions about its molecular mechanism of action (Zulkipli et al., 2017). Therefore, further studies are needed because the effectiveness of this herb's prophylactic action has not been proven, especially in cancer studies.

18.8 SUMMARY POINTS

- CN has been consumed and cultivated by Asians for its various medical applications.
- Studies have shown that CN extract can reduce the toxicity of human cancer cells.
- Several compounds have been isolated from the plant's various parts, including the leaves and stems.
- The study revealed that CN ethanolic extract had potent tumoricidal effects on mice by inducing caspase-3 expression.
- Dichloromethane extracts induced cell cycle arrest in the S phase in HeLa cells.
- CN hexane extract elevated the levels of the antioxidant enzymes in cancer cell lines, leading to cell death.
- CN promotes angiogenesis by regulating a major pro-angiogenic factor. The effect of CN on the vascular cell outgrowth was observed in the rat ring assay.

18.9 ACKNOWLEDGMENT

This work was supported by Research University Top-Down Grant Scheme, Universiti Sains Malaysia with Project No: 1001/CIPPT/8070019, Project Code: NO0060 (Reference No: 2021/0318).

REFERENCES

Alam, Ariful, Sahena Ferdosh, Kashif Ghafoor, Abdul Hakim, Abdul Shukor Juraimi, Alfi Khatib, and Zaidul I. Sarker. 2016. "*Clinacanthus nutans*: A Review of the Medicinal Uses, Pharmacology and Phytochemistry." *Asian Pacific Journal of Tropical Medicine* 9 (4): 402–409. Elsevier (Singapore) Pte Ltd.

Aliyu, Abdullahi, Mohd Rosly Shaari, Nurul Syahirah Ahmad Sayuti, Mohd Farhan Hanif Reduan, Shanmugavelu Sithambaram, Mustapha Mohamed Noordin, Khozirah Shaari, and Hazilawati Hamzah. 2020. "Subacute Oral Administration of *Clinacanthus nutans* Ethanolic Leaf Extract Induced Liver and Kidney Toxicities in ICR Mice." *Molecules* 25 (11). MDPI AG.

Arullappan, Sangeetha, Prabu Rajamanickam, Naadeirmuthu Thevar, and Clara Carol Kodimani. 2014. "In Vitro Screening of Cytotoxic, Antimicrobial and Antioxidant Activities of *Clinacanthus nutans* (Acanthaceae) Leaf Extracts." *Tropical Journal of Pharmaceutical Research* 13 (9). University of Benin: 1455–1461.

Bracci, L., G. Schiavoni, A. Sistigu, and F. Belardelli. 2014. "Immune-Based Mechanisms of Cytotoxic Chemotherapy: Implications for the Design of Novel and Rationale-Based Combined Treatments against Cancer." *Cell Death and Differentiation* 21 (1): 15–25.

Cheng, Angelina Ying Fang, Peik Lin Teoh, Lalith Jayasinghe, and Bo Eng Cheong. 2021. "Volatile Profiling Aided in the Isolation of Anti-Proliferative Lupeol from the Roots of *Clinacanthus nutans* (Burm. f.) Lindau." *Processes* 9 (8): 1–14.

Chiu, Hock Ing, Che Nurul Azieyan Che Mood, Nur Nadhirah Mohamad Zain, Muggundha Raoov Ramachandran, Noorfatimah Yahaya, Nik Nur Syazni Nik Mohamed Kamal, Wai Hau Tung, Yoke Keong Yong, Chee Keong Lee, and Vuanghao Lim. 2021. "Biogenic Silver Nanoparticles of *Clinacanthus nutans* as Antioxidant with Antimicrobial and Cytotoxic Effects." *Bioinorganic Chemistry and Applications* 2021: 1–11.

Choudhari, Amit S., Pallavi C. Mandave, Manasi Deshpande, Prabhakar Ranjekar, and Om Prakash. 2020. "Phytochemicals in Cancer Treatment: From Preclinical Studies to Clinical Practice." *Frontiers in Pharmacology* 10 (January): 1–17.

Danforth, David N. 2021. "The Role of Chronic Inflammation in the Development of Breast Cancer." *Cancers* 13 (15): 3918.

Dayem, Ahmed Abdal, Mohammed Kawser Hossain, Soo bin Lee, Kyeongseok Kim, Subbroto Kumar Saha, Gwang Mo Yang, Hye Yeon Choi, and Ssang Goo Cho. 2017. "The Role of Reactive Oxygen Species (ROS) in the Biological Activities of Metallic Nanoparticles." *International Journal of Molecular Sciences* 18 (1): 120. MDPI AG.

Devasvaran, Kogilavanee, Nabilah Hanim Baharom, Hui Wen Chong, Rozi Nuraika Ramli, Hock Ing Chiu, Chee Keong Lee, and Vuanghao Lim. 2020. "Quality Assessment of *Clinacanthus nutans* Leaf Extracts by GC-MS-Based Metabolomics." *Current Science* 119 (4): 641–648.

Diao, Hong Zhang, Wen Hao Chen, Jian Cao, Tai Ming Shao, Xiao Ping Song, and Chang Ri Han. 2019. "Furofuran Lignans and Alkaloids from *Clinacanthus nutans.*" *Natural Product Research* 33 (9): 1317–1321.

Disis, Mary L. 2010. "Immune Regulation of Cancer." *Journal of Clinical Oncology* 28 (29): 4531–4538.

Fong, Siat Yee, Dilani Wimalasiri, Terrence Piva, Chaitali Dekiwadia, Sylvia Urban, and Tien Huynh. 2019. "Evaluation of Cytotoxic and Apoptotic Activities of *Clinacanthus nutans* (Burm. f.) Lindau Leaves against D24 Human Melanoma Cells." *Journal of Herbal Medicine* 17–18 (June 2018). Elsevier: 100285.

Haron, Nor Hasyimah, Zaleha Md Toha, Rafedah Abas, Mohammad Razak Hamdan, Nizuwan Azman, Melati Khairuddean, and Hasni Arsad. 2019. "In Vitro Cytotoxic Activity of *Clinacanthus nutans* Leaf Extracts against HeLa Cells." *Asian Pacific Journal of Cancer Prevention* 20 (2): 601–609.

Huang, Danmin, Wenjie Guo, Jing Gao, Jun Chen, and Joshua Opeyemi Olatunji. 2015. "*Clinacanthus nutans* (Burm. f.) Lindau Ethanol Extract Inhibits Hepatoma in Mice through Upregulation of the Immune Response." *Molecules* 20: 17405–17428.

Kamarudin, Muhamad Noor Alfarizal, Md Moklesur Rahman Sarker, Habsah Abdul Kadir, and Long Chiau Ming. 2017. "Ethnopharmacological Uses, Phytochemistry, Biological Activities, and Therapeutic Applications of *Clinacanthus nutans* (Burm. f.) Lindau: A Comprehensive Review." *Journal of Ethnopharmacology* 206: 245–266. Elsevier Ireland Ltd.

Khoo, Leng Wei, Siew Audrey Kow, Ming Tatt Lee, Chin Ping Tan, Khozirah Shaari, Chau Ling Tham, and Faridah Abas. 2018. "A Comprehensive Review on Phytochemistry and Pharmacological Activities of *Clinacanthus nutans* (Burm.f.) Lindau." *Evidence-Based Complementary and Alternative Medicine* 2018: 1–39. Hindawi Limited.

Lin, Chung Ming, Hsin Han Chen, Chi Wen Lung, and Hui Jye Chen. 2021. "Recent Advancement in Anticancer Activity of *Clinacanthus nutans* (Burm. f.) Lindau." *Evidence-Based Complementary and Alternative Medicine.* 2021: 1–13. Hindawi Limited.

Lu, Mei Chin, Tsung Yuan Li, Yu Chun Hsieh, Pao Chuan Hsieh, and Yung Lin Chu. 2018. "Chemical Evaluation and Cytotoxic Mechanism Investigation of *Clinacanthus nutans* Extract in Lymphoma SUP-T1 Cells." *Environmental Toxicology* 33 (12): 1229–1236.

Ma, Li, Mengmeng Zhang, Rong Zhao, Dan Wang, Yuerong Ma, and Li Ai. 2021. "Plant Natural Products: Promising Resources for Cancer Chemoprevention." *Molecules* 26 (4).

Mohd Rosli, Nur Hasnieza, Kok Meng Chan, Fariza Juliana Nordin, Lek Mun Leong, Nur Syazwani Abdul
    Aziz, and Nor Fadilah Rajab. 2018. "Assessment of Cytotoxicity Potency of Paclitaxel in Combination
    with *Clinacanthus nutans* Extracts on Human MDA-MB-231 Breast Cancer Cells." *Jurnal Sains
    Kesihatan Malaysia* 16 (Special Issue): 95–103.

Murugesu, Suganya, Alfi Khatib, Qamar Uddin Ahmed, Zalikha Ibrahim, Bisha Fathamah Uzir, Khaled
    Benchoula, Nik Idris Nik Yusoff, et al. 2019. "Toxicity Study on *Clinacanthus nutans* Leaf Hexane
    Fraction Using Danio Rerio Embryos." *Toxicology Reports* 6 (January). Elsevier Inc.: 1148–1154.

Mutazah, Roziasyahira, Hazrulrizawati Abd Hamid, Aizi Nor Mazila Ramli, Mohd Fadhlizil Fasihi Mohd
    Aluwi, and Mashitah M. Yusoff. 2020. "In Vitro Cytotoxicity of *Clinacanthus nutans* Fractions on Breast
    Cancer Cells and Molecular Docking Study of Sulphur Containing Compounds against Caspase-3." *Food
    and Chemical Toxicology* 135 (September 2019). Elsevier: 110869.

Ng, Chin Theng, Lai Yen Fong, Jun Jie Tan, Nor Fadilah Rajab, Faridah Abas, Khozirah Shaari, Kok Meng
    Chan, Fariza Juliana, and Yoke Keong Yong. 2018. "Water Extract of *Clinacanthus nutans* Leaves
    Exhibits in Vitro, Ex Vivo and in Vivo Anti-Angiogenic Activities in Endothelial Cell via Suppression of
    Cell Proliferation." *BMC Complementary and Alternative Medicine* 18 (1). BMC Complementary and
    Alternative Medicine: 1–12.

Ng, Pei Ying, Soi Moi Chye, Chew Hee Ng, Rhun Yian Koh, Yee Lian Tiong, Liew Phing Pui, Yong Hui
    Tan, Crystale Siew Ying Lim, and Khuen Yen Ng. 2017. "*Clinacanthus nutans* Hexane Extracts Induce
    Apoptosis through a Caspase-Dependent Pathway in Human Cancer Cell Lines." *Asian Pacific Journal
    of Cancer Prevention* 18 (4): 917–926.

Nik Abd Rahman, Nik Mohd Afizan, M.Y. Nurliyana, M.N.F. Natasha Nur Afiqah, Mohd Azuraidi Osman,
    Muhajir Hamid, and Mohd Azmi Mohd Lila. 2019. "Antitumor and Antioxidant Effects of *Clinacanthus
    nutans* Lindau in 4 T1 Tumor-Bearing Mice." *BMC Complementary and Alternative Medicine* 19 (1).
    BMC Complementary and Alternative Medicine: 1–9.

Nordin, Fariza Juliana, Lishantini Pearanpan, Kok Meng Chan, Endang Kumolosasi, Yoke Keong Yong,
    Khozirah Shaari, and Nor Fadilah Rajab. 2021. "Immunomodulatory Potential of *Clinacanthus
    nutans* Extracts in the Co-Culture of Triple negative Breast Cancer Cells, MDA-MB-231, and THP-1
    Macrophages." *PLoS ONE* 16 (8 August): 1–19.

Rashidi, Bahman, Mehrnoush Malekzadeh, Mohammad Goodarzi, Aria Masoudifar, and Hamed Mirzaei.
    2017. "Green Tea and Its Anti-Angiogenesis Effects." *Biomedicine and Pharmacotherapy* 89. Elsevier
    Masson SAS: 949–956.

Reczek, Colleen R., and Navdeep S. Chandel. 2017. "The Two Faces of Reactive Oxygen Species in Cancer."
    Annual Review of Cancer Biology 1. Annual Reviews Inc.: 79–98.

Roslan, S.N.F.M., Y. Zakaria, and H. Abdullah. 2018. "Cytotoxicity of *Clinacanthus nutans* and Mechanism of
    Action of Its Active Fraction towards Human Cervical Cancer Cell Line, HeLA." *Jurnal Sains Kesihatan
    Malaysia* 16 (02): 39–50.

Sakdarat, Santi, Sujittapron Sittiso, Tipaya Ekalaksananan, Chamsai Pientong, Nicha Charoensri, and Bunkerd
    Kongyingyoes. 2018. "Study on Effects of Compounds from *Clinacanthus nutans* on Dengue Virus Type
    2 Infection." *SSRN Electronic Journal* 25: 272–275.

Samad, Nozlena Abdul, Ahmad Bustamam Abdul, Heshu Sulaiman Rahman, Abdullah Rasedee, Tengku Azmi
    Tengku Ibrahim, and Yeap Swee Keon. 2017. "Zerumbone Suppresses Angiogenesis in HepG2 Cells through
    Inhibition of Matrix Metalloproteinase-9, Vascular Endothelial Growth Factor, and Vascular Endothelial Growth
    Factor Receptor Expressions." *Pharmacognosy Magazine* 13 (52). Medknow Publications: S731–S736.

Steiger, S., S. Kuhn, F. Ronchese, and J.L. Harper. 2015. "Monosodium Urate Crystals Induce Upregulation of
    NK1.1-Dependent Killing by Macrophages and Support Tumor-Resident NK1.1+ Monocyte/Macrophage
    Populations in Antitumor Therapy." *The Journal of Immunology* 195 (11): 5495–5502.

St. Paul, Michael, and Pamela S. Ohashi. 2020. "The Roles of CD8+ T Cell Subsets in Antitumor Immunity."
    Trends in Cell Biology 30 (9). Elsevier Ltd: 695–704.

Tan, Loh Teng Hern, Kooi Yeong Khaw, Yong Sze Ong, Tahir Mehmood Khan, Learn Han Lee, Wai Leng
    Lee, and Bey Hing Goh. 2020. "An Overview of *Clinacanthus nutans* (Burm. f.) Lindau as a Medicinal
    Plant with Diverse Pharmacological Values." In *Plant-Derived Bioactives: Production, Properties and
    Therapeutic Applications*, 461–491. Springer, Singapore.

Teoh, Peik Lin, Angelina Ying, Fang Cheng, Monica Liau, Fui Fui Lem, P Grace, Fern Nie Chua, et al. 2017.
    "Chemical Composition and Cytotoxic Properties of *Clinacanthus nutans* Root Extracts." *Pharmaceutical
    Biology* 55 (1). Taylor 8 Francis: 394–401.

Wang, K., C. Chan, A. Ahmad Hidayat, Y. Kadir, and H. Wong. 2019. "*Clinacanthus nutans* Induced Reactive Oxygen Species-Dependent Apoptosis and Autophagy in HCT116 Human Colorectal Cancer Cells." *Pharmacognosy Magazine* 15: 87–97.

Whittaker, Steven R., Aurélie Mallinger, Paul Workman, and Paul A. Clarke. 2017. "Inhibitors of Cyclin-Dependent Kinases as Cancer Therapeutics." *Pharmacology and Therapeutics* 173: 83–105. Elsevier Inc.

Xiu Wen, P'ng, Gabriel Akyirem Akowuah, and Jin Han Chin. 2012. "Acute Oral Toxicity Study of *Clinacanthus nutans* in Mice." *IJPSR* 3 (11): 4202–4205.

Yong, Marilyn Jane, Ahmad Zaidi Tani, Falah Abass Mohamed Salih, Rahmawati Pare, Rina Norgainathai, and Siat Yee Fong. 2020. "Aqueous Leaf Extract of *Clinacanthus nutans* Inhibits Growth and Induces Apoptosis via the Intrinsic and Extrinsic Pathways in MDA-MB-231 Human Breast Cancer Cells." *Pharmacognosy Magazine* 16 (72). Medknow: 689.

Yong, Yoke Keong, Jun Jie Tan, Soek Sin Teh, Siau Hui Mah, Gwendoline Cheng Lian Ee, Hoe Siong Chiong, and Zuraini Ahmad. 2013. "Clinacanthus Nutans Extracts Are Antioxidant with Antiproliferative Effect on Cultured Human Cancer Cell Lines." *Evidence-Based Complementary and Alternative Medicine*.

Zainuddin, Nik Aina Syazana Nik, Nik Fakhuruddin Nik Hassan, Yusmazura Zakaria, Hussin Muhammad, and Nor Hayati Othman. 2019. "Semi-Purified Fraction of *Clinacanthus nutans* Induced Apoptosis in Human Cervical Cancer, SiHa Cells via up-Regulation of Bax and down-Regulation of Bcl-2." *Sains Malaysiana* 48 (9). Penerbit Universiti Kebangsaan Malaysia: 1997–2006.

Zakaria Khairun Najwa, Azura Amid, Zubaidah Zakaria, Parveen Jamal, and Azli Ismail. 2019. "Anti-Proliferative Activity of Triterpenes Isolated from *Clinicanthus nutans* on Hep-G2 Liver Cancer Cells." *Asian Pac J Cancer Prev* 20 (2): 563–567.

Zulkapli, Rahayu, and Fathilah Abdul Razak. 2019. "The Preliminary Cytotoxicity Study: Anti-Proliferative Activity of Aqueous Extract of *Clinacanthus nutans, Strobilanther crispa* and *Pereskia bleo* on Oral Squamous Carcinoma Cells Orl-48/Rahayu Zulkapli and Fathilah Abdul Razak." *Proceedings of 9th Dental Student Scientific Symposium, Malaysia (Malaysia, 2019)* 1: 1–2.

Zulkipli, Ihsan N., Rajan Rajabalaya, Adi Idris, Nurul Atiqah Sulaiman, R. David, Rajan Rajabalaya, Adi Idris, Nurul Atiqah Sulaiman, and Sheba R. David. 2017. "*Clinacanthus nutans*: A Review on Ethnomedicinal Uses, Chemical Constituents and Pharmacological Properties." *Pharmaceutical Biology* 55 (1). Informa Healthcare USA, Inc: 1093–1113.

19 The Antiproliferative Effects of *Cakile maritima* Scop. (Sea Rocket) in Cancer Prevention and Treatment

Ian Edwin Cock and Matthew James Cheesman

ABBREVIATIONS

AMPK	AMP-activated protein kinase
Bax	Bcl-2 associated X apoptosis regulator
Bcl-2	B-cell lymphoma 2
bFGF	basic fibroblast growth factor
CAT	catalase
CDK	cyclin-dependent kinase
COX	cyclooxygenase
GSH-Px	glutathione peroxidase
LPS	lipopolysaccharide
LOX	lipooxygenase
MAPK	mitogen-activated protein kinase
NF-κB	nuclear factor kappa B
NO	nitric oxide
PGE$_2$	prostaglandin E$_2$
ROS	reactive oxygen species
SOD	superoxide dismutase
THx	thioredoxin
TNF-α	tumor necrosis factor alpha
VEGF	vascular endothelial growth factor

19.1 INTRODUCTION

Cakile maritima Scop. (family Brassicaceae; commonly known as European sea rocket) is an annual succulent halophyte plant that is native to coastal regions of Europe, northern Africa, and western Asia, although it has been naturalized globally. It thrives in harsh, sandy areas, particularly regions with high salt content, and can tolerate transient seawater inundation (Arbelet-Bonnin et al. 2020). Indeed, high salinity may be beneficial for this species as it stimulates polyphenol synthesis and the accumulation of antioxidant compounds that provide an antioxidant defense against reactive oxygen species (ROS) (Ksouri et al. 2007). *Cakile maritima* has a multi-branched stem and grows in clumps/mounds up to 40 cm high and up to 45 cm in diameter (Figure 19.1A). Small white, lilac, or purple flowers (Figure 19.1B) are produced in the summer months, which develop into yellow/brown seeds (Figure 19.1C).

DOI: 10.1201/9781003260028-21

All parts of the plant are consumed and are valued for their high antioxidant content (Fuochi et al. 2019; Omer et al. 2019; Meot-Duros et al. 2008). The mature leaves are relatively tough and fibrous and are usually cooked prior to consumption, while the young leaves may be consumed raw in salads. Powdered *C. maritima* roots may also be baked into a bread for consumption. Additionally, the whole plant has been used in several traditional medicine systems as a digestive, diuretic, and a dandruff treatment (Placines et al. 2020). It produces several noteworthy phytochemicals with medicinal bioactivities including flavonoids, terpenoids, tannins, and phenolic acids (Omer et al. 2019; Placines et al. 2020; Sheikh et al. 2020; Omer et al. 2016; Rabi and Bishayee 2009) and it has been reported to have a high antioxidant capacity (Stambouli-Essassi et al. 2020). The high levels of antioxidants in this plant have attracted substantial recent attention and have been linked with anticancer (Fuochi et al. 2019; Omer et al. 2019; Aboul-Enein et al. 2012), antibacterial (Fuochi et al. 2019; Meot-Duros et al. 2008; Omer et al. 2016), anti-inflammatory (Fuochi et al. 2019), and antidiabetic (Fuochi et al. 2019; Placines et al. 2020) activities.

19.2   TRADITIONAL USES TO TREAT AND PREVENT CANCER

Cakile maritima was noted for its chemotherapeutic potential as early as the 12th century by physician Moses Maimonides (Casal and Casal 2004). Interestingly, little is known of its traditional use as an antiproliferative agent. The plant is edible and can be consumed either raw or cooked (Guil-Guerrero et al. 1999), indicating that it was primarily used for dietary rather than antiproliferative purposes, despite the plant now being identified as containing a diverse mixture of bioactive molecules with antiproliferative activity (Ksouri et al. 2007). Instead, traditional uses are derived from its antioxidant properties due to the abundance of vitamin C, iron, and iodine in the plant (Fuochi et al. 2019). The flowers are also used to prepare a digestive and diuretic herbal tea that treats lymphatic disturbances (Davy et al. 2006). Thus, while a definitive ethnomedicinal basis for the use of *C. maritima* in the treatment of cancer cannot be established, antiproliferative effects of *C. maritima* have now been identified through the

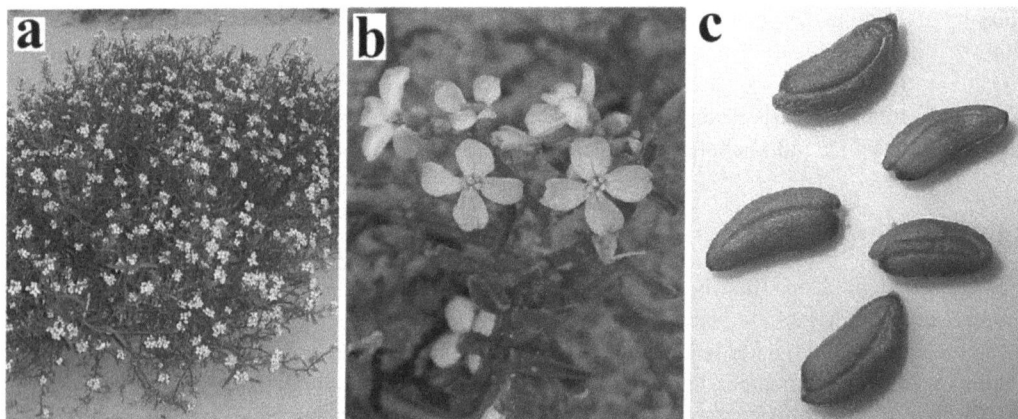

FIGURE 19.1   *Cakile maritima*: (A) whole plant, (B) flowers, and (C) seeds.

Source: All figures are available under Creative Commons License (https://commons.wikimedia.org/wiki/File:Cakile-maritima-(eurMeersenf)_1.jpg; https://commons.wikimedia.org/wiki/File:C.maritima-seeds-1.jpg) and are reproduced here with all relevant permissions.

advent of modern science, which has revealed compounds from the plant with potential anti-cancer applications.

19.3   ANTICANCER VERIFICATION STUDIES

Despite its therapeutic uses, there have been relatively few studies into the anticancer properties of *C. maritima* preparations. Instead, most studies have either evaluated the phytochemical composition of *C. maritima* preparations or have tested individual extract components without verifying the activity in the crude preparation (the activity of individual *C. maritima* components will be discussed in detail later in this chapter). However, plant extracts may have substantially higher biological activities than the sum of their individual components (Cheesman et al. 2017). Often, the "bioactive" component(s) in extracts require potentiator molecule(s) to increase their activity to therapeutic levels. Therefore, studies that only test individual components and neglect to screen crude plant extracts (and/or enriched fractions) may overlook clinically relevant activities. Furthermore, several compounds may function against different anticancer targets, allowing the therapy to bypass resistance mechanisms in some cell lines, thereby not only increasing the potency of the therapy but also increasing the range of cancer cells that the therapy is useful against. It is therefore important that future studies do not neglect screening against crude extracts and fractions.

A recent study from our group screened solvent extracts prepared from *C. maritima* against human Caco2 colorectal and cervical HeLa cancer cell lines and reported potent activity for a hexane extract (12 and 126 µg/mL, respectively) (Omer et al. 2019). That study also reported strong activity for an ethyl acetate extract (185 and 468 µg/mL against Caco2 and HeLa cells, respectively), indicating that the main anticancer components may be mid- to low polarity. Of further note, that study also correlated the anticancer activity with antioxidant content and highlighted several monoterpenoids including 2-hydroxy-1,8-cineole, limonene, and citronellal. However, while that study did identify the contribution of antioxidant mechanisms, it did not establish detail about how the extracts and components achieved the activity. Indeed, while the authors of that study postulated that the *C. maritima* extracts exerted their effects via both cytostatic and cytotoxic mechanisms, details of these pathways and mechanisms were not reported in that study.

Another study tested extracts prepared from *C. maritima* stems, seeds, leaves, and flowers and reported that all of the extracts substantially inhibited the expression of pro-inflammatory cytokines in human U937 lymphoma cells following lipopolysaccraride (LPS) treatment (Fuochi et al. 2019). Additionally, that study also reported that the extracts were potent inhibitors of human U266 multiple myeloma cells yet were nontoxic towards normal cells. The authors also correlated the therapeutic properties with the antioxidant contents of the extracts. In contrast, a different study reported that a *C. maritima* extract did not significantly alter the proliferation of murine RAW cells (Ghonime et al. 2015). However, that study reported several bioactivities relevant to anticancer therapy. In particular, the *C. maritima* extract significantly altered TFN-α release and decreased COX-2 production in RAW cells.

Further *in vivo* studies have also reported anticancer activity for *C. maritima* ethanol and water extracts against Ehrlich ascites carcinoma cells (EACC) and HepG3 human liver carcinoma cells (~90% inhibition of proliferation) (Aboul-Enein et al. 2012). However, that study only tested single extract concentrations and did not quantify the potency, making comparisons with other studies impossible. In addition, *C. maritima* extracts inhibit human MDA-MB-231 epithelial breast cancer cell proliferation, although only with relatively weak activity (Nasr et al. 2018). Substantially more work is required to screen *C. maritima* preparations against a wider panel of cancer cell lines.

19.4   ANTIOXIDANT CONTENT

There are numerous reports of the antioxidant contents of *C. maritima* extracts. Leaf extracts, extracted with a 1:1 water-methanol solution, possess high radical cation scavenging activity as well as total antioxidant activity (Meot-Duros et al. 2008), while ethanolic extracts of the aerial organs of the plant have significant radical cation scavenging and ferric-reducing capacities (Placines et al. 2020). Interestingly, the antioxidant activities of leaf extracts are increased by greater salinity levels during plant growth (Ksouri et al. 2007), which includes the elevation of antioxidant enzymes such as superoxide dismutase (SOD), catalase (CAT), and peroxidases (Ellouzi et al. 2011; Ben Amor et al. 2020; Houmani et al. 2016). This indicates that *C. maritima* regulates its antioxidant mechanisms in response to salt levels. All parts of the plant possess antioxidant activity, including the stems, seeds, flowers, and leaves (Fuochi et al. 2019).

19.5   OXIDATIVE STRESS AND CANCER

A disturbance in the balance between antioxidants and prooxidants leads to oxidative stress. Intracellular enzymes including SOD, CAT, thioredoxin (THx), and glutathione peroxidase (GSH-Px), as well as vitamin-based antioxidants (e.g., vitamins C and E) are essential in neutralizing ROS (reactive oxygen species) and assist in the repair of various cellular components that have become oxidized during normal or toxic metabolic processes (Shang et al. 2006). Failure in these enzyme systems results in excessive ROS production, which leads to ROS-mediated attack on proteins, lipids, RNA, and DNA. Oxidative stress significantly contributes to the pathogenesis of a myriad of diseases, including cancer (Hayes et al. 2020). Mechanisms to decrease cellular ROS levels are recognized as targets for treating cancer (Cock and Cheesman 2021).

19.6   PHYTOCHEMISTRY OF *C. MARITIMA* SCOP.

Despite the traditional uses and medicinal properties of *C. maritima*, the majority of studies to date have focused on the classes of the phytochemical constituents without identifying the individual components. These studies have identified flavonoids, terpenoids, coumarins, sterols, alkaloids, and sulfur glycosides as major classes of compounds (Radwan et al. 2008). Several of these classes of compounds may contribute to the anticancer activities of this species. However, several recent studies have reported relatively high levels of a diversity of flavonoids, with multiple kaempferol and quercetin glycosides identified as major components (Fuochi et al. 2019; Sheikh et al. 2020; Lozada-García et al. 2017; Sertel et al. 2010; Shamshoum et al. 2017; Schindler and Mentlein 2006; Lee et al. 2002). Similarly, a variety of terpenoids (particularly monoterpenoids) have also been identified (Omer et al. 2019; Sheikh et al. 2020; Omer et al. 2016; Rabi et al. 2009). Notably, several of these compounds have verified anticancer properties (summarized in Table 19.1). Additionally, several glucosinolates and isothiocyanates have also been identified (Iranshahi 2012).

19.6.1   FLAVONOIDS

Phenolic compounds, and in particular the flavonoids, have been identified as the major class of antioxidant compounds in *C. maritima*. Some flavonoids have been linked to the induction of cellular

TABLE 19.1

Important Phytoconstituents Identified in *Cakile maritima* Extracts and Their Anticancer Mechanisms (Where Known)

Compound Class	Compound	Known Anticancer Activities	References
Antioxidants	α-Tocopherol γ-Tocopherol	Inhibition of ROS via activation of cellular antioxidant systems and by direct scavenging.	Sheik et al. 2020
Terpenoids	Citronellal Homomyrtenol 2-Hydroxy-1,8-cineole Levomenthol D-Limonene Linalool α-Copaene *trans*-β-Damascenone *cis*-α-Bergamotene Guaia-6,9-diene Caryophyllene β-Farnesene Guaia-1(10),11-diene α-Curcumene 6-Epishyobunone Myristicin Spathulenol	Increases levels of detoxifying enzymes, inhibits ROS levels via activation of cellular antioxidant systems and by direct scavenging, induces apoptosis, inhibits angiogenesis, inhibits isoprenylation of G-proteins (including p21). Upregulates Bax expression and release of cytochrome c from the mitochondria as well as caspase-3 and caspase-9 cleavage. Regulates cell cycle progression. Upregulation of NF-κB mediates TNF-α. Activation of MAPK and signaling pathways for autophagy. Enhances Fas expression and caspase stimulation.	Sheik et al. 2020; Omer et al. 2019; Omer et al. 2016; Rabi and Bishayee 2009
Flavonoids	Isorhamnetin-dHex	Similar to other flavonoids including kaempferol and quercetin.	Sheik et al. 2020; Placines et al. 2020; Lozada-García et al. 2017; Sertel et al. 2010; Schindler and Mentlein 2006; Lee et al. 2002
	Kaempferol-Rut	May be similar to kaempferol.	
	Kaempferol-dHex	May be similar to kaempferol.	
	Kaempferol-Hex	May be similar to kaempferol.	
	Kaempferol-Hex-Rut	May be similar to kaempferol.	
	Kaempferol-dHex-Hex	May be similar to kaempferol.	
	Quercetin-Rut	May be similar to quercetin.	
	Quercetin-dHex	May be similar to quercetin.	
	Quercetin-di-Hex-dHex	May be similar to quercetin.	
	Quercetin-Hex-dHex	May be similar to quercetin.	
	Isosakuranetin Kaempferol Kaempferol-7-O-glucoside Luteolin Luteolin-7-glucoside Prenylnarigenine Scutellarein Quercetin-3-O-rhamnoside Quercetin	Stimulates apoptosis, cell cycle arrest (G1 and G2/M phases) via modulation of CDKs, inhibition of oxidative enzyme, inhibition of ROS via activation of cellular antioxidant systems, inhibition of angiogenesis. Upregulation of NF-κB mediated TNF-α. Activation of MAPK and signaling pathways for autophagy.	Sheik et al. 2020; Fuochi et al. 2019; Lozada-García et al. 2017; Sertel et al. 2010; Schindler and Mentlein 2006; Lee et al. 2002

(Continued)

TABLE 19.1
(Continued)

Compound Class	Compound	Known Anticancer Activities	References
Tannins	Ellagic acid	Inhibition of ROS via activation of cellular antioxidant systems and by direct scavenging, induces apoptosis, modulates Bax and decreases Bcl-2 expression, regulation of NF-κB and TNF-α levels, increases p27, p21, and p53 levels, stimulates release of cytochrome c from the mitochondria as well as caspase-3 and caspase-9 cleavage. Regulates cell cycle progression.	Cock and Cheesman 2021; Youness et al. 2021; Fuochi et al. 2019; Cai et al. 2017
	Gallic acid		
Other polyphenolics	Disinapoyl-Hex	Unknown	Placines et al. 2020
	Caffeic acid	Inhibition of ROS via activation of cellular antioxidant systems and by direct scavenging, induces apoptosis, inhibits DNA methylation. Upregulation of NF-κB mediated TNF-α.	Sheik et al. 2020; Fuochi et al. 2019
	Chlorogenic acid		
	Cinnamic acid		
	Cumaric acid		
	Fertaric acid		
	Ferulic acid		
	Oleuropein	Induces apoptosis via caspase-3 activation, increases Bax and decreases Bcl-2, decreases cell proliferation and angiogenesis, upregulates the tumor suppressor p21. Inhibits cell cycle progression via reduction of cyclin D1 levels.	Placines et al. 2020; Shamshoum et al. 2017
	Bergaptene	Induces apoptosis via increasing Bax and decreasing Bcl-2 expression, decreases cell proliferation and angiogenesis. Upregulation of NF-κB mediated TNF-α. G0/G1 cell cycle arrest.	Fuochi et al. 2019
	Esculetine		
	Resveratrol	Inhibition of ROS via activation of cellular antioxidant systems and by direct scavenging, induces apoptosis by modulating Bax/Bcl-2 ratio. Potent inhibitor of NF-κB activation and induction of TNF-α and IL-1β. Blocks cell proliferation (and metastasis) by disrupting microtubule formation. Blocks cell cycle progression in M phase. Stimulates caspase 3 activation.	Cock and Cheesman 2021; Fuochi et al. 2019; Wang et al. 2019

mechanisms that affect cancer cell progression and proliferation, as well as inhibiting tumor invasion. Flavonoids exert their anticancer effects via several mechanisms (Figure 19.2):

- Stimulation of apoptosis (Lee et al. 2002).
- Cell cycle arrest in G1 or G2/M phases by modulation of cyclin-dependent kinases (CDKs) (Sheikh et al. 2020; Fuochi et al. 2019; Cock 2013).
- Inhibition of proliferation (Sheikh et al. 2020; Fuochi et al. 2019; Cock 2013).
- Inhibition of enzymes that induce inflammation and/or cytochromes P450, thereby decreasing the activation of carcinogens (Sheikh et al. 2020).
- Decreasing reactive oxygen species (ROS) levels via activation of cellular antioxidant systems and by direct scavenging (Sheikh et al. 2020; Fuochi et al. 2019; Cock 2013).
- Blocking angiogenesis by inhibition of vascular endothelial growth factor (VEGF) and basic fibroblast growth factor (bFGF) (Schindler and Mentlein 2006).

Of the identified *C. maritima* flavonoid components, kaempferol, quercetin, and their glycosides are the dominant components (Sheik et al. 2020; Placines et al. 2020; Fuochi et al. 2019). The authors of those studies linked these compounds to the anticancer activity of *C. maritima* extracts. Furthermore, a recent study reported good antiproliferative properties for isolated dihydrokaempferol and quercetin (Zhang et al. 2008). When tested at a concentration of 100 μg/mL against human CAL-27 and KB oral carcinoma cell lines, HT29 and HCT-116 colorectal cancer cells, and LNCaP and DU145 prostate cancer cells, these flavonoids inhibited

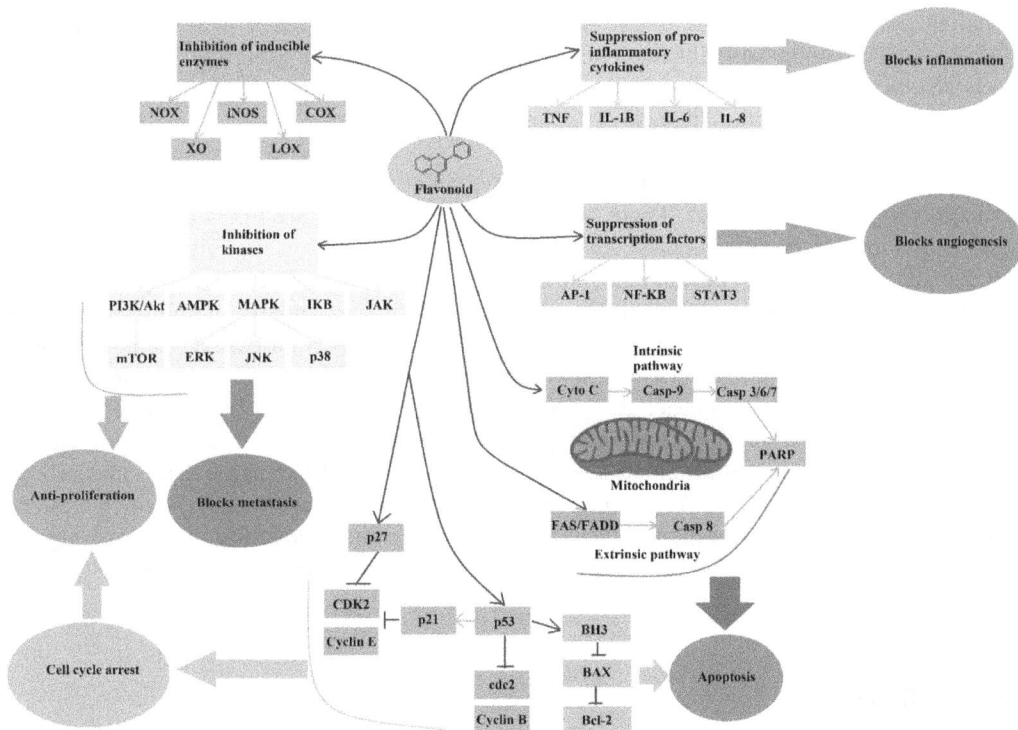

FIGURE 19.2 An overview of cytostatic and cytotoxic anticancer activities of *Cakile maritima* flavonoids.

cell proliferation by as much as 80% of the untreated cell proliferation rate. Unfortunately, this study did not report IC_{50} values, making it difficult to compare the efficacy with other compounds/other studies. A different study reported that kaempferol induces apoptosis in human LNCaP prostate cancer and MDA-MB-231 breast cancer cells (Brusselmans et al. 2005). That study noted a strong relationship between the induction of apoptosis and an inhibition in fatty acid synthesis. When exogenous palmitate was added to the treated cells, apoptosis was supressed, indicating that the mechanism by which flavonoids induce apoptosis is associated with their inhibition of fatty acid synthesis. Quercetin and kaempferol also inhibit glutathione S-transferase P1–1 and GS-X pump activity in MCF7 cells, with IC_{50} values between 0.8 and 8 μM, indicating that these flavonoids may be useful for potentiating apoptosis in multidrug resistant cells (van Zanden et al. 2004).

Similarly, luteolin contributes to the anticancer properties of *C. maritima* via multiple mechanisms and has both cytostatic and cytotoxic effects (Seelinger et al. 2008). It inhibits proliferation of multiple cancer cell lines *in vitro* (Woerdenbag et al. 1994; Selvendiran et al. 2006; Chiu and Lin 2008) and can induce cell cycle arrest at both the G1 or G2/M phases (Lim et al. 2007; Chang et al. 2005). Additionally, luteolin can also induce apoptosis via multiple mechanisms, including increasing Bax and decreasing Bcl-2 expression (Selvendiran et al. 2006; Cheng et al. 2005). It also induces cytochrome c release from the mitochondria (Cheng et al. 2005; Lee et al. 2005), thereby activating caspases 3 and 9 (Kim et al. 2006; Lim et al. 2007) and triggering the intrinsic pathway of apoptosis. The anticancer effects of luteolin are well established and have been reviewed in substantial detail in Seelinger et al. (2008). For a complete discussion of the anticancer activities of luteolin, the reader is referred to that study.

The antioxidant capacity of flavonoids is important for many of the anticancer properties of flavonoids. Indeed, high antioxidant levels modulate cellular levels of transcription factors including nuclear factor kappa B (NF-κB), thereby stimulating tumor necrosis factor alpha (TNF-α)–induced apoptosis (Sheikh et al. 2020; Fuochi et al. 2019). Similarly, high antioxidant levels also activate several kinase enzymes, including AMPK, ERK, JAK, JNK, MAPK, and p38, and therefore modulate the cell cycle and cell proliferation (Sheikh et al. 2020; Ahmad et al. 1998).

Recent studies have reported that many flavonoids also have potent anti-inflammatory activities (Nijveldt et al. 2001). These anti-inflammatory effects are likely due to the inhibition of the enzymes cyclooxygenase and lipoxygenase, resulting in the inhibition of prostaglandin and leukotriene synthesis and the downstream release of cytokines (Ferrandiz and Alcaraz 1991; Laughton et al. 1991). Quercetin has particularly potent inhibitory effects on both cyclooxygenase and lipoxygenase enzyme activities via its antioxidant activity, resulting in diminished eicosanoid biosynthesis (Kim et al. 1998). These effects are exerted via a downregulation of cyclooxygenase-2 (COX-2) and 5-lipoxygenase (5-LOX), tumor necrosis factor alpha (TNF-α), and interleukin-6 (IL-6) (Nijveldt et al. 2001). This downregulation results in the inhibition of inflammatory mediators including nitric oxide (NO) and prostaglandin E_2 (PGE_2) production. As mitogen-activated protein kinases (MAPKs), which regulate inflammatory and immune responses, may be activated by the production of reactive oxygen species (ROS), it is likely that the inhibition of ROS via quercetin is also responsible for its anti-inflammatory activity.

19.6.2 TERPENOIDS

Another noteworthy aspect of the phytochemistry of *C. maritima* is the diversity of mono- and sesquiterpenoids that have been identified (Sheik et al. 2020; Omer et al. 2019; Omer et al. 2016; Rabi and Bishayee 2009). Multiple monoterpenoids with anticancer properties were identified and they have been reported to function via multiple mechanisms. These mechanisms are summarized in Figure 19.3. Many of these mechanisms are similar to or complement those already discussed in the flavonoids section of this chapter. In particular, terpenoids may:

- Decrease the levels of ROS by direct scavenging of free radicals and by regulating cellular antioxidant systems (Huang et al. 2013; Cock 2013).
- Inhibit cellular proliferation by suppressing the levels of transcription factors including NF-κB, JAK-STAT, and AP-1 (Huang et al. 2013; Jain et al. 2016).
- Arrest cell cycle progression in G1 or G2/M phases via decreasing the production and activation of cyclins and CDKs (Huang et al. 2013; Sharma et al. 2017).
- Stimulate apoptosis by several mechanisms. Some terpenoids can induce increases in Bax expression while decreasing Bcl-2 expression (Huang et al. 2013; Sharma et al. 2017). Additionally, terpenoids can trigger the intrinsic pathway of apoptosis by stimulating mitochondrial cytochrome c release and activating caspases 3 and. They can also stimulate the extrinsic apoptotic pathways by activating caspase 8 (Huang et al. 2013; Sharma et al. 2017).
- Decrease the release of pro-inflammatory cytokines including TNF-α, IL-6, and IL-8 via inhibition of pro-inflammatory enzymes (Huang et al. 2013; Sharma et al. 2017).
- Direct inhibition of angiogenesis systems via modulation of oxidative stress (Huang et al. 2013).

Linalool has cytotoxic effects in SW620, T-47D, A549, and Hep G2 cells via a stimulation of TFN-α secretion (Chang and Shen 2014). It also activates p53 and cyclin dependent kinase inhibitors, suggesting that they induce apoptosis as well as arresting the cell cycle in a panel of leukemia cell lines (Gu et al. 2010). Furthermore, linalool exposure reverses doxorubicin resistance in MCF7

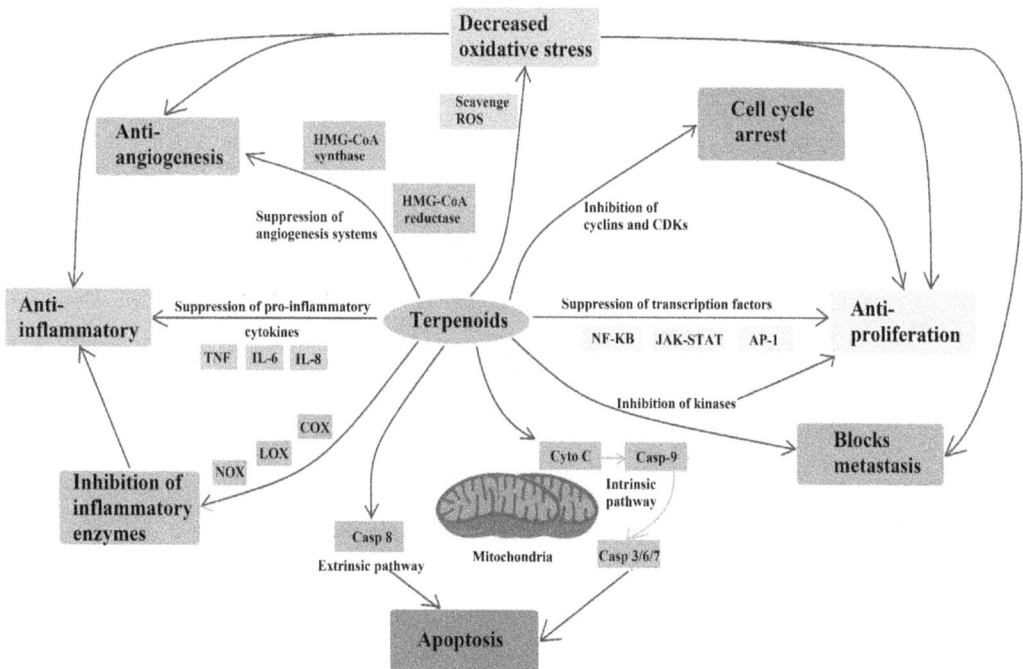

FIGURE 19.3 An overview of cytostatic and cytotoxic anticancer activities of *Cakile maritima* terpenoids.

AdrR multidrug resistant human breast adenocarcinoma cells, thereby improving the therapeutic index of doxorubicin (Ravizza et al. 2008).

Another study reported the presence of an abundance of 2-hydroxy-1,8-cineole, limonene, and citronellal in *C. maritima* extracts (Omer et al. 2019). Additionally, *C. maritima* also contained several other terpenoids, including safranal, cymene, and citral in lower abundance. Many of these monoterpenoids also have anticancer properties via several mechanisms. For example, limonene has been reported to be useful in the prevention and treatment of cancer in a murine test model, reducing stomach tumor formation by approximately 60% (Wattenberg et al. 1989). Similarly, both geraniol and iosgeraniol inhibit murine leukemia, hepatoma, and melanoma proliferation *in vitro* (Yu et al. 1995; Shoff et al. 1991). Cineole and 2-hydroxy-1,8-cineole activate p38 and caspase-3 in HCT116 and RKO human colon carcinoma cells, thereby inducing apoptosis. In addition, they also inactivate Akt (Murata et al. 2013). Interestingly, Akt is a protein kinase that is overexpressed and/or its activation is stimulated in ovarian, lung, and pancreatic cancer. Therefore, the inactivation of Akt by these terpenoids may inhibit both proliferation and stimulate apoptosis in multiple cancer cell lines. Additionally, α-pinene stimulates ROS production in metastatic melanoma cells by disrupting their mitochondrial membrane potential (Matsuo et al. 2011). The increased levels of ROS stimulate caspase-3 activation, resulting in DNA fragmentation, which subsequently induces apoptosis (Matsuo et al. 2011).

In addition to monoterpenoids, sesquiterpenoids, diterpenoids, and triterpenoids have also been identified in *C. maritima* extracts (Omer et al. 2019). Multiple sesquiterpenoids also have anticancer properties via several mechanisms. For example, the sesquiterpenoid caryophyllene inhibits progression of the cell cycle in human PC-3 prostate and MCF-7 breast cancer cells progression *in vitro* and also induces apoptosis (Park et al. 2011). Zingiberene (Togar et al. 2015) and phytol (Komiya et al. 1999) induce apoptosis in N2a-NB neuroblastoma cells and Molt 4B human leukemia cells, respectively. Furthermore, monoterpenoids, sesquiterpenoids, diterpenoids, and triterpenoids inhibit NF-κB signaling pathways and thereby inhibit cell cycle progression and cell proliferation and stimulate apoptosis (Jain et al. 2016).

19.6.3   Other Compounds

The presence of the tannin compounds gallic acid and ellagic acid is noteworthy as tannins have antiproliferative effects against a variety of carcinoma cell lines. Gallic acid can inhibit cellular growth by binding cell surface molecules including lipoteichoic acid and proline-rich cell surface proteins (Buzzini et al. 2008; Wolinsky et al. 1984), and by inhibiting glucosyltransferase enzymes (Wu-Yuan et al. 1988). Ellagic acid is also a potent inhibitor of cell growth and functions via several mechanisms including interaction with cytoplasmic oxidoreductases (Buzzini et al. 2008; Hogg and Embery 1982).

The stilbene resveratrol, which was identified in *C. maritima* extracts, has been particularly well studied and has been reported to be useful in the prevention and treatment of cancer (Cock and Cheesman 2021). Readers are referred to that study for an in-depth analysis of the anticancer mechanisms of resveratrol. Briefly, resveratrol is a potent specific inhibitor of NF-κB activation via its induction by TFN-α and IL-1β (Elmali et al. 2007). Thus, resveratrol treatment directly blocks cytokine production and inflammation via its inhibition of NF-κB activation. As inhibition of NF-κB potentiates apoptosis (Pikarsky et al. 2004; Wang et al. 1996), resveratrol is useful in the prevention and treatment of some cancers (Athar et al. 2007; Boocock et al. 2007; Jang et al. 1997). Resveratrol has also been shown to block IL-17 production in stimulated human mononuclear cells (Lanzilli et al. 2012). Additionally, resveratrol inhibits the cell cycle, cell proliferation, and metastasis by inhibiting cellular microtubule polymerization. It acts by a similar mechanism to that of colchicine

(N-[(7S)-1, 2, 3, 10-tetramethoxy-9-oxo-5, 6, 7, 9-tetrahydrobenzo[a]heptlen-7-yl] acetamide) by binding the colchicine binding site on the tubulin peptide (Bhardwaj et al. 2010). Additionally, resveratrol suppresses NF-κB binding to DNA, thus inhibiting multiple cancer cell processes (Huang et al. 2013).

19.7   FUTURE DIRECTIONS

While the anticancer properties of *C. maritima* extracts are promising, mechanistic studies into this species are limited. Instead, most anticancer mechanistic studies relevant to this species involve pure compounds that have been identified in *C. maritima* extracts, despite those compounds generally being isolated from different sources. Those studies report a number of diverse mechanisms from *C. maritima* constituents and indicate that *C. maritima* preparations may therefore be thought of as effective combinational therapies that function against multiple anticancer targets. Interestingly, despite the range of anticancer activities reported for *C. maritima* constituents, their individual activities are generally relatively modest. Therefore, combinational therapy utilizing several *C. maritima* components should be optimal for clinical usage. Despite this, studies testing the individual components in combination to screen for potentiating activity are relatively lacking, and much more research is needed in this area.

19.8   TOXICITY AND CAUTIONARY NOTES

Few studies have examined the toxicity of *C. maritima* extracts, with substantially more work required before they can be adapted for clinical usage. Some studies have reported that several different *C. maritima* preparations were nontoxic in several toxicity models. Placines et al. (2020) reported that extracts of both the aerial vegetative organs and the fruits were nontoxic in several mammalian cell lines including RAW 264.7, HEK 293, and HepG2. Additionally, studies indicate that *C. maritima* extracts are nontoxic towards *Artemia franciscana* nauplii (Omer et al. 2016) and HeLa and CaCo2 cells (Omer et al. 2019). However, further investigation is required to test *C. maritima* preparations against a variety of other cell lines, and against *in vivo* models, to further validate the safety of *C. maritima* for therapeutic use. Until these studies are completed, caution is advised when using *C. maritima* preparations.

19.9   SUMMARY POINTS

- *C. maritima* Scop. (commonly known as sea rocket) is used in several traditional medicine systems to treat multiple medical conditions.
- Several noteworthy phytochemicals including flavonoids, terpenoids, tannins, and phenolic acids have been identified in *C. maritima*, and it has a high antioxidant capacity.
- The high antioxidant contents are associated with antiproliferative effects.
- *C. maritima* flavonoids and terpenoids have direct antiproliferative and apoptotic effects. They also block cell cycle progression.
- Several tannins with antiproliferative and pro-apoptotic effects have also been identified in *C. maritima* extracts.
- Resveratrol (which mediates cellular proliferation via inhibition of tubulin polymerization) is also present in *C. maritima* leaves.
- Several other compounds with anticancer properties have also been identified in *C. maritima* extracts.
- This chapter reviews the current phytochemical knowledge and the previous studies into the anticancer properties of *C. maritima*.

REFERENCES

Aboul-Enein, Ahmed M., Faten Abu El-Ela, Emad A. Shalaby, and Hany A. El-Shemy. 2012. Traditional medicinal plants research in Egypt: Studies of antioxidant and anticancer activities. Journal of Medicinal Plants Research 6:689–703.

Ahmad, Nihal, Hala Gali, Seema Javed, and Rajesh Agarwal. 1998. Skin cancer chemopreventive effects of a flavonoid antioxidant silymarin are mediated via impairment of receptor tyrosine kinase signaling and perturbation in cell cycle progression. Biochemical and Biophysical Research Communications 247:294–301.

Arbelet-Bonnin, Delphine, Camille Blasselle, Emily Rose Palm, Mirvat Redwan, Maharajah Ponnaiah, Patrick Laurenti, Patrice Meimoun et al. 2020. Metabolism regulation during salt exposure in the halophyte *Cakile maritima*. Environmental and Experimental Botany 177:104075.

Athar, Mohammad, Jung Ho Back, Xiuwei Tang, Kwang Ho Kim, Levy Kopelovich, David R. Bickers, and Arianna L. Kim. 2007. Resveratrol: A review of preclinical studies for human cancer prevention. Toxicology and Applied Pharmacology 224:274–283.

Ben Amor, N., A. Jiménez, M. Boudabbous, F. Sevilla, and C. Abdelly. 2020. Chloroplast implication in the tolerance to salinity of the halophyte *Cakile maritima*. Russian Journal of Plant Physiology 67:507–514.

Bhardwaj, Sakshi, Sarabjeet Bakshi, Bhawna Chopra, Ashwani Dhingra, and K.L. Dhar. 2010. Synthesis of combretastatin analogues with their potent anticancer activity. International Journal of Research in Pharmaceutical Sciences 1:414–416.

Boocock, David J., Guy E.S. Faust, Ketan R. Patel, Anna M. Schinas, Victoria A. Brown, Murray P. Ducharme, Tristan D. Booth et al. 2007. Phase I dose escalation pharmacokinetic study in healthy volunteers of resveratrol, a potential cancer chemopreventive agent. Cancer Epidemiology and Prevention Biomarkers 16:1246–1252.

Brusselmans, Koen, Ruth Vrolix, Guido Verhoeven, and Johannes V. Swinnen. 2005. Induction of cancer cell apoptosis by flavonoids is associated with their ability to inhibit fatty acid synthase activity. Journal of Biological Chemistry 280:5636–5645.

Buzzini, Pietro, Panagiotis Arapitsas, Marta Goretti, Eva Branda, Benedetta Turchetti, Patrizia Pinelli, F. Ieri, and Annalisa Romani. 2008. Antimicrobial and antiviral activity of hydrolysable tannins. Mini-Reviews in Medicinal Chemistry 8: 1179–1187.

Cai, Yuee, Jinming Zhang, Nelson G. Chen, Zhi Shi, Jiange Qiu, Chengwei He, and Meiwan Chen. 2017. Recent advances in anticancer activities and drug delivery systems of tannins. Medicinal Research Reviews 37:665–701.

Casal, M.T., and M. Casal. 2004. Maimonides and the chemotherapy of infectious diseases. Revista Espanola Quimioterapia 17:289–294.

Chang, Jung San, Ya Ling Hsu, Po Lin Kuo, Yu Chun Kuo, Lien Chai Chiang, and Chun Ching Lin. 2005. Increase of Bax/Bcl-XL ratio and arrest of cell cycle by luteolin in immortalized human hepatoma cell line. Life Sciences 76:1883–1893.

Chang, Mei-Yin, and Yi-Ling Shen. 2014. Linalool exhibits cytotoxic effects by activating antitumor immunity. Molecules 19:6694–6706.

Cheesman, Matthew J., Aishwarya Ilanko, Baxter Blonk, and Ian E. Cock. 2017. Developing new antimicrobial therapies: Are synergistic combinations of plant extracts/compounds with conventional antibiotics the solution? Pharmacognosy Reviews 11:57–72.

Cheng, An-Chin, Tzou-Chi Huang, Ching-Shu Lai, and Min-Hsiung Pan. 2005. Induction of apoptosis by luteolin through cleavage of Bcl-2 family in human leukemia HL-60 cells. European Journal of Pharmacology 509:1–10.

Chiu, Feng-Lan, and Jen-Kun Lin. 2007. Downregulation of androgen receptor expression by luteolin causes inhibition of cell proliferation and induction of apoptosis in human prostate cancer cells and xenografts. The Prostate 68:61–71.

Cock, I.E. 2013. The phytochemistry and chemotherapeutic potential of *Tasmannia lanceolata* (Tasmanian pepper): A review. Pharmacognosy Communications 3:13–25.

Cock, I.E., and M. Cheesman. 2021. Plants of the genus *Terminalia*: Phytochemical and antioxidant profiles, proliferation, and cancer. In: Cancer (Second Edition). Preedy, V.R., Patel, V.B. (editors); Academic Press, USA: 495–503.

Davy, Anthony John, Red Scott, and César Vieira Cordazzo. 2006. Biological flora of the British Isles: *Cakile maritima* Scop. Journal of Ecology 94:695–711.

Ellouzi, Hasna, Karim Ben Hamed, Jana Cela, Sergi Munné-Bosch, and Chedly Abdelly. 2011. Early effects of salt stress on the physiological and oxidative status of *Cakile maritima* (halophyte) and *Arabidopsis thaliana* (glycophyte). Physiologia Plantarum 142:128–143.

Elmali, Nurzat, O. Baysal, Ahmet Harma, I. Esenkaya, and Bülent Mizrak. 2007. Effects of resveratrol in inflammatory arthritis. Inflammation 30:1–6.

Ferrandiz, M.L., and M. José Alcaraz. 1991. Anti-inflammatory activity and inhibition of arachidonic acid metabolism by flavonoids. Agents and Actions 32:283–288.

Fuochi, V., I. Barbagallo, A. Distefano, F. Puglisi, R. Palmeri, M. Di Rosa, C. Giallongo et al. 2019. Biological properties of *Cakile maritima* Scop. (Brassicaceae) extracts. European Review for Medical and Pharmacological Sciences 23:2280–2292.

Ghonime, Mohammed, Mohamed Emara, Riham Shawky, Hesham Soliman, Ramadan El-Domany, and Ahmed Abdelaziz. 2015. Immunomodulation of RAW 264.7 murine macrophage functions and antioxidant activities of 11 plant extracts. Immunological Investigations 44:237–252.

Gu, Ying, Zhang Ting, Xi Qiu, Xuzhao Zhang, Xiaoxian Gan, Yongming Fang, Xiaohua Xu, and Rongzhen Xu. 2010. Linalool preferentially induces robust apoptosis of a variety of leukemia cells via upregulating p53 and cyclin-dependent kinase inhibitors. Toxicology 268:19–24.

Guil-Guerrero, José Luis, Juan José Giménez-Martínez, and María Esperanza Torija-Isasa. 1999. Nutritional composition of wild edible crucifer species. Journal of Food Biochemistry 23:283–294.

Hayes, John D., Albena T. Dinkova-Kostova, and Kenneth D. Tew. 2020. Oxidative stress in cancer. Cancer Cell 38:167–197.

Hogg, S.D., and G. Embery. 1982. Blood-group-reactive glycoprotein from human saliva interacts with lipotcichoic acid on the surface of *Streptococcus sanguis* cells. Archives of Oral Biology 27:261–268.

Houmani, Hayet, Marta Rodríguez-Ruiz, José M. Palma, Chedly Abdelly, and Francisco J. Corpas. 2016. Modulation of superoxide dismutase (SOD) isozymes by organ development and high long-term salinity in the halophyte *Cakile maritima*. Protoplasma:885–894.

Huang, C., Y. Wang, J. Wang, W. Yao, X. Chen, and W. Zhang. 2013. 2-O-β-D-glucoside suppresses induction of proinflammatory factors by attenuating the binding activity of nuclear factor-κB in microglia. Journal of Neuroinflammation 10:129.

Iranshahi, Mehrdad. 2012. A review of volatile sulfur-containing compounds from terrestrial plants: Biosynthesis, distribution and analytical methods. Journal of Essential Oil Research 24:393–434.

Jain, H., N. Dhingra, T. Narsinghani, and R. Sharma. 2016. Insights into the mechanism of natural terpenoids as NF-κB inhibitors: An overview on their anticancer potential. Experimental Oncology 38:158–168.

Jang, Meishiang, Lining Cai, George O. Udeani, Karla V. Slowing, Cathy F. Thomas, Christopher W.W. Beecher, Harry H.S. Fong et al. 1997. Cancer chemopreventive activity of resveratrol, a natural product derived from grapes. Science 275:218–220.

Kim, H.P., I. Mani, L. Iversen, and V.A. Ziboh. 1998. Effects of naturally-occurring flavonoids and biflavonoids on epidermal cyclooxygenase and lipoxygenase from guinea-pigs. Prostaglandins, Leukotrienes and Essential Fatty Acids 58:17–24.

Kim, Jin-Hyung, Eun-Ok Lee, Hyo-Jung Lee, Jin-Sook Ku, Min-Ho Lee, Deok-Chun Yang, and Sung-Hoon Kim. 2006. Caspase activation and extracellular signal-regulated kinase/akt inhibition were involved in luteolin-induced apoptosis in Lewis lung carcinoma cells. Annals of the New York Academy of Sciences 1090:147–160.

Komiya, T., M. Kyohkon, S. Ohwaki, J. Eto, H. Katsuzaki, K. Imai, T. Kataoka, K. Yoshioka, Y. Ishii, and H. Hibasami. 1999. Phytol induces programmed cell death in human lymphoid leukemia Molt 4B cells. International Journal of Molecular Medicine 4:377–457.

Ksouri, Riadh, Wided Megdiche, Ahmed Debez, Hanen Falleh, Claude Grignon, and Chedly Abdelly. 2007. Salinity effects on polyphenol content and antioxidant activities in leaves of the halophyte *Cakile maritima*. Plant Physiology and Biochemistry 45:244–249.

Lanzilli, Giulia, Andrea Cottarelli, Giuseppe Nicotera, Serena Guida, Giampiero Ravagnan, and Maria Pia Fuggetta. 2012. Anti-inflammatory effect of resveratrol and polydatin by *in vitro* IL-17 modulation. Inflammation 35:240–248.

Laughton, Miranda J., Patricia J. Evans, Michele A. Moroney, J.R.S. Hoult, and Barry Halliwell. 1991. Inhibition of mammalian 5-lipoxygenase and cyclo-oxygenase by flavonoids and phenolic dietary additives: Relationship to antioxidant activity and to iron ion-reducing ability. Biochemical Pharmacology 42:1673–1681.

Lee, Herng-Jiun, Chau-Jong Wang, Hsing-Chun Kuo, Fen-Pi Chou, Lian-Fwu Jean, and Tsui-Hwa Tseng. 2005. Induction apoptosis of luteolin in human hepatoma HepG2 cells involving mitochondria translocation of Bax/Bak and activation of JNK. Toxicology and Applied Pharmacology 203:124–131.

Lee, Woan-Rouh, Shing-Chuan Shen, Hui-Yi Lin, Wen-Chi Hou, Ling-Ling Yang, and Yen-Chou Chen. 2002. Wogonin and fisetin induce apoptosis in human promyeloleukemic cells, accompanied by a decrease of reactive oxygen species, and activation of caspase 3 and Ca^{2+}-dependent endonuclease. Biochemical Pharmacology 63:225–236.

Lim, Do Y., Yoonhwa Jeong, Angela L. Tyner, and Jung H.Y. Park. 2007. Induction of cell cycle arrest and apoptosis in HT-29 human colon cancer cells by the dietary compound luteolin. American Journal of Physiology-Gastrointestinal and Liver Physiology 292:G66–G75.

Lozada-García, María Concepción, Raúl G. Enríquez, Teresa O. Ramírez-Apán, Antonio Nieto-Camacho, Juan Francisco Palacios-Espinosa, Zeltzin Custodio-Galván, Olivia Soria-Arteche, and Jaime Pérez-Villanueva. 2017. Synthesis of curcuminoids and evaluation of their cytotoxic and antioxidant properties. Molecules 22:633.

Matsuo, Alisson L., Carlos R. Figueiredo, Denise C. Arruda, Felipe V. Pereira, Jorge A. Borin Scutti, Mariana H. Massaoka, Luiz R. Travassos, Patricia Sartorelli, and João HG Lago. 2011. α-Pinene isolated from Schinus terebinthifolius Raddi (Anacardiaceae) induces apoptosis and confers antimetastatic protection in a melanoma model. Biochemical and Biophysical Research Communications 411:449–454.

Meot-Duros, Laetitia, Gaëtan Le Floch, and Christian Magné. 2008. Radical scavenging, antioxidant and antimicrobial activities of halophytic species. Journal of Ethnopharmacology 116:258–262.

Murata, Soichiro, Risa Shiragami, Chihiro Kosugi, Tohru Tezuka, Masato Yamazaki, Atsushi Hirano, Yukino Yoshimura et al. 2013. Antitumor effect of 1,8-cineole against colon cancer. Oncology Reports 30:2647–2652.

Nasr, Fahd A., Nael Abutaha, Mohammad Al-Zahrani, Muhammad Farooq, and Mohammad A. Wadaan. 2018. Anticancer potential of plant extracts from Riyadh (Saudi Arabia) on MDA-MB-231 breast cancer cells. African Journal of Traditional, Complementary and Alternative Medicines 15:46–53.

Nijveldt, Robert J., E.L.S. Van Nood, Danny E.C. van Hoorn, Petra G. Boelens, Klaske Van Norren, and Paul A.M. Van Leeuwen. 2001. Flavonoids: A review of probable mechanisms of action and potential applications. The American Journal of Clinical Nutrition 74:418–425.

Omer, Elsayed, Abdelsamed Elshamy, Abdel Nasser El Gendy, Xin Cai, Joseph Sirdaarta, Alan White, and Ian Edwin Cock. 2016. Cakile maritima Scop. extracts inhibit the growth of some bacterial triggers of autoimmune diseases: GC-MS analysis of an inhibitory extract. Pharmacognosy Journal 8:361–374.

Omer, Elsayed, Abdelsamed Elshamy, Rihab Taher, Walaa El-Kashak, Joseph Shalom, Alan White, and Ian Cock. 2019. Cakile maritima Scop. extracts inhibit CaCo2 and HeLa human carcinoma cell growth: GC-MS analysis of an anti-proliferative extract. Pharmacognosy Journal 11:258–266.

Park, Kyung-Ran, Dongwoo Nam, Hyung-Mun Yun, Seok-Geun Lee, Hyeung-Jin Jang, Gautam Sethi, Somi K. Cho, and Kwang Seok Ahn. 2011. β-Caryophyllene oxide inhibits growth and induces apoptosis through the suppression of PI3K/AKT/mTOR/S6K1 pathways and ROS-mediated MAPKs activation. Cancer Letters 312:178–188.

Pikarsky, Eli, Rinnat M. Porat, Ilan Stein, Rinat Abramovitch, Sharon Amit, Shafika Kasem, Elena Gutkovich-Pyest, Simcha Urieli-Shoval, Eithan Galun, and Yinon Ben-Neriah. 2004. NF-κB functions as a tumor promoter in inflammation-associated cancer. Nature 431:461–466.

Placines, Chloé, Viana Castañeda-Loaiza, Maria João Rodrigues, Catarina G. Pereira, Azzurra Stefanucci, Adriano Mollica, Gokhan Zengin, Eulogio J. Llorent-Martínez, Paula C. Castilho, and Luísa Custódio. 2020. Phenolic profile, toxicity, enzyme inhibition, in silico studies, and antioxidant properties of Cakile maritima Scop. (Brassicaceae) from southern Portugal. Plants 9:142.

Rabi, Thangaiyan, and Anupam Bishayee. 2009. d-Limonene sensitizes docetaxel-induced cytotoxicity in human prostate cancer cells: Generation of reactive oxygen species and induction of apoptosis. Journal of Carcinogenesis 8:9.

Radwan, H.M., Kh A. Shams, W.A. Tawfik, and A.M. Soliman. 2008. Investigation of the glucosinolates and lipids constituents of Cakile maritima (Scope) growing in Egypt and their biological activity. Research Journal of Medical Sciences 3:182–187.

Ravizza, Raffaella, Marzia B. Gariboldi, Roberta Molteni, and Elena Monti. 2008. Linalool, a plant-derived monoterpene alcohol, reverses doxorubicin resistance in human breast adenocarcinoma cells. Oncology Reports 20:625–630.

Schindler, Rainer, and Rolf Mentlein. 2006. Flavonoids and vitamin E reduce the release of the angiogenic peptide vascular endothelial growth factor from human tumor cells. The Journal of Nutrition 136:1477–1482.

Seelinger, Günter, Irmgard Merfort, Ute Wölfle, and Christoph M. Schempp. 2008. Anti-carcinogenic effects of the flavonoid luteolin. Molecules 13:2628–2651.

Selvendiran, Karuppaiyah, Hironori Koga, Takato Ueno, Takafumi Yoshida, Michiko Maeyama, Takuji Torimura, Hirohisa Yano, Masamichi Kojiro, and Michio Sata. 2006. Luteolin promotes degradation in signal transducer and activator of transcription 3 in human hepatoma cells: An implication for the antitumor potential of flavonoids. Cancer Research 66:4826–4834.

Sertel, Serkan, Tolga Eichhorn, Sebastian Sieber, Alexandra Sauer, Johanna Weiss, Peter K. Plinkert, and Thomas Efferth. 2010. Factors determining sensitivity or resistance of tumor cell lines towards artesunate. Chemico-Biological Interactions 185:42–52.

Shamshoum, Hesham, Filip Vlavcheski, and Evangelia Tsiani. 2017. Anticancer effects of oleuropein. Biofactors 43:517–528.

Shang, Ya-Zhen, Bo-Wen Qin, Jian-Jun Cheng, and Hong Miao. 2006. Prevention of oxidative injury by flavonoids from stems and leaves of *Scutellaria baicalensis* Georgi in PC12 cells. Phytotherapy Research 20:53–57.

Sharma, Sharada H., Senthilkumar Thulasingam, and Sangeetha Nagarajan. 2017. Terpenoids as anti-colon cancer agents: A comprehensive review on its mechanistic perspectives. European Journal of Pharmacology 795:169–178.

Sheikh, Imran, V. Sharma, Hardeep Singh Tuli, Diwakar Aggarwal, Atul Sankhyan, Pritesh Vyas, Anil K. Sharma, and Anupam Bishayee. 2020. Cancer chemoprevention by flavonoids, dietary polyphenols and terpenoids. Biointerface Research in Applied Chemistry 11:8502–8537.

Shoff, Suzanne M., Mary Grummer, Milton B. Yatvin, and Charles E. Elson. 1991. Concentration-dependent increase of murine P388 and B16 population doubling time by the acyclic monoterpene geraniol. Cancer Research 51:37–42.

Stambouli-Essassi, Sondes, Faiza Mejri, Manel Dhoueibi, Yassine Mrabet, Fethia Harzallah-Skhiri, and Karim Hosni. 2020. *Cakile maritima* subsp. *maritima* Scop. Fruit. Journal of Animal and Plant Sciences 43:7366–7379.

Togar, Basak, Hasan Turkez, Abdulgani Tatar, Ahmet Hacimuftuoglu, and Fatime Geyikoglu. 2015. Cytotoxicity and genotoxicity of zingiberene on different neuron cell lines in vitro. Cytotechnology 67:939–946.

van Zanden, Jelmer J., Liesbeth Geraets, Heleen M. Wortelboer, Peter J. van Bladeren, Ivonne M.C.M. Rietjens, and Nicole H.P. Cnubben. 2004. Structural requirements for the flavonoid-mediated modulation of glutathione S-transferase P1–1 and GS-X pump activity in MCF7 breast cancer cells. Biochemical Pharmacology 67:1607–1617.

Wang, Cun-Yu, Marty W. Mayo, and Albert S. Baldwin. 1996. TNF-and cancer therapy-induced apoptosis: Potentiation by inhibition of NF-κB. Science 274:784–787.

Wang, Xiaodong, Chunlan Yang, Qian Zhang, Chunjing Wang, Xiaohui Zhou, Xiaoling Zhang, and Sixi Liu. 2019. *In vitro* anticancer effects of esculetin against human leukemia cell lines involves apoptotic cell death, autophagy, G0/G1 cell cycle arrest and modulation of Raf/MEK/ERK signalling pathway. Journal of the Balkan Union of Oncology 24:1686–1691.

Wattenberg, Lee W., Velta L. Sparnins, and George Barany. 1989. Inhibition of N-nitrosodiethylamine carcinogenesis in mice by naturally occurring organosulfur compounds and monoterpenes. Cancer Research 49:2689–2692.

Woerdenbag, Herman J., Irmgard Merfort, Claus M. Paßreiter, Thomas J. Schmidt, Günter Willuhn, Wim van Uden, Niesko Pras, Harm H. Kampinga, and Antonius W.T. Konings. 1994. Cytotoxicity of flavonoids and sesquiterpene lactones from *Arnica* species against the GLC4 and the COLO 320 cell lines. Planta Medica 60:434–437.

Wolinsky, L.E., and E.O. Sote. 1984. Isolation of natural plaque-inhibiting substances from 'Nigerian chewing sticks'. Caries Research 18:216–225.

Wu-Yuan, C.D., C.Y. Chen, and R.T. Wu. 1988. Gallotannins inhibit growth, water-insoluble glucan synthesis, and aggregation of mutans streptococci. Journal of Dental Research 67:51–55.

Youness, Rana, Rabab Kamel, Nermeen A. Elkasabgy, Ping Shao, and Mohamed A. Farag. 2021. Recent advances in tannic acid (gallotannin) anticancer activities and drug delivery systems for efficacy improvement; A comprehensive review. Molecules 26:1486.

Yu, Suzanne G., Leslie A. Hildebrandt, and Charles E. Elson. 1995. Geraniol, an inhibitor of mevalonate biosynthesis, suppresses the growth of hepatomas and melanomas transplanted to rats and mice. The Journal of Nutrition 125:2763–2767.

Zhang, Yanjun, Navindra P. Seeram, Rupo Lee, Lydia Feng, and David Heber. 2008. Isolation and identification of strawberry phenolics with antioxidant and human cancer cell antiproliferative properties. Journal of Agricultural and Food Chemistry 56:670–675.

20 Self-Heal (*Prunella vulgaris* L.) In Vitro *and* In Vivo *Aspects of Anticancer Activity in Different Cancers*

Zeynep Dogan, Vahap Murat Kutluay and Iclal Saracoglu

ABBREVIATIONS

A-549	human lung carcinoma
ABAE	adult bovine aortic endothelial cell
ABTS	2,2'-azinobis 3-ethyl benzothiazoline-6-sulfonic acid
AgNOR	silver stained nucleolar organizer region
AHR	aryl hydrocarbon receptor
ATP	adenosine triphosphate
Bad	B-cell lymphoma-2 associated agonist of cell death
Bax	B-cell lymphoma-2 associated X protein
Bcl-2	B-cell lymphoma-2
Caspase	cysteine-dependent aspartate-specific protease
CYP1A1	cytochrome P450 family 1 subfamily A member 1
CYP1B1	cytochrome P450 family 1 subfamily B member 1
DHURS	2α,3α-dihydroxy urs-12-ene-28-oic acid
DPPH	1,1-diphenyl-1-picrylhydrazyl
ECC-1	endometrial cancer cell
ERK	extracellular signal-related kinase
Fas	apoptosis antigen 1
FRAP	ferric-reducing antioxidant power
FTC-133	follicular thyroid cancer cell line
HA22T	human hepatoma
HCT-8	human ileocecal carcinoma
HeLa	human cervical carcinoma
HepG2	human hepatocellular carcinoma
HPLC	high-performance liquid chromatography
HT-1080	human fibrosarcoma
HT29	human colorectal adenocarcinoma
Huh-7	human hepatoma
IC_{50}	half-maximal inhibitory concentration
IFN-γ	interferon gamma
Jurkat T cell	human acute leukemia cell
K1	human papillary thyroid carcinoma
KB	human epithelial carcinoma
L-1210	lymphoid leukemia
LPS	lipopolysaccharide

DOI: 10.1201/9781003260028-22

MCF-5	human breast carcinoma
MCF-7	mammary gland carcinoma
MDA-MB-231	human breast adenocarcinoma
MDA-MB-231BO	human bonehoming breast cancer cell
MKN-45	human gastric carcinoma
MMP-2	matrix metalloproteinase 2
MMP-9	matrix metalloproteinase 9
MTT	3-(4,5-dimethylthiazol-2-yl)-2,5-di-phenyltetrazolium bromide
NF-κB	nuclear factor kappa B
P-388	lymphocytic leukemia
PCNA	proliferating cell nuclear antigen
PMA	12-phorbol 13-myristate acetate
RA	rosmarinic acid
RANKL	receptor activator of nuclear factor kappa B ligand
SKBr-3	human breast cancer cell
SKOV-3	human ovarian adenocarcinoma
SMMC-7721	human hepatocarcinoma
SPC-A1	human lung cancer cell
ST-2	murine bone marrow stromal cell
STAT3	signal transducer and activator of transcription 3
SW579	human squamous thyroid cancer cell line
TPA	12-O-tetradecanoylphorbol-13-acetate
TPC-1	human thyroid papillary cancer cell line
VEGF	vascular endothelial growth factor
VEGF-A	vascular endothelial growth factor A
VEGFR2	vascular endothelial growth factor receptor 2

20.1　INTRODUCTION

Plants are important sources for discovering new drug molecules. Plant-derived therapeutics for the treatment of several disorders have significantly increased recently. *Prunella vulgaris* L., a perennial plant belonging to the Lamiaceae family, is widely distributed in Asia and Europe (Lin et al. 2015).

This species has a short rhizome; a freely branching, angular 30 cm stem; and the leaf blades are lanceolate to ovate and glabrous to sparsely villous. The flowers are purple in color with spikes at top of the stem (Figure 20.1). The spike is nearly cylindrical with many bracts and calyxes attached, 3 cm to 6 cm in length and 10 mm to 15 mm in diameter. Each bract is cordate to eccentric and exhibits white hairs on the vein (Lin et al. 2015). It is traditionally used as a medicinal plant for various disorders.

20.2　BACKGROUND

The plant is commonly known as "self-heal" and "heal-all." The name *Prunella* came from *Brunellen*, a German word meaning "inflammation of the mouth." German military physicians used this plant for treatment of contagious fever characterized by sore throat and a brown-coated tongue. Therefore, the name of the plant was derived from this kind of usage (Patel and Sharma 2019).

P. vulgaris is very popular medicinal plant in European, Asian, and traditional Chinese medicine. It is commonly used in northeastern Asia, especially in Korea, Japan, and China to treat throat infections, to reduce fever, and for wound healing (Figure 20.2).

The plant is dried after the summer solstice; therefore the Chinese name of the plant is *Xia-Ku-Cao* (*Xiakucao*), which means "grass perished at the end of the summer." Traditionally, the action of xiakucao is to quench liver fire and eye inflammation, reduce thyroid nodulation, and prevent swelling. It is mainly used in Chinese medicine for treatment of eye inflammations, nighttime eye pain

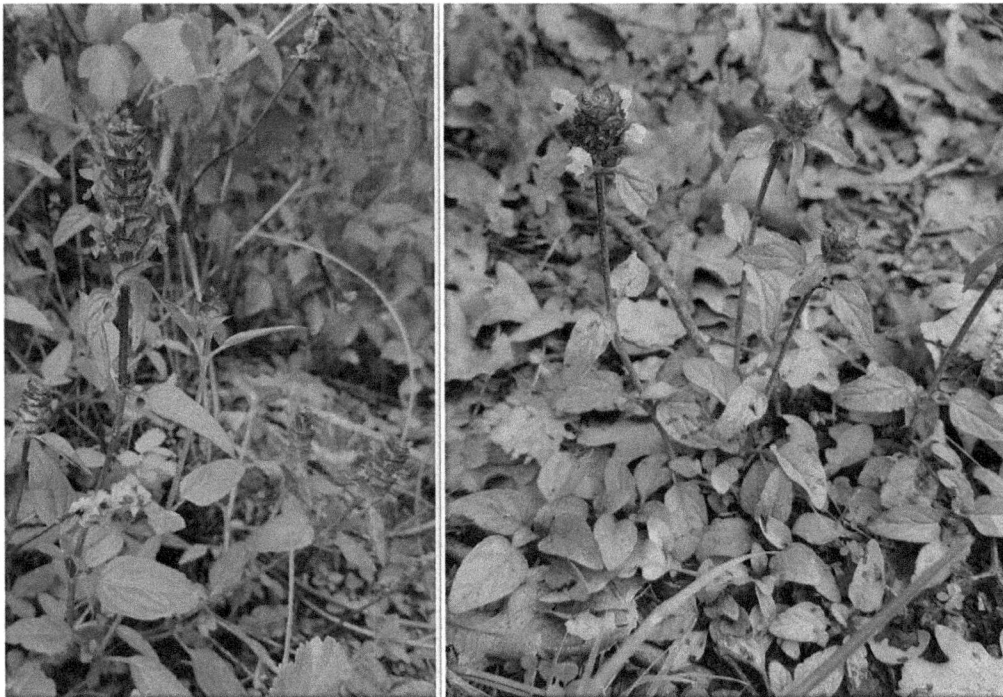

FIGURE 20.1   *Prunella vulgaris* L.

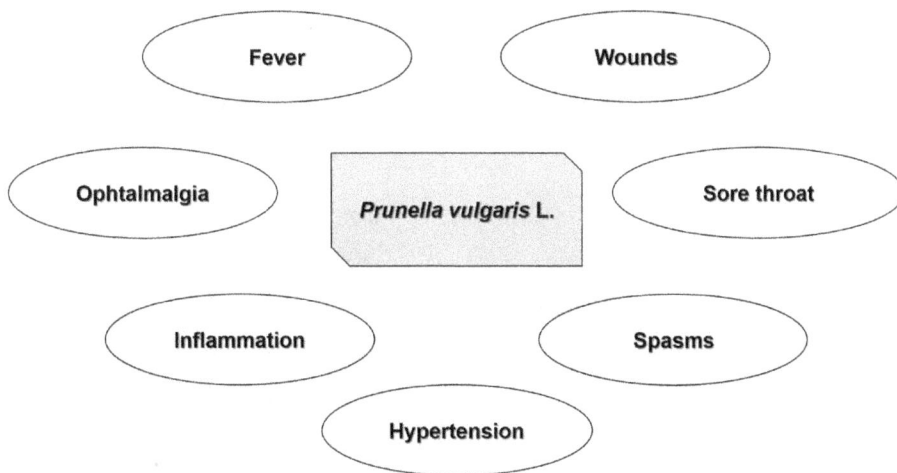

FIGURE 20.2   The traditional usages of *Prunella vulgaris.*

(ophthalmalgia), headache and dizziness, sore throat, spasms, wounds, scrofula, goiter, mastitis with swelling and pain, breast hyperplasia, and hypertension (Lin et al. 2015; Patel and Sharma 2019; Rasool and Ganai 2013; Wang et al. 2019). The plant is one of the active ingredients of traditional medicine which is used in Kashmir for bathing pregnant women after delivery (Patel and Sharma 2019).

The spikes, leaves, and stems of *P. vulgaris* are rich in a variety of active chemical components. It has been reported that triterpenoids, mainly ursolic and oleanolic acids and their esters, and flavonoids are the main chemical components (Table 20.1). Also present in *P. vulgaris* are coumarins, phenylpropanoids, long-chain fatty acids, volatile oils, carbohydrates, alkaloids, inorganic salts, vitamins, resins, bitter taste, tannic acid, and proteins (Lin et al. 2015; Patel and Sharma 2019; Wang et al. 2019).

Therefore, the plant possesses various pharmacological activities such as antioxidant, antiinflammatory, antirheumatic, anticancer, antimetastatic, antidiabetic, neuroprotective, anticolitic, anti-estrogenic, antimicrobial, wound healing, antiseptic, antipyretic, antispasmodic, astringent, anti-allergic, carminative, diuretic, hypotensive, anti-arrhythmic, antidiarrhoeic, antistomachic, tonic, and vermifuge (Figure 20.3). Additionally, the plant is also used as a health-promoting food

TABLE 20.1

Main Phytochemical Content of *Prunella vulgaris*

Metabolite	Compound Name
Carbohydrates	*Monosaccharides*: rhamnose, glucose, xylose, arabinose, mannose, galactose *Disaccharides*: sucrose and fructose *Polysaccharides*
Fatty acids	Palmitic acid, ethyl palmitate, tetracosanoic acid, stearic acid 6,9-Octodecadienoic acid, 3,6,7-eicosatrienoic acid Oleic acid, moringoic acid, lauric acid, myristic acid, linolenic acid, linoleic acid
Volatile oils	1,8-Eucalyptol, β-pinene, myrcene, linalylacetate, α-phellandene, linalool 1,6-Cyclononone, palmitic acid, trihexadecane
Flavonoids	Rutin, hyperoside, luteolin, homoorinetin, cinaroside Quercetin-3-*O*-β-D-galactoside, quercetin-3-*O*-β-D-glucoside, kaempferol-3-*O*-β-D-glucoside
Phenylpropanoids	*p*-Coumaric acid, *cis*-caffeic acid, *trans*-caffeic acid, rosmarinic acid Methyl rosmarine, ethyl rosmarine, *E*-butyl rosmarine 3,4α-Trihydroxy-methyl-phenyl propionate, 3,4α-trihydroxy-butyl-phenyl propionate
Coumarins	Umbelliferone, scopoletin, and esculetin
Triterpenoids	Ursolic and oleanolic acids and their esters (methyl oleanolate, methyl ursolate, methyl maslinate) Prunelloside A, pravulosides A, B, vulgarsaponins A, B
Sterols	β-Sitosterol, stigmasterol, α-spinolol, and stigmast-7-en-3β-ol, ducosterol, α-spinasterol α-Spinasterolyl-β-D-glucopyranose glucoside, stigmasterolyl-β-D-glucopyranose glucoside

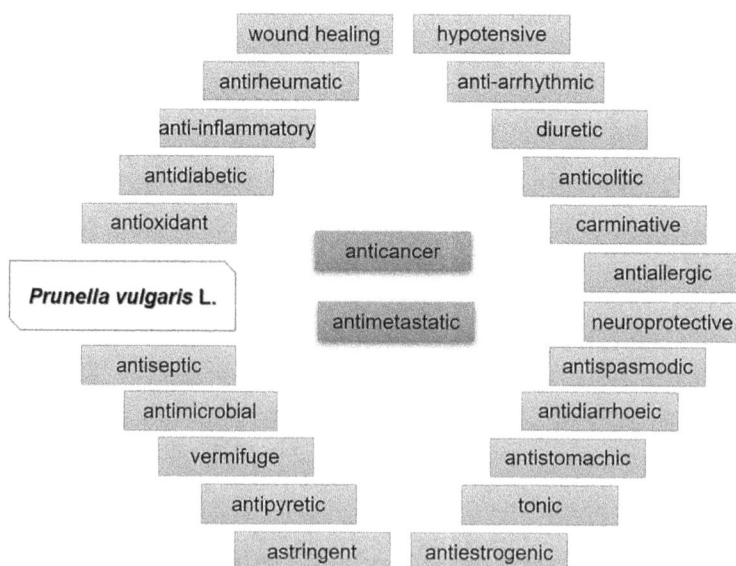

FIGURE 20.3 The pharmacological activities of Prunella vulgaris.

or tea extensively in China and Europe (Lin et al. 2015; Patel and Sharma 2019; Rasool and Ganai 2013; Wang et al. 2019; Harput et al. 2006; Health Canada 2009a, 2009b; Yesilada et al. 1993).

The present chapter mainly focuses on the *in vitro*, *in vivo*, and clinical studies on anticancer activity of *P. vulgaris*.

20.3 *IN VITRO* STUDIES: CYTOTOXIC EFFECTS

In vitro cytotoxic effect studies on *P. vulgaris* extracts are represented by classifying them according to cancer types. The mechanisms of action of the extracts in various cancer cell lines are summarized in Table 20.2.

20.3.1 BREAST CANCER

The cytotoxic effect of methanol extract of *P. vulgaris* root on MCF-5 cell line was investigated by MTT method. Cell survival rates were significantly reduced in the concentration range of

TABLE 20.2
Possible Mechanisms of Actions of Different *Prunella vulgaris* Extracts on Various Cell Lines

Extract	Cell Line	Action of Mechanism	References
PV-Root-Methanol	MCF-5	↑ Bax ↓ Bcl2 Induction of apoptosis G2/M phase arrest	(Gao et al. 2019)
PV-Water	MDA-MB-231, SKOV-3	Inhibition of EMT Inhibition of NF-κB	(Cho et al. 2015)
PV-Spike-Ethanol	HCT-8	Induction of apoptosis ↑ miR-34a ↓ Bcl2, Notch1, Notch2	(Fang et al. 2017)
PV-Water	HT-1080	↓ MMP-9 ↓ PMA-stimulated NF-κB activity	(Choi et al. 2010)
PV-Water	HepG2, Huh-7	Inhibition of cell invasion and migration ↓ MMP-2, MMP-9	(Kim et al. 2012)
PV-Water	Huh-7, HA22T	↓ MMP-9, VEGF Inhibition of AP-1, NF-κB Inhibition of TPA ↓ ERK, p38 gene	(Su et al. 2016)
PV-Spike-60% Ethanol	SPC-A-1	G0/G1 phase arrest Induction of apoptosis	(Feng et al. 2010)
PV-Spike-50% Ethanol	TPC-1	↓ Colony formation, cell migration	(Yu et al. 2021)
PV	TPC-1, FTC-133	↑ Bax, caspase-3 ↓ Bcl2 Induction of apoptosis	(Yin et al. 2017)
PV-Whole part-70% ethanol and water	A-549	↑ p53, Bax and Fas	(Hwang et al. 2013)
PV-Ethanol	ECC-1	↓ Alkaline phosphatase activity ↓ CYR61 ↑ CYP1A1, CYP1B1, AHR	(Collins et al. 2009)

Abbreviation: PV = Prunella vulgaris.

3.12–100 µg/mL. The extract induced apoptosis by increasing the Bax/Bcl2 ratio and triggering DNA damage. The extract also inhibited angiogenesis and arrested G2/M phase (Gao et al. 2019).

Total phenol content, antioxidant capacity, and cytotoxic effects of *Prunella* species grown in Turkey were compared by Sahin et al. (2014). The total phenol content of the methanol extract of whole parts of *P. vulgaris* was determined as 97 mg gallic acid equivalent per g of extract (mg GAE/g extract). The cytotoxic effects of the extracts against MCF-7 (estrogen receptor +) and MDA-MB-231 (estrogen receptor –) cells were determined by ATP method, and the IC_{50} value of the *P. vulgaris* methanol extract was determined as >20 µg/mL for both cells. *P. laciniata* possessed strong cytotoxic activity with IC_{50} of 17.5 µg/mL on MCF-7 cells, and *P. orientalis* with IC_{50} of 10 µg/mL on MDA-MB-231 cells (Sahin et al. 2014). According to Grosan et al., 70% methanol extract of *P. vulgaris* spike possessed significant inhibition on cell viability of MDA-MB-231 cells after 72 hours of treatment with the extract of 250 µg/mL concentration (Grosan et al. 2020).

P. vulgaris extracts are known to have an anti-estrogenic effect (Collins et al. 2009). As a result of the studies carried out for the isolation of effective compounds from 70% ethanol extract of the spikes, it was thought that betulinic acid and ursolic acid may be responsible for the anti-estrogenic effect. It has been determined that betulinic acid and ursolic acid inhibit the synthesis of ERα (estrogen receptor α), both via the ER signaling pathway and by reducing the protein level, instead of directly affecting the ER (Kim et al. 2014).

The effects of *P. vulgaris* decoction on the epithelial–mesenchymal transition (EMT), which plays an important role in the invasion and metastasis of tumor cells, were investigated in LPS-stimulated cancer cells, MDA-MB-231 and SKOV-3. It was observed that decoction inhibits EMT through inhibition of NF-κB. *P. vulgaris* decoction was thought to be a potent candidate for inhibiting cancer invasion and migration (Cho et al. 2015).

Polysaccharides and compounds isolated from *P. vulgaris* were also tested *in vitro* for their cytotoxic activities. In a study by Hao et al., it was observed that *P. vulgaris* polysaccharides inhibited cell growth and migration, induced apoptosis and arrested the G0 phase in SKBr-3 cells, by inhibiting the expression of basic fibroblast growth factor (bFGF) (Hao et al. 2020).

The cytotoxic effect of four compounds from *P. vulgaris* spike on MCF-7 cells were determined by cell counting kit-8 assay. Protocatechuic acid and rosmarinic acid have IC_{50} values over 100 µM, while protocatechualdehyde and caffeic acid have IC_{50} values of 10.9 and 26.8 µg/mL, respectively (Yang et al. 2020). The effect of rosmarinic acid (RA) obtained from the aqueous extract of *P. vulgaris* spike on bone metastasis of breast cancer and its possible mechanism of action were investigated. Cytotoxic effect was determined by MTT method on MDA-MB-231BO and ST-2 cells. IC_{50} values of RA were found as 118.04 µg/mL and 279.32 µg/mL for MDA-MB-231BO and ST-2 cells, respectively. RA significantly reduced cell migration in MDA-MB-231BO cells at concentrations of ≥7.5 µg/mL. RA decreased alkaline phosphatase level in ST-2 cells more potently than positive control, zoledronic acid. It has been observed that the antimetastatic effect of RA was not due to its selective cytotoxicity, but via the receptor activator of NF-κB ligand (RANKL)/RANK/osteoprotegerin pathway (Xu et al. 2010).

20.3.2 COLON CANCER

The ethanol extract of *P. vulgaris* spike was applied to HCT-8 cells for determination of cytotoxic activity by MTT assay, and the IC_{50} value was found as 770 µg/mL. Extract also inhibited colony formation when compared to control group in a concentration-dependent manner. To determine the mechanism of action, the cells were treated with the extract at the concentration of IC_{50} and the extract induced apoptosis. It was observed that upregulation of the tumor suppressor gene (miR-34a) played an important role in the effect of the extract by suppression of expression of Bcl-2 and Notch1 with Notch2, which play roles in the formation of malignant tumors (Fang et al. 2017).

20.3.3 LIVER CANCER

Matrix metalloproteinases plays critical role in metastasis of cancer cells through degrading extracellular matrix components. The inhibition of MMP-9, which plays an important role in angiogenesis and tumor invasion, was investigated by Choi et al., and *P. vulgaris* aqueous extract (PVAE) reported to inhibit MMP-9 expression through downregulation of PMA-stimulated NF-κB activity. Findings showed that PVAE reduced metastasis and invasion in HT-1080 cells in a concentration-dependent manner at the range of 10–200 μg/mL (Choi et al. 2010). In another study examining cytotoxic effects of PVAE on hepatocellular carcinoma cells (HepG2 and Huh-7), it was observed that the extract concentration dependently inhibited cell invasion and migration by downregulation of MMP-2 and MMP-9 expression (Kim et al. 2012). In another study by Su et al., inhibition of MMP-9 and VEGF was found to be dependent on the inhibition of activator protein-1 (AP-1) with NF-κB. In the same study, the mechanism of action of PVAE was studied on Huh-7 and HA22T cells. TPA inhibition was found to play a role in the activity. Inhibition of the TPA-mediated NF-κB signaling pathway was found to be via IκB, while inhibition of AP-1 was due to inhibition of ERK expression and suppression of the p38 gene (Su et al. 2016).

In a study by Li et al., a heteropolysaccharide, P1, that isolated from the water extract of *P. vulgaris* fruits, possessed potent immunomodulatory effect by a significant increase in nitric oxide, tumor necrosis factor alpha (TNF-α), and interleukin-6 (IL-6) levels in macrophage cells (Li et al. 2015). Additionally, P1-Zn complex was prepared and its effects on HepG2 cells were investigated. P1-Zn complex significantly reduced cell viability at 500 μg/mL concentration on HepG2 cells. It has been determined that the cytotoxic effect was depend on inducing apoptosis through G0/G1 phase arrest, formation of reactive oxygen species, and caspase activity (Li et al. 2016).

20.3.4 LUNG CANCER

The cytotoxic effects of 60% ethanol, 30% ethanol, and aqueous extracts of *P. vulgaris* spike on SPC-A-1 cells were investigated by MTT method and 60% ethanol extract showed the highest cytotoxic effect, with the IC_{50} value of 650 μg/mL. The 60% ethanol extract arrested G0/G1 phase at 250 μg/mL and induced apoptosis at 500 μg/mL, at the 48th hour of treatment (Feng, Jia, et al. 2010b). Oleanolic acid isolated from the 60% ethanol extract showed similar effects with the extract in terms of cytotoxic effects on SPC-A-1 cells. Oleanolic acid induced apoptosis at 8 μM via suppression of Bcl-2 expression and stimulation of Bax and Bad expression (Feng et al. 2011).

20.3.5 THYROID CANCER

The cytotoxic effect of 50% ethanol extract of *P. vulgaris* spikes was investigated in TPC-1, SW579, and FTC-133 cells by MTT method. While the extract had an IC_{50} value of 5–10 mg/mL in SW579 and TPC-1 cells, the extract significantly reduced colony formation in TPC-1 cells at 500 μg/mL and cell migration at 1 mg/mL (Yu et al. 2021).

In another study by Yin et al., *P. vulgaris* extract also inhibited proliferation of TPC-1 and FTC-133 cells and induced apoptosis by downregulation of Bcl-2, and induction of Bax and caspase-3 expression (Yin et al. 2017).

20.3.6 OTHER CANCERS

Total phenol content, antioxidant capacity and cytotoxic effects of whole parts of *P. vulgaris* var. *lilacina* 70% ethanol, water, hexane, chloroform, and butanol extracts were investigated. It was observed that 70% ethanol and aqueous extracts have high phenolic content and potent scavenging effects on DPPH, ABTS, and FRAP radicals compared to other extracts, correlating each other. Total phenolic content of 70% ethanol and aqueous extracts were 303.7 and 322.8 mg GAE/g extract, respectively. When the cytotoxic effects of 70% ethanol and aqueous extracts against various cancer cells (HepG2, HT29, A-549, MKN-45, HeLa) were screened, the highest cytotoxic effect was observed on A-549 cells, with the inhibition values of 32.4% and 28.7%, respectively. These active extracts induced apoptosis by increasing p53, Bax, and Fas expression (Hwang et al. 2013).

It was observed that *P. vulgaris* ethanol extract decreased alkaline phosphatase activity in ECC-1 cell and decreased estrogen-induced cell growth by blocking expression of estrogen induced protein, CYR61 without inhibition of estrogen signaling at 5 µg/mL and higher concentrations. When the relevance of this effect to the aryl hydrocarbon receptor (AHR), which is indicated as responsible of anti-estrogenic effects of many herbal drugs, was examined, it was observed that the extract stimulated the expression of CYP1A1, CYP1B1, and AHR at 50 µg/mL (Collins et al. 2009).

Basic fibroblast growth factor (bFGF) plays a critical role in tumor growth, blocking this target by competitive binding is one of the ways to decrease proliferation of tumor. Sulfated polysaccharides from *P. vulgaris* (SPPV) revealed competitive binding to bFGF resulting in bFGF-SPPV complex. Moreover, SPPV induced apoptosis concentration dependently at 10–100 µg/mL on ABAE cells (Wu et al. 2011).

The cytotoxic effects of ursolic acid isolated from methanol extract of *P. vulgaris* fruiting spikes on different cancer cells were investigated and it was found that ursolic acid is one of the active compounds of the extract (Lee et al. 1988). Ursolic acid was treated with cells for 72 hours, and the growth in the cells was followed by hemocytometer at the end of the period. The IC_{50} values of ursolic acid against KB, P-388, L-1210, A-549, HCT-8, and MCF-7 cells were found to be 6.6, 3.18, 4.0, 4.0, 4.5, and 4.9 µg/mL, respectively (Lee et al. 1988). 2α,3α-Dihydroxy urs-12-ene-28-oic acid (DHURS) isolated from spikes of *P. vulgaris* methanolic extract indicated cytotoxic activity on Jurkat T cells with an IC_{50} value of 22 µg/mL, and human peripheral T cells with 25 µg/mL. DHURS induced apoptosis by regulating mitochondrial cytochrome c release and caspase cascade (Woo et al. 2011).

20.4   *IN VIVO* STUDIES: ANTITUMOR EFFECTS

20.4.1   BREAST CANCER

Methanol extract of *P. vulgaris* root significantly reduced cell survival rates on MCF-5 cell line in a concentration range of 3.12–100 µg/mL. In the MCF-5 induced mice breast cancer model, the treatment group received 25 mg/kg of the extract. Significant reductions in tumor volume and mass were observed in the treatment group compared to the control group (Gao et al. 2019).

20.4.2   LIVER CANCER

P. vulgaris total flavonoid extract inhibited the proliferation of SMMC 7721 cells. However, in H22 tumor bearing mice model, total flavonoid extract significantly reduced tumor volume and tumor weight at the doses of 100 and 200 mg/kg. At the same doses, the extract induced apoptosis by expression of caspases 3 and 9, upregulation of Bax and downregulation of Bcl-2. The extract induced autophagy via the PI3K/Akt/mTOR pathway, which is known pathway for autophagy induction. The extract also significantly increased IL-6, TNF-α, and IFN-γ due to the immunomodulatory effect of the extract. The extract can be considered as a drug candidate due to both its antitumor effect on liver cancer and its immunomodulatory effect in *in vivo* experiments (Song, Kang, et al. 2021).

20.4.3   LUNG CANCER

The inhibitory effect on lung metastasis of the aqueous extract of *P. vulgaris* aerial parts was found to be due to the activation of natural killer (NK) cells (Lee et al. 2009).

The pretreatment with 60% ethanol extract of *P. vulgaris* spike (PVS-60, 10 g/kg) for 24 weeks was investigated in the benzo[a]pyrene-induced lung tumor model in mice. The PVS-60 treated group possessed a significant reduction in tumor formation compared to the control group (Feng, Jia, et al. 2010b). In another study by Feng et al., PVS-60 inhibited tumor growth by 63% in a Lewis cell–induced lung cancer model in mice at 10 g/kg. It was thought that the antitumor effect of the extract might be due to its contribution to the balance in the antioxidant mechanism by increasing SOD and reducing MDA levels in tumor tissue (Feng, Jia, et al. 2010a).

The cytotoxic effects of 95% ethanol extracts of various *Prunella* spikes collected from different regions were investigated *in vitro* by the MTT method against A-549 and SPC-A-1 cells. *P. vulgaris* extract (PVS-95) was one of the active extracts. PVS-95 extract at a dose of 10 g/kg reduced tumor formation by 63% in Lewis cells–induced lung cancer in mice. In addition, PVS-95 significantly increased TNF-α levels in the tumor compared to control group. When the contents of the active extracts were examined and compared by HPLC, it was observed that the active extracts contain some compounds in similar proportions. These compounds were triterpenes (ursolic acid and olea-nolic acid) and phenolics (caffeic acid, rosmarinic acid, rutin, and quercetin). The total triterpenoid and total phenolic compounds which were obtained from 95% ethanol and 60% ethanol extracts, respectively, were analyzed separately in cytotoxic and antitumor activity studies. It was determined that combination of total triterpenoids and total phenolics showed higher cytotoxic and antitumor effect than application of these compounds separately. Therefore, it was stated that the phytochemi-cal components of the extract, the ratios of the compounds, and synergism of the compounds were important for the antitumor effect (Feng, Jia, Jiang, et al. 2010).

P. vulgaris aqueous extract (PVAE) and the polysaccharide (P32) isolated from PVAE reduced tumor weight significantly in Lewis cell–induced lung cancer model in mice at 10 g/kg. However, at the same doses, P32 and PVAE possessed immunomodulatory effects by increasing the thymus and spleen weights, which play an important role in body defense against cancer (Feng, Jia, Shi, et al. 2010).

20.4.4 Thyroid Cancer

The aqueous extract of *P. vulgaris* spike significantly reduced cell proliferation in the K1 cell line at a concentration of 100 μg/mL. In the thyroid cancer model induced by K1 cells in the mouse, the tumor weight was significantly reduced without any change in body weight when the extract was administered at 50 mg/kg. Autophagy was induced in both cell culture studies and the mouse thyroid cancer model, with upregulation of LC3-II, BECN1, and p62 through the AMPK/mTOR/ULK1 pathway (Song, Zhang, et al. 2021).

The 50% ethanol extract of *P. vulgaris* spikes significantly reduced tumor weight at 125 mg/mL without changing body weight in a TPC-1–induced mouse model of thyroid cancer. In immunob-lotting assays performed on tumor tissue, expressions of MK167, PCNA, and CDH1 significantly decreased at the concentration of 500 mg/mL (0.4 mL every day for 14 days) (Yu et al. 2021).

20.4.5 Other Cancers

In a study to examine the effects of *P. vulgaris* tea (PV tea, aqueous extract) on endometriosis in a knockout mouse model, it was observed that tea significantly reduced implant formation com-pared to mice treated with estradiol alone. In addition, immunohistochemical studies conducted to analyze the effects of tea at the biochemical level displayed that MKI67, one of the mark-ers of cell growth, decreased significantly. Considering the anti-estrogenic effect of PV tea, the tea could be beneficial for breast, uterine, and other estrogen-dependent cancers. Additionally, the possible effects of tea on fertility due to its anti-estrogenic effect were investigated, and it has been observed that the plant has few side effects on fertility (Collins et al. 2009). An 85% ethanol extract of *Prunella* spike reduced tumor weight without changing body weight in the HT29-induced mouse model. In the *in vitro* MTT assay performed on HT29 cells, the extract significantly reduced cell survival at 500 μg/mL. According to immunohistochemistry studies on tumor tissues, the extract increased Bax expression and decreased the expressions of cyclin D1 and CDK4, which play important roles in the cell cycle, with Bcl-2, VEGF-A, and VEGFR-2 by inhibiting the STAT3 pathway (Lin et al. 2013).

20.5 CLINICAL STUDIES

In the case study conducted by Chang et al., a 29-year-old male patient with a vocal fold polyp had administrated the herbal medicines containing *P. vulgaris* for 14 days, and it was observed that the hoarseness was improved and the inflammation level in the larynx was decreased, but the polyp did not disappear initially. Then, the herbal mixture was used for 3 months and it was observed that the polyp disappeared and all the symptoms were healed (Chang et al. 2021).

In the case report by Lee et al., breast cancer (stage III) of a 46-year-old female patient metastasized and relapsed after the treatments. The patient preferred the Korean medicine. The patient initially administrated some herbal medicines, but at the end of the sixth month, with the recurrence of metastatic tissues as lymphadenopathies, the patient was offered for *P. vulgaris* pharmacopuncture (300 g decoction of plant in 2000 mL) in addition to other Korean medicines because she refused chemotherapy. After 5 months of treatment, the patient was found to be stable and remained stable for 6 months. Pharmacopuncture is the application of aqueous solutions of herbal medicines in the form of acupuncture. The authors concluded that *P. vulgaris* pharmacopuncture plays an important role in reducing the size of lymphadenopathies due to its anti-inflammatory, anti-estrogenic, and antitumor effects (Lee et al. 2015).

The placebo-controlled study conducted by Zhao et al. is a clinical trial comparing standard treatment and standard treatment together with *P. vulgaris* oral solution (decoction of *P. vulgaris*). A total of 424 patients with breast cancer were included in the study, and all patients received standard treatment procedures. *P. vulgaris* oral solution was given to the treatment group at 10 mL twice a day. The control group and the treatment group continued to be administered docetaxel and taxane. The patients were followed up for 41 months. In the treatment group, a significant decrease in the side effects of chemotherapy and an increase in the long-term survival rate and in the pathological response were observed. Major compounds of the solution were detected as caffeic acid and rosmarinic acid by HPLC. Consequently, it was concluded that it would be beneficial and safe for combination of *P. vulgaris* extract and adjuvant therapy (Zhao et al. 2018). In another study on *P. vulgaris* oral solution, the use of the solution in combination with antibiotics in chronic breast cancer patients was compared with the use of antibiotics alone. A significant improvement was observed in the *P. vulgaris*–treated group compared to the control group, while the recurrence rate of the disease was significantly reduced (Wang et al. 2019; Li et al. 2017).

In a randomized, placebo-controlled study involving 120 patients, the therapeutic effect of ZengShengPing mixture (ZSP) containing *P. vulgaris* aqueous extract was tested against oral leukoplakia, which has a high incidence of transforming into oral cancer. The experimental group was given four tablets of ZSP three times a day for 8–12 weeks, and the control group was given placebo. The patients were followed for 3 months. Improvement was observed in 67% of the lesions in the experimental group, while 83% of the control group remained stable. However, AgNOR level and PCNA-labeling index decreased significantly in the experimental group (Sun et al. 2010).

In a study investigating the role of *P. vulgaris* tablets in benign prostatic hyperplasia, the use of PV in combination with finasteride was compared with the use of finasteride alone. A significant decrease in side effects and prostate volume was observed when compared with the control group (Wang et al. 2019; Gong et al. 2014).

The placebo-controlled clinical studies are needed for the activities of the effective parts of the plant, which are also proven by *in vivo* experiments.

20.6 OTHER FOODS, HERBS, SPICES, AND BOTANICALS USED IN CANCER

Results of quantitative analysis to uncover the phytochemical content of *P. vulgaris* reported that rosmarinic acid is one of the major components of the aerial parts (Liu et al. 2014). In several studies, antioxidant, anti-inflammatory, antidiabetic, anticancer, antimutagenic, antiviral, and antibacterial effects of rosmarinic acid were reported (Nadeem et al. 2019). Rosmarinic acid is firstly identified from *Rosmarinus officinalis* (rosemary) and found mainly in the Lamiaceae family. Rosemary is a major source of rosmarinic acid and is used widely as food. Literature survey also indicates the potential of rosemary extract in cancer through *in vitro* and *in vivo* experiments performed (Moore et al. 2016). Rosemary extract was reported to inhibit cell proliferation on several cell lines including HT29, MCF-7, SKBr-3, and A549 cells, in which *P. vulgaris* also showed cytotoxic activity (Moore et al. 2016).

20.7 TOXICITY AND CAUTIONARY NOTES

The air-dried aerial parts of *P. vulgaris* and its preparations are used orally, buccally, and topically. Powdered plant material, infusions, and tinctures are administrated by the oral route and infusions for rinse or gargle by the buccal route. On the other hand, infusions, creams, and ointments are applied by the topical route. As given in Table 20.3, oral doses of infusions and decoctions up to 6–15 g/day and topical doses up to 30 g/day are accepted as safe for adults. Tinctures are used safely in doses of 1 g dried herb equivalent, two to three times per day (1:5, 40% ethyl alcohol, 5 mL) and 0.25–0.5 g, three times per day (1:4, 30% ethyl alcohol, 1–2 mL). No side effects, toxicity, or contraindications are reported with the use of the drug in these proper doses (Health Canada 2009a, 2009b, 2015). When used in excessive doses or inappropriately, patients may suffer from diarrhea (Lin et al. 2015).

It is recommended not to use without consulting a qualified healthcare practitioner, particularly if one is pregnant, nursing, or on any medications.

During the treatment, if symptoms persist or worsen, or if new symptoms develop, one should discontinue use and consult a health care practitioner (Health Canada 2009a, 2009b; Lin et al. 2015).

20.8 SUMMARY POINTS

- This chapter focuses on cytotoxic and antitumor effects of *P. vulgaris*.
- *P. vulgaris* is known as "self-heal" and "heal-all."
- It has a wide distribution in Asia and Europe.
- *P. vulgaris* is used for the treatment of diseases such as throat infections and fever and to treat wounds.
- Aerial parts of the plant are rich in triterpenoids, flavonoids, coumarins, and phenylpropanoids.
- Spikes are the most commonly used part of *P. vulgaris* in all experimental models.
- Aqueous and ethanolic extracts have active cytotoxic effects against breast and thyroid cancer cells.
- The mechanism of action of the extracts was found to be the induction of apoptosis by upregulation of Bax and downregulation of Bcl2.
- In *in vivo* mouse cancer models, studies focused on lung cancer.
- There were promising clinical studies on the aqueous extract.

TABLE 20.3
Safe Daily Amounts for *Prunella vulgaris* Extracts for Different Applications

Plant Material	Type of Preparation	Daily Amount
Dried aerial parts of *P. vulgaris*	Oral doses of infusions and decoctions	Up to 6–15 g/day
	Topical doses	Up to 30 g/day
	Tinctures	1 g dried herb equivalent, two to three times per day (1:5, 40% ethyl alcohol, 5 mL)
		0.25–0.5 g, three times per day (1:4, 30% ethyl alcohol, 1–2 mL)

REFERENCES

Chang, C. H., C. P. Lin, I. MacDonald, T. W. Chiu, and S. T. Huang. 2021. "Resolution of a vocal fold polyp treated with Chinese herbal medicine: One case report with literature review." *Journal of Herbal Medicine* 29. doi:10.1016/j.hermed.2021.100486

Cho, I. H., E. H. Jang, D. Hong, B. Jung, M. J. Park, and J. H. Kim. 2015. "Suppression of LPS-induced epithelial-mesenchymal transition by aqueous extracts of *Prunella vulgaris* through inhibition of the NF-kappa B/Snail signaling pathway and regulation of EMT-related protein expression." *Oncology Reports* 34 (5):2445–2450. doi:10.3892/or.2015.4218

Choi, J. H., E. H. Han, Y. P. Hwang, J. M. Choi, C. Y. Choi, Y. C. Chung, J. K. Seo, and H. G. Jeong. 2010. "Suppression of PMA-induced tumor cell invasion and metastasis by aqueous extract isolated from *Prunella vulgaris* via the inhibition of NF-kappa B-dependent MMP-9 expression." *Food and Chemical Toxicology* 48 (2):564–571. doi:10.1016/j.fct.2009.11.033

Collins, N. H., E. C. Lessey, C. D. DuSell, D. P. McDonnell, L. Fowler, W. A. Palomino, M. J. Illera, X. Z. Yu, B. L. Mo, A. M. Houwing, and B. A. Lessey. 2009. "Characterization of antiestrogenic activity of the Chinese herb, *Prunella vulgaris*, using *in vitro* and *in vivo* (mouse xenograft) models." *Biology of Reproduction* 80 (2):375–383. doi:10.1095/biolreprod.107.065375

Fang, Y., L. Zhang, J. Y. Feng, W. Lin, Q. Y. Cai, and J. Peng. 2017. "Spica Prunellae extract suppresses the growth of human colon carcinoma cells by targeting multiple oncogenes via activating miR-34a." *Oncology Reports* 38 (3):1895–1901. doi:10.3892/or.2017.5792

Feng, L. A., W. Au-yeung, Y. H. Xu, S. S. Wang, Q. Zhu, and P. Xiang. 2011. "Oleanolic acid from *Prunella vulgaris* L. induces SPC-A-1 cell line apoptosis via regulation of Bax, Bad and Bcl-2 expression." *Asian Pacific Journal of Cancer Prevention* 12 (2):403–408.

Feng, L. A., X. B. Jia, J. Jiang, M. M. Zhu, Y. Chen, X. B. Tan, and F. Shi. 2010. "Combination of active components enhances the efficacy of *Prunella* in prevention and treatment of lung cancer." *Molecules* 15 (11):7893–7906. doi:10.3390/molecules15117893

Feng, L. A., X. B. Jia, F. Shi, and Y. Chen. 2010. "Identification of two polysaccharides from *Prunella vulgaris* L. and evaluation on their anti-lung adenocarcinoma activity." *Molecules* 15 (8):5093–5103. doi:10.3390/molecules15085093

Feng, L. A., X. B. Jia, M. M. Zhu, Y. Chen, and F. Shi. 2010a. "Antioxidant activities of total phenols of *Prunella vulgaris* L. *in vitro* and in tumor-bearing mice." *Molecules* 15 (12):9145–9156. doi:10.3390/molecules15129145

Feng, L. A., X. B. Jia, M. M. Zhu, Y. Chen, and F. Shi. 2010b. "Chemoprevention by *Prunella vulgaris* L. extract of non–small cell lung cancer via promoting apoptosis and regulating the cell cycle." *Asian Pacific Journal of Cancer Prevention* 11 (5):1355–1358.

Gao, W., H. Liang, Y. L. Li, Y. Y. Liu, and Y. X. Xu. 2019. "Root extract of *Prunella vulgaris* inhibits in vitro and in vivo carcinogenesis in MCF-5 human breast carcinoma cells via suppression of angiogenesis, induction of apoptosis, cell cycle arrest and modulation of PI3K/AKT signalling pathway." *Journal of Buon* 24 (2):549–554.

Gong, X. J., W. G. Liu, and H. Zhong. 2014. "*Prunella* tablets treatment of benign prostatic hyperplasia in 40 cases." *Journal of Practice in Traditional Chinese Medicine* 30:964–965.

Grosan, A., C. E. Vari, R. Stefanescu, C. Danciu, I. Z. Pavel, C. Dehelean, A. Man, R. E. David, L. Vlase, and L. D. Muntean. 2020. "Antibacterial and antitumor activity of the species *Prunella vulgaris* L." *Revista Romana De Medicina De Laborator* 28 (4):405–417. doi:10.2478/rrlm-2020-0031

Hao, J., X. L. Ding, X. Yang, and X. Z. Wu. 2020. "*Prunella vulgaris* polysaccharide inhibits growth and migration of breast carcinoma-associated fibroblasts by suppressing expression of basic fibroblast growth factor." *Chinese Journal of Integrative Medicine* 26 (4):270–276. doi:10.1007/s11655-016-2587-x

Harput, U. S., I. Saracoglu, and Y. Ogihara. 2006. "Effects of two *Prunella* species on lymphocyte proliferation and nitric oxide production." *Phytotherapy Research* 20 (2):157–159. doi:10.1002/ptr.1805

Health Canada. 2009a. "Drugs and Health Products, Natural Health Products Ingredients Database Monograph: Heal-all-Topical." accessed February 25, 2022. http://webprod.hc-sc.gc.ca/nhpid-bdipsn/monoReq.do?id=115&lang=eng.

Health Canada. 2009b. "Drugs and Health Products, Natural Health Products Ingredients Database Monograph: Heal-all-Oral." accessed February 25, 2022. http://webprod.hc-sc.gc.ca/nhpid-bdipsn/monoReq.do?id=114&lang=eng.

Health Canada. 2015. "Natural Health Product, Natural Chinese Medicine Ingredients (TCMI)." accessed January 25, 2022. https://webprod.hc-sc.gc.ca/nhpid-bdipsn/dbImages/mono_traditional-chinese-medicine-ingredients_english.pdf.

Hwang, Y. J., E. J. Lee, H. R. Kim, and K. A. Hwang. 2013. "In vitro antioxidant and anticancer effects of solvent fractions from *Prunella vulgaris* var. *lilacina*." *Bmc Complementary and Alternative Medicine* 13. doi:10.1186/1472-6882-13-310

Kim, H. I., F. S. Quan, J. E. Kim, N. R. Lee, H. J. Kim, S. J. Jo, C. M. Lee, D. S. Jang, and K. S. Inn. 2014. "Inhibition of estrogen signaling through depletion of estrogen receptor alpha by ursolic acid and betulinic acid from *Prunella vulgaris* var. *lilacina*." *Biochemical and Biophysical Research Communications* 451 (2):282–287. doi:10.1016/j.bbrc.2014.07.115

Kim, S. H., C. Y. Huang, C. Y. Tsai, S. Y. Lu, C. C. Chiu, and K. Fang. 2012. "The aqueous extract of *Prunella vulgaris* suppresses cell invasion and migration in human liver cancer cells by attenuating matrix metalloproteinases." *American Journal of Chinese Medicine* 40 (3):643–656. doi:10.1142/s0192415x12500486

Lee, D. H., S. S. Kim, S. Seong, N. Kim, and J. B. Han. 2015. "Korean Medicine Therapy as a substitute for chemotherapy for metastatic breast cancer: A case report." *Case Reports in Oncology* 8 (1):63–70. doi:10.1159/000375292

Lee, J. B., T. B. Kang, S. H. Choi, U. Lee, A. J. Kim, C. J. Jeong, H. C. Lee, Y. S. Cho, J. G. Won, J. C. Lim, and T. J. Yoon. 2009. "Effect of *Prunella vulgaris* Labiatae extract on innate immune cells and anti-metastatic effect in mice." *Food Science and Biotechnology* 18 (1):218–222.

Lee, K. H., Y. M. Lin, T. S. Wu, D. C. Zhang, T. Yamagishi, T. Hayashi, I. H. Hall, J. J. Chang, R. Y. Wu, and T. H. Yang. 1988. "Antitumor agents. 88: The cytotoxic principles of *Prunella vulgaris, Psychotria serpens*, and *Hyptis capitata* – Ursolic acid and related derivatives." *Planta Medica* (4):308–311. doi:10.1055/s-2006-962441

Li, C., Q. Huang, J. Xiao, X. Fu, L. J. You, and R. H. Liu. 2016. "Preparation of *Prunella vulgaris* polysaccharide-zinc complex and its antiproliferative activity in HepG2 cells." *International Journal of Biological Macromolecules* 91:671–679. doi:10.1016/j.ijbiomac.2016.06.012

Li, C., L. You, X. Fu, Q. Huang, S. Yu, and R. H. Liu. 2015. "Structural characterization and immunomodulatory activity of a new heteropolysaccharide from *Prunella vulgaris*." *Food & Function* 6 (5):1557–1567. doi:10.1039/c4fo01039f

Li, X., W. Liu, and B. Niu. 2017. "Clinical observation of *Prunella* oral liquid and cefdinir dispersible tablets in treating chronic mastitis." *Pharmacology Clinical Traditional Chinese Medicine* 33:190–192.

Lin, L. M., H. M. Gao, and J. J. Zhu. 2015. "*Prunella vulgaris* L. (Xiakucao, Common Selfheal)." In *Dietary Chinese Herbs, Chemistry, Pharmacology and Clinical Evidence*, edited by Y. Liu, Z. Wang, and J. Zhang, 469–475. Wien: Springer.

Lin, W., L. P. Zheng, Q. C. Zhuang, J. Y. Zhao, Z. Y. Cao, J. W. Zeng, S. Lin, W. Xu, and J. Peng. 2013. "Spica Prunellae promotes cancer cell apoptosis, inhibits cell proliferation and tumor angiogenesis in a mouse model of colorectal cancer via suppression of stat3 pathway." *Bmc Complementary and Alternative Medicine* 13. doi:10.1186/1472-6882-13-144

Liu, J. P., L. Feng, J. F. Gu, R. S. Wang, M. H. Zhang, J. Jiang, D. Qin, X. B. Jia, Y. Chen, S. X. Chen, R. Sataer, X. Zhang, and M. M. Zhu. 2014. "Simultaneous determination of ten characteristic antioxidant compounds for inhibiting cancer cell proliferation in *Prunella vulgaris* L. from different regions using HPLC-UV coupled with MS identification." *Analytical Methods* 6 (9):3139–3146. doi:10.1039/c3ay41754a

Moore, J., M. Yousef, and E. Tsiani. 2016. "Anticancer effects of rosemary (*Rosmarinus officinalis* L.) extract and rosemary extract polyphenols." *Nutrients* 8 (11). doi:10.3390/nu8110731

Nadeem, M., M. Imran, T. A. Gondal, A. Imran, M. Shahbaz, R. M. Amir, M. W. Sajid, T. B. Qaisrani, M. Atif, G. Hussain, B. Salehi, E. A. Ostrander, M. Martorell, J. Sharifi-Rad, W. C. Cho, and N. Martins. 2019. "Therapeutic potential of rosmarinic acid: A comprehensive review." *Applied Sciences-Basel* 9 (15). doi:10.3390/app9153139

Patel, J. K., and M. K. Sharma. 2019. "A review on ethno botanical, phytochemistry, bioactivities and medicinal potential of *Prunella vulgaris* (mint family/common self-heal)." *East African Scholars Journal of Biotechnology and Genetics* 1 (5):99–105. doi:10.36349/EASJBG.2019.v01i05.001

Rasool, R., and B. A. Ganai. 2013. "*Prunella vulgaris* L.: A literature review on its therapeutic potentials." *Pharmacologia* 4 (6):441–448. doi:10.5567/pharmacologia.2013.441.448

Sahin, S., F. Ari, C. Demir, and E. Ulukaya. 2014. "Isolation of major phenolic compounds from the extracts of *Prunella* L. species grown in Turkey and their antioxidant and cytotoxic activities." *Journal of Food Biochemistry* 38 (2):248–257. doi:10.1111/jfbc.12043

Song, J., Z. B. Zhang, Y. K. Hu, Z. Y. Li, Y. Wan, J. F. Liu, X. W. Chu, Q. Z. Wei, M. Zhao, and X. F. Yang. 2021. "An aqueous extract of *Prunella vulgaris* L. inhibits the growth of papillary thyroid carcinoma by inducing autophagy in vivo and in vitro." *Phytotherapy Research* 35 (5):2691–2702. doi:10.1002/ptr.7015

Song, Y. G., L. Kang, S. Tian, L. L. Cui, Y. Li, M. Bai, X. Y. Fang, L. H. Cao, K. Coleman, and M. S. Miao. 2021. "Study on the anti-hepatocarcinoma effect and molecular mechanism of *Prunella vulgaris* total flavonoids." *Journal of Ethnopharmacology* 273:113891. doi:10.1016/j.jep.2021.113891

Su, Y. C., I. H. Lin, Y. M. Siao, C. J. Liu, and C. C. Yeh. 2016. "Modulation of the tumor metastatic microenvironment and multiple signal pathways by *Prunella vulgaris* in human hepatocellular carcinoma." *American Journal of Chinese Medicine* 44 (4):835–849. doi:10.1142/s0192415x16500464

Sun, Z., X. B. Guan, N. Li, X. Y. Liu, and X. X. Chen. 2010. "Chemoprevention of oral cancer in animal models, and effect on leukoplakias in human patients with ZengShengPing, a mixture of medicinal herbs." *Oral Oncology* 46 (2):105–110. doi:10.1016/j.oraloncology.2009.06.004

Wang, S. J., X. H. Wang, Y. Y. Dai, M. H. Ma, K. Rahman, H. Nian, and H. Zhang. 2019. "*Prunella vulgaris*: A comprehensive review of chemical constituents, pharmacological effects and clinical applications." *Current Pharmaceutical Design* 25 (3):359–369. doi:10.2174/1381612825666190313121608

Woo, H. J., D. Y. Jun, J. Y. Lee, M. H. Woo, C. H. Yang, and Y. H. Kim. 2011. "Apoptogenic activity of 2 alpha,3 alpha-dihydroxyurs-12-ene-28-oic acid from *Prunella vulgaris* var. *lilacina* is mediated via mitochondria-dependent activation of caspase cascade regulated by Bcl-2 in human acute leukemia Jurkat T cells." *Journal of Ethnopharmacology* 135 (3):626–635. doi:10.1016/j.jep.2011.03.067

Wu, X. Z., S. X. Zhang, C. Zhu, and D. Chen. 2011. "Effects of sulfated polysaccharide extracted from *Prunella vulgaris* on endothelial cells." *Journal of Medicinal Plants Research* 5 (17):4218–4223. doi:10.5897/JMPR.9000541

Xu, Y. C., Z. J. Jiang, G. A. Ji, and J. W. Liu. 2010. "Inhibition of bone metastasis from breast carcinoma by rosmarinic acid." *Planta Medica* 76 (10):956–962. doi:10.1055/s-0029-1240893

Yang, A. P., Z. G. Zheng, F. Liu, J. Liu, R. X. Wang, H. Yang, Z. J. Huang, P. Y. Huang, and H. Liu. 2020. "Screening for potential antibreast cancer components from Prunellae spica using MCF-7 cell extraction coupled with HPLC-ESI-MS/MS." *Natural Product Communications* 15 (6). doi:10.1177/1934578x20931965

Yesilada, E., G. Honda, E. Sezik, M. Tabata, K. Goto, and Y. Ikeshiro. 1993. "Traditional medicine in Turkey 4: Folk medicine in the Mediterranean subdivision." *Journal of Ethnopharmacology* 39 (1):31–38. doi:10.1016/0378-8741(93)90048-A

Yin, D. T., M. Y. Lei, J. H. Xu, H. Q. Li, Y. F. Wang, Z. Liu, R. S. Ma, K. Yu, and X. H. Li. 2017. "The Chinese herb *Prunella vulgaris* promotes apoptosis in human well-differentiated thyroid carcinoma cells via the B-cell lymphoma-2/Bcl-2-associated X protein/caspase-3 signaling pathway." *Oncology Letters* 14 (2):1309–1314. doi:10.3892/ol.2017.6317

Yu, F. Q., L. L. Zhang, R. S. Ma, C. G. Liu, Q. D. Wang, and D. T. Yin. 2021. "The antitumor effect of *Prunella vulgaris* extract on thyroid cancer cells *in vitro* and *in vivo*." *Evidence-Based Complementary and Alternative Medicine* 2021. doi:10.1155/2021/8869323

Zhao, J. X., D. G. Ji, X. J. Zhai, L. R. Zhang, X. Luo, and X. Fu. 2018. "Oral administration of *Prunella vulgaris* L improves the effect of taxane on preventing the progression of breast cancer and reduces its side effects." *Frontiers in Pharmacology* 9. doi:10.3389/fphar.2018.00806

21 Lichen, *Pseudevernia furfuracea* (L.) Zopf
Analytical Compositional Features, Biological Activity and Use in Cancer Studies

Martin Kello and Michal Goga

ABBREVIATIONS

8-OH-dG	8-hydroxy-2′-deoxyguanosine
Akt	protein kinase B
α-SMA	smooth muscle alpha-actin
ATM	ataxia–telangiectasia mutated kinase
BAD	BCL2 associated agonist of cell death gene
BAG3	BAG family molecular chaperone regulator 3 gene
BAK1	BCL2 antagonist/killer 1 gene
BCL2	B-cell lymphoma 2 apoptosis regulator gene
BrdU	5-bromo-2′-deoxyuridine
CAM	chorioallantoic membrane
CASP3,5,6,7,8	caspase 3, 5, 6, 7, 8 gene
CHEK1	checkpoint kinase 1 gene
DDR	DNA damage response
DFFA	DNA fragmentation factor subunit alpha gene
EMT	epithelial–mesenchymal transition
ER+	estrogen receptor positive
FADD	Fas-associated via death domain gene
FAS	Fas cell surface death receptor
FASLG	Fas ligand
HER2–	human epidermal growth factor receptor 2 negative
IARC	International Agency for Research on Cancer
IC_{50}	half-maximal inhibitory concentration
JNK	c-Jun N-terminal kinase
MAPK	mitogen-activated protein kinase
MMP-9	matrix metallopeptidase 9
MTT	3-(4,5-dimethylthiazol-2-yl)-2,5-diphenyl-tetrazolium bromide
PARP	poly (ADP-ribose) polymerase
PI	propidium iodide
PI3K	phosphoinositide 3-kinase
PR+	progesterone receptor positive
Rb	retinoblastoma protein
Slug	recombinant protein of human snail homolog 2
SMC1	structural maintenance of chromosomes 1

DOI: 10.1201/9781003260028-23

Smad2/3	human SMAD family member 2/3
TME	tumor microenvironment
TNF	tumor necrosis factor
TP63	tumor protein P63 gene
VEGF	vascular endothelial growth factor

21.1 *PSEUDEVERNIA FURFURACEA*

Lichen *P. furfuracea* belongs to the family Parmeliaceae and was first described by Zopf. Parmeliaceae is the largest family of lichenized fungi with approximately 2700 species which are distributed in about 80 genera (Gomez-Serranillos et al. 2014). *P. furfuracea*, also known as "tree moss," represents foliose lichen thallus, which usually lies on the branch in the young stages and is often clearly fruticose in an older stage. It forms lobes that grow dorsiventrally and are well branched. Lobes are quite variable and depend on environmental conditions. The length of the thallus can be up to 15 cm in diameter and up to 1 cm wide. The color of the thallus can be distinguished at the upper and lower surfaces (Figure 21.1).

The upper surface is light to dark gray and the lower surface is ridged and typically mainly black. On the upper surface are soralia (reproductive structures) but more often isidia, coral-like structures which can break off and grow into new lichens containing mycobiont and photobiont (Stenroos et al. 2016; Thell and Moberg 2011). *P. furfuracea* often grows in the same habitat as *Evernia prunastri*. In younger stages, these lichens can be exchanged, but chemical variation and tests can serve for taxonomic recognition.

21.2 CHEMISTRY AND SECONDARY METABOLITES OF *P. FURFURACEA*

Lichens are a unique example of symbiosis because they produce specific secondary metabolites, and their greatest benefit is their mass yield and stability (Galun and Shomer-Ilan 1988; Goga et al. 2018; Solhaug et al. 2009; Stocker-Worgotter 2008). Secondary metabolites are produced by mycobiont, which is a fungal partner of lichen, and that is the reason why lichens are known as lichenized fungi. Secondary metabolites are crystals deposited on the surface of fungal cells called hyphae. These crystals are interesting from the perspective that they can be stored and remain stable for a very long time. The analyses of secondary metabolites from deposited herbarium specimens are an example (Rundel 1978).

Lichen secondary metabolites are synthesized by the acetyl-malonate pathway, shikimate pathway, and mevalonate pathway (Culberson and Elix 1989). By the acetyl-malonate pathway are synthesized most of the secondary metabolites, which belong to the classes of lichen substances as dibenzofurans, anthraquinones, chromones, xanthones, depsides, and depsidones. Because each step ends with a decarboxylation reaction, the formation of the polyketide chain could be envisioned as a series of Claisen reactions between the starting acetyl-CoA and a variable number of malonyl-CoA. The main

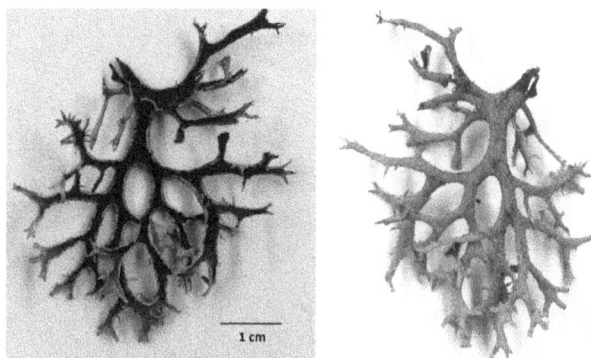

FIGURE 21.1 *Pseudevernia furfuracea* thallus. Lower surface (black) and upper surface (greenish) of *P. furfuracea* lichen thallus.

intermediate in the biosynthesis of depsides and depsidones, orsellinic acid, is formed by an intra-molecular aldol reaction of a polyketide containing four keto groups, followed by enolization and hydrolysis. Atranorin is a member of the depsides class as a result of the esterification of two orsellinic acid molecules. The most well-known orcinol-type depsidones have a keto group in the first ring's side chain. Because enol lactones form easily, this functional group has a strong effect on the ester linkage between the two rings. The 2-hydroxyl of ring A and the 5-position of ring B are usually joined during oxidative cyclization of depsides to depsidones (Figure 21.2) (Goga et al. 2018).

P. furfuracea produces secondary metabolites, which belong to the depsides (atranorin, chlo-ratranorin, olivetoric acid) and depsidones (physodic acid, 3-hydroxyphysodic acid, physodalic acid) classes (Figure 21.3). The biological potential of these secondary metabolites cannot be

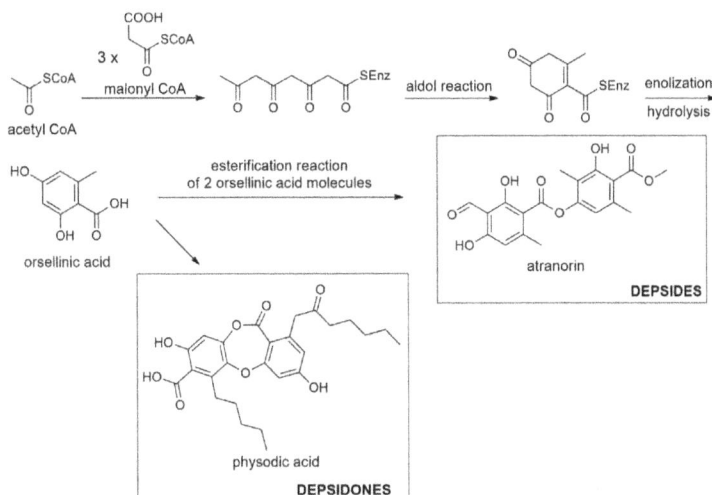

FIGURE 21.2 Synthesis pathway of lichen secondary metabolites. Classes of depsides and depsidones derived by acetyl-malonate pathway.

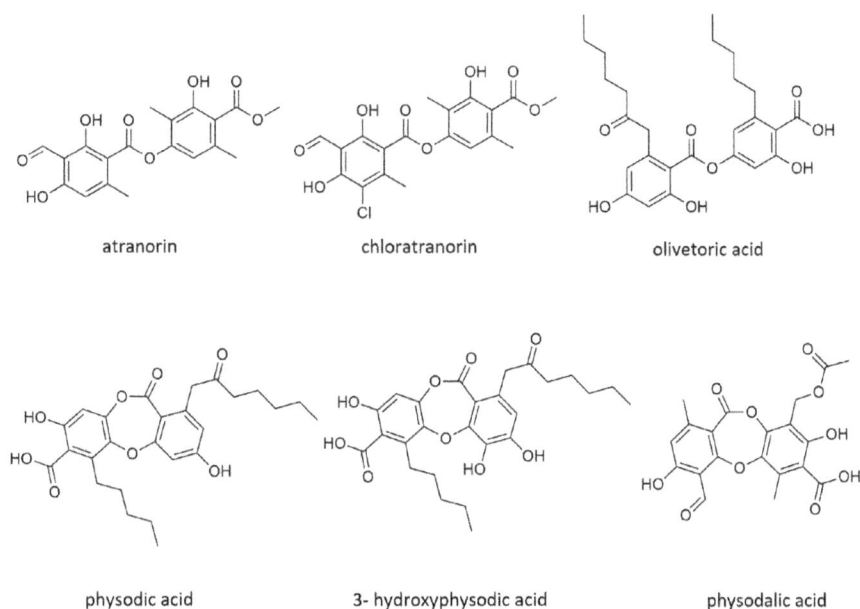

FIGURE 21.3 Secondary metabolites belong to the depsides and depsidones classes.

TABLE 21.1
Biological Activities of Secondary Metabolites from the Lichen *Pseudevernia furfuracea*

P. furfuracea	Secondary Metabolites		
Types of Activity	**Atranorin**	**Physodic Acid**	**Olivetoric Acid**
Allelopathy	(Rucova et al. 2019)	(Rucova et al. 2019)	
Antiangiogenic			(Kello et al. 2021; Koparal et al. 2010; Petrova et al. 2021; Ulus 2021)
Antibiofilm			(Mitrovic et al. 2014)
Antifungal activity	(Tekiela et al. 2021)		
Antiinflammatory	(Ingelfinger et al. 2020)	(Ingelfinger et al. 2020)	
Antimicrobial	(Turk et al. 2006)	(Urena-Vacas et al. 2021)	(Mitrovic et al. 2014; Turk et al. 2006)
Antioxidant		(Emsen et al. 2017; Urena-Vacas et al. 2021)	(Emsen et al. 2017; Mitrovic et al. 2014)
Antitumor			(Emsen et al. 2016)
Apoptotic		(Emsen et al. 2020)	
Cytotoxic		(Emsen et al. 2020; Ingelfinger et al. 2020; Urena-Vacas et al. 2021)	(Emsen et al. 2018)
Genotoxic		(Emsen et al. 2020)	(Emsen et al. 2018)
Inhibition of enzymes	(Proksa et al. 1994)		
Oxidative		(Emsen et al. 2020)	
Photoprotective	(Varol et al. 2015)		

ignored, which was proved in considerable research works for in recent decades. The pharmaceutical potential of secondary metabolites known from lichen *P. furfuracea* is shown in Table 21.1.

21.3 MEDICAL USES AND FOLKLORE

Lichens grow around the world from the North Pole to Antarctica in all climate zones. The cultures inhabiting these regions have collected knowledge about the medicinal uses of lichens for centuries. In traditional medicine lichens were used for their curative effects but also the storage of carbohydrates (Crawford 2019).

During the 15th century, the *Doctrine of Signatures* was written, where people believed that diseases can be treated by a plant that looked like an organ. This theory established the basics of the science-based medical practice called phytotherapy. Phytotherapeutic practices are known around the world from Asia as traditional Chinese medicine, traditional Indian medicine, Unani medicine, the traditional system of medicine in Indonesia, the Koryo system of medicine in DPR Korea, Ayurveda, and Chinese acupuncture–moxibustion (Chaudhury and Rafei 2002). European traditional medicine also has a very long history (Firenzuoli and Gori 2007). From the Western part of the world, this traditional knowledge is known as Western herbal medicine or Western medicinal herbalism (Bown 2001; Niemeyer et al. 2013). All of these traditional medicines are accepted by the World Health Organization (WHO).

Lichens as medical plants were used a long time ago in folklore as well. The lichen *Evernia furfuracea* (L.), today known as *Pseudevernia furfuracea* (L.) Zopf, was first used as a drug in the Egypt 18th dynasty in 1700–1800 BC (Launert 1981). Lichens and especially their secondary compounds were used for coughs, jaundice, hair restoration, and to treat rabies (Pereira 1853), skin disorders, respiratory and digestive issues, and obstetric and gynecological concerns (Crawford 2019). During the middle ages, the sanipractors or healers tried the effects of lichens as herbs (Malhotra et al. 2007). It was the age when the success or mistake of unknown herbs formed modern phytotherapeutics. The decoction of lichen *P. furfuracea* was used in Spanish folk medicine against respiratory illness (González-Tejero et al. 1995). *P. furfuracea* is used in traditional medicine in Turkey as a treatment for wounds, eczema, anticatarrhal, a hypotensive drug, or against hemorrhoids (Guvenc et al. 2012; Mitrovic et al. 2014; Shukla et al. 2018; Zambare and Christopher 2012).

Few reviews about the lichens in Europe (Llano 1948; Richardson 1974; Smith 1921), India (Upreti and Chatterjee 2007), and China (Wang and Qian 2013) as medicinal or traditional use plants were published. In the present review, the medical uses of lichen *P. furfuracea* as well as their secondary metabolites are summarized.

Lichen *P. furfuracea* was commonly used in traditional medicine mostly in Europe and North Africa. In the late 1600s in Europe, there was a popular hair powder called Cyprus which contained aromatic ingredients (Bauhin and Cherler 1650; Zwelfer 1672). People called it "oak moss," probably because of the substrate where was collected. At the time in Europe, the botanists were able to discern genera of several lichens in Cyprus powder. France is one of the biggest producers of perfumes. At that time, *P. furfuracea* and *E. prunastri* were the most preferred lichens in the perfumery industry (Amoreux 1787). Nowadays, *E. prunastri* (later oak moss) and *P. furfuracea* (tree moss) are the most harvested lichen species used for perfume. Extracts of lichens have good fixative properties and give also bass notes in perfume while the top notes give floral essences. The bass notes evaporate slowly and can be perceived after some time after application (Joulain and Tabacchi 2009a, 2009b; Moxham 1986). It is also important to mention that some lichens can cause also negative dermatologic reactions in people with sensitive skin.

In the culture of the ancient Greeks, there was a traditional medical herb called *splanchon*. It was a mixture of *E. prunastri*, *P. furfuracea*, and some *Usnea* species. This lichen began to be used in European pharmacy around the 1500s, where all fruticose lichens were included. Later in the 1700s, only *Usnea* species were recognized as the main effect of *splanchon*. The decoction of this lichen showed application against styptic, as a treatment for drying skin lesions, as an anti-inflammatory, as a skin moisturizer, for nausea, diarrhea, whooping cough, smallpox, insomnia, umbilical hernias, and as uterine medicine (Lebail 1853). *P. furfuracea* was also used in ointments as an astringent. The decoction could be used cold or hot for washing the vulva for womb diseases, or it could be used against fatigue (López Eire et al. 2006).

In Libyan folk medicine, the lichens *P. furfuracea*, *Ramalina calicaris* and *R. farinacea* were used as ingredients in a medicinal decoction called *scíba*. Italian botanist Alessandro Trotter described lichens as belonging to the genera *Evernia* (today *Pseudevernia*) and *Ramalina*. It was known that they were used as dyes, perfumes, or in traditional medicine along with the secondary metabolite usnic acid. Unfortunately, he did not mention the therapeutic application for this decoction (De Natale and Pollio 2012).

In Ancient Egypt, the lichen *P. furfuracea* was found in a vase from the 16th to 14th centuries BC with other medicinal plants (Müller 1881). During the New Kingdom (1549–1069 BC) and the Third Intermediate Period (1069–656 BC) in Egypt, lichens were used in the mummification process, in which bodies were stuffed with lichens and other botanicals (Baumann 1960; Schmull and Brown 2009). At that time, *P. fufuracea* did not grow in Egypt because the country was too dry, so it is assumed that lichen was probably a result of trading and came from Lebanon or the hills of Macedonia, which was not proven.

In Europe during the early modern era, a mixture of *E. prunastri* and *P. furfuracea* known as lichen quercinus virdes became popular drug (Llano 1948; Senft 1911). Both lichens were probably taken together because of their appearance, but their chemical composition is different.

21.4 ANTICANCER POTENTIAL

The latest International Agency for Research on Cancer (IARC) GLOBOCAN cancer statistics update for the year 2020 revealed that with 2.26 million new cases, breast cancer has now become the most commonly diagnosed cancer worldwide, followed by lung cancer (2.21 million). Lung cancer remains the most common cause of cancer death (1.80 million deaths), followed by liver (0.83 million) and stomach cancers (0.77 million) (Ferlay et al. 2021). The need for new treatments and approaches in cancer research and therapy stays actual and challenging nowadays. Despite advances in cancer research, surgical operation, radiotherapy, and chemotherapy represent standard treatment options for newly diagnosed patients or in remission. The biggest disadvantage of chemotherapy is the inability to distinguish between cancer cells and normal cells, followed by side effects and system toxicities. There has been enormous progress in cancer treatment in past decades from standard cytotoxic chemotherapy to targeted therapy (Bedard et al. 2020). Still, the identification of novel natural or synthetic anticancer substances with reduced toxicity and drug resistance or increased efficiency represents the hallmark in cancer research. It is known that more than 70% of anticancer drugs have a natural origin or were synthesized or constructed (semi-synthetic drugs) based on natural substances (Katz and Baltz 2016). Commonly, phytochemicals are found to be effective against various types of cancer by alteration of initial and progress cell mechanisms like proliferation, differentiation, cell death, angiogenesis, or metastasis (Atanasov et al. 2021). In light of this knowledge, lichens show a broad spectrum of biological potential for cancer research (Dar et al. 2021; Goga et al. 2018; Solarova et al. 2020). The secondary metabolites of lichens have gained attention worldwide recently for their cytotoxic, anticancer, antiproliferative, anti-invasive, antimigratory, antimetastatic, and pro-apoptotic effects. In the past decade, the tree moss lichen *P. furfuracea* (L.) Zopf extract and its metabolites (atranorin, chloratranorin, physodic acid, olivetoric acid, lecanoric acid, protocetraric acid, and geopyxins) have been analyzed for their anticancer potential. In this subchapter, we summarized recently published data based on cancer types. Although the anticancer research with *P. furfuracea* or secondary metabolites directly isolated from extract represents a new area, the progress accelerates every year.

21.4.1 Breast Cancer

The antiproliferative effect of *P. furfuracea* acetone extract was tested on the human breast adenocarcinoma MCF-7 (ER+, PR+, HER2−) line by using MTT (3-(4,5-dimethylthiazol-2-yl)-2,5-diphenyl-tetrazolium bromide) colorimetric assay (Tas et al. 2019). The results clearly showed that *P. furfuracea* extract with high atranorin content possesses cytotoxic potential against MCF-7 cells with an IC_{50} value set at 146.5 µg/mL. Based on these preliminary data, the mechanisms of anticancer potential mediated by *P. furfuracea* or their metabolites should be elucidated. First inside view to the mechanisms brought the paper discussing the effect of lichen extract *P. furfuracea* and metabolite physodic acid on tumor microenvironment (TME) modulation in normal human mammary epithelial cells (MCF-10A) as an *in vitro* model system (Petrova et al. 2021). Understanding the regulatory mechanisms affecting the tumor microenvironment can reveal new therapeutic options in cancer research. TME contains the mass of heterogenic cells including tumor and stromal cells (fibroblasts, cancer-associated fibroblasts, endothelial and immune cells), and the secretome of these cells initiates processes like carcinogenesis, the epithelial–mesenchymal transition (EMT), angiogenesis, and metastasis (Hanahan and Coussens 2012). Petrova et al. (2021) for the first time demonstrated that *P. furfuracea* extract and metabolite physodic acid significantly modulated TME processes in the MCF-10A cell system. The low IC_{10} concentrations of both substances indicated the prevention potential of extract as well as physodic acid in breast cancer initiation or progression. Several EMT-associated proteins, such as Slug, Smad2/3, N-cadherin, fibronectin, and α-SMA were mediated and downregulated by *P. furfuracea* extract and physodic acid in a concentration- and time-dependent manner in MCF-10A cells. It is known that stromal-derived mesenchymal stem cells or mesenchymal-like cells derived from EMT transformation in breast cancer are precursors of cancer-associated fibroblasts (Weber et al. 2015). Therefore, *P. furfuracea* extract or physodic acid treatment could be beneficial in the inhibition of breast cancer induction, progression, or metastasis as a result of inhibition or downregulation of mesenchymal markers.

21.4.2 COLON CANCER

The cytotoxic activity of *P. furfuracea* extract or physodic acid was studied on several colon cancer lines in the past decade. Moreover, a different extraction approach was used in the preparing of *P. furfuracea* extract. The methanol, acetone, and ethyl acetate extracts of *P. furfuracea* were tested on the HCT116 and SW480 colon cancer cells, whereas all the treatments considerably decreased cell viability in a dose- and time-dependent manner (Seklic et al. 2018). The ethyl acetate extract of *P. furfuracea* showed the most significant cytotoxic effect on HCT116 cells with IC_{50} 21.2 µg/mL. On the other side, acetone extract had the highest cytotoxic effect on SW480 cells (51.3 µg/mL). Methanol extract showed the lowest cytotoxic effect. Acetone extract of *P. furfuracea* was also tested on colon adenocarcinoma cell line HT-29 using colorimetric metabolic WST1 assay. The results showed the inhibitory effect of the extract in a dose-dependent manner (IC_{50} 57.1 µg/mL). Moreover, cell viability loss was in accordance with morphological changes (enlarged shape and a formation of blebs in the cell's membranes) and with the appearance of apoptotic bodies, large vacuoles in the cell cytoplasm, and rounded shape of the cells that start to detach (Aoussar et al. 2020). The approximately same IC_{50} value (56.9 µg/mL) was calculated for the growth inhibitory effect of *P. furfuracea* acetone extract on colon cancer LS174 cell line. In addition, in this paper isolated physodic acid from *P. furfuracea* revealed a stronger cytotoxic effect (IC_{50} 17.9 µg/mL) compared with crude extract (Kosanic et al. 2013). Annexin V/PI staining on HCT116 and SW480 colon cancer cells also evaluated the pro-apoptotic potential of *P. furfuracea* extract (Seklic et al. 2018). The results showed that apoptotic effects depend on the concentration of treatment and time of exposure. The ethyl acetate extract of *P. furfuracea* showed the strongest significant apoptotic effect on HCT116 cells at 72 hours after both tested concentrations caused up to 20.12% (10 µg/mL) and 75.39% (100 µg/mL) occurrences of late apoptotic cells. Furthermore, methanol and acetone extracts of *P. furfuracea* had the highest pro-apoptotic effects on SW480 cells after 72 hours. Consistent with the induced apoptosis, the extracts of *P. furfuracea* could be arranged as follows: ethyl acetate > acetone > methanol (HCT116) and acetone > methanol > ethyl acetate (SW480). Among others, the significant antimigratory effects revealed *P. furfuracea* methanol extract (50 µg/mL) on both tested cell lines (Seklic et al. 2022). Migration of tumor cells is a critical process in cancer progression and is crucial for cancer cell dissemination from a primary tumor to distant metastasis (Campbell and Casanova 2016). Seklic et al. (2022) described that the antimigratory/anti-invasive effects of *P. furfuracea* methanol extract are connected with reduction of pro-migratory and pro-invasive markers at genes and proteins levels in colorectal cancer. *P. furfuracea* methanol extract significantly increased E-cadherin expression, decreased N-cadherin expression, significantly reduced the level of nuclear β-catenin, and reduced vimentin expression that correlated with the antimigratory effects of this treatment in both cell lines (HCT116, SW480). Moreover, *P. furfuracea* methanol extract reduced Snail protein as the basic regulator of EMT that results in a lower expression of mesenchymal and migratory markers (N-cadherin, Vimentin) (Vu and Datta 2017). Furthermore, anti-invasive effects of *P. furfuracea* methanol extract was documented by decreased gene and protein expression of MMP-9.

21.4.3 HEPATIC CANCER

The acetone extract of *P. furfuracea* and two isolated metabolites, physodic and olivetoric acid, were analyzed as potential antiproliferative or pro-apoptotic agents in the hepatic adenocarcinoma model. The metabolic WST1 or MTT test revealed the cytotoxic potential of acetone extract on human hepatocellular carcinoma (HepG2, IC_{50} 68.6 µg/mL) (Aoussar et al. 2020) and more resistant HepG2/C3A clone (IC_{50} 184.3 µg/mL) (Tas et al. 2019). The secondary metabolites physodic acid (Emsen et al. 2020) and olivetoric acid (Emsen et al. 2021) isolated from *P. furfuracea* showed effective IC_{50} concentrations, inhibited metabolic activity and proliferation of HepG2 cells on levels of 400 µg/mL or 129.4 µg/mL, respectively. Regarding the cytotoxic effect of physodic and olivetoric acid on HepG2 cells, the genotoxicity determined by oxidative DNA damage levels was evaluated. The results with both metabolites clearly showed increased 8-hydroxy-2′-deoxyguanosine (8-OH-dG) levels, a product of oxidative damage to 2′-deoxyguanosine (Emsen et al. 2020, 2021). Moreover, qPCR analysis of mRNA samples obtained from HepG2 cells treated with physodic acid revealed significant expression changes in 31 out of 83 apoptosis-related genes (Emsen et al. 2020). The downregulated genes were not statistically changed, and the top five apoptotic genes most affected by physodic acid were CASP5, BAG3, DFFA, TP63, and CHEK1. In addition, physodic acid manifests apoptotic effect through both intrinsic and extrinsic pathways. It was demonstrated the activation of TNF receptor and CASP8, CASP7, and CASP3 genes (extrinsic pathway) and BCL2, BAX, and BAK genes (intrinsic pathway) by physodic acid treatment. The similar quantitative PCR analyses for olivetoric acid showed upregulation of pro-apoptotic genes BAK, CASP6, CASP7, CASP8, FADD, FAS, and FASLG in HepG2 cells (Emsen et al. 2021). Related genes are of great importance in the apoptotic process.

21.4.4 Glioblastoma

The rapid growth glioblastoma (GB) is one of the nervous system cancers most difficult to treat. Side effects of radiotherapy and chemotherapy treatments of GB require an alternative approach carried out by the combination of plant-based products. Therefore, cytotoxic, antioxidative, pro-oxidative, and genotoxic potentials of physodic and olivetoric acid isolated from *P. furfuracea* were evaluated on healthy (PRCC) and glioblastoma (U87MG) brain cells (Emsen et al. 2016). The metabolic MTT assay was used to test the cell viability of PRCC and U87MG cells treated by physodic and olivetoric acid. The results showed that both physodic and olivetoric acid highly inhibited U87MG cell proliferation in the concentration range 20–40 μg/mL. Based on this screening, 50% inhibition (IC_{50}) should be achieved for U87MG cells by 17.5 μg/mL olivetoric acid and 410.7 μg/mL physodic acid. The healthy PRCC brain cells showed increased cytotoxic effects after a higher concentration of olivetoric (IC_{50} 125.7 μg/mL) and physodic acid (698.1 μg/mL). Moreover, 8-OH-dG activities as a marker of DNA damage increased in a concentration-dependent manner for both cells treated with olivetoric or physodic acid, suggesting that oxidative stress could be one of the pro-apoptotic stimuli. DNA damage in healthy brain cells was induced by the highest tested concentration (40 μg/mL) compared to U87MG cells, where all tested concentrations (2.5–40 μg/mL) had the effect.

21.4.5 Leukemia

Recently, a pivotal study was published in the field of antileukemic research and lichen potential. The main challenge in acute lymphoblastic leukemia is mitigation of the main side effects of conventional therapy. The use of natural compounds with antileukemic potential and minimal side effects might be helpful to address these problems. At the end of 2021, *P. furfuracea* extract and physodic acid were tested as antileukemic agents (Kello et al. 2021). The preliminary screening revealed efficient antiproliferative IC_{50} concentration for *P. furfuracea* extract as 45 μg/mL and physodic acid as 60 μM in Jurkat cells. Moreover, both the extract and physodic acid disrupted the mitochondrial membrane potential (ΔΨm) that represents a sign of initiated cell death. The cell cycle analyses revealed that *P. furfuracea* extract caused S-phase arrest while physodic acid G1-phase cell cycle arrest in a time-dependent manner. The contribution of *P. furfuracea* extract and physodic acid treatment on the apoptosis induction in Jurkat cells was confirmed by a significant increase of externalized phosphatidyl serine on the cell membrane surface; release of cytochrome *c* from mitochondria to cytosol and caspase-9 and caspase-3 activation with subsequent PARP cleavage. The cytotoxic effects of *P. furfuracea* extract and physodic acid were linked with oxidative stress and DNA damage in Jurkat cells. Kello et al. (2021) documented significant increases in superoxide and total ROS accumulation observed shortly after 6 hours of *P. furfuracea* extract and physodic acid treatment. Moreover, the analyses of DNA damage response (DDR) mechanisms represented by the activation of ATM (ataxia–mutated kinase), SMC1 protein (structural maintenance of chromosome 1), and histone H2A.X clearly showed DNA single- or double-strand breaks in the presence of *P. furfuracea* extract or physodic acid. In addition, both treatment-mediated DNA damage and cell cycle arrest caused the activation of cell cycle checkpoint proteins including p53, p21, p27, and deactivation of Rb protein in time-dependent manner. For the first time, Kello et al. (2021) demonstrated precise mechanisms connected in *P. furfuracea* extract or physodic acid-mediated apoptosis. In Jurkat cells, both treatments led to the phosphorylation of MAPK kinases, including p38 MAPK, JNK, and PI3K/Akt as the results of oxidative stress, and the activation of these kinases correspond to the pro-apoptotic effect of *P. furfuracea* extract or physodic acid.

21.4.6 Minor Screenings Data

In addition, the pivotal basic cytotoxic data were obtained from the human melanoma FemX (Kosanic et al. 2013) and human prostate cancer 22RV1 cells (Aoussar et al. 2020) exposed to *P. furfuracea* acetone extract or isolated physodic acid. The screening clearly showed that *P. furfuracea* extract inhibited proliferation of prostate and melanoma cancer cells in a dose-dependent manner with IC_{50} 42.3 µg/mL (22RV1) and 55.1 µg/mL (FemX). Moreover, the melanoma FemX cells showed a higher sensitivity to physodic acid exposure with IC_{50} 19.5 µg/mL. It has also been proven by cell cycle analyses that both extract (22.8%) and physodic acid (27.1%) increased the number of melanoma cells in the sub-G0/G1 population with fragmented DNA that are considered as apoptotic cells.

The basic broader screening of cytotoxic and pro-apoptotic potential of *P. furfuracea* extract or isolated secondary metabolites should be considered for future evaluation.

21.5 ANTI-ANGIOGENIC POTENTIAL

Angiogenesis, in term of new blood vessel formation, represents one of the crucial processes involved in solid tumor microenvironment development. Tumor cells, stromal cells, and secreted cytokines provide an environment that supports the growth and development of tumors (Jiang et al. 2020; Lugano et al. 2020). The therapies based on angiogenesis inhibition, involving substances that reduce blood vessel formation in malignant tumors, have attracted great interest as potential anticancer therapy (Teleanu et al. 2020). In the past decades, several substances were isolated from natural compounds that are able to modulate the angiogenesis process. The lichens and their secondary metabolites have been included in this group of potential anti-angiogenic agents (Ulus 2021).

From the several lichens species with proven anticancer effect, *P. furfuracea* has been conducted also with anti-angiogenic potential (Koparal et al. 2010; Petrova et al. 2021). Koparal et al. (2010) performed the first study on the anti-angiogenic activity of a *P. furfuracea* secondary metabolite olivetoric acid. The Matrigel tube formation assay revealed that olivetoric acid inhibited tube formation in a dose-dependent manner. As the main cause, the significant dose-dependent decrease in cell viability and proliferation of endothelial cells after olivetoric acid treatment was considered. Moreover, the depolymerization of actin stress fibers and inhibition of their formation occurred after a 200 µM dose of olivetoric acid. Therefore, olivetoric acid has been considered as actin and tubulin cytoskeleton disrupting agents and may exhibit anti-angiogenic activity *in vitro*.

Besides that, the potential anti-angiogenic effect of *P. furfuracea* acetone extract and isolated physodic acid was tested using the *ex ovo* CAM (chorioallantoic membrane) assay (Petrova et al. 2021). It was demonstrated that both extract and physodic acid reduced blood vessel density, total vessel network length, and total branching points on VEGF (vascular endothelial growth factor) induced vascularization of fertilized quail eggs (*Coturnix coturnix japonica*). In addition, the impact of *P. furfuracea* extract and physodic acid on HUVEC (primary human umbilical cord vein endothelial cells) proliferation was evaluated by metabolic MTT and BrdU incorporating assay. Both tests revealed that VEGF-stimulated HUVECs proliferation was inhibited by *P. furfuracea* extract and physodic acid treatment in a dose-dependent manner. Non-stimulated HUVECs showed no significant proliferation changes after treatment with extract and physodic acid, suggesting that VEGF stimulus sensitized endothelial cells.

21.6 CONCLUSIONS

Under the impact of published data, several findings uncover the potential of *P. furfuracea* extract and isolated secondary metabolites and their mechanics as anticancer or anti-angiogenic agents. Despite these facts, more associated mechanisms of the anticancer action of the lichen should be revealed. The lichen use limitations such as rarity in nature, extraction, and purity exist, but these issues will be eliminated in the near future. In this regard, many of these substances may be applied and provide reasonable clinical use.

21.7 OTHER FOODS, HERBS, SPICES, AND BOTANICALS USED IN CANCER

Nowadays, lichens are used as an ingredient in foods and diets and are consumed around the world. Several reviews deal with health-promoting effects of edible lichens (Zhao et al. 2021). For example, *Cetraria islandica* is used in Scandinavia and Baltic countries in salads, mush or ingredients of bread which prevent the diseases of lung, kidney, or the gastrointestinal tract (Airaksinen et al. 1986; Kalle and Soukand 2012). The lichen *Cladina ragniferina*, which contain other secondary metabolites, is used in salads (Huang et al. 2018) or as a treatment of inflammation in the United States (Wang et al. 2001). In India lichens are used often with vegetables, spices, or as flavoring agents (Kekuda et al. 2011). *Lethariella* species in China have wide use and can be found in teas, wines, or other beverages, where the applications include reduce inflammation (Ju et al. 2013). In Balkan countries the lichen *Lobaria pulmonaria* is used as a mush or ingredients of bread, where again compounds which contain this lichen are anti-inflammatory, antiseptic, and can be used to treat pulmonary diseases (Huang et al. 2018; Simkova and Polesny 2015; Suleyman et al. 2003).

The lichen *P. furfuracea* is very popular in the Balkan region but also in Turkey, Nepal, Spain, and in Europe in general. This lichen can be used as an ingredient of bread or mush (Simkova and Polesny 2015). The tea from this lichen can treat respiratory diseases, hypertension, or asthma (Emsen et al. 2018). The lichen *Platismatia glauca*, which also contains atranorin and chloratranorin, is used as a spice in India and Middle Eastern countries (Seklic and Jovanovic 2022). One of the most studied lichens, *Usnea longissima*, which is very rare in Europe, is consumed in China at meals and also has anti-inflammatory activity (Bai et al. 2014).

Besides lichen sources, natural plant molecules, herbs, and spices could provide therapeutic effects against tumor cells. A broad spectrum of plant-derived substances such as flavonoids, carotenoids, phenolic acids, and organosulfur compounds possess chemoprevention activity by suppressing the initiation and progression of carcinogenesis with minimal side effects. For example, several animal studies, focused on plant food diets, demonstrated significantly reduce risk of experimental breast cancer. Rosemary extract (Singletary et al. 1996), blueberries (Kubatka et al. 2016a), caraway (Chen et al. 2015), pomegranate (Bishayee et al. 2016), *Origanum vulgare L.* (Kubatka et al. 2017a), *Syzygium aromaticum L.* (Kubatka et al. 2017b), *Thymus vulgaris L.* (Kubatka et al. 2019), young barley (Kubatka et al. 2016b), chlorella (Kubatka et al. 2015), *Rhus coriaria* L. (sumac) (Kubatka et al. 2021), and cinnamon (Kubatka et al. 2020) clearly show the tumor-suppressive effects *in vivo* in breast cancer model. Regarding isolated phytochemicals, only curcumin (Masuelli et al. 2013) and epigallocatechin-3-gallate (Gu et al. 2013) showed significant anticancer potential. However, well-designed clinical trials are needed to establish individualized treatment and optimal conditions for use of dietary phytochemicals in chemoprevention.

21.8   TOXICITY AND CAUTIONARY NOTES

Lichen chemistry and production of secondary metabolites is somewhat related to toxicity. The pharmaceutical potential of lichen substances was described in several reviews (Goga et al. 2018; Solarova et al. 2020), and the toxicity especially on animals or human health was mentioned. One of the most studied secondary metabolites of lichen is usnic acid. This dibenzofuran is synthesized only by lichens and cannot be found in another organisms (Ingolfsdottir 2002). There is still a lack of information about degradation or absorption of usnic acid; nevertheless its toxic effect on the human liver is well-known (Wegrzyn et al. 2019). The mechanism of usnic acid toxicity was described *in vitro* by uncoupling of oxidative phosphorylation in liver mitochondria (Araujo et al. 2015). There is still a lack of information about usnic acid metabolism *in vivo*. There are only few studies on human liver fraction after incubation with indication of the presence oxidized metabolites and two glucuronide conjugates (Foti et al. 2008). Another *in vitro* study on human, rat, and mouse microsomes showed that usnic acid changed into two reactive metabolites and formed a product with glutathione (Piska et al. 2018). Another metabolite, atranorin, has been shown to have no toxicity in animal models (de Melo et al. 2011). The metabolic, pharmacokinetic, and pharmacodynamic parameters of lichen secondary metabolites in animals or human body need further studies.

21.9   SUMMARY POINTS

- This chapter focuses on the anticancer potential of the lichen *P. furfuracea.*
- Lichens are used nowadays around the world as ingredients in food, teas, or as herbs.
- *P. furfuracea* has historical use in traditional medicine.
- *P. furfuracea* extract or identified secondary metabolites possess anticancer or anti-angiogenic potential.
- *P. furfuracea* extract led to the phosphorylation of MAPK kinases, including p38 MAPK, JNK, and PI3K/Akt as the results of oxidative stress, and the activation of these kinases corresponds to the pro-apoptotic effect in cancer models.

REFERENCES

Airaksinen, M.M., Peura, P., Ala-Fossi-Salokangas, L., Antere, S., Lukkarinen, J., Saikkonen, M., Stenback, F., 1986. Toxicity of plant material used as emergency food during famines in Finland. Journal of Ethnopharmacology, 18(3), 273–296.

Amoreux, P.J., 1787. Recherches et Expe´rences sur les Diverses Especies de Lichens, Dont on peut faire usage en Me´decine et dans les Arts. In: G.F. Hoffmann (Ed.), Mémoires sur l'utilité des lichens dans la médecine et dans les arts. Chez Piestre et Delamollie're, Lyon, pp. 1–103.

Aoussar, N., Laasri, F.E., Bourhia, M., Manoljovic, N., Mhand, R.A., Rhallabi, N., Ullah, R., Shahat, A.A., Noman, O.M., Nasr, F.A., Almarfadi, O.M., El Mzibri, M., Vasiljevic, P., Benbacer, L., Mellouki, F., 2020. Phytochemical analysis, cytotoxic, antioxidant, and antibacterial activities of lichens. Evidence-Based Complementary and Alternative Medicine, 2020, 1–11.

Araujo, A.A., de Melo, M.G., Rabelo, T.K., Nunes, P.S., Santos, S.L., Serafini, M.R., Santos, M.R., Quintans-Junior, L.J., Gelain, D.P., 2015. Review of the biological properties and toxicity of usnic acid. Natural Product Research, 29(23), 2167–2180.

Atanasov, A.G., Zotchev, S.B., Dirsch, V.M., International Natural Product Sciences, T., Supuran, C.T., 2021. Natural products in drug discovery: Advances and opportunities. Nat Rev Drug Discov, 20(3), 200–216.

Bai, L., Bao, H.Y., Bau, T., 2014. Isolation and identification of a new benzofuranone derivative from *Usnea longissima*. Natural Product Research, 28(8), 534–538.

Bauhin, J., Cherler, J.H., 1650. Historiae plantarum universalis. Tomus I [section 2]. Liber VII, 2. Typographia Caldoriana, Ebroduni, pp. 1–449.

Baumann, B.B., 1960. The botanical aspects of Ancient Egyptian embalming and burial. Economic Botany, 14, 84–104.

Bedard, P.L., Hyman, D.M., Davids, M.S., Siu, L.L., 2020. Small molecules, big impact: 20 years of targeted therapy in oncology. Lancet, 395(10229), 1078–1088.

Bishayee, A., Mandal, A., Bhattacharyya, P., Bhatia, D., 2016. Pomegranate exerts chemoprevention of experimentally induced mammary tumorigenesis by suppression of cell proliferation and induction of apoptosis. Nutrition and Cancer, 68(1), 120–130.

Bown, D., 2001. Encyclopedia of Herbs and Their Uses. Dorling Kindersley, London, pp. 1–424.

Campbell, K., Casanova, J., 2016. A common framework for EMT and collective cell migration. Development, 143(23), 4291–4300.

Chaudhury, R.R., Rafei, U.M., 2002. Traditional Medicine in Asia. Volume 39. World Health Organization Publications, Regional Office for South-East Asia, New Delhi, India, pp. 1–309.

Chen, X.Y., Zhou, J., Luo, L.P., Han, B., Li, F., Chen, J.Y., Zhu, Y.F., Chen, W., Yu, X.P., 2015. Black rice anthocyanins suppress metastasis of breast cancer cells by targeting RAS/RAF/MAPK pathway. BioMed Research International, 2015, 414250.

Crawford, S.D., 2019. Lichens used in traditional medicine. In: B. Ranković (Ed.), Lichen Secondary Metabolites: Bioactive Properties and Pharmaceutical Potential. Springer International Publishing, Cham, pp. 31–97.

Culberson, C.F., Elix, J.A., 1989. Lichen substances. In: J.B. Harbone (Ed.), Methods in Plant Biochemistry. Academic Press, London, pp. 509–535.

Dar, T.U.H., Dar, S.A., Islam, S.U., Mangral, Z.A., Dar, R., Singh, B.P., Verma, P., Haque, S., 2021. Lichens as a repository of bioactive compounds: An open window for green therapy against diverse cancers. Semin Cancer Biol, 86, 1120–1137.

de Melo, M.G.D., Araujo, A.A.D., Serafini, M.R., Carvalho, L.F., Bezerra, M.S., Ramos, C.S., Bonjardim, L.R., Albuquerque-Junior, R.L.C., Lima, J.T., Siqueira, R.S., Fortes, V.S., Fonseca, M.J.V., Quintans-Junior, L.J., 2011. Anti-inflammatory and toxicity studies of atranorin extracted from *Cladina kalbii* Ahti in rodents. Braz J Pharm Sci, 47(4), 861–872.

De Natale, A., Pollio, A., 2012. A forgotten collection: The Libyan ethnobotanical exhibits (1912–14) by A. Trotter at the Museum O. Comes at the University Federico II in Naples, Italy. Journal of Ethnobiology and Ethnomedicine, 8(4), 1–19.

Emsen, B., Aslan, A., Togar, B., Turkez, H., 2016. In vitro antitumor activities of the lichen compounds olivetoric, physodic and psoromic acid in rat neuron and glioblastoma cells. Pharm Biol, 54(9), 1748–1762.

Emsen, B., Sadi, G., Bostanci, A., Aslan, A., 2020. In vitro evaluation of cytotoxic, oxidative, genotoxic, and apoptotic activities of physodic acid from *Pseudevernia furfuracea* in HepG2 and THLE2 cells. Plant Biosyst, 155(6), 1111–1120.

Emsen, B., Sadi, G., Bostanci, A., Gursoy, N., Emsen, A., Aslan, A., 2021. Evaluation of the biological activities of olivetoric acid, a lichen-derived molecule, in human hepatocellular carcinoma cells. Rendiconti Lincei-Scienze Fisiche E Naturali, 32(1), 135–148.

Emsen, B., Togar, B., Turkez, H., Aslan, A., 2018. Effects of two lichen acids isolated from *Pseudevernia furfuracea* (L.) Zopf in cultured human lymphocytes. Zeitschrift für Naturforschung Section C – A Journal of Biosciences, 73(7–8), 303–312.

Emsen, B., Turkez, H., Togar, B., Aslan, A., 2017. Evaluation of antioxidant and cytotoxic effects of olivetoric and physodic acid in cultured human amnion fibroblasts. Hum Exp Toxicol, 36(4), 376–385.

Ferlay, J., Colombet, M., Soerjomataram, I., Parkin, D.M., Piñeros, M., Znaor, A., Bray, F., 2021. Cancer statistics for the year 2020: An overview. International Journal of Cancer, 149(4), 778–789.

Firenzuoli, F., Gori, L., 2007. European traditional medicine – International Congress – Introductory statement. Evidence-Based Complementary and Alternative Medicine, 4(S1), 3–4.

Foti, R.S., Dickmann, L.J., Davis, J.A., Greene, R.J., Hill, J.J., Howard, M.L., Pearson, J.T., Rock, D.A., Tay, J.C., Wahlstrom, J.L., Slatter, J.G., 2008. Metabolism and related human risk factors for hepatic damage by usnic acid containing nutritional supplements. Xenobiotica; The Fate of Foreign Compounds in Biological Systems, 38(3), 264–280.

Galun, M., Shomer-Ilan, A., 1988. Secondary metabolic products. In: M. Galun (Ed.), CRC Handbook of Lichenology. CRC Press, Boca Raton, p. 6.

Goga, M., Elecko, J., Marcincinova, M., Rucova, D., Backorova, M., Backor, M., 2018. Lichen metabolites: An overview of some secondary metabolites and their biological potential. In: J.M. Merillon, K.G. Ramawat (Eds.), Co-Evolution of Secondary Metabolites. Reference Series in Phytochemistry. Springer Nature, Cham, pp. 1–36.

Gomez-Serranillos, M.P., Fernandez-Moriano, C., Gonzalez-Burgos, E., Divakar, P.K., Crespo, A., 2014. Parmeliaceae family: Phytochemistry, pharmacological potential and phylogenetic features. Rsc Advances, 4(103), 59017–59047.

González-Tejero, M.R., Martínez-Lirola, M.J., Casares-Porcel, M., Molero-Mesa, J., 1995. Three lichens used in popular medicine in Eastern Andalucia (Spain). Economic Botany, 49(1), 96–98.

Gu, J.W., Makey, K.L., Tucker, K.B., Chinchar, E., Mao, X.W., Pei, I., Thomas, E.Y., Miele, L., 2013. EGCG, a major green tea catechin suppresses breast tumor angiogenesis and growth via inhibiting the activation of HIF-1 alpha and NF kappa B, and VEGF expression. Vasc Cell, 5(9), 1–10.

Guvenc, A., Akkol, E.K., Suntar, I., Keles, H., Yildiz, S., Calis, I., 2012. Biological activities of *Pseudevernia furfuracea* (L.) Zopf extracts and isolation of the active compounds. Journal of Ethnopharmacology, 144(3), 726–734.

Hanahan, D., Coussens, L.M., 2012. Accessories to the crime: Functions of cells recruited to the tumor microenvironment. Cancer Cell, 21(3), 309–322.

Huang, X.J., Ma, J.B., Wei, L.X., Song, J.Y., Li, C., Yang, H.X., Du, Y.Z., Gao, T.T., Bi, H.T., 2018. An antioxidant alpha-glucan from *Cladina rangiferina* (L) Nyl. and its protective effect on alveolar epithelial cells from Pb2+-induced oxidative damage. Int J Biol Macromol, 112, 101–109.

Ingelfinger, R., Henke, M., Roser, L., Ulshofer, T., Calchera, A., Singh, G., Parnham, M.J., Geisslinger, G., Furst, R., Schmitt, I., Schiffmann, S., 2020. Unraveling the pharmacological potential of lichen extracts in the context of cancer and inflammation with a broad screening approach. Front Pharmacol, 11(1322).

Ingolfsdottir, K., 2002. Usnic acid. Phytochemistry, 61(7), 729–736.

Jiang, X., Wang, J., Deng, X., Xiong, F., Zhang, S., Gong, Z., Li, X., Cao, K., Deng, H., He, Y., Liao, Q., Xiang, B., Zhou, M., Guo, C., Zeng, Z., Li, G., Li, X., Xiong, W., 2020. The role of microenvironment in tumor angiogenesis. J Exp Clin Cancer Res, 39(1), 204.

Joulain, D., Tabacchi, R., 2009a. Lichen extracts as raw materials in perfumery. Part 1: Oakmoss. Flavour and Fragrance Journal, 24(2), 49–61.

Joulain, D., Tabacchi, R., 2009b. Lichen extracts as raw materials in perfumery. Part 2: Treemoss. Flavour and Fragrance Journal, 24(3), 105–116.

Ju, Y., Zhuo, J.X., Liu, B., Long, C.L., 2013. Eating from the wild: Diversity of wild edible plants used by Tibetans in Shangri-la region, Yunnan, China. Journal of Ethnobiology and Ethnomedicine, 9(28), 1–22.

Kalle, R., Soukand, R., 2012. Historical ethnobotanical review of wild edible plants of Estonia (1770s–1960s). Acta Soc Bot Pol, 81(4), 271–281.

Katz, L., Baltz, R.H., 2016. Natural product discovery: Past, present, and future. J Ind Microbiol Biotechnol, 43(2–3), 155–176.

Kekuda, T.R.P., Vinayaka, K.S., Swathi, D., Suchitha, Y., Venugopal, T.M., Mallikarjun, N., 2011. Mineral composition, total phenol content and antioxidant activity of a macrolichen *Everniastrum cirrhatum* (Fr.) Hale (Parmeliaceae). E-J Chem, 8(4), 1886–1894.

Kello, M., Kuruc, T., Petrova, K., Goga, M., Michalova, Z., Coma, M., Rucova, D., Mojzis, J., 2021. Pro-apoptotic potential of *Pseudevernia furfuracea* (L.) Zopf extract and isolated physodic acid in acute lymphoblastic leukemia model in vitro. Pharmaceutics, 13(12), 2173.

Koparal, A.T., Ulus, G., Zeytinoglu, M., Tay, T., Turk, A.O., 2010. Angiogenesis inhibition by a lichen compound olivetoric acid. Phytother Res, 24(5), 754–758.

Kosanic, M., Manojlovic, N., Jankovic, S., Stanojkovic, T., Rankovic, B., 2013. *Evernia prunastri* and *Pseudevernia furfuraceae* lichens and their major metabolites as antioxidant, antimicrobial and anticancer agents. Food Chem Toxicol, 53, 112–118.

Kubatka, P., Kapinova, A., Kello, M., Kruzliak, P., Kajo, K., Vybohova, D., Mahmood, S., Murin, R., Viera, T., Mojzis, J., Zulli, A., Pec, M., Adamkov, M., Kassayova, M., Bojkova, B., Stollarova, N., Dobrota, D., 2016a. Fruit peel polyphenols demonstrate substantial anti-tumor effects in the model of breast cancer. Eur J Nutr, 55(3), 955–965.

Kubatka, P., Kapinova, A., Kruzliak, P., Kello, M., Vybohova, D., Kajo, K., Novak, M., Chripkova, M., Adamkov, M., Pec, M., Mojzis, J., Bojkova, B., Kassayova, M., Stollarova, N., Dobrota, D., 2015. Antineoplastic effects of *Chlorella pyrenoidosa* in the breast cancer model. Nutrition, 31(4), 560–569.

Kubatka, P., Kello, M., Kajo, K., Kruzliak, P., Vybohova, D., Mojzis, J., Adamkov, M., Fialova, S., Veizerova, L., Zulli, A., Pec, M., Statelova, D., Grancai, D., Busselberg, D., 2017a. Oregano demonstrates distinct tumor-suppressive effects in the breast carcinoma model. Eur J Nutr, 56(3), 1303–1316.

Kubatka, P., Kello, M., Kajo, K., Kruzliak, P., Vybohova, D., Smejkal, K., Marsik, P., Zulli, A., Gonciova, G., Mojzis, J., Kapinova, A., Murin, R., Pec, M., Adamkov, M., Przygodzki, R.M., 2016b. Young Barley indicates antitumor effects in experimental breast cancer in vivo and in vitro. Nutrition and Cancer, 68(4), 611–621.

Kubatka, P., Kello, M., Kajo, K., Samec, M., Jasek, K., Vybohova, D., Uramova, S., Liskova, A., Sadlonova, V., Koklesova, L., Murin, R., Adamkov, M., Smejkal, K., Svajdlenka, E., Solar, P., Samuel, S.M., Kassayova, M., Kwon, T.K., Zubor, P., Pec, M., Danko, J., Busselberg, D., Mojzis, J., 2020. Chemopreventive and therapeutic efficacy of *Cinnamomum zeylanicum* L. bark in experimental breast carcinoma: Mechanistic in vivo and in vitro analyses. Molecules, 25(6), 1399.

Kubatka, P., Kello, M., Kajo, K., Samec, M., Liskova, A., Jasek, K., Koklesova, L., Kuruc, T., Adamkov, M., Smejkal, K., Svajdlenka, E., Solar, P., Pec, M., Busselberg, D., Sadlonova, V., Mojzis, J., 2021. *Rhus coriaria* L. (Sumac) demonstrates oncostatic activity in the therapeutic and preventive model of breast carcinoma. Int J Mol Sci, 22(1), 183.

Kubatka, P., Uramova, S., Kello, M., Kajo, K., Kruzliak, P., Mojzis, J., Vybohova, D., Adamkov, M., Jasek, K., Lasabova, Z., Zubor, P., Fialova, S., Dokupilova, S., Solar, P., Pec, M., Adamicova, K., Danko, J., Adamek, M., Busselberg, D., 2017b. Antineoplastic effects of clove buds (*Syzygium aromaticum* L.) in the model of breast carcinoma. J Cell Mol Med, 21(11), 2837–2851.

Kubatka, P., Uramova, S., Kello, M., Kajo, K., Samec, M., Jasek, K., Vybohova, D., Liskova, A., Mojzis, J., Adamkov, M., Zubor, P., Smejkal, K., Svajdlenka, E., Solar, P., Samuel, S.M., Zulli, A., Kassayova, M., Lasabova, Z., Kwon, T.K., Pec, M., Danko, J., Busselberg, D., 2019. Anticancer activities of *Thymus vulgaris* L. in experimental breast carcinoma in vivo and in vitro. Int J Mol Sci, 20(7), 1749.

Launert, E., 1981. Edible and Medicinal Plants. Hamlyn, London, pp. 1–288.

Lebail, J.B.E.F., 1853. Des lichens, considérés sous le point de vue é conomique, médical, et physiologique (nutrition). M.D. thesis, pp. 1–42.

Llano, G.A., 1948. Economic uses of lichens. Economic Botany, 2, 15–45.

López Eire, A., Cortés Gabaudan, F., Gutiérrez Rodilla, B.M., Vázquez de Benito, M.C., 2006. Estudios y Traducción. Dioscórides. Sobre los remedios medicinales Manuscrito de Salamanca. Ediciones Universidad, Spain, Salamanca, pp. 1–498.

Lugano, R., Ramachandran, M., Dimberg, A., 2020. Tumor angiogenesis: Causes, consequences, challenges and opportunities. Cell Mol Life Sci, 77(9), 1745–1770.

Malhotra, S., Subban, R., Singh, A., 2007. Lichens- role in traditional medicine and drug discovery. The Internet Journal of Alternative Medicine, 5(2), 1–6.

Masuelli, L., Benvenuto, M., Fantini, M., Marzocchella, L., Sacchetti, P., Di Stefano, E., Tresoldi, I., Izzi, V., Bernardini, R., Palumbo, C., Mattei, M., Lista, F., Galvano, F., Modesti, A., Bei, R., 2013. Curcumin induces apoptosis in breast cancer cell lines and delays the growth of mammary tumors in neu transgenic mice. J Biol Reg Homeos Ag, 27(1), 105–119.

Mitrovic, T., Stamenkovic, S., Cvetkovic, V., Radulovic, N., Mladenovic, M., Stankovic, M., Topuzovic, M., Radojevic, I., Stefanovic, O., Vasic, S., Comic, L., 2014. *Platismatia glauca* and *Pseudevernia furfuracea* lichens as sources of antioxidant, antimicrobial and antibiofilm agents. Excli Journal, 13, 938–953.

Moxham, T.H., 1986. The commercial exploitation of lichens for the perfume industry. In: E.J. Brunke (Ed.), Progress in Essential Oil Research. Walter de Gruyter, Berlin, pp. 491–503.

Müller, J., 1881. Lichenologische Beiträge. In: P. Poschlod (Ed.), Flora oder Allgemeine Botanische Zeitung. Regensburgische Botanische Gesellschaft, Regensburg, pp. 512–527.

Niemeyer, K., Bell, I.R., Koithan, M., 2013. Traditional knowledge of Western herbal medicine and complex systems science. J Herb Med, 3(3), 112–119.

Pereira, J., 1853. The Elements of Material Medica and Therapeutics. 2, Lea and Blanchard, Philadelphia, pp. 1–852.

Petrova, K., Kello, M., Kuruc, T., Backorova, M., Petrovova, E., Vilkova, M., Goga, M., Rucova, D., Backor, M., Mojzis, J., 2021. Potential effect of *Pseudevernia furfuracea* (L.) Zopf extract and metabolite physodic acid on tumor microenvironment modulation in MCF-10A cells. Biomolecules, 11(3), 420.

Piska, K., Galanty, A., Koczurkiewicz, P., Zmudzki, P., Potaczek, J., Podolak, I., Pekala, E., 2018. Usnic acid reactive metabolites formation in human, rat, and mice microsomes: Implication for hepatotoxicity. Food Chem Toxicol, 120, 112–118.

Proksa, B., Adamcova, J., Sturdikova, M., Fuska, J., 1994. Metabolites of *Pseudevernia furfuracea* (L.) Zopf and their inhibition potential of proteolytic enzymes. Pharmazie, 49(4), 282–283.

Richardson, D.H.S., 1974. The Vanishing Lichens: Their History and Importance. Hafner Press, New York, pp. 1–231.

Rucova, D., Goga, M., Sabovljevic, M., Vilkova, M., Petrulova, V., Backor, M., 2019. Insights into physiological responses of mosses *Physcomitrella patens* and *Pohlia drummondii* to lichen secondary metabolites. Protoplasma, 256(6), 1585–1595.

Rundel, P.W., 1978. Ecological role of secondary lichen substances. Biochemical Systematics and Ecology, 6(3), 157–170.

Schmull, M., Brown, D.L., 2009. *Pseudevernia furfuracea*, the mummy's lichen at the Farlow Herbarium. Opuscula Philolichenum, 6, 45–50.

Seklic, D.S., Jovanovic, M.M., 2022. *Platismatia glauca* – lichen species with suppressive properties on migration and invasiveness of two different colorectal carcinoma cell lines. Journal of Food Biochemistry, e14096.

Seklic, D.S., Jovanovic, M.M., Virijevic, K.D., Grujic, J.N., Zivanovic, M.N., Markovic, S.D., 2022. *Pseudevernia furfuracea* inhibits migration and invasion of colorectal carcinoma cell lines. Journal of Ethnopharmacology, 284, 114758.

Seklic, D.S., Obradovic, A.D., Stankovic, M.S., Zivanovic, M.N., Mitrovic, T.L.J., Stamenkovic, S.M., Markovic, S.D., 2018. Proapoptotic and antimigratory effects of *Pseudevernia furfuracea* and *Platismatia glauca* on colon cancer cell lines. Food Technology and Biotechnology, 56(3), 421–430.

Senft, E., 1911. The so-called "Lichen Quercinus virides." Pharmazeutische Post, 43, 1017–1019.

Shukla, I., Azmi, L., Gautam, A., Shukla S.K., Rao C.V., 2018. Lichens are the next promising candidates for medicinally active compounds. Int J Phytopharm, 8(4), 31–38.

Simkova, K., Polesny, Z., 2015. Ethnobotanical review of wild edible plants used in the Czech Republic. J Appl Bot Food Qual, 88, 49–67.

Singletary, K., MacDonald, C., Wallig, M., 1996. Inhibition by rosemary and carnosol of 7,12-dimethylbenz[a] anthracene (DMBA)-induced rat mammary tumorigenesis and in vivo DMBA-DNA adduct formation. Cancer Letters, 104(1), 43–48.

Smith, A.L., 1921. Lichens. Cambridge University Press, London, pp. 1–492.

Solarova, Z., Liskova, A., Samec, M., Kubatka, P., Busselberg, D., Solar, P., 2020. Anticancer Potential of Lichens' Secondary Metabolites. Biomolecules, 10(1), 87.

Solhaug, K.A., Lind, M., Nybakken, L., Gauslaa, Y., 2009. Possible functional roles of cortical depsides and medullary depsidones in the foliose lichen *Hypogymnia physodes*. Flora, 204(1), 40–48.

Stenroos, S., Velmala, S., Pykälä, J., Ahi, T., 2016. Lichens of Finland. Norrlinia, 30, Finnish Museum of Natural History, Helsinki, Finland, pp. 1–896.

Stocker-Worgotter, E., 2008. Metabolic diversity of lichen-forming ascomycetous fungi: Culturing, polyketide and shikimate metabolite production, and PKS genes. Natural Product Reports, 25(1), 188–190.

Suleyman, H., Odabasoglu, F., Aslan, A., Cakir, A., Karagoz, Y., Gocer, F., Halici, M., Bayir, Y., 2003. Anti-inflammatory and antiulcerogenic effects of the aqueous extract of *Lobaria pulmonaria* (L.) Hoffm. Phytomedicine: International Journal of Phytotherapy and Phytopharmacology, 10(6–7), 552–557.

Tas, I., Yildirim, A.B., Ozkan, E., Ozyigitoglu, G.C., Yavuz, M.Z., Turker, A.U., 2019. Biological Evaluation and Phytochemical Profiling of Some Lichen Species. Acta Alimentaria, 48(4), 457–465.

Tekiela, A., Furmanek, Ł., Andrusiewicz, M., Bara, G., Seaward, M.R.D., Kapusta, I., Czarnota, P., 2021. Can lichen secondary compounds impact upon the pathogenic soil fungi *Fusarium oxysporum* and *F. avenaceum*? Folia Cryptogamica Estonica, 58, 165–181.

Teleanu, R.I., Chircov, C., Grumezescu, A.M., Teleanu, D.M., 2020. Tumor angiogenesis and anti-angiogenic strategies for cancer treatment. Journal of Clinical Medicine, 9(1), 84.

Thell, A., Moberg, R., 2011. Nordic Lichen Flora. Parmeliaceae, 4. Nordic Lichen Society, Göteborg, Sweden, pp. 1–184.

Turk, H., Yilmaz, M., Tay, T., Turk, A.O., Kivanc, M., 2006. Antimicrobial activity of extracts of chemical races of the lichen *Pseudevernia furfuracea* and their physodic acid, chloroatranorin, atranorin, and olivetoric acid constituents. Z Naturforsch C, 61(7–8), 499–507.

Ulus, G., 2021. Antiangiogenic properties of lichen secondary metabolites. Phytother Res, 35(6), 3046–3058.

Upreti, D.K., Chatterjee, S., 2007. Significance of lichens and their secondary metabolites: A review. In: B.N. Ganguli, S.K. Deshmukh (Eds.), Fungi: Multifaceted Microbes. Anamaya Publishers, Lado Sarai, Delhi, pp. 169–188.

Urena-Vacas, I., Gonzalez-Burgos, E., Divakar, P.K., Gomez-Serranillos, M.P., 2021. Lichen depsidones with biological interest. Planta Med, 1–26.

Varol, M., Tay, T., Candan, M., Turk, A., Koparal, A.T., 2015. Evaluation of the sunscreen lichen substances usnic acid and atranorin. Biocell, 39(1), 25–31.

Vu, T., Datta, P.K., 2017. Regulation of EMT in colorectal cancer: A culprit in metastasis. Cancers (Basel), 9(12), 171.

Wang, L.S., Qian, Z.G., 2013. Zhong guo yao yong di yi tu jian [Illustrated Medicinal Lichens of China]. Yunnan Science and Technology Press, Yunnan, China, pp. 1–200.

Wang, T., Bengtsson, G., Karnefelt, I., Bjorn, L.O., 2001. Provitamins and vitamins D-2 and D-3 in *Cladina* spp. over a latitudinal gradient: possible correlation with UV levels (vol 62, pg 118, 2001). J Photoch Photobio B, 65(1), 85.

Weber, C.E., Kothari, A.N., Wai, P.Y., Li, N.Y., Driver, J., Zapf, M.A., Franzen, C.A., Gupta, G.N., Osipo, C., Zlobin, A., Syn, W.K., Zhang, J., Kuo, P.C., Mi, Z., 2015. Osteopontin mediates an MZF1-TGF-beta1-dependent transformation of mesenchymal stem cells into cancer-associated fibroblasts in breast cancer. Oncogene, 34(37), 4821–4833.

Wegrzyn, M.H., Wietrzyk-Pelka, P., Galanty, A., Cykowska-Marzencka, B., Sundset, M.A., 2019. Incomplete degradation of lichen usnic acid and atranorin in Svalbard reindeer (*Rangifer tarandus platyrhynchus*). Polar Res, 38.

Zambare, V.P., Christopher, L.P., 2012. Biopharmaceutical potential of lichens. Pharm Biol, 50(6), 778–798.

Zhao, Y.S., Wang, M.F., Xu, B.J., 2021. A comprehensive review on secondary metabolites and health-promoting effects of edible lichen. J Funct Foods, 80.

Zwelfer, J., 1672. Pharmacopoeia augustana. Apud Vincentium Caimax, Dordrechti, Italy, pp. 1–239.

22 Turmeric (*Curcuma longa*) and Applications to Cancer Studies

A Focus on the Molecular Effects of Curcumin in Colorectal Cancer

Fereshteh Asgharzadeh and Maryam Moradi Binabaj

ABBREVIATIONS

CDK	cyclin-dependent kinase
COX-2	cyclooxygenase-2
CRC	colorectal cancer
EMT	epithelial–mesenchymal transition
ER	endoplasmic reticulum
erythroid-derived 2-related factor 2	nuclear factor NRF-2
HIF-1	hypoxia-inducible factor 1
IL	interleukin
iNOS	inducible nitric oxide synthesis
MMP	matrix-degrading proteinase
NF-κB	nuclear factor kappa B
ROS	reactive oxygen species
Th	helper T
Treg	regulatory T
VEGF	vascular endothelial growth factor

22.1 INTRODUCTION

22.1.1 COLORECTAL CANCER

Colorectal cancer (CRC) is one of the most common type of cancers worldwide and one of the most common causes of cancer mortality in the general population (Bahrami, Moradi Binabaj, and Ferns 2021). The 5-year survival rate of patients with CRC is 64.9%, and the length of survival is dependent on several factors including age, race/ethnicity, and stage of diagnosis. There are different treatment options for CRC treatment including surgery, chemotherapy, and radiotherapy. However, the prognosis of CRC patients is still unsatisfactory because of the numerous drug-induced side effects and toxicity (Asgharzadeh et al. 2018). Clearly, further research and effective therapeutic approaches are needed for a successful treatment.

22.2 CURCUMIN

22.2.1 Chemical Composition and Properties

Turmeric (*Curcuma longa*), also called *C. domestica*, is a perennial herbaceous plant that belongs to the ginger family (Zingiberaceae). Its major bioactive component is the yellow pigment curcumin (Figure 22.1) (Priyadarsini 2014).

Curcumin (diferuloylmethane), a hydrophobic polyphenol phytochemical, is the main active compound of the turmeric herb rhizome (*C. longa*). The chemical structure of curcumin was first identified in 1910 with the molecular formula of $C_{21}H_{20}O_6$ and molecular weight of 368.37 g/mol (Figure 22.2) (Aggarwal, Kumar, and Bharti 2003).

It has been shown that natural extracts of *C. longa* contain three different curcuminoids including curcumin (77%), demethoxycurcumin (17%), and bis-demethoxycurcumin (3%).

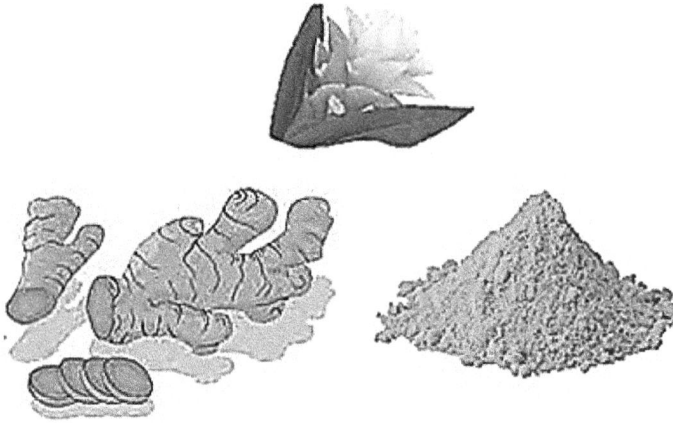

FIGURE 22.1 Turmeric (*Curcuma longa*) and its bioactive component, curcumin.

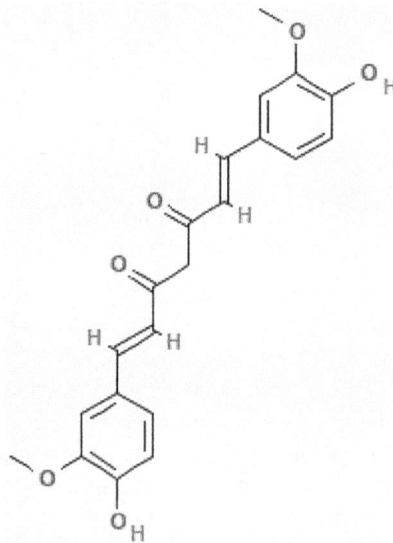

FIGURE 22.2 Chemical structure of curcumin.

Curcumin is typically yellow in color, which is due to the presence of curcuminoids. Curcumin is used in food industries widely as a food color additive and a popular spice and food flavoring agent (de Porras, Layos, and Martínez-Balibrea 2021). It also contains different mineral elements as well as organic molecules including carbohydrates, proteins, and fats (Shehzad, Wahid, and Lee 2010).

Due to the hydrophobic nature of curcumin, it can diffuse inside the cell through the cell membrane and be distributed in different cellular compartments such as the endoplasmic reticulum, mitochondria, and nucleus, where it can exert its biological activity (Jaruga et al. 1998).

22.2.2 Delivery of Curcumin

There are various routes of curcumin delivery which modulate the efficacy of its absorption, biodistribution, and bioavailability. It has been shown that oral delivery of curcumin has different biological properties, especially anticancer effects (Ryan et al. 2013). In subcutaneous delivery, the observed level of curcumin in tissue is maintained (Shahani et al. 2010). In intraperitoneal delivery form, curcumin injection exerts antitumor activity via decreasing inflammatory fibrotic marker levels *in vivo* (Tu et al. 2012). The other forms of curcumin delivery are topical and nasal administration (Sun, Zhao, and Hu 2013).

22.2.3 Curcumin Formulation

There are different studies showing that curcumin has low absorption, biodistribution, and bioavailability. Thus, in seeking to find novel ways to overcome these barriers, numerous studies are in progress. There are now different formulation approaches and techniques to optimize and solve such problems including nanoparticles, liposomes, micelles, and phospholipid complexes of curcumin (Prasad, Tyagi, and Aggarwal 2014). A nanoparticle drug delivery–based system increases curcumin solubility and dispersion in aqueous solution in comparison to curcumin suspension (Guzman-Villanueva et al. 2013). Moreover, the nanoparticle form of curcumin increases its concentration in plasma (i.e., bioavailability) (Cheng, Yeung, et al. 2013). Another example of curcumin formulation is polylactic-co-glycolic acid resulting in more enhanced cellular uptake, half-life, and bioavailability (Khalil et al. 2013). In the liposome encapsulated form of curcumin, its bioavailability and uptake is increased in comparison to free curcumin (Zhang et al. 2012). The other delivery forms of curcumin are cyclodextrin and piperine (Figure 22.3) (Rachmawati, Edityaningrum, and Mauludin 2013).

22.2.4 Molecular Targets of Curcumin

Curcumin and its main biological active components have been shown to exert various antitumoral effects against via modulating different signaling pathways including oxidative stress and angiogenesis (Moradi-Marjaneh et al. 2018), metastasis (Zhang et al. 2018), and inflammation (Porro et al. 2019). It also regulates different targets and process involved in cellular pathways such as cell cycle (Zhang et al. 2015), proliferation (Teiten et al. 2011), apoptosis (Khan et al. 2020), migration (Wang et al. 2020), and invasion (Lu et al. 2021) (Figure 22.4).

It is well established that curcumin has chemoprevention and chemotherapy potential in different types of cancer, including gastrointestinal (Hashemzehi et al. 2018), ovarian (Weir et al. 2007), leukemia (Li et al. 2018), and prostate (Mukhopadhyay et al. 2001). Moreover, several published studies have been shown that curcumin has synergistic effects in combination with other anticancer drugs (DiMarco-Crook et al. 2020; Patra et al. 2021; Xu et al. 2020). As a result, there is currently extensive interest toward clinical development of curcumin as an anticancer compound.

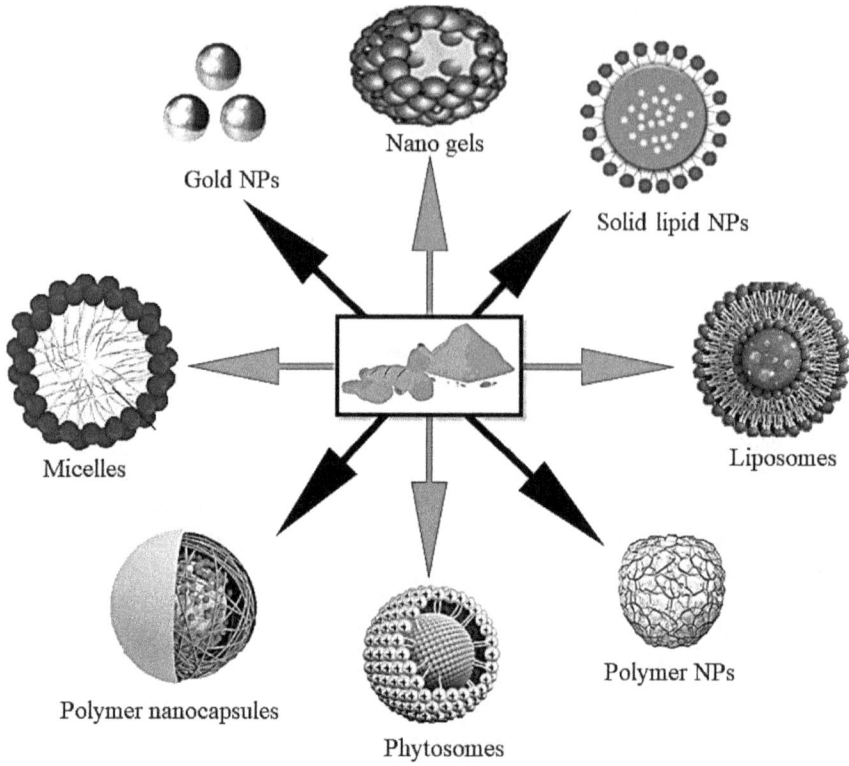

FIGURE 22.3   Nano formulations of curcumin used in colorectal cancer.

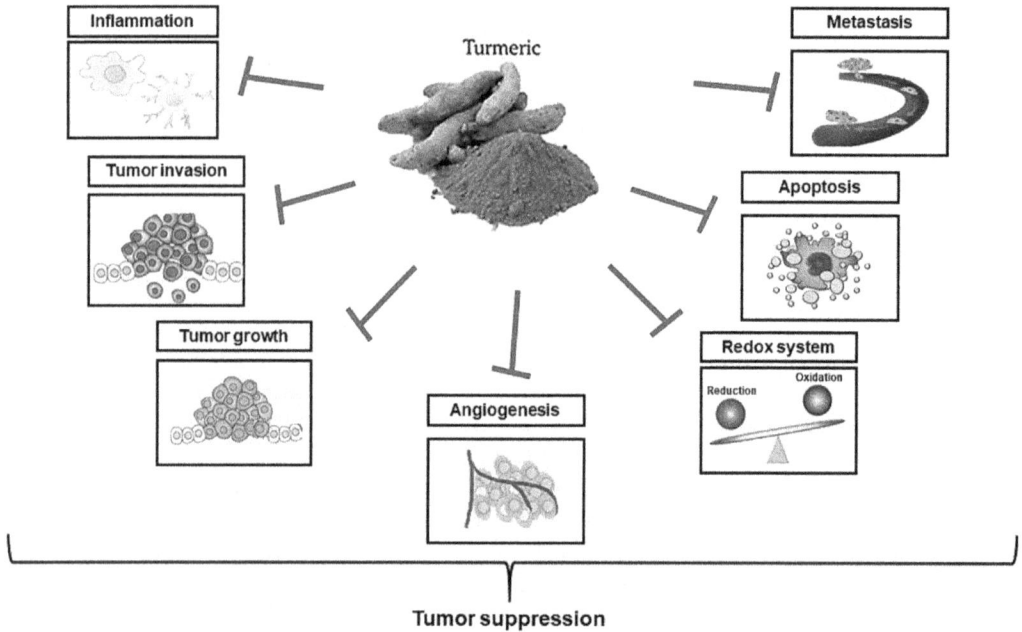

FIGURE 22.4   An overview of molecular pathways modulated by curcumin in colorectal cancer.

22.3 ANTI-CARCINOGENIC PROPERTIES OF CURCUMIN ON CRC

22.3.1 INFLAMMATION

The three phases of carcinogenesis are initiation, promotion, and progression (Park and Conteas 2010) (Figure 22.5).

CRC development is known to be influenced by inflammation (de Porras, Layos, and Martínez-Balibrea 2021). Chronic inflammation and oxidative stress are responsible for cancer initiation via inducing proliferating signals and apoptosis inhibition (Surh et al. 2005). Inflammation plays a key role in the initiation and progression of cancer through cytokine production (Park and Conteas 2010). Tumor cells can proliferate, invade, and metastasize as a result of cytokines, antigenic factors, and matrix-degrading proteases release by leukocytes. Lymphocytes infiltrating from tumors produce a matrix-degrading proteinase (MMP-9), which increases growth and invasion of tumor cells (Park and Conteas 2010). Tumor growth and proliferation are affected by the pathways activated by NF-κB upregulators, as well as resistance to anticancer drugs, radiation, and death cytokines (Luo, Kamata, and Karin 2005). Inhibition of NF-κB, as well as other molecular targets, is thought to be the mechanism by which curcumin inhibits carcinogenesis (Table 22.1).

The effects of curcumin on tumor initiation are multifaceted. NF-κB or its inhibition seems to be a common component of many of these treatments. The fact is that curcumin's ability to inhibit the NF-κB pathway activation (Shanmugam et al. 2015) is largely responsible for its anti-inflammatory and antitumor properties, which have been reported to cause drug resistance in CRC representing a major causative factor for drug resistance (Patel et al. 2018). Curcumin inhibits NF-κB activity in CRC by downregulating thymidylate synthase, the receptor for 5-fluorouracil (Rajitha et al. 2016).

Chronic inflammation accelerates epithelial tumorigenesis, with NF-κB activation as the major mechanism (De Visser and Coussens 2005). The curcumin inhibits cell proliferation and cytokine production by inhibiting NF-κB targets involved in T cells and interleukin-2 production, and the production of nitric oxide in response to mitogens. Curcumin inhibits NF-κB induction and therefore reduces cytokine production induced by reduction in IL-10, IL-6, and IL-18 expression (Grandjean-Laquerriere et al. 2002).

Cancer cells infiltrate the colon as a result of a heterogeneous population of immune cells. These immune cells include pro-inflammatory cells like CD8+ cytotoxic T cells, type 1 CD4+ helper T

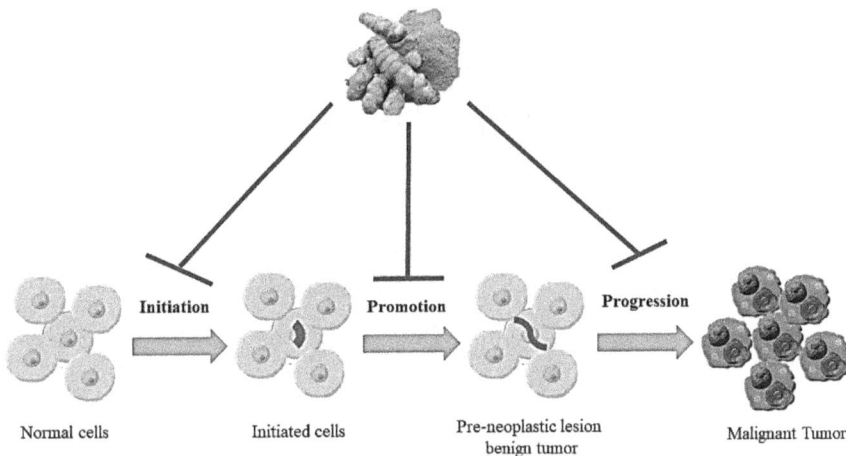

Fig 5

FIGURE 22.5 Curcumin inhibited the initiation, promotion, and progression processes of carcinogenesis of colorectal cancer.

TABLE 22.1

Antitumoral Activities of Curcumin in Colorectal Cancer

Biological Effects	Mechanisms of Action
Pro-Apoptotic	AMPK increase
	APC decrease
	Bax increase
	Bcl-2 decrease
	Bcl-xL decrease
	Caspase-3 activation
	Caspase-7 activation
	COX-2 decrease
	Cyclin D1 decrease
	DR5 upregulation
	E-cadherin decrease
	Fas-mediated caspase-8 activation
	IAP-2 decrease
	Mitochondrial [Ca^{2+}] increase
	Mitochondrial cytochrome c release
	Mitochondrial membrane potential reduction
	pAKT decrease
	β-catenin decrease
Antiproliferative	CDK2 decrease
	Cell cycle arrest at G1 phase
	Cell cycle arrest at G2/M phase
	Cell viability decrease
	Cyclin A decrease
	E2F4 decrease
	p21 and p27 increase
	p53 increase
	ROS increase
Antimetastatic	MMP2 decrease
	MMP9 decrease
	NF-κB signaling pathway inhibition
	TIMP-2 increase
Anti-Inflammation	Nf-κB inhibition
	5-lipoxygenase inhibition
	COX-1 and COX-2 inhibition
	ROS inhibition
	Cytokine decrease
Pro-Oxidant	Mitochondrial membranes lysis
	ROS increase
	MDA increase
	Total thiol increase
	SOD decrease
	CAT decrease
	Nrf2 decrease

(Th1) cells, NK cells, and M1 macrophages; and anti-inflammatory cells like regulatory T (Treg) cells, type 2 helper T (Th2) cells, M2 macrophages, and myeloid-derived suppressor cells (Väyrynen et al. 2013). A good prognosis is associated with the infiltration of the former. The latter are thought to negatively regulate the immune response. Treg cells are one of the most critical components in suppressing CD8$^+$ T cells and Th1 cells in tumor immune tolerance and evasion (Sakaguchi et al. 2008). PD-1/PD-L1 and CTLA-4 inhibitors may also be more effective if Treg cells are depleted. Therefore, depleting Treg cells are being studied as a possible medical treatment against cancer (Hoos 2016). Curcumin has been shown to modulate the expression of CTLA-4 and forkhead box protein while generating interferon gamma in Treg cells that possess antitumor effects (Sahebkar and Mohammadi 2019). In addition, Xiao and colleagues recently showed that curcumin increases antitumor T cell infiltration, greatly improving the antitumor immune response (Xiao et al. 2020).

22.3.2 OXIDATIVE STRESS

Reactive oxygen species (ROS, free radicals) create an environment that disrupts the balance between antioxidant defenses and ROS. Oxidative stress can be caused by accumulation of ROS and can affect cancer cell behavior via increasing the rate of mutation (Huang et al. 2017). It should be noted that cancer cells are more prone to acute induction of oxidative stress because they have higher basal levels of oxidative stress than normal cells (Cairns, Harris, and Mak 2011). High ROS levels can promote various pro-apoptotic signaling pathways, such as endoplasmic reticulum (ER) stress and mitochondrial dysfunction, resulting in impaired cell apoptosis or necrosis (Circu and Aw 2010). Different types of cancer cells are induced to apoptosis by ROS-mediated pathways (Huang et al. 2017). According to results, curcumin potentiate the efficacy of irinotecan-induced apoptosis, through changes in redox pathway proteomics. Furthermore, the combination of curcumin and irinotecan induced ROS production in LoVo/HT-29 cells in comparison to curcumin or irinotecan alone (Carini et al. 2017). The *N*-acetylcysteine pretreatment reversed almost perfectly the inhibition of cell growth and apoptosis in CRC cells, induced by ROS generation.

Activated neutrophils and macrophages produce ROS and reactive nitrogen species, leading to mutations and carcinogenesis (Park and Conteas 2010). There have been numerous studies showing that curcumin reduces inflammation. Considering that chronic inflammation is the result of oxidative stress, antioxidant compounds can help prevent and treat inflammatory disease. Similarly, curcumin's anti-inflammatory activity is unlikely to be dependent on its antioxidant activity, as it has a high antioxidant activity (Mansouri et al. 2020). It does not appear likely that curcumin's anti-inflammatory effects are as result of only antioxidant properties, since many of the antioxidants have been reported to have no anti-inflammatory qualities. Several mechanisms are involved in the action of curcumin as an anti-inflammatory factor. For instance, NF-κB activation is inhibited by curcumin (Wilken et al. 2011). NF-κB activity has been reported to be restored by curcumin in lab studies where it neutralizes oxidative stress caused by tumor formation. Curcumin inhibits TNF-α production, thus T-cell apoptosis caused by tumor will be minimized (Bhattacharyya et al. 2007). Researchers have shown that curcumin reduces the level of inducible nitric oxide synthesis (iNOS). Inhibition of nitric oxide synthase by curcumin and scavenger of free radicals such as nitric oxide is one of the benefits of curcumin. The activation of NF-κB induces the production of iNOS, one of the causes of oxidative stress, which plays a role in tumor initiation. Turmeric blocks NF-κB phosphorylation and degradation, which inhibits iNOS gene transcription by preventing the phosphorylation and degradation of inhibitor κBα (Park and Conteas 2010).

Phase II studies have shown that curcumin increases conjugation enzyme expression and suppress ROS-mediated activation of ROS-activated NF-κB, activator protein 1, and the mitogen-activated protein kinase. Sulfotransferases and glutathione-s-transferases, for example, conjugate toxic metabolites (through phase I enzymatic action) and eliminate them (Feng et al. 2005). In chemical carcinogenesis, turmeric inhibits the formation of aflatoxin B1-DNA adducts, an inhibitory step that plays an important role in cytochrome p450 functions. The levels of ornithine decarboxylase, glutathione, antioxidant enzymes, and phase II metabolic enzymes were found to be increased by curcumin when applied to various cancer models. The antioxidative effects of curcumin are mediated through its effect on nuclear factor (erythroid-derived 2)–related factor 2 (NRF-2) and NF-κB and can help reduce oxidative stress (Table 22.1) (Park and Conteas 2010).

It has been shown that colon cancer is a result of the subsequent progression of an adenoma to a carcinoma as a result of oxidative stress. There is still controversy about the effect of antioxidants on oxidative stress and CRC, but antioxidants have been implicated in promoting health in CRC studies for decades. Therefore, patients with CRC should consume antioxidants on almost a daily basis (Carini et al. 2017). For further understanding of dietary antioxidants and the development of CRC, larger studies involving CRC patients are required.

22.3.3 Apoptosis, Proliferation, and Progression

CRC is still largely treated with chemotherapy. Transcriptional and replication blockade by cytotoxic agents leads to repair of DNA damage and/or initiation of cell death (Agarwal et al. 2018).

Various signaling pathways are regulated by curcumin, causing tumor cell death. In summary, curcumin regulates intracellular ROS levels, promotes autophagy and apoptosis, induces G1 and G2 cell cycle arrests, and activates p53 through p21 mediated senescence (Pricci et al. 2020). Apoptosis is therefore triggered through intrinsic and extrinsic pathways (Ismail et al. 2019).

The expression of Bcl-2 family molecules has been impaired in many cancer isotypes, including CRC (Pricci et al. 2020). Through phosphorylation of Ser15 and activation of p53, curcumin promotes Bax expression and reduces Bcl-2 in colon adenocarcinomas (Song et al. 2005). Neoplastic cells may exhibit increased Bcl-2/Bax or Bcl-xL, which will ultimately lead to cell death. Colon cancer line proliferation was also found to be inhibited by curcumin-induced Bax upregulation (Table 22.1).

In various cell lines including colon carcinoma, curcumin induces apoptosis both p53 dependently and p53 independently (Zhou, S Beevers, and Huang 2011). Curcumin also appears to modulate the MEK/ERK proliferative signaling pathway through the p38 MAPK/JNK1 pathway, which is activated by phosphorylation of p53 and transactivation of BAX and Bcl-2 binding component 3 (PUMA) genes, leading to the promotion of CRC cell death (Jalili-Nik et al. 2018). Curcumin might also promote apoptosis by increasing the expression of p53 in colon cancer cells, as well as by downregulating survival genes such as EGR-1 (early growth response), c-myc, Bcl-2, and Bcl-xL (Ismail et al. 2019).

Apart from its capacity to induce apoptosis, curcumin is also able to inhibit the proliferation of CRC cells via modulation of cell cycle progression. This can be achieved by overexpressing cyclin dependent kinase (CDK) inhibitors such as p16, p21, p27, and inhibiting CDK2, CDK4, cyclin B, E, and D1 (Dasiram et al. 2017). Curcumin attenuates the proliferation of CRC cells by inhibiting expression of cyclooxygenase-2 (COX-2) via inhibition of NF-κB (de Porras, Layos, and Martínez-Balibrea 2021) or the AMP-activated protein kinase-AKT signaling pathway (Lee et al. 2009). Moreover, curcumin suppresses the Wnt/β-catenin (Dou et al. 2017) and Notch (Howells et al. 2011) pathways, which are altered in almost all CRCs, demonstrating that it has an antiproliferative effect (Table 22.1).

Curcumin also has been demonstrated to induce apoptosis in CRC. However, its effectiveness as an apoptotic inducer is limited due to its low bioavailability and poor absorption by the gastrointestinal tract, and preclinical and clinical research should be conducted.

Cancer develops and progresses as a result of proliferation, and a number of signal transduction pathways are simultaneously activated (Feitelson et al. 2015). Research shows that curcumin inhibits colorectal cancer growth *in vitro* via several mechanisms (Table 22.1; Song et al. 2019). It is generally thought that curcumin regulates cell cycle progression, protein kinase activity, and transcription factor expression in order to reduce proliferation (Pricci et al. 2020).

The effects of curcumin on proliferation and apoptosis have been shown in both wild type and mutant CRC cells, suggesting that p53 mutational status does not influence curcumin potency (Howells, Mitra, and Manson 2007).

22.3.4 ANGIOGENESIS

Angiogenesis, also known as the growth of new blood vessels from preexisting vessels, is a process that depends largely on a price equilibrium between anti-angiogenic and antigenic factors. Hypoxia usually occurs in tumor sites. Using hypoxia-inducible factor 1 (HIF-1), tumor cells overcome hypoxia through their regulation of genes related to angiogenesis, cell cycle, metastasis, and drug resistance (Jahani et al. 2019). There are several studies demonstrating that HIF-1 activates genes such as vascular endothelial growth factor (VEGF) and NF-κB to promote angiogenesis in tumor cells (Mansouri et al. 2016).

In CRC cells, curcumin exerts its anti-angiogenic effects via inhibiting the expression of VEGF, FGF, and COX-2 pathways which are regulated by NF-κB (de Porras, Layos, and Martínez-Balibrea 2021). Also, curcumin inhibits HIF-1α, which is involved in the regulation of VEGF expression (de Porras, Layos, and Martínez-Balibrea 2021). Additionally, STAT3 increases VEGF expression, thereby increasing CRC cell angiogenesis, survival, and growth (de Porras, Layos, and Martínez-Balibrea 2021). Curcumin also inhibits the JAK/STAT3/IL-8 pathway in CRC cells (Jin et al. 2017).

22.3.5 METASTASIS

The main reason for treatment withdrawals is the development of resistance to treatment and toxicity in metastatic tumors (Jin et al. 2017). CRC patients with metastatic disease often require consecutive treatments for 3 to 5 years (Jin et al. 2017). When curcumin is used with existing drugs, it could widen the range of options available to patients (Jin et al. 2017).

Curcumin inhibited the expression of molecules that are contributed to cellular adhesion and metastasis, such as intercellular adhesion and MMPs (Sa and Das 2008). Further, curcumin induces the expression of several antimetastatic proteins, including tissue inhibitor of metalloproteinases 2, non-metastatic protein 23, and E-cadherin, among others. Metastasis is more likely to occur without E-cadherin, and adhesion between cells is maintained by E-cadherin (Table 22.1; Chatterjee et al. 2003).

In general, curcumin can be used in combination with other drugs to inhibit and control tumor growth, improve clinical symptoms and prevent metastasis (Jin et al. 2017).

Besides its antiproliferative and anti-invasion properties, curcumin has antimetastatic properties as well (Kim et al. 2020). The epithelial–mesenchymal transition (EMT) is responsible for cell migration and cell dissociation from the primary tumor site, enabling metastatic spread to distant organs and tissues (Gao et al. 2018).

The MMP enzymes that degrade extracellular matrix proteins are responsible for the invasion and metastasis of cancer cells, allowing them to migrate and invade the extracellular compartment (Irani 2019).

NF-κB is one of several signaling pathways influenced by curcumin which exerts antimetastatic effects. The transcriptional regulation of Twist family BHLH transcription factor 1, SLUG (the protein product of SNAI2), and Smad interacting protein 1 by NF-κB/p65 results in the upregulation of E-cadherin, and mesenchymal markers N-cadherin and MMP-11, which may be used for EMT progression (Pires et al. 2017). Table 22.1 shows the mechanisms of action by which curcumin inhibits colorectal cancer metastasis through different mechanisms.

In studies with curcumin, the membrane-anchored serine protease matriptase, one of the key tumor types, was significantly reduced (Cheng, Chen, et al. 2013). Recent studies have demonstrated that increasing dosages of curcumin led to a downregulation of proteins associated with cell migration, including MMP-9 and claudin-3 (Xiang et al. 2020). In addition, curcumin prevents invasiveness and migration of human metastatic CRC cells (Calibasi-Kocal et al. 2019). The activation of STAT3 has been shown to contribute to the formation of metastases in several kinds of cancer (Jin 2020). Curcumin also decreased the expression of STAT3-regulated genes that contribute to tumor invasion, including ICAM, VEGF, MMP2, and MMP7 (Yang et al. 2012).

22.4 OTHER FOODS, HERBS, SPICES, AND BOTANICALS USED IN COLORECTAL CANCER

Herbal and natural-based medicine has been attracting great interest and public popularity in recent years because it is increasingly gaining widespread acceptance and has positively influenced healthcare professionals. This growing interest is due to the reported advancements over the years that delineated the underlying molecular mechanisms by which herbal compounds are positively linked to good health status outcomes and higher quality of life. Based on World Health Organization (WHO) data, globally around 80% of the world population utilizes natural products from medicinal plants as a source for their health care (Suroowan and Mahomoodally 2015).

Regarding the supportive evidence about the therapeutic effects of medicinal plants, there is a global trend toward the use of natural products for prevention and treatment of CRC (Aiello et al. 2019). Increasing evidence has confirmed that herbal remedies could be used as effective chemopreventive therapies to reduce the incidence of CRC in high-risk populations (Ye et al. 2015).

Medicinal herbs have various bioactive secondary metabolites, and different studies show that these metabolites (also known as phytochemicals) exert therapeutic effects and could improve human health. Many studies have been done to develop different drugs originating from plants.

More than 2000 plants have been recorded in the traditional medicine system (Rajalakshmy, Pydi, and Kavimani 2011), and some of these have been shown to help patients obtain adequate relief of CRC-related complications and have been linked to better management of disease. To decrease the adverse effects of CRC, more studies should be done to better investigate the protective and therapeutic effects of bioactive components derived from food and plant resources.

22.5 TOXICITY AND CAUTIONARY NOTES

The results of fertility, reproductive performance, and multigenerational investigations revealed that curcumin up to 2000 mg/kg (in rats) and 8400 mg/kg (in mice) did not induce any adverse effects (Bhavanishankar and Sreenivasa Murthy 1987). In toxicity study models, it has been shown that curcumin is biologically safe up to 100 mg/day in humans and up to 6 g/day in rats (Commandeur and Vermeulen 1996), and its Acceptable Daily Intake is 1–3 mg/kg body weight (Meeting, Additives, and Organization 2004).

It is important to note that uptake and distribution of curcumin has a major role in its biological activity. The liver and intestine are the major sites of curcumin metabolism (Ireson et al. 2002), and it has been shown that curcumin has the highest bioavailability in the gastrointestinal tract, especially in the colon. This could be expected to be associated with preventive and therapeutic properties of curcumin against CRC (de Porras, Layos, and Martínez-Balibrea 2021).

22.6 CONCLUSION

In conclusion, the active ingredient in turmeric, curcumin, inhibits carcinogenic pathways including CRC. It therefore acts to prevent or delay cancer development. Because of curcumin's quick excretion, its retention time in the body is short, causing its therapeutic effects to be restricted and the long-term effects of curcumin to be limited. Meanwhile, various delivery strategies (such as nanoparticles, liposomes, or synthetic analogues) can be adapted to improve curcumin absorption and bioavailability, which may eventually lead to relevant outcomes. A golden spice revolution cannot be ignored in light of so many efforts.

22.7   SUMMARY POINTS

- An overview of the effect of curcumin as an active component of turmeric on the molecular mechanisms underlying colorectal cancer is presented in this chapter.
- Curcumin, a hydrophobic polyphenol phytochemical, is the main active compound of turmeric herb rhizome (*C. longa*).
- The anticarcinogenic properties of curcumin may be explained by its effects on multiple pathways via modulating different signaling pathways including oxidative stress, metastasis, inflammation, and angiogenesis.
- Curcumin could diffuse inside the cell through the cell membrane and be distributed into different cellular compartments due to its hydrophobic nature.
- Various delivery strategies of curcumin (such as nanoparticles, liposomes, or synthetic analogs) can be used to improve its absorption and bioavailability.

REFERENCES

Agarwal, Ayushi, Akiladdevi Kasinathan, Ramamoorthi Ganesan, Akhila Balasubramanian, Jahnavi Bhaskaran, Samyuktha Suresh, Revanth Srinivasan, KB Aravind, and Nageswaran Sivalingam. 2018. "Curcumin induces apoptosis and cell cycle arrest via the activation of reactive oxygen species: Independent mitochondrial apoptotic pathway in Smad4 and p53 mutated colon adenocarcinoma HT29 cells." *Nutrition Research* 51:67–81.

Aggarwal, Bharat B, Anushree Kumar, and Alok C Bharti. 2003. "Anticancer potential of curcumin: preclinical and clinical studies." *Anticancer Research* 23 (1/A):363–398.

Aiello, Paola, Maedeh Sharghi, Shabnam Malekpour Mansourkhani, Azam Pourabbasi Ardekan, Leila Jouybari, Nahid Daraei, Khadijeh Peiro, Sima Mohamadian, Mahdiyeh Rezaei, and Mahdi Heidari. 2019. "Medicinal plants in the prevention and treatment of colon cancer." *Oxidative Medicine and Cellular Longevity* 2019:2072614.

Asgharzadeh, Fereshteh, Seyed M Hassanian, Gordon A Ferns, Majid Khazaei, and Malihe Hasanzadeh. 2018. "The therapeutic potential of angiotensin-converting enzyme and angiotensin receptor inhibitors in the treatment of colorectal cancer: Rational strategies and recent progress." *Current Pharmaceutical Design* 24 (39):4652–4658.

Bahrami, Afsane, Maryam Moradi Binabaj, and Gordon A Ferns. 2021. "Exosomes: Emerging modulators of signal transduction in colorectal cancer from molecular understanding to clinical application." *Biomedicine & Pharmacotherapy* 141:111882.

Bhattacharyya, Sankar, Debaprasad Mandal, Gouri Sankar Sen, Suman Pal, Shuvomoy Banerjee, Lakshmishri Lahiry, James H Finke, Charles S Tannenbaum, Tanya Das, and Gaurisankar Sa. 2007. "Tumor-induced oxidative stress perturbs nuclear factor-κB activity-augmenting tumor necrosis factor-α–mediated T-cell death: Protection by curcumin." *Cancer Research* 67 (1):362–370.

Bhavanishankar, TN, and V Sreenivasa Murthy. 1987. "Reproductive response of rats fed turmeric (*Curcuma longa* L.) and its alcoholic extract." *Journal of Food Science and Technology* 24 (1):45–49.

Cairns, Rob A, Isaac S Harris, and Tak W Mak. 2011. "Regulation of cancer cell metabolism." *Nature Reviews Cancer* 11 (2):85–95.

Calibasi-Kocal, Gizem, Ahu Pakdemirli, Serdar Bayrak, Nazli Mert Ozupek, Tolga Sever, Yasemin Basbinar, Hulya Ellidokuz, and Turkan Yigitbasi. 2019. "Curcumin effects on cell proliferation, angiogenesis and metastasis in colorectal cancer." *Journal of the Balkan Union of Oncology* 24 (4):1482–1487.

Carini, Francesco, Margherita Mazzola, Francesca Rappa, Abdo Jurjus, Alice Gerges Geagea, Sahar Al Kattar, Tarek Bou-Assi, Rosalyn Jurjus, Provvidenza Damiani, and Angelo Leone. 2017. "Colorectal carcinogenesis: Role of oxidative stress and antioxidants." *Anticancer Research* 37 (9):4759–4766.

Chatterjee, Amitava, Aparna Mitra, Subrata Ray, Nibedita Chattopadhyay, and Maqsood Siddiqi. 2003. "Curcumin exhibits antimetastatic properties by modulating integrin receptors, collagenase activity, and expression of Nm23 and E-cadherin." *Journal of Environmental Pathology, Toxicology and Oncology* 22 (1).

Cheng, Kwok Kin, Chin Fung Yeung, Shuk Wai Ho, Shing Fung Chow, Albert HL Chow, and Larry Baum. 2013. "Highly stabilized curcumin nanoparticles tested in an in vitro blood: Brain barrier model and in Alzheimer's disease Tg2576 mice." *The AAPS Journal* 15 (2):324–336.

Cheng, Tai-Shan, Wen-Chi Chen, Ya-Yun Lin, Chin-Hsien Tsai, Chia-I Liao, Hsin-Yi Shyu, Chun-Jung Ko, Sheue-Fen Tzeng, Chun-Yin Huang, and Pan-Chyr Yang. 2013. "Curcumin-targeting pericellular serine protease matriptase role in suppression of prostate cancer cell invasion, tumor growth, and metastasis." *Cancer Prevention Research* 6 (5):495–505.

Circu, Magdalena L, and Tak Yee Aw. 2010. "Reactive oxygen species, cellular redox systems, and apoptosis." *Free Radical Biology and Medicine* 48 (6):749–762.

Commandeur, JNM, and NPE Vermeulen. 1996. "Cytotoxicity and cytoprotective activities of natural compounds: The case of curcumin." *Xenobiotica* 26 (7):667–680.

Dasiram, Jade Dhananjay, Ramamoorthi Ganesan, Janani Kannan, Venkatesan Kotteeswaran, and Nageswaran Sivalingam. 2017. "Curcumin inhibits growth potential by G1 cell cycle arrest and induces apoptosis in p53-mutated COLO 320DM human colon adenocarcinoma cells." *Biomedicine & Pharmacotherapy* 86:373–380.

de Porras, Vicenç Ruiz, Laura Layos, and Eva Martínez-Balibrea. 2021. "Curcumin: A therapeutic strategy for colorectal cancer?" *Seminars in Cancer Biology* 73:321–330.

De Visser, KE, and LM Coussens. 2005. "The interplay between innate and adaptive immunity regulates cancer development." *Cancer Immunology, Immunotherapy* 54 (11):1143–1152.

DiMarco-Crook, Christina, Kanyasiri Rakariyatham, Zhengze Li, Zheyuan Du, Jinkai Zheng, Xian Wu, and Hang Xiao. 2020. "Synergistic anticancer effects of curcumin and 3′, 4′-didemethylnobiletin in combination on colon cancer cells." *Journal of Food Science* 85 (4):1292–1301.

Dou, Huiqiang, Renhui Shen, Jianxin Tao, Longchang Huang, Haoze Shi, Hang Chen, Yixin Wang, and Tong Wang. 2017. "Curcumin suppresses the colon cancer proliferation by inhibiting Wnt/β-catenin pathways via miR-130a." *Frontiers in Pharmacology* 8:877.

Feitelson, Mark A, Alla Arzumanyan, Rob J Kulathinal, Stacy W Blain, Randall F Holcombe, Jamal Mahajna, Maria Marino, Maria L Martinez-Chantar, Roman Nawroth, and Isidro Sanchez-Garcia. 2015. "Sustained proliferation in cancer: Mechanisms and novel therapeutic targets." *Seminars in Cancer Biology* 35:S25–S54.

Feng, Rentian, Yongju Lu, Linda L Bowman, Yong Qian, Vincent Castranova, and Min Ding. 2005. "Inhibition of activator protein-1, NF-κB, and MAPKs and induction of phase 2 detoxifying enzyme activity by chlorogenic acid." *Journal of Biological Chemistry* 280 (30):27888–27895.

Gao, Dingcheng, Vivek Mittal, Yi Ban, Ana Rita Lourenco, Shira Yomtoubian, and Sharrell Lee. 2018. "Metastatic tumor cells: Genotypes and phenotypes." *Frontiers in Biology* 13 (4):277–286.

Grandjean-Laquerriere, Alexia, Sophie C Gangloff, Richard Le Naour, Chantal Trentesaux, William Hornebeck, and Moncef Guenounou. 2002. "Relative contribution of NF-κB and AP-1 in the modulation by curcumin and pyrrolidine dithiocarbamate of the UVB-induced cytokine expression by keratinocytes." *Cytokine* 18 (3):168–177.

Guzman-Villanueva, Diana, Ibrahim M El-Sherbiny, Dea Herrera-Ruiz, and Hugh DC Smyth. 2013. "Design and in vitro evaluation of a new nano-microparticulate system for enhanced aqueous-phase solubility of curcumin." *BioMed Research International* 2013:1–9.

Hashemzehi, Milad, Reihane Behnam-Rassouli, Seyed Mahdi Hassanian, Maryam Moradi-Binabaj, Reyhaneh Moradi-Marjaneh, Farzad Rahmani, Hamid Fiuji, Mahdi Jamili, Mahdi Mirahmadi, and Nadia Boromand. 2018. "Phytosomal-curcumin antagonizes cell growth and migration, induced by thrombin through AMP-Kinase in breast cancer." *Journal of Cellular Biochemistry* 119 (7):5996–6007.

Hoos, Axel. 2016. "Development of immuno-oncology drugs: From CTLA4 to PD1 to the next generations." *Nature Reviews Drug Discovery* 15 (4):235–247.

Howells, Lynne M, Anita Mitra, and Margaret M Manson. 2007. "Comparison of oxaliplatin-and curcumin-mediated antiproliferative effects in colorectal cell lines." *International Journal of Cancer* 121 (1):175–183.

Howells, Lynne M, Stewart Sale, Sathya Neelature Sriramareddy, Glen RB Irving, Donald JL Jones, Christopher J Ottley, D Graham Pearson, Christopher D Mann, Margaret M Manson, and David P Berry. 2011. "Curcumin ameliorates oxaliplatin-induced chemoresistance in HCT116 colorectal cancer cells in vitro and in vivo." *International Journal of Cancer* 129 (2):476–486.

Huang, Yan-Feng, Da-Jian Zhu, Xiao-Wu Chen, Qi-Kang Chen, Zhen-Tao Luo, Chang-Chun Liu, Guo-Xin Wang, Wei-Jie Zhang, and Nv-Zhu Liao. 2017. "Curcumin enhances the effects of irinotecan on colorectal cancer cells through the generation of reactive oxygen species and activation of the endoplasmic reticulum stress pathway." *Oncotarget* 8 (25):40264.

Irani, Soussan. 2019. "Emerging insights into the biology of metastasis: A review article." *Iranian Journal of Basic Medical Sciences* 22 (8):833.

Ireson, Christopher R, Donald JL Jones, Samantha Orr, Michael WH Coughtrie, David J Boocock, Marion L Williams, Peter B Farmer, William P Steward, and Andreas J Gescher. 2002. "Metabolism of the cancer chemopreventive agent curcumin in human and rat intestine." *Cancer Epidemiology and Prevention Biomarkers* 11 (1):105–111.

Ismail, Nor Isnida, Iekhsan Othman, Faridah Abas, Nordin H Lajis, and Rakesh Naidu. 2019. "Mechanism of apoptosis induced by curcumin in colorectal cancer." *International Journal of Molecular Sciences* 20 (10):2454.

Jahani, Mozhgan, Mehri Azadbakht, Hassan Rasouli, Reza Yarani, Davood Rezazadeh, Nader Salari, and Kamran Mansouri. 2019. "L-arginine/5-fluorouracil combination treatment approaches cells selectively: Rescuing endothelial cells while killing MDA-MB-468 breast cancer cells." *Food and Chemical Toxicology* 123:399–411.

Jalili-Nik, Mohammad, Arash Soltani, Soussan Moussavi, Majid Ghayour-Mobarhan, Gordon A Ferns, Seyed Mahdi Hassanian, and Amir Avan. 2018. "Current status and future prospective of curcumin as a potential therapeutic agent in the treatment of colorectal cancer." *Journal of Cellular Physiology* 233 (9):6337–6345.

Jaruga, Ewa, Adam Sokal, Slawomir Chrul, and Grzegorz Bartosz. 1998. "Apoptosis-independent alterations in membrane dynamics induced by curcumin." *Experimental Cell Research* 245 (2):303–312.

Jin, G, Y Yang, K Liu, J Zhao, X Chen, H Liu, R Bai, X Li, Y Jiang, and X Zhang. 2017. "Combination curcumin and (–)-epigallocatechin-3-gallate inhibits colorectal carcinoma microenvironment-induced angiogenesis by JAK/STAT3/IL-8 pathway." *Oncogenesis* 6 (10):e384.

Jin, Wook. 2020. "Role of JAK/STAT3 signaling in the regulation of metastasis, the transition of cancer stem cells, and chemoresistance of cancer by epithelial-mesenchymal transition." *Cells* 9 (1):217.

Khalil, Najeh Maissar, Thuane Castro Frabel do Nascimento, Diani Meza Casa, Luciana Facco Dalmolin, Ana Cristina de Mattos, Ivonete Hoss, Marco Aurélio Romano, and Rubiana Mara Mainardes. 2013. "Pharmacokinetics of curcumin-loaded PLGA and PLGA–PEG blend nanoparticles after oral administration in rats." *Colloids and Surfaces B: Biointerfaces* 101:353–360.

Khan, Abdul Q, Eiman I Ahmed, Noor Elareer, Hamna Fathima, Kirti S Prabhu, Kodappully S Siveen, Michal Kulinski, Fouad Azizi, Said Dermime, and Aamir Ahmad. 2020. "Curcumin-mediated apoptotic cell death in papillary thyroid cancer and cancer stem-like cells through targeting of the JAK/STAT3 signaling pathway." *International Journal of Molecular Sciences* 21 (2):438.

Kim, Mi Ju, Ki-Su Park, Kyoung-Tae Kim, and Eun Young Gil. 2020. "The inhibitory effect of curcumin via fascin suppression through JAK/STAT3 pathway on metastasis and recurrence of ovary cancer cells." *BMC Women's Health* 20 (1):1–9.

Lee, Yun-Kyoung, Song Yi Park, Young-Min Kim, and Ock Jin Park. 2009. "Regulatory effect of the AMPK-COX-2 signaling pathway in curcumin-induced apoptosis in HT-29 colon cancer cells." *Annals of the New York Academy of Sciences* 1171 (1):489–494.

Li, Yanyan, Aaron Domina, Gi Lim, Teralyn Chang, and Tao Zhang. 2018. "Evaluation of curcumin, a natural product in turmeric, on Burkitt lymphoma and acute myeloid leukemia cancer stem cell markers." *Future Oncology* 14 (23):2353–2360.

Lu, Ko-Hsiu, Heng-Hsiung Wu, Renn-Chia Lin, Ya-Chiu Lin, Peace Wun-Ang Lu, Shun-Fa Yang, and Jia-Sin Yang. 2021. "Curcumin analogue L48H37 suppresses human osteosarcoma U2OS and MG-63 cells' migration and invasion in culture by inhibition of uPA via the JAK/STAT signaling pathway." *Molecules* 26 (1):30.

Luo, Jun-Li, Hideaki Kamata, and Michael Karin. 2005. "IKK/NF-κB signaling: Balancing life and death: A new approach to cancer therapy." *The Journal of Clinical Investigation* 115 (10):2625–2632.

Mansouri, Kamran, Ali Mostafie, Davood Rezazadeh, Mohsen Shahlaei, and Mohammad Hossein Modarressi. 2016. "New function of TSGA10 gene in angiogenesis and tumor metastasis: A response to a challengeable paradox." *Human Molecular Genetics* 25 (2):233–244.

Mansouri, Kamran, Shna Rasoulpoor, Alireza Daneshkhah, Soroush Abolfathi, Nader Salari, Masoud Mohammadi, Shabnam Rasoulpoor, and Shervin Shabani. 2020. "Clinical effects of curcumin in enhancing cancer therapy: A systematic review." *BMC Cancer* 20 (1):1–11.

Meeting, Joint FAO/WHO Expert Committee on Food Additives, Joint FAO/WHO Expert Committee on Food Additives, and World Health Organization. 2004. *Evaluation of Certain Food Additives and Contaminants: Sixty-First Report of the Joint FAO/WHO Expert Committee on Food Additives.* Vol. 61: World Health Organization.

Moradi-Marjaneh, Reyhaneh, Seyed M Hassanian, Farzad Rahmani, Seyed H Aghaee-Bakhtiari, Amir Avan, and Majid Khazaei. 2018. "Phytosomal curcumin elicits anti-tumor properties through suppression of angiogenesis, cell proliferation and induction of oxidative stress in colorectal cancer." *Current Pharmaceutical Design* 24 (39):4626–4638.

Mukhopadhyay, Asok, Carlos Bueso-Ramos, Devasis Chatterjee, Panayotis Pantazis, and Bharat B Aggarwal. 2001. "Curcumin downregulates cell survival mechanisms in human prostate cancer cell lines." *Oncogene* 20 (52):7597–7609.

Park, Jung, and Chris N Conteas. 2010. "Anti-carcinogenic properties of curcumin on colorectal cancer." *World Journal of Gastrointestinal Oncology* 2 (4):169.

Patel, Meera, Paul G Horgan, Donald C McMillan, and Joanne Edwards. 2018. "NF-κB pathways in the development and progression of colorectal cancer." *Translational Research* 197:43–56.

Patra, Srimanta, Biswajita Pradhan, Rabindra Nayak, Chhandashree Behera, Laxmidhar Rout, Mrutyunjay Jena, Thomas Efferth, and Sujit Kumar Bhutia. 2021. "Chemotherapeutic efficacy of curcumin and resveratrol against cancer: Chemoprevention, chemoprotection, drug synergism and clinical pharmacokinetics." *Seminars in Cancer Biology* 47:7209–7228.

Pires, Bruno RB, Andre L Mencalha, Gerson M Ferreira, Waldemir F de Souza, José A Morgado-Díaz, Amanda M Maia, Stephany Corrêa, and Eliana SFW Abdelhay. 2017. "NF-kappaB is involved in the regulation of EMT genes in breast cancer cells." *PLoS One* 12 (1):e0169622.

Porro, Chiara, Antonia Cianciulli, Teresa Trotta, Dario Domenico Lofrumento, and Maria Antonietta Panaro. 2019. "Curcumin regulates anti-inflammatory responses by JAK/STAT/SOCS signaling pathway in BV-2 microglial cells." *Biology* 8 (3):51.

Prasad, Sahdeo, Amit K Tyagi, and Bharat B Aggarwal. 2014. "Recent developments in delivery, bioavailability, absorption and metabolism of curcumin: The golden pigment from golden spice." *Cancer Research and Treatment: Official Journal of Korean Cancer Association* 46 (1):2.

Pricci, Maria, Bruna Girardi, Floriana Giorgio, Giuseppe Losurdo, Enzo Ierardi, and Alfredo Di Leo. 2020. "Curcumin and colorectal cancer: From basic to clinical evidences." *International Journal of Molecular Sciences* 21 (7):2364.

Priyadarsini, Kavirayani Indira. 2014. "The chemistry of curcumin: From extraction to therapeutic agent." *Molecules* 19 (12):20091–20112.

Rachmawati, Heni, Citra Ariani Edityaningrum, and Rachmat Mauludin. 2013. "Molecular inclusion complex of curcumin–β-cyclodextrin nanoparticle to enhance curcumin skin permeability from hydrophilic matrix gel." *Aaps Pharmscitech* 14 (4):1303–1312.

Rajalakshmy, I, R Pydi, and S Kavimani. 2011. "Cardioprotective medicinal plants – A review." *International Journal of Pharmaceutical Science Invention* 1:24–41.

Rajitha, Balney, Astrid Belalcazar, Ganji Purnachandra Nagaraju, Walid L Shaib, James P Snyder, Mamoru Shoji, Subasini Pattnaik, Afroz Alam, and Bassel F El-Rayes. 2016. "Inhibition of NF-κB translocation by curcumin analogs induces G0/G1 arrest and downregulates thymidylate synthase in colorectal cancer." *Cancer Letters* 373 (2):227–233.

Ryan, Julie L, Charles E Heckler, Marilyn Ling, Alan Katz, Jacqueline P Williams, Alice P Pentland, and Gary R Morrow. 2013. "Curcumin for radiation dermatitis: A randomized, double-blind, placebo-controlled clinical trial of thirty breast cancer patients." *Radiation Research* 180 (1):34–43.

Sa, Gaurisankar, and Tanya Das. 2008. "Anti cancer effects of curcumin: Cycle of life and death." *Cell Division* 3 (1):1–14.

Sahebkar, Amirhossein, and Asadollah Mohammadi. 2019. "Targeting the balance of T helper cell responses by curcumin in inflammatory and autoimmune states." *Autoimmunity Reviews* 18:738–748.

Sakaguchi, Shimon, Tomoyuki Yamaguchi, Takashi Nomura, and Masahiro Ono. 2008. "Regulatory T cells and immune tolerance." *Cell* 133 (5):775–787.

Shahani, Komal, Suresh Kumar Swaminathan, Diana Freeman, Angela Blum, Linan Ma, and Jayanth Panyam. 2010. "Injectable sustained release microparticles of curcumin: A new concept for cancer chemoprevention." *Cancer Research* 70 (11):4443–4452.

Shanmugam, Muthu K, Grishma Rane, Madhu Mathi Kanchi, Frank Arfuso, Arunachalam Chinnathambi, ME Zayed, Sulaiman Ali Alharbi, Benny KH Tan, Alan Prem Kumar, and Gautam Sethi. 2015. "The multifaceted role of curcumin in cancer prevention and treatment." *Molecules* 20 (2):2728–2769.

Shehzad, Adeeb, Fazli Wahid, and Young Sup Lee. 2010. "Curcumin in cancer chemoprevention: molecular targets, pharmacokinetics, bioavailability, and clinical trials." *Archiv der Pharmazie* 343 (9):489–499.

Song, G, YB Mao, QFl Cai, LM Yao, GL Ouyang, and SD Bao. 2005. "Curcumin induces human HT-29 colon adenocarcinoma cell apoptosis by activating p53 and regulating apoptosis-related protein expression." *Brazilian Journal of Medical and Biological Research* 38 (12):1791–1798.

Song, Xinqiang, Mu Zhang, Erqin Dai, and Yuan Luo. 2019. "Molecular targets of curcumin in breast cancer." *Molecular Medicine Reports* 19 (1):23–29.

Sun, Jun, Yi Zhao, and Jinhong Hu. 2013. "Curcumin inhibits imiquimod-induced psoriasis-like inflammation by inhibiting IL-1beta and IL-6 production in mice." *PLoS One* 8 (6):e67078.

Surh, Young-Joon, Joydeb Kumar Kundu, Hye-Kyung Na, and Jeong-Sang Lee. 2005. "Redox-sensitive transcription factors as prime targets for chemoprevention with anti-inflammatory and antioxidative phytochemicals." *The Journal of Nutrition* 135 (12):2993S-3001S.

Suroowan, Shanoo, and Fawzi Mahomoodally. 2015. "Common phyto-remedies used against cardiovascular diseases and their potential to induce adverse events in cardiovascular patients." *Clinical Phytoscience* 1 (1):1–13.

Teiten, Marie-Helene, Francois Gaascht, Marcus Cronauer, Estelle Henry, Mario Dicato, and Marc Diederich. 2011. "Anti-proliferative potential of curcumin in androgen-dependent prostate cancer cells occurs through modulation of the Wingless signaling pathway." *International Journal of Oncology* 38 (3):603–611.

Tu, Shui Ping, Huanyu Jin, Jin Dong Shi, Li Ming Zhu, Ya Suo, Gang Lu, Anna Liu, Timothy C Wang, and Chung S Yang. 2012. "Curcumin induces the differentiation of myeloid-derived suppressor cells and inhibits their interaction with cancer cells and related tumor growth." *Cancer Prevention Research* 5 (2):205–215.

Väyrynen, JP, A Tuomisto, K Klintrup, J Mäkelä, TJ Karttunen, and MJ Mäkinen. 2013. "Detailed analysis of inflammatory cell infiltration in colorectal cancer." *British Journal of Cancer* 109 (7):1839–1847.

Wang, Naizhi, Tao Feng, Xiaona Liu, and Qin Liu. 2020. "Curcumin inhibits migration and invasion of non–small cell lung cancer cells through up-regulation of miR-206 and suppression of PI3K/AKT/mTOR signaling pathway." *Acta Pharmaceutica* 70 (3):399–409.

Weir, Nathan M, Karuppaiyah Selvendiran, Vijay Kumar Kutala, Liyue Tong, Shilpa Vishwanath, Murugesan Rajaram, Susheela Tridandapani, Shrikant Anant, and Periannan Kuppusamy. 2007. "Curcumin induces G2/M arrest and apoptosis in cisplatin-resistant human ovarian cancer cells by modulating Akt and p38 MAPK." *Cancer Biology & Therapy* 6 (2):178–184.

Wilken, Reason, Mysore S Veena, Marilene B Wang, and Eri S Srivatsan. 2011. "Curcumin: A review of anti-cancer properties and therapeutic activity in head and neck squamous cell carcinoma." *Molecular Cancer* 10 (1):1–19.

Xiang, Lei, Bin He, Qiang Liu, Dongdong Hu, Wenjing Liao, Ruochan Li, Xinyi Peng, Qian Wang, and Gang Zhao. 2020. "Antitumor effects of curcumin on the proliferation, migration and apoptosis of human colorectal carcinoma HCT-116 cells." *Oncology Reports* 44 (5):1997–2008.

Xiao, Zecong, Zhenwei Su, Shisong Han, Jinsheng Huang, Liteng Lin, and Xintao Shuai. 2020. "Dual pH-sensitive nanodrug blocks PD-1 immune checkpoint and uses T cells to deliver NF-κB inhibitor for antitumor immunotherapy." *Science Advances* 6 (6):eaay7785.

Xu, Ting, Pu Guo, Chao Pi, Yingmeng He, Hongru Yang, Yi Hou, Xianhu Feng, Qingsheng Jiang, Yumeng Wei, and Ling Zhao. 2020. "Synergistic effects of curcumin and 5-Fluorouracil on the Hepatocellular Carcinoma in vivo and vitro through regulating the expression of COX-2 and NF-κB." *Journal of Cancer* 11 (13):3955.

Yang, Cheng-Liang, Yong-Yu Liu, Ye-Gang Ma, Yi-Xue Xue, De-Gui Liu, Yi Ren, Xiao-Bai Liu, Yao Li, and Zhen Li. 2012. "Curcumin blocks small cell lung cancer cells migration, invasion, angiogenesis, cell cycle and neoplasia through Janus kinase-STAT3 signalling pathway." *PLoS One* 7 (5):e37960.

Ye, Lin, Yongning Jia, KE Ji, Andrew J Sanders, Kan Xue, Jiafu Ji, Malcolm D Mason, and Wen G Jiang. 2015. "Traditional Chinese medicine in the prevention and treatment of cancer and cancer metastasis." *Oncology Letters* 10 (3):1240–1250.

Zhang, Hao, Weili Xu, Baolin Li, Kai Zhang, Yudong Wu, Haidong Xu, Junyong Wang, Jun Zhang, Rui Fan, and Jinxing Wei. 2015. "Curcumin promotes cell cycle arrest and inhibits survival of human renal cancer cells by negative modulation of the PI3K/AKT signaling pathway." *Cell Biochemistry and Biophysics* 73 (3):681–686.

Zhang, Hui-Hui, Ying Zhang, Yan-Na Cheng, Fu-Lian Gong, Zhan-Qi Cao, Lu-Gang Yu, and Xiu-Li Guo. 2018. "Metformin in combination with curcumin inhibits the growth, metastasis, and angiogenesis of hepatocellular carcinoma in vitro and in vivo." *Molecular Carcinogenesis* 57 (1):44–56.

Zhang, Lu, Cui-Tao Lu, Wen-Feng Li, Jin-Guo Cheng, Xin-Qiao Tian, Ying-Zheng Zhao, Xing Li, Hai-Feng Lv, and Xiao-Kun Li. 2012. "Physical characterization and cellular uptake of propylene glycol liposomes in vitro." *Drug Development and Industrial Pharmacy* 38 (3):365–371.

Zhou, Hongyu, Christopher S Beevers, and Shile Huang. 2011. "The targets of curcumin." *Current Drug Targets* 12 (3):332–347.

Section III

Resources

23 Recommended Resources on Cancer in Relation to Foods, Plants, Herbs and Spices in Human Health

Rajkumar Rajendram, Daniel Gyamfi,
Vinood B. Patel and Victor R. Preedy

23.1 INTRODUCTION

The management of cancer is driven by multi-disciplinary teams of specialists. These teams, led by oncologists, usually administer a cocktail of therapies including surgery, chemotherapy, radiotherapy, and immunotherapy. Because of the side effects of such interventions, alternative approaches are necessary, and these include lifestyle modifications as well as the investigation of plant-based materials.

Up to 80% of the world's population use traditional remedies alone for the initial treatment of any symptoms they develop (Hossain et al., 2022a, 2022b). The reasons for this include concerns about the effectiveness and safety of pharmaceuticals (Hossain et al., 2022a, 2022b), as well as the cost and availability of such medications. Thus, natural remedies have gained tremendous importance as sources of polypharmacological drugs for several diseases including cancer (Hossain et al., 2022a, 2022b).

Yet, many diseases treated with natural remedies are inherently self-limiting. So, many physicians have fundamental questions pertaining to the scientific evidence for the use of traditional remedies in the treatment of cancer. The knowledge that ancient religious texts have recommended the use of plants for the treatment of diverse ailments has encouraged researchers to evaluate the scientific validity of these claims (Hossain et al., 2016, 2022a). Indeed, it must be remembered that some treatments based on traditional remedies also have side effects or may be ineffective.

The potential anticancer activity of chemicals derived from natural remedies (i.e., nutraceuticals) has been previously investigated. For example, the role of spices and herbs in the inhibition of the growth of cancer cells has been described (Jaksevicius et al., 2017; Khor et al., 2018; Hallajzadeh et al., 2020).

We have previously raised awareness of the fact that experienced researchers and clinicians must stay up to date. Such specialists are often guided by regulatory bodies and professional societies. Those embarking on research into the interrelationships between foods, plant-based extracts, and cancer need guidance on starting points from which to begin their explorations. To address this, we have produced tables containing resources as recommended by active researchers and experts, and we acknowledge their contributions below.

23.2 RESOURCES

Tables 23.1–23.5 list the most up-to-date information on the regulatory bodies (Table 23.1), professional societies (Table 23.2), books (Table 23.3), emerging technologies and platforms (Table 23.4), and other resources of interest (Table 23.5) that are relevant to an evidence-based approach to the

DOI: 10.1201/9781003260028-26

TABLE 23.1

Regulatory Bodies and Organizations Relevant to the Study of Foods, Plants, Herbs, Spices, and Cancer or Related Fields and Areas

Regulatory Body or Organization	Web Address
Academy of Nutrition and Dietetics	www.eatrightpro.org/
American Congress of Rehabilitation Medicine	https://acrm.org/
American Institute for Cancer Research	www.aicr.org
Biodiversity and Food Sovereignty Action, Thailand	www.biothai.org/
Botanical Safety Consortium	https://botanicalsafetyconsortium.org/
Cancer Australia	www.canceraustralia.gov.au/
Cancer Index	www.cancerindex.org/
Cancer League of the Slovak Republic	www.lpr.sk/
Cancer Research Foundation, Slovak	www.nvr.sk/
Cancer Research UK	www.cancerresearchuk.org/
Cancer Support Community	www.cancersupportcommunity.org/
Cancer.Net	www.cancer.net/
Centers for Disease Control and Prevention	www.cdc.gov/
Consortium for Globalization of Chinese Medicine (CGCM)	www.tcmedicine.org/
European Commission's Food Safety	https://ec.europa.eu/food/overview_en/
European Food Safety Authority (EFSA)	www.efsa.europa.eu/en
Food and Agriculture Organization of the United Nations (FAO)	www.fao.org/
Food and Drug Administration, Thailand	www.fda.moph.go.th/
Food and Drug Administration: Center for Food Safety and Applied Nutrition	www.fda.gov/food/
Food with Health Claims, Food for Special Dietary Uses, and Nutrition Labeling, Japan	www.mhlw.go.jp/english/topics/foodsafety/fhc/
International Institute of Anticancer Research	https://iiar-anticancer.org/
Linus Pauling Institute: Oregon State University	https://lpi.oregonstate.edu
Majlis Kanser Nasional (MAKNA): Cancer Matters	https://makna.org.my/
MD Anderson Cancer Center: University of Texas	www.mdanderson.org/cancerwise.html
Memorial Sloan Kettering Cancer Center, USA	www.mskcc.org/
National Academy of Medicine	https://nam.edu/
National Agency for Food and Drug Administration and Control	www.nafdac.gov.ng
National Cancer Institute (NIH)	www.cancer.gov/
National Cancer Institute of Thailand	www.nci.go.th/
National Cancer Institute, Malaysia	www.ppj.gov.my/en/second-menu/institut-kanser-negara
National Center for Complementary and Integrative Health (NCCIH)	www.nccih.nih.gov/
National Health and Medical Research Council (NHMRC), Australia	www.nhmrc.gov.au/
National Health Service (NHS) England	www.england.nhs.uk/
National Health Service (NHS), UK	www.nhs.uk/
National Institute on Aging	www.nia.nih.gov/
National Institutes of Health	www.nih.gov/
National Institutes of Health (NIH): National Cancer Institute	www.cancer.gov/
National Oncology Institute	www.noisk.sk/en
National Pharmaceutical Control Bureau, Malaysia	https://npra.gov.my/index.php/en/
National Research Centre, Egypt	www.nrc.sci.eg/
Nestlé Nutrition Institute	https://nnia.nestlenutrition-institute.org/

TABLE 23.1
(Continued)

Regulatory Body or Organization	Web Address
Nutrition.gov: US Department of Agriculture	www.nutrition.gov/
Office of Dietary Supplements: National Institutes of Health	https://ods.od.nih.gov/
Physicians Committee for Responsible Medicine	www.pcrm.org/
Royal Botanic Gardens, UK	https://mpns.science.kew.org/
Swedish Nutrition Foundation	https://snf.ideon.se/
US Department of Agriculture (USDA)	www.usda.gov/
US Food and Drug Administration	www.fda.gov/
United Nations System Standing Committee on Nutrition	www.unscn.org/
World Food Safety Organisation (WFSO)	https://worldfoodsafety.org/
World Health Organization (WHO)	www.who.int/

Note: This table lists the regulatory bodies and organizations involved with the study of foods, plants, herbs, spices and cancer. Some of the links have indirect references to this topic. The links were accurate at the time of going to press but may move or alter. In these cases, the use of the search tabs should be explored at the parent address or site. See also Table 23.2.

TABLE 23.2
Professional Societies Relevant to Foods, Plants, Herbs, Spices, and Cancer or Related Fields and Areas

Society Name	Web Address
American Cancer Society	www.cancer.org/
American Nutrition Association	https://theana.org/
American Society for Nutrition	https://nutrition.org/
American Society for Parenteral and Enteral Nutrition	www.nutritioncare.org
American Society of Pharmacognosy	www.pharmacognosy.us/
Canadian Cancer Society	https://cancer.ca/en/
Canadian Nutrition Society	www.cns-scn.ca/
Chinese Nutrition Society	www.cnsoc.org/
Complementary Medical Association, UK	www.the-cma.org.uk/
Complementary Medicine Association, Australia	https://cma.asn.au/
Czech Society for Nutrition	www.vyzivaspol.cz/
Danish Nutrition Society	www.sfe.dk/dansk1
European Society for Clinical Nutrition and Metabolism	www.espen.org/
Federation of African Nutrition Society	http://fanus.org/
Federation of European Nutrition Societies	https://fensnutrition.org/
German Society for Nutritional Medicine	www.dgem.de
Good Practice in Traditional Chinese Medicine Research Association (GP-TCM RA)	www.gp-tcm.org/
Herb Society of America	www.herbsociety.org/
Hong Kong Nutrition Association	www.hkna.org.hk/
International and American Association of Clinical Nutritionists	www.iaacn.org
International Association for Plant Taxonomy (IAPT)	www.iaptglobal.org/
International Confederation of Dietetic Associations (ICDA)	www.internationaldietetics.org/
International Practitioners of Holistic Medicine	www.iphm.co.uk/

(Continued)

TABLE 23.2

(Continued)

Society Name	Web Address
International Society for Horticultural Science	www.ishs.org/
International Union of Nutritional Sciences (IUNS)	https://iuns.org/
Malaysian Natural Products Society	www.mymnps.org/
Modernized Chinese Medicine International Association (MCMIA)	https://mcmia.org/en/
National Association of Nutrition Professionals	https://nanp.org/
National Children's Cancer Society	https://thenccs.org/
Nutrition Society	www.nutritionsociety.org
Slovak Myeloma Society	http://myelom.sk/
Slovak Oncological Society	http://onkologia.sk/
Society for Integrative Oncology	https://integrativeonc.org/
Society for Medicinal Plant and Natural Product Research (GA)	https://ga-society.org/
Society for Nutrition Education and Behavior	www.sneb.org/
Swiss Society for Clinical Nutrition	www.sfkn.se/
Thai Cancer Society	https://thaicancersociety.com/
Thai Gynecologic Cancer Society	www.tgcsthai.com/
Thai Society of Clinical Oncology	www.thethaicancer.com/
Thai Women's Medical Association	www.tmwa.or.th/
Universal Society of Food and Nutrition	www.usfn.net

Note: This table lists the professional societies involved with the study of foods, plants, herbs, spices and cancer in human health. Some of the links have indirect references to this topic. See also Table 23.1.

TABLE 23.3

Books on Foods, Plants, Herbs, Spices, and Cancer or Related Fields and Areas of Study

Book Title	Authors or Editors	Publisher	Year of Publication
Active Phytochemicals from Chinese Herbal Medicines	Ho WS	CRC Press	2016
Beat Back Cancer Naturally	Brandy DA	Natural Insights into Cancer	2019
Bioactive Compounds and Cancer	Milner JA, Romagnolo DF	Humana Press	2010
Bioactive Foods and Extracts Cancer Treatment and Prevention	Watson RR	CRC Press	2010
Biodiversity, Natural Products and Cancer Treatment	Kuete V, Efferth T	World Scientific	2014
Botanical Medicine and Clinical Practice	Watson RR, Preedy VR	CABI	2008
Cancer Genetics and Therapeutics – Focus on Phytochemicals	Roy M, Datta A	Springer	2019
Cancer: Oxidative Stress and Dietary Antioxidants	Preedy VR	Elsevier Science	2021
Cell Signalling and Molecular Targets in Cancer	Chatterjee M, Kashfi K	Springer	2012
Critical Dietary Factors in Cancer Chemoprevention	Ullah FM, Ahmad A	Springer	2016

TABLE 23.3
(Continued)

Book Title	Authors or Editors	Publisher	Year of Publication
Edible Medicinal and Non-Medicinal Plants Volume 1, Fruits	Lim TK	Springer, Dordrecht	2012
Encyclopedia of Herbs and Spices	Ravindran PN	CABI	2017
Evidence-Based Validation of Herbal Medicine: Translational Research on Botanicals	Mukherjee PK	Elsevier	**2022**
Flavonoidy a ich biologické účinky	Mojžiš J, Mojžišová G	Vienala (Košice)	2001
Food Code	College Park	Public Health Service Food and Drug Administration	2017
Food Phytochemicals for Cancer Prevention II (Teas, Spices, and Herbs)	Ho C-T, Osawa T, Huang M-T, Rosen RT	American Chemical Society	1994
Food Quality: Balancing Health and Disease	Grumezescu AM, Holban AM	Academic Press	2018
Food Security and Safety: African Perspectives	Babalola OO	Springer	2021
Functional Foods in Cancer Prevention and Therapy	Kabir Y	Academic Press	2020
Handbook of Herbs and Spices	Peter KV	Woodhead	2012
Handbook of Medicinal Herbs	Duke JA	CRC Press	2002
Herbal Medicine: Biomolecular and Clinical Aspects. 2nd edition	Benzie IFF, Sissi Wachtel-Galor S	CRC Press	2011
Herbs and Natural Supplements, Volume 2: An Evidence-Based Guide, 4th edition	Braun L, Cohen M	Churchill Livingstone	**2015**
Herbs, Spices, and Medicinal Plants for Human Gastrointestinal Disorders	Goyal MR, Birwal P, Chauhan DN	Apple Academic Press	2022
Inflammation, Oxidative Stress, and Cancer Dietary Approaches for Cancer Prevention	Kong ANT	CRC Press	2014
Lead Compounds from Medicinal Plants for the Treatment of Cancer	Wiart C	Elsevier	2013
Medicinal Herbs in Primary Care: An Evidence-Guided Reference for Healthcare Providers	Bokelmann JM	Elsevier	2021
Natural Cancer Cure: How I Beat Cancer Through Diet and Herbs and Found a Life of Health and Hope	Lawson R	School of Natural Healing	2018
Natural Products for Cancer Chemoprevention: Single Compounds and Combinations	Pezzuto JM, Vang O	Springer	2020
Natural Substances for Cancer Prevention	Xu JP	CRC Press	2018
Nature's Medicine: A Collection of Medicinal Plants from Malaysia's Rainforest	Hussain AG, Hussin K, Mohd Noor N	Landskap Malaysia	2018
Protinádorové účinky rastlinných funkčných potravín v modeli karcinómu prsníka.	Kubatka P, Kapinová A, Kello M, Mojžiš J, Péč M	Academic Press Bratislava	2017
Resistance to Targeted ABC Transporters in Cancer	Efferth T	Springer	2014
Traditional Malay Medicinal Plants	Zakaria M, Mohd MA	Oxford Fajar Sdn. Bhd.	2010
Treating Cancer with Herbs: An Integrative Approach	Tierra M	Lotus Press	2003
Understanding Cancer Therapies	Srinivasan P, Shanmugam T	Taylor and Francis	2018

Note: This table lists books relevant to the study of foods, plants, herbs, spices, and cancer in human health.

TABLE 23.4

Emerging Techniques, Instruments, and Analytical Platforms or Devices for Investigating Foods, Plants, Herbs, Spices, and Cancer or Related Fields and Areas

Organization or Company Name	Web Address
Al-innovate	https://ai-innovate.com/
Biological Procedures Online	https://biologicalproceduresonline.biomedcentral.com/articles/10.1186/s12575-022-00166-y
BioMed Central (BMC) Biotechnology	www.ncbi.nlm.nih.gov/pmc/articles/PMC3849190/
Bio-Rad	www.bio-rad.com/
Central Laboratory (Thailand) Company Limited	www.centrallabthai.com/
Frontiers in Genetics	www.frontiersin.org/articles/10.3389/fgene.2021.742095/full
LI-COR: Biotechnology and Environmental	www.licor.com/
National Science and Technology Development Agency	www.nstda.or.th/
Precision X-Ray Irradiation	https://precisionxray.com/
Thailand Institute of Scientific and Technological Research	www.tistr.or.th/
ThermoFisher Scientific: Cancer Metabolomics	www.thermofisher.com/my/en/home/industrial/mass-spectrometry/mass-spectrometry-learning-center/mass-spectrometry-applications-area/metabolomics-mass-spectrometry/metabolomics-applications/cancer-metabolomics.html
Veerasense: Artificial Intelligence Company	https://veerasense.com/
Waters	www.waters.com/nextgen/us/en.html
ZOE: In-Depth Nutrition	https://joinzoe.com/

Note: This table lists technologies or platforms relevant to the study of foods, plants, herbs, spices, and cancer in human health. Please note, occasionally the location of the website or Web address changes.

TABLE 23.5

Other Resources of Interest or Relevance for Health Care Professionals or Patients Related to the Study of Foods, Plants, Herbs, Spices, and Cancer or Related Fields and Areas

Name of Resource or Organization	Web Address
American Society of Clinical Oncology (ASCO): Cancer.Net	www.cancer.net/navigating-cancer-care/cancer-basics/cancer-care-team/oncology-team
Australian Regulatory Guidelines for Listed Medicines and Registered Complementary Medicines	www.tga.gov.au/publication/australian-regulatory-guidelines-listed-medicines-and-registered-complementary-medicines
Cancer Australia: Cancer Support Organisations	www.canceraustralia.gov.au/impacted-cancer/cancer-support-organisations
Cancer Research UK: General Cancer Organisations	www.cancerresearchuk.org/about-cancer/coping/general-books-links/general-cancer-organisations
Center for Advanced Functional Foods Research and Entrepreneurship: Ohio State University	https://u.osu.edu/caffre/
Children's Cancer Hospital Egypt 57357(CCHE)	www.57357.org/en/home-page/?
Department for the Development of Thai Traditional and Alternative Medicine	www.dtam.moph.go.th/index.php/en/

TABLE 23.5
(Continued)

Name of Resource or Organization	Web Address
European Federation of Pharmaceutical Industries and Associations: Working with Patient Groups	www.efpia.eu/relationships-code/patient-organisations/
European Food Safety Authority: Material on Botanicals	www.efsa.europa.eu/en/topics/topic/botanicals
Fort Worth Botanic Garden and the Botanical Research Institute of Texas	https://brit.org/
Foundation for Cancer Care Siriraj Hospital	www.si.mahidol.ac.th/office_m/foundation/
Global Biodiversity Information Facility	www.gbif.org/
Global Plants Database	https://plants.jstor.org/
I Had Cancer	www.ihadcancer.com
International Plant Name Index	www.ipni.org/
Medical Oncology	www.springer.com/journal/12032
Memorial Sloan Kettering Cancer Center: Herbs, Botanicals and Other Products	www.mskcc.org/cancer-care/diagnosis-treatment/symptom-management/integrative-medicine/herbs
Micronutrient Forum	https://micronutrientforum.org/
Micronutrient Information Center: Oregon State University	https://lpi.oregonstate.edu/mic
National Cancer Institute: Complementary and Alternative Medicine	www.cancer.gov/about-cancer/treatment/cam
National Center for Complementary and Integrative Health: Resources for Health Care Providers	www.nccih.nih.gov/health/providers
National Center for Complementary and Integrative Health: Clinical Practice Guidelines	www.nccih.nih.gov/health/providers/clinicalpractice
National Center for Natural Products Research: The University of Mississippi	https://pharmacy.olemiss.edu/ncnpr/research-programs/medicinal-plant-research/
National Institute of Neurological Disorders and Stroke: Patient Organizations	www.ninds.nih.gov/Disorders/Support-Resources/Patient-Organizations
Natural and Non-Prescription Health Products Directorate: Government of Canada	www.canada.ca/en/health-canada/corporate/about-health-canada/branches-agencies/health-products-food-branch/natural-non-prescription-health-products-directorate.html
Natural Health Products Regulations: Government of Canada	https://laws-lois.justice.gc.ca/eng/regulations/SOR-2003-196/page-1.html
Nestlé Health Science	www.nestlehealthscience.com/
Nutrition and Cancer	www.tandfonline.com/journals/hnuc20
Parkinson's UK	www.parkinsons.org.uk/
Patient Associations and Partners	https://onkoinfo.sk/
Plant Identification: University of Massachusetts	https://extension.umass.edu/plant-identification/common/all
Queen Sirikit Centre for Breast Cancer	https://qscbc.org/
Regulatory Frameworks for Nutraceuticals: Australia, Canada, Japan, and the United States	https://pubmed.ncbi.nlm.nih.gov/34345505/
Regulatory Frameworks for Nutraceuticals: Different Countries of the World	https://pubmed.ncbi.nlm.nih.gov/32427089/
Tang Center for Herbal Medicine Research: University of Chicago	www.uchicago.edu/education-and-research/center/tang_center_for_herbal_medicine_research/
The Patients Association	www.patients-association.org.uk/
The Plant List	www.theplantlist.org/
Trends in Pharmaceutical Sciences	www.cell.com/trends/pharmacological-sciences/home
UMass Amherst Plant Identification	https://extension.umass.edu/plant-identification/
UniProt Taxonomy	www.uniprot.org/taxonomy/
USDA Forest Service	www.fs.usda.gov/
Verywell Health	www.verywellhealth.com/
World Cancer Research Fund/American Institute for Cancer Research: Cancer Prevention	www.paho.org/hq/dmdocuments/2011/nutrition-AICR-WCR-food-physical-activ.pdf

(Continued)

TABLE 23.5
(Continued)

Name of Resource or Organization	Web Address
World Flora Online	www.worldfloraonline.org/
World Health Organization: International Regulatory Cooperation for Herbal Medicines (IRCH)	www.who.int/initiatives/international-regulatory-cooperation-for-herbal-medicines#:~:text=International%20Regulatory%20Cooperation%20for%20Herbal%20Medicines%20(IRCH)%20is%20a%20global,improved%20regulation%20for%20herbal%20medicines
World Health Organization: Nutrition	www.who.int/health-topics/nutrition

Note: This table lists other resources of interest or relevance to foods, plants, herbs, spices, and cancer in human health. Please note, occasionally the location of the websites or Web address changes.

study of foods, plants, herbs, spices and cancer. Some organizations are listed in more than one table as they occasional fulfill multiple roles.

23.3 OTHER RESOURCES

The Wellcome Collection (https://wellcomecollection.org/collections) and The British Library (www.bl.uk/) also hold material on biomedical topics.

Other chapters on resources relevant to nutrition or cancer (recommended by authors and practitioners) may also be relevant to the study of foods, plants, herbs, spices, and cancer (Alzaid et al., 2015; Rajendram et al., 2014, 2015, 2016, 2017, 2019a, 2019b, 2020, 2022a, 2022b, 2013a, 2013b).

This list of material in these tables is included to provide general information only. It does not constitute any recommendation or endorsement of the activities of these sites, facilities, or other resources listed in this chapter, by the authors or editors of this book.

23.4 SUMMARY POINTS

A significant proportion of the world's population use only use traditional remedies for the initial treatment of any symptoms they develop.

There are fundamental questions pertaining to the scientific evidence for the use of traditional remedies in modern medicine.

Cancer is one of the most common causes of morbidity and mortality worldwide.

Natural remedies have gained tremendous importance as sources of drugs for several diseases including cancer.

This chapter lists resources relevant to foods, plants, herbs, spices, and cancer in human health.

23.5 ACKNOWLEDGMENTS

We thank the following authors for their contributions to the development of this resource. We apologize if some of the suggested material was not included in this chapter or has been moved to different sections.

Asgharzadeh, Fereshteh
Dogan, Zeynep
Efferth, Thomas

Fang, Yujiang
Hafez Ghoran, Salar
Hegazy, Mohamed-Elamir F
Kantapan, Jiraporn
Kello, Martin
Lee, Hayden
Lim, Vuanghao
Nabih, Heba K.
Shahdadian, Farnaz
Taktaz, Fatemeh
Tang, Trien Trey

REFERENCES

Alzaid, F., Rajendram, R., Patel, V.B., Preedy, V.R. (2015). Expanding the Knowledge Base in Diet, Nutrition and Critical Care: Electronic and Published Resources. In Rajendram, R., Preedy, V.R., Patel, V.B. (Editors). Diet and Nutrition in Critical Care. Springer, Germany.

Hallajzadeh, J., Maleki Dana, P., Mobini, M., Asemi, Z., Mansournia, M. A., Sharifi, M., & Yousefi, B. (2020). Targeting of oncogenic signaling pathways by berberine for treatment of colorectal cancer. *Medical oncology* (Northwood, London, England), 37(6), 49.

Hossain, M.S., Kader, M.A., Goh, K.W., et al. (2022a). Herb and Spices in Colorectal Cancer Prevention and Treatment: A Narrative Review. Front. Pharmacol. 13, 865801

Hossain, M.S., Karuniawati, H., Jairoun, A.A., Urbi, Z., Ooi, J., John, A., et al. (2022b). Colorectal Cancer: A Review of Carcinogenesis, Global Epidemiology, Current Challenges, Risk Factors, Preventive and Treatment Strategies. Cancers (Basel) 14 (7), 1732.

Hossain, M.S., Urbi, Z., Evamoni, F.Z., Zohora, F.T., Rahman, K.M.H. (2016). A Secondary Research on Medicinal Plants Mentioned in the Holy Qur'an. J. Med. Plants 3 (59), 81–97.

Jaksevicius, A., Carew, M., Mistry, C., Modjtahedi, H., Opara, E.I. (2017). Inhibitory Effects of Culinary Herbs and Spices on the Growth of HCA-7 Colorectal Cancer Cells and Their COX-2 Expression. Nutrients 9 (10), 1051.

Khor, K.Z., Lim, V., Moses, E.J., Abdul Samad, N. (2018). The In Vitro and In Vivo Anticancer Properties of Moringa Oleifera. Evid. Based Complement. Altern. Med. 2018, 1071243. doi:10.1155/2018/1071243

Rajendram, R., Gyamfi, D., Patel, V.B., Preedy, V.R. (2022a). Recommended Resources for Biomarkers of Nutrition. In Preedy, V.R., Patel, V.B. (Editors). Biomarkers of Nutrition. Elsevier, USA.

Rajendram, R., Gyamfi, D., Patel, V.B., Preedy, V.R. (2022b). Recommended Resources for Biomarkers in Diabetes: Methods, Discoveries, and Applications. In Patel, V.B., Preedy, V.R. (Editors). Biomarkers in Diabetes. Biomarkers in Disease: Methods, Discoveries and Applications. Springer, Cham. doi:10.1007/978-3-030-81303-1_58-2

Rajendram, R., Patel, V.B., Preedy, V.R. (2014). Web Based Resources and Suggested Reading. In Rajendram, R., Patel, V.B., Preedy, V.R. (Editors). Glutamine in Health and Disease (pp. 527–532). Springer, USA.

Rajendram, R., Patel, V.B., Preedy, V.R. (2015). Web Based Resources and Suggested Reading. In Rajendram, R., Patel, V.B., Preedy, V.R. (Editors). Branched Chain Amino Acids in Health and Disease. Springer, USA.

Rajendram, R., Patel, V.B., Preedy, V.R. (2016). Recommended Resources on Biomarkers in Cancer. In Patel, V., Preedy, V. (Editors). Biomarkers in Cancer. Springer, Dordrecht. doi:10.1007/978-94-007-7741-5_52-1

Rajendram, R., Patel, V.B., Preedy, V.R. (2017). Recommended Resources on Maternal Nutrition. In Rajendram, R., Patel, V.B., Preedy, V.R. (Editors). Nutrition and Diet in Maternal Diabetes (pp. 495–500). Springer, USA.

Rajendram, R., Patel, V.B., Preedy, V.R. (2019a). Resources in Famine, Starvation, and Nutrient Deprivation. In Patel, V.B., Preedy, V.R. (Editors). Famine, Starvation, and Nutrient Deprivation (pp. 2399–2406). Springer, USA.

Rajendram, R., Patel, V.B., Preedy, V.R. (2019b). Resources in Diet, Nutrition and Epigenetics. In Patel, V.B., Preedy, V.R. (Editors). Nutrition and Epigenetics (pp. 2309–2314). Springer, USA.

Rajendram, R., Patel, V.B., Preedy, V.R. (2020). Recommended Resources for Nutrition, Oxidative Stress, and Dietary Antioxidants. In Martin, C.R., Preedy, V.R. (Editors). Nutrition, Oxidative Stress, and Dietary Antioxidants (pp. 393–397). Elsevier, USA.

Rajendram, R., Rajendram, R., Patel, V.B., Preedy, V.R. (2013a). Interlinking Diet, Nutrition, the Menopause and Recommended Resources. In Hollins-Martin, C.J., Watson, R.R., Preedy, V.R. (Editors). Nutrition and Diet in Menopause. Springer, Germany.

Rajendram, R., Rajendram, R., Patel, V.B., Preedy, V.R. (2013b). Diet Quality: What More Is There to Know? In Preedy, V.R., Hunter, L.-A., Patel, V.B. (Editors). Diet Quality: An Evidence-Based Approach (pp. 397–401). Springer, Germany.

Index

Note: **Boldfaced** page references indicate tables. *Italic* references indicate figures.

For Product Safety Concerns and Information please contact our EU
representative GPSR@taylorandfrancis.com
Taylor & Francis Verlag GmbH, Kaufingerstraße 24, 80331 München, Germany